Titles of related inte

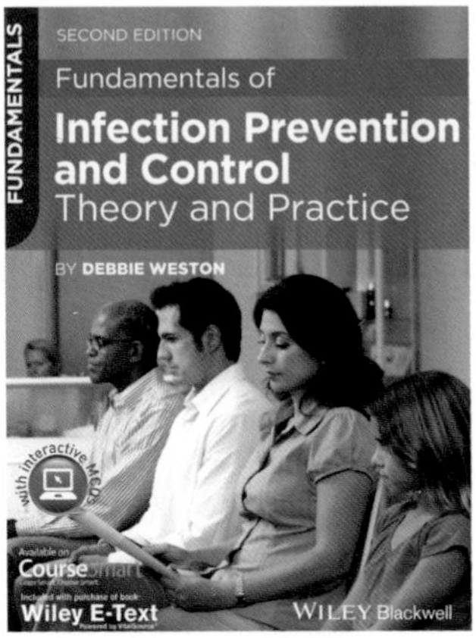

ISBN: 978-1-118-30665-9
Review of the first edition: "Interesting and readable . . . the most important book any healthcare professional or healthcare student can own." (Amazon reviewer)

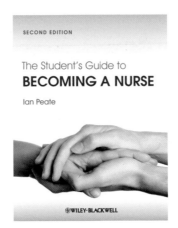

ISBN: 978-0-470-67270-9
"This comprehensive book will be indispensable throughout a student's education." (Nursing Standard by Sarah Lovie, nursing student, Royal Cornhill Hospital)

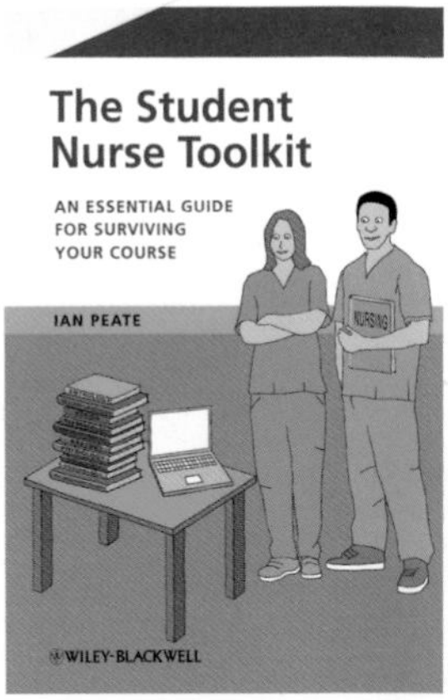

ISBN: 978-1-1183-9378-9
"I instantly felt like I could relate to the book and to the ideas of the author in a way that really built trust between me as the reader and what the book was teaching me." (Second year adult nursing student, University of Nottingham)

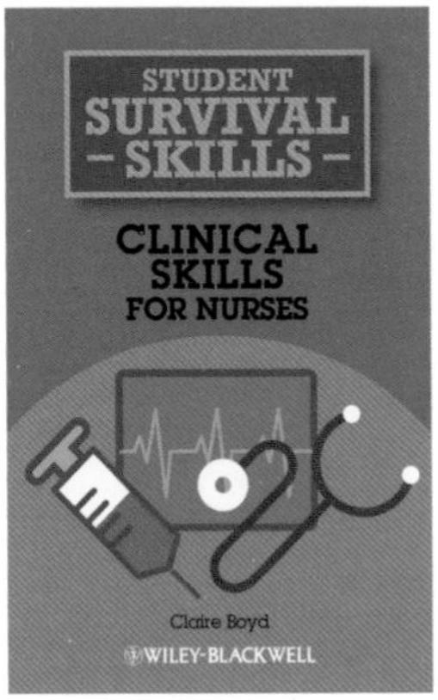

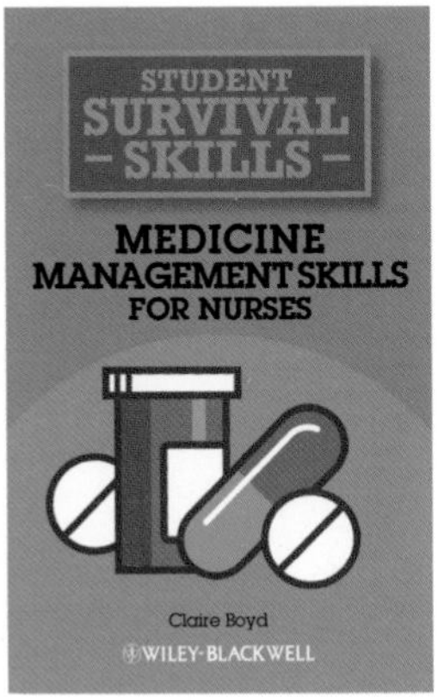

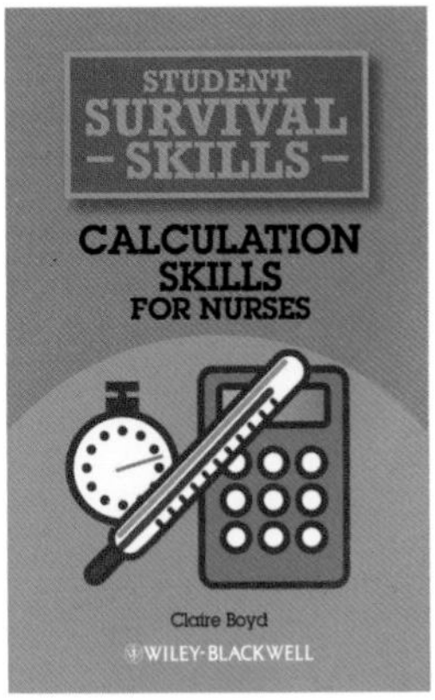

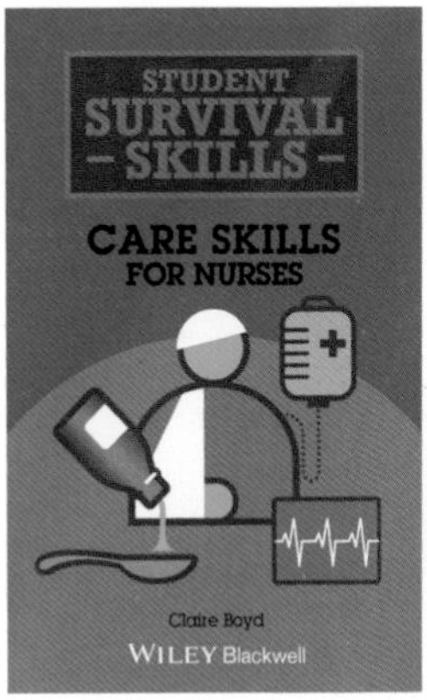

ISBN: 978-1-1184-4877-9 ISBN: 978-1-1184-4885-4 ISBN: 978-1-1184-4889-2 ISBN: 978-1-118-65738-6

"I love this series. . . . I am truly looking forward to them being published as I can't wait to get my hands on them." (Second year nursing student, University of Abertay, Dundee)

Fundamentals of Medical-Surgical Nursing: A Systems Approach

EDITED BY
ANNE-MARIE BRADY
CATHERINE McCABE
MARGARET McCANN
Trinity College Dublin, Dublin, Ireland

WILEY Blackwell

This edition first published 2014 © 2014 by John Wiley & Sons, Ltd

Registered office: John Wiley & Sons, Ltd, The Atrium, Southern Gate, Chichester, West Sussex, PO19 8SQ, UK

Editorial offices: 9600 Garsington Road, Oxford, OX4 2DQ, UK
The Atrium, Southern Gate, Chichester, West Sussex, PO19 8SQ, UK
111 River Street, Hoboken, NJ 07030-5774, USA

For details of our global editorial offices, for customer services and for information about how to apply for permission to reuse the copyright material in this book please see our website at www.wiley.com/wiley-blackwell

Library of Congress Cataloging-in-Publication Data
ISBN 9780470658239
Fundamentals of medical-surgical nursing : a systems approach / edited by Anne-Marie Brady, Catherine McCabe, Margaret McCann.
p. ; cm.
Includes bibliographical references and index.
ISBN 978-0-470-65823-9 (pbk. : alk. paper) – ISBN 978-1-118-49091-4 (mobi) – ISBN 978-1-118-49092-1 (ePDF) – ISBN 978-1-118-49093-8 (ePub) – ISBN 978-1-118-51479-5 – ISBN 978-1-118-51478-8
I. Brady, Anne-Marie, 1965–, editor of compilation. II. McCabe, Catherine, editor of compilation. III. McCann, Margaret, editor of compilation.
[DNLM: 1. Perioperative Nursing. WY 161]
RD99.24
617'.0231–dc23

2013017938

A catalogue record for this book is available from the British Library.

Wiley also publishes its books in a variety of electronic formats. Some content that appears in print may not be available in electronic books.

Cover image: Veer/Alloy Photography
Cover design by Visual Philosophy

Set in 9.5/11 pt Calibri by Toppan Best-set Premedia Limited
Printed and bound in Malaysia by Vivar Printing Sdn Bhd

1 2014

Contents

About the series ix
Preface x
About the editors xii
Contributors xiii
How to get the best out of your textbook xviii
About the companion website xxi

Part 1: Common Principles Underlying Medical and Surgical Nursing Practice 1

Chapter 1 Principles of nursing assessment 2
Naomi Elliott

Chapter 2 Principles of drug administration 12
Sue Jordan

Chapter 3 Principles of intravenous therapy 26
Lisa Dougherty

Chapter 4 Principles of nutritional care 44
Carolyn Best and Helen Hitchings

Chapter 5 Principles of infection prevention and control 58
Sile Creedon and Maura Smiddy

Chapter 6 Principles of acute care for older people 78
Louise Daly, Debbie Tolson and Anna Ayton

Chapter 7 Principles of end of life care 90
Kevin Connaire

Chapter 8 Principles of perioperative nursing 104
Joy O'Neill, Bernie Pennington and Adele Nightingale

Chapter 9 Principles of high-dependency nursing 124
Tina Day

Chapter 10 Principles of emergency nursing 142
Valerie Small, Gabrielle Dunne and Catherine McCabe

Part 2: Adult Medical and Surgical Nursing 155

Chapter 11 Nursing care of conditions related to the skin 156
Zena Moore and Julie Jordan O'Brien

Chapter 12 Nursing care of conditions related to the respiratory system 176
Anne Marie Corroon and Geralyn Hynes

Chapter 13 Nursing care of conditions related to the circulatory system 210
Kate Olson and Tracey Bowden

Chapter 14 Nursing care of conditions related to the digestive system 240
Joanne Cleary-Holdforth and Therese Leufer

Chapter 15 Nursing care of conditions related to the urinary system 262
Margaret McCann, Ciara White and Louisa Fleure

Chapter 16 Nursing care of conditions related to the endocrine system 298
David Chaney and Anna Clarke

Chapter 17 Nursing care of conditions related to the neurological system 326
Elaine Pierce and Mary E. Braine

Chapter 18 Nursing care of conditions related to the immune system 364
Michael Coughlan and Mary Nevin

Chapter 19 Nursing care of conditions related to haematological disorders 386
Mairead Ni Chonghaile and Laura O'Regan

Chapter 20 Nursing care of conditions related to the musculoskeletal system 422
Sonya Clarke and Julia Kneale

Chapter 21 Nursing care of conditions related to the ear, nose, throat and eye 448
Dympna Tuohy, Jane McCarthy, Carmel O'Sullivan and Niamh Hurley

Chapter 22 Nursing care of conditions related to reproductive health 478
Debra Holloway and Louisa Fleure

Index 510

About the series

Wiley's *Fundamentals* series are a wide-ranging selection of textbooks written to support pre-registration nursing and other healthcare students throughout their course. Packed full of useful features such as learning objectives, activities to test knowledge and understanding, and clinical scenarios, the titles are also highly illustrated and fully supported by interactive MCQs, and each one includes access to a **Wiley E-Text: powered by VitalSource** – an interactive digital version of the book including downloadable text and images and highlighting and note-taking facilities. Accessible on your laptop, mobile phone or tablet device, the *Fundamentals* series is *the* most flexible, supportive textbook series available for nursing and healthcare students today.

Preface

The impetus for this book came from the experience of teaching undergraduate and postgraduate nursing students and the realisation that a comprehensive textbook on medical and surgical nursing was needed to inform and guide learning related to the nursing care of adults. This book is designed to provide a broad overview and a practical understanding of the principles related to adult nursing. It examines the principles underpinning medical and surgical nursing and includes contemporary developments in clinical care, drawing extensively on national and international evidence. Using a systems approach, the book is designed to provide a comprehensive application of the relevant anatomy and physiology, which will inform medical and surgical nursing practice.

The book comprises 22 chapters and is presented in two sections that are designed to guide readers so they can reach an understanding of the context and the key aspects of medical and surgical nursing practice.

- Part 1: Common Principles Underlying Medical and Surgical Nursing Practice
- Part 2: Adult Medical and Surgical Nursing

Part 1 addresses common principles that underpin medical and surgical nursing practice. Chapter 1 presents an overview of the principles underlying the comprehensive nursing assessment of patient care needs. The management of medications is a major component of the everyday work of the nurse in a medical-surgical environment, and Chapters 2 and 3 provide a comprehensive overview of the principles underlying care and the nurses' responsibilities in relation to drug administration, both oral and parental. Nutritional assessment and support is a key responsibility of medical-surgical nursing care and is given detailed consideration in Chapter 4. The prevention and control of infection is discussed in Chapter 5 as this a fundamental element of all healthcare practice. Influenced by changing demographics, caring for the older person represents a significant proportion of everyday medical-surgical nursing practice, and Chapter 6 seeks to develop an understanding of the unique care needs of this population. Chapter 7 aims to develop the nurse's ability to provide appropriate and individualised care to families at the final stage of life. Chapter 8 provides students with an overview of the principles of perioperative nursing. High-dependency care is an increasing feature of medical and surgical care environments and is addressed in Chapter 9. The final chapter in this section gives the reader an overview of emergency department nursing and an understanding of the diverse nature of presenting medical/surgical emergencies, trauma and shock.

In Part 2, a systems approach is taken to afford an overview of adult nursing in medical and surgical acute care environments. The nursing care related to all the systems is discussed in Chapters 11–22 and covers topics related to the skin and the respiratory, cardiovascular, digestive, urinary, endocrine, neurology, immune, haematological, musculoskeletal, eye/ear,/nose/throat and reproductive systems. Each chapter presents a brief overview of the related anatomy and physiology to enhance students' understanding. All of the main conditions are considered, with a focus on relating the main concerns and priorities of medical and surgical nursing. Each chapter is associated with **additional sources of information** such as further reading, professional organisations and online resources.

To be used in addition to the traditional text, learning outcomes, conclusion and references, the website provides a series of **reflective questions** to prompt further discussion in both the classroom and the work setting. **Case studies** are employed where possible to enable the reader to engage with the content from a service provider/user perspective. **Multiple choice questions** are also provided to enable self-evaluation.

The primary market for this textbook is undergraduate students in general nursing at the 3rd level in Ireland and the UK. The book should, however, be of interest to all students undertaking nursing degrees and courses in which general nursing skills are an expectation for professional performance. It will also be relevant to students of other nursing disciplines undertaking health service professional degrees who wish to understand the comorbidities of clients in their care. In additional, it will be a resource for staff already working in medical and surgical nursing.

Anne-Marie Brady
Catherine McCabe
Margaret McCann

Acknowledgements

The editors wish to acknowledge and thank all of the contributors for their commitment, time and effort in sharing their professional clinical and academic expertise. We also wish to thank the reviewers who have provided us with valuable critique as we have developed this work.

About the editors

Anne-Marie Brady PhD BSN MSc PG Dip CHSE PG Dip Stats RGN RNT
Anne-Marie Brady is an assistant professor at Trinity College Dublin and has been involved in undergraduate and postgraduate education since 2000. She has completed a PhD, PG Diploma in Clinical Health Sciences Education and in Statistics at Trinity College Dublin, and a MSc and BSN at Northeastern University Boston, Massachusetts, USA. Her particular areas of research and teaching interest are general nursing and healthcare management She has considerable international nursing experience, having worked in the UK, USA and Irish Republic.

Catherine McCabe PhD MSc BSc RGN RNT
Catherine McCabe has been an assistant professor at Trinity College Dublin since 2002. Her particular area of interest in teaching is general nursing and advanced nursing practice. The focus of her research is primarily exploring the effect of technology and multimedia systems on enhancing communications systems and quality of life for patients with chronic and life-threatening illnesses both in acute care settings and in the home. She has written a great deal on communication in nursing and published a number of papers on her research on communication and technology in healthcare.

Margaret McCann MSc BSc RGN RNT FFNMRCSI
Margaret McCann has been an assistant professor in the School of Nursing and Midwifery, Trinity College Dublin since 2005 and was previously employed as a lecturer in the Faculty of Nursing and Midwifery, Royal College of Surgeons in Ireland. She obtained an MSc in Nursing from the University of Manchester and Royal College of Nursing in 2001. She has been involved in nurse education since 1996. Margaret's primary teaching and research interests lie in the area of urology and renal care. The focus of her research is on the prevention and control of vascular access infection in haemodialysis, and she has published a number of papers on issues relating to renal care and vascular access.

Contributors

Part 1 Common Principles Underlying Medical and Surgical Nursing Practice

Chapter 1 Principles of nursing assessment

Naomi Elliott, PhD, RGN, RNT, Assistant Professor
School of Nursing and Midwifery
Trinity College Dublin, Dublin, Ireland

Chapter 2 Principles of drug administration

Sue Jordan, MB, BCh, PhD, PGCE (FE), Reader
College of Human and Health Science
Swansea University
Swansea, West Glamorgan, UK

Chapter 3 Principles of intravenous therapy

Lisa Dougherty, OBE, RN, MSc, DClinP, Nurse Consultant
Royal Marsden NHS Foundation Trust
Sutton, Surrey, UK

Chapter 4 Principles of nutritional care

Carolyn Best, BSc (Hons), RGN, Nutrition Nurse Specialist
Royal Hampshire Country Hospital
Winchester, Hampshire, UK

Helen Hitchings, BSc (Hons), RD, Nutrition Support Dietician
Royal Hampshire Country Hospital
Winchester, Hampshire, UK

Chapter 5 Principles of infection prevention and control

Sile Creedon, PhD, MSc, BNS, RMT, RNT, RGN, Lecturer
School of Nursing and Midwifery
Brookfield Health Sciences Complex
University College Cork, Cork, Ireland

Maura Smiddy, Doctoral Student
Department of Epidemiology and Public Health
Western Gateway Building
University College Cork, Cork, Ireland

Chapter 6 Principles of acute care for older people
Louise Daly, PhD, MSc, BNS, RNT, RGN, Assistant Professor
School of Nursing and Midwifery
Trinity College Dublin, Dublin, Ireland

Debbie Tolson, PhD, MSc, BSc (Hons), RGN, FRCN, Professor
School of Nursing, Midwifery and Community Health
Glasgow Caledonian University, Glasgow, UK

Anna Ayton, MSc, BNS, RGN, Assistant Professor
School of Nursing and Midwifery
Trinity College Dublin/St James's Hospital, Dublin, Ireland

Chapter 7 Principles of end of life care
Kevin Connaire, MSc, FFNMRCSI, PhD, BNS, RPN, RNT, RGN, Director of Education
Centre for Continuing Education
St Francis Hospice, Dublin, Ireland

Chapter 8 Principles of perioperative nursing
Joy O'Neill, RGN, BSc (Hons) Nursing Studies, Dip Business Studies, Cert Ed, Senior Lecturer
Faculty of Health
Edge Hill University, Manchester, UK

Bernie Pennington, RGN, RODP, BA (Hons), MA Ed, Senior Lecturer
Faculty of Health
Edge Hill University, Manchester, UK

Adele Nightingale, RODP, PGCE, BSc (Hons), Senior Lecturer
Faculty of Health
Edge Hill University, Manchester, UK

Chapter 9 Principles of high-dependency nursing
Tina Day, PhD, MSc, BSc, RN, Cert Ed. RNT, ENB100, Lecturer
Florence Nightingale School of Nursing and Midwifery
Kings College London, London, UK

Chapter 10 Principles of emergency nursing
Valerie Small, MSc, PG Dip CHSE, A&E Cert, RGN, RNT, RNP, RANP, Advanced Nursing Practitioner (Emergency)
Emergency Department
St James's Hospital, Dublin, Ireland

Gabrielle Dunne, MSc, FFNMRCSI, RGN, RANP, Advanced Nursing Practitioner (Emergency)
Emergency Department
St James's Hospital, Dublin, Ireland

Catherine McCabe, PhD, MSc, BNS, RNT, RGN, Assistant Professor
School of Nursing and Midwifery
Trinity College Dublin, Dublin, Ireland

Part 2 Adult Medical and Surgical Nursing

Chapter 11 Nursing care of conditions related to the skin

Zena Moore, PhD, MSc, FFNMRCSI, PG Dip, Dip Management, RGN, Lecturer
Faculty of Nursing and Midwifery
Royal College of Surgeons in Ireland, Dublin, Ireland

Julie Jordan O'Brien, MSc, RGN, Tissue Viability Nurse Specialist
Beaumont Hospital, Dublin, Ireland

Chapter 12 Nursing care of conditions related to the respiratory system

Anne Marie Corroon, MSc, PGDip Ed, RGN, Assistant Professor
School of Nursing and Midwifery
Trinity College Dublin, Dublin, Ireland

Geralyn Hynes, PhD, FFNMRCSI, MSc, RGN, RM, Associate Professor
Faculty of Nursing and Midwifery
Royal College of Surgeons in Ireland, Dublin, Ireland

Chapter 13 Nursing care of conditions related to the circulatory system

Kate Olson, MA, PG Dip, RN, RNT, Senior Lecturer
Adult Years Division
School of Health Sciences
City University London, London, UK

Tracey Bowden, MSc, PGDip Ed, BSc, RN, RNT, Senior Lecturer
School of Health Sciences
City University London, London, UK

Chapter 14 Nursing care of conditions related to the digestive system

Joanne Cleary-Holdforth, MSc, BSc, RGN, RM, Lecturer
School of Nursing
Dublin City University, Dublin, Ireland

Therese Leufer, PGDip Ed, BSc, RGN, Lecturer
School of Nursing
Dublin City University, Dublin, Ireland

Chapter 15 Nursing care of conditions related to the urinary system

Margaret McCann, MSc, FFNMRCSI, BNS (Hons), Certificate Nephrology Dialysis & Transplantation, RNT, RGN, Assistant Professor
School of Nursing and Midwifery
Trinity College Dublin, Dublin, Ireland

Ciara White, MSc Nursing (Renal), Graduate Certificate Nurse Education, RNT, RGN, Renal Nurse Education Facilitator
Centre of Education
Beaumont Hospital, Dublin, Ireland

Louisa Fleure, MSc, PgDip, BSc (Hons), RN, Prostate Cancer Specialist Nurse
Urology Centre
Guy's Hospital, London, UK

Chapter 16 Nursing care of conditions related to the endocrine system

David Chaney, PhD, PG Dip CHSE, MSc, BNS (Hons), DPSN, RNT, RGN, Lecturer
Nursing Research Institute
School of Nursing
University of Ulster
Derry~Londonderry, Northern Ireland, UK

Anna Clarke, PhD (diabetes education), MSc, Higher Diploma Diabetes Nursing, SCM, RGN, Health Promotion & Research Manager
Diabetes Federation of Ireland, Dublin, Ireland

Chapter 17 Nursing care of conditions related to the neurological system

Elaine Pierce, PhD, BSc (Hons), RCNT, ENB148 Neuromedical and Neurosurgical Nursing, RN (RSA), RM, RGN, Principal Lecturer
London South Bank University, London, UK

Mary E. Braine, D.Prof, PGCert HEPR, MSc, BSc (Hons), RN, Lecturer
School of Nursing and Midwifery
College of Health and Social Care
University of Salford, Manchester, UK

Chapter 18 Nursing care of conditions related to the immune system

Michael Coughlan, MEd. BNS, RNT, RGN, RPN, Assistant Professor
School of Nursing and Midwifery
Trinity College Dublin, Dublin, Ireland

Mary Nevin, MSc, BNS (Hons), RNT, RGN, Clinical Nurse Tutor
School of Nursing and Midwifery
Trinity College Dublin, Dublin, Ireland

Chapter 19 Nursing care of conditions related to haematological disorders

Mairead Ni Chonghaile, MSc, BNS, RGN, Transplant Co-ordinator
Hope Directorate
St James' Hospital, Dublin, Ireland

Laura O'Regan, MA (Med Law & Ethics), Cert Tropical Med, Dip Physiology & Counselling, BSc in Cancer Nursing, RGN, BMT Coordinator
Faculty of Health and Social Care
St George's, University of London, and Kingston University, London, UK

Chapter 20 Nursing care of conditions related to the musculoskeletal system

Sonya Clarke, MSc, PGCE (Higher Education), PG Cert (Pain Management), BSc (Hons) Specialist Practitioner in Orthopaedic Nursing, RCN, RGN, Teaching Fellow
School of Nursing and Midwifery
Queen's University Belfast
Belfast, Northern Ireland, UK

Julia Kneale, MSc, BSc, RN, Senior Lecturer
School of Nursing and Caring Sciences
Faculty of Health
University of Central Lancashire
Preston, Lancashire, UK

Chapter 21 Nursing care of conditions related to the ear, nose, throat and eye

Dympna Tuohy, MSc Nursing, Graduate Diploma Medical-Surgical Nursing, BNS (Hons), ICU Certificate, RNT, RGN, Lecturer
Department of Nursing and Midwifery
University of Limerick, Limerick, Ireland

Jane McCarthy, MSc, BNS, RNT, RM, RGN, Lecturer
Department of Nursing and Midwifery
University of Limerick, Limerick, Ireland

Carmel O'Sullivan, RGN, Clinical Nurse Manager 2
ENT Ward
Mid-Western Regional Hospital, Limerick, Ireland

Niamh Hurley, MHSc (Nursing), ENB 998, ENB 346, RGN, Clinical Nurse Manager 2
Eye Ward
Mid-Western Regional Hospital, Limerick, Ireland

Chapter 22 Nursing care of conditions related to reproductive health

Debra Holloway, MSc, BA (Hons), RGN, Nurse Consultant in Gynaecology
McNair Centre
Guy's Hospital, London, UK

Louisa Fleure, MSc, PgDIp, BSc (Hons), RN, Prostate Cancer Specialist Nurse
Urology Centre
Guy's Hospital, London, UK

How to get the best out of your textbook

Welcome to the new edition of *Fundamentals of Medical-Surgical Nursing: A Systems Approach*. Over the next few pages you will be shown how to make the most of the learning features included in the textbook.

The anytime, anywhere textbook

Wiley E-Text

For the first time, your textbook comes with free access to a **Wiley E-Text: Powered by VitalSource** – a digital, interactive version of this textbook which you own as soon as you download it.

Your **Wiley E-Text** allows you to:
Search: Save time by finding terms and topics instantly in your book, your notes, even your whole library (once you've downloaded more textbooks)
Note and Highlight: Colour code, highlight and make digital notes right in the text so you can find them quickly and easily
Organize: Keep books, notes and class materials organized in folders inside the application
Share: Exchange notes and highlights with friends, classmates and study groups
Upgrade: Your textbook can be transferred when you need to change or upgrade computers
Link: Link directly from the page of your interactive textbook to all of the material contained on the companion website

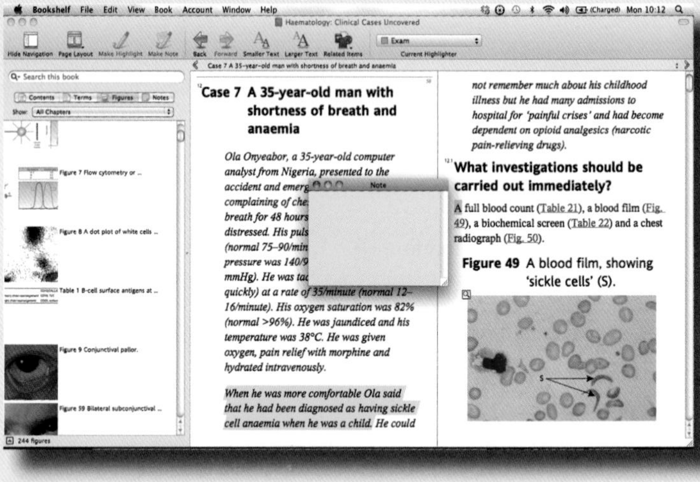

Wiley E-Text
Powered by VitalSource®

To access your Wiley E-Text:

- Find the redemption code on the inside front cover of this book and carefully scratch away the top coating of the label. Visit **www.vitalsource.com/software/bookshelf/downloads** to download the Bookshelf application to your computer, tablet, laptop or mobile device.
- If you have purchased this title as an e-book, access to your Wiley E-Text Edition is available with proof of purchase within 90 days. Visit **http://support.wiley.com** to request a redemption code via the 'Live Chat' or 'Ask A Question' tabs.
- Open the Bookshelf application on your computer and register for an account.
- Follow the registration process and enter your redemption code to download your digital book.
- Find the full access instructions at **www.wileyfundamentalseries.com/medicalnursing.**

The VitalSource Bookshelf can now be used to view your Wiley E-Text on iOS, Android and Kindle Fire!

- **For iOS:** Visit the app store to download the VitalSource Bookshelf: **https://itunes.apple.com/gb/app/vitalsource-bookshelf/id389359495?mt=8**
- **For Android:** Visit the Google Play Market to download the VitalSource Bookshelf: **http://support.vitalsource.com/kb/android/getting-started**
- **For Kindle Fire, Kindle Fire 2 or Kindle Fire HD:** Simply install the VitalSource Bookshelf onto your Fire (see how at **http://support.vitalsource.com/kb/Kindle-Fire/app-installation-guide**). You can now sign in with the email address and password you used when you created your VitalSource Bookshelf Account.

Full E-Text support for mobile devices is available at: **http://support.vitalsource.com**.

CourseSmart

CourseSmart gives you instant access (via computer or mobile device) to this Wiley eTextbook and its extra electronic functionality, at 40% off the recommended retail print price. See all the benefits at **www.coursesmart.com/students**.

Instructors . . . receive your own digital desk copies!

It also offers instructors an immediate, efficient, and environmentally-friendly way to review this textbook for your course.

For more information visit **www.coursesmart.com/instructors**.

With CourseSmart, you can create lecture notes quickly with copy and paste, and share pages and notes with your students. Access your Wiley CourseSmart digital textbook from your computer or mobile device instantly for evaluation, class preparation, and as a teaching tool in the classroom.

Simply sign in at **http://instructors.coursesmart.com/bookshelf** to download your Bookshelf and get started. To request your desk copy, hit 'Request Online Copy' on your search results or book product page.

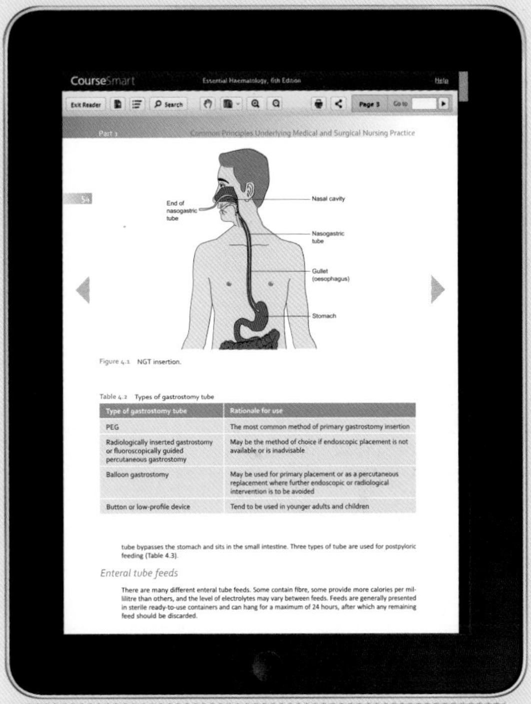

CourseSmart
Learn Smart. Choose Smart.

Features contained within your textbook

Every chapter begins with a **contents list** and **learning outcomes** that you should aim to achieve by the end of the chapter.

Your textbook is full of useful illustrations, boxes, photographs and tables.

1

Principles of nursing assessment

Naomi Elliott

School of Nursing and Midwifery, Trinity College Dublin, Dublin, Ireland

Contents

Introduction	3
The purpose of nursing assessment	3
Assessment frameworks	4
Methods of assessment	6
Rapid assessment of the acutely ill patient	8
Documenting patient assessment and record-keeping	9
Conclusion	10
References	10

Learning outcomes

This chapter will examine the WHY, WHAT, HOW questions of nursing assessment. It will enable you to ask:

- **Why** – to explain the purpose of nursing assessment and why it is vital to quality patient care
- **What** – to consider what patient information is collected and the rationale for using an assessment framework
- **How** – to identify a range of methods available to assess patients and collect information that support clinical decision-making and individualised patient care plans.

Part 1 Common Principles Underlying Medical and Surgical Nursing Practice

54

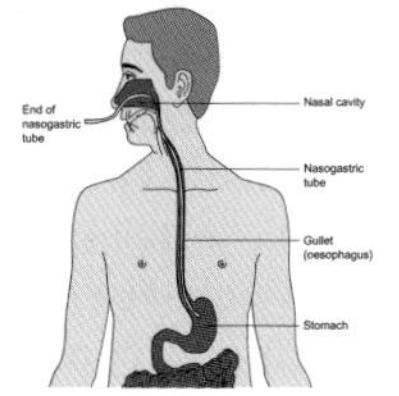

Figure 4.1 NGT insertion.

Table 4.2 Types of gastrostomy tube

Type of gastrostomy tube	Rationale for use
PEG	The most common method of primary gastrostomy insertion
Radiologically inserted gastrostomy or fluoroscopically guided percutaneous gastrostomy	May be the method of choice if endoscopic placement is not available or is inadvisable
Balloon gastrostomy	May be used for primary placement or as a percutaneous replacement where further endoscopic or radiological intervention is to be avoided
Button or low-profile device	Tend to be used in younger adults and children

tube bypasses the stomach and sits in the small intestine. Three types of tube are used for postpyloric feeding (Table 4.3).

Enteral tube feeds

Standard precautions

Standard precautions are taken by healthcare workers to protect themselves and patients against exposure to blood and/or body fluid. Implementation of standard precautions minimises the risk of transmission of infectious agents. These precautions are based on the principle that all blood, body fluids, secretions, excretions except sweat, non-intact skin and mucous membranes may contain transmissible infectious agents.

Standard precautions apply to **ALL** patients at **ALL** times regardless of their diagnosis.

Definition

Polypharmacy is 'the prescription, administration, or use of more medications than are clinically indicated in a given patient' (Charles & Lehman 2010, p. 262).

Box 5.1 The cycle of infection (adapted from Health Protection Surveillance Centre 2009)

- **Infectious agent:** an organism that causes disease (e.g. a bacterium, virus, fungus or protozoon)
- **Reservoir or source of infectious agent:** the place where an infectious agent lives and grows (e.g. the gastrointestinal and upper respiratory tracts for the normal flora)
- **Portal of exit:** any body opening that allows the infectious agent to leave (e.g. the mouth, nose, rectum or breaks in the skin)
- **Means of transmission:** how the infectious agent travels from the infected person to another person. The principle routes of transmission are contact (indirect and direct), droplet and airborne. The mode of transmission varies by type of infectious agent, and some may be transmitted by more than one route
- **Portal of entry:** any body opening that allows the infectious agent to enter (e.g. the nose, mouth, eyes, mucous membranes, a surgical or non surgical break in the skin or medical devices such as urethral catheters that bypass the body's natural defences)
- **A susceptible host:** a non-infected person who could get infected. The factors that influence the acquisition and severity of the infection are related to the virulence of the infectious agent and host factors such as extremes of age, underlying disease, treatment for complex diseases, immunosuppression and whether the patient is the recipient of an organ and tissue transplants

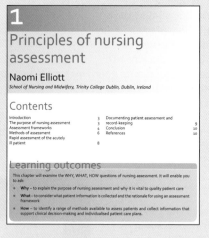

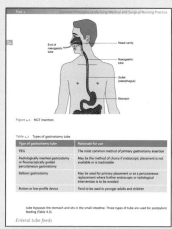

Each chapter ends with a **conclusion** to consolidate learning, a reminder to test yourself on the **website** and a list of **references**.

Conclusion

The nursing assessment of the patient is complex as it involves using different methods to gather information on diverse aspects of patient care across a range of acute and chronic healthcare situations. Nursing assessment generates information that is used to inform nursing actions and interventions. From this information, the patient's problems are identified, further investigations to determine the cause of the problem are selected, and decisions are made about what observations need to be tracked and which referrals to other healthcare professionals are needed.

The pace at which nursing assessment is carried out is determined by the patient's condition and whether it is an emergency, the level of patient distress, how quickly the patient's condition is deteriorating, whether the patient's condition is stable or unstable, and whether the patient is presenting with an acute or chronic illness. The principles of nursing assessment in this chapter are intended to serve as a framework to guide nurses in organising their patient assessment. The key to nursing assessment, however, is to listen to the patient and work towards an understanding the nature of the healthcare problem from the patient's perspective.

Now visit the companion website and test yourself on this chapter:
www.wileyfundamentalseries.com/medicalnursing

References

Bailey, D.G. (2010) Fruit juice inhibition of uptake transport: a new type of food-drug interaction. *British Journal of Clinical Pharmacology*, **70**(5):645–55.
British National Formulary (2011) *British National Formulary* 61. London: British Medical Association/Royal Pharmaceutical Society of Great Britain.
Buxton, I. (2006) Pharmacokinetics and pharmacodynamics. In: Brunton, L., Lazo, J. & Parker K. (eds), *Goodman & Gilman's The Pharmacological Basis of Therapeutics*, 11th edn (pp. 1–39). New York: McGraw-Hill.
Chappell, B. (1993) Implications of switching antiepileptic drugs. *Prescriber*, **4**(18):37–8.
Currier, G. & Simpson, G. (2001) Risperidone liquid concentrate and oral lorazepam versus intramuscular haloperidol and intramuscular lorazepam for treatment of psychotic patients. *Journal of Clinical Psychiatry*, **62**(3):153–7.

A useful **glossary** can be found at the end of Chapter 2 (Principles of drug administration).

Glossary

This chapter contains some difficult terminology. Rather than disrupt the text with explanations, we have added a short glossary.

Angiotensin-converting enzyme (ACE) inhibitors	ACEs, e.g. enalapril and lisinopril, are prescribed for hypertension or heart failure (see Jordan 2008)
Adverse drug reactions (ADRs)	ADRs are any untoward and unintended responses in patients or investigational subjects to a medicinal product that is related to any dose administered. Serious ADRs are those that result

Look out for **website information boxes** throughout the book – they indicate that you can find extra learning resources on the website.

Visit www.wileyfundamentalseries.com/medicalnursing and read Reflective Question 1.1 to think more about this topic.

Now visit the companion website and test yourself on this chapter:
www.wileyfundamentalseries.com/medicalnursing

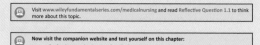

We hope you enjoy your new textbook. Good luck with your studies!

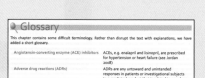

About the companion website

Don't forget to visit the companion website for this book:

www.wileyfundamentalseries.com/medicalnursing

You'll find valuable material designed to enhance your learning, including:

- Interactive multiple-choice questions
- Reflective questions
- Case studies
- Links to online resources

Part 1

Common Principles Underlying Medical and Surgical Nursing Practice

Chapter 1	Principles of nursing assessment	2
Chapter 2	Principles of drug administration	12
Chapter 3	Principles of intravenous therapy	26
Chapter 4	Principles of nutritional care	44
Chapter 5	Principles of infection prevention and control	58
Chapter 6	Principles of acute care for older people	78
Chapter 7	Principles of end of life care	90
Chapter 8	Principles of perioperative nursing	104
Chapter 9	Principles of high-dependency nursing	124
Chapter 10	Principles of emergency nursing	142

1

Principles of nursing assessment

Naomi Elliott

School of Nursing and Midwifery, Trinity College Dublin, Dublin, Ireland

Contents

Introduction 3
The purpose of nursing assessment 3
Assessment frameworks 4
Methods of assessment 6
Rapid assessment of the acutely ill patient 8
Documenting patient assessment and record-keeping 9
Conclusion 10
References 10

Learning outcomes

This chapter will examine the WHY, WHAT, HOW questions of nursing assessment. It will enable you to ask:

- **Why** – to explain the purpose of nursing assessment and why it is vital to quality patient care
- **What** – to consider what patient information is collected and the rationale for using an assessment framework
- **How** – to identify a range of methods available to assess patients and collect information that support clinical decision-making and individualised patient care plans.

Fundamentals of Medical-Surgical Nursing: A Systems Approach, First Edition. Edited by Anne-Marie Brady, Catherine McCabe, and Margaret McCann.

Introduction

Assessment is the first step in determining the condition of the patient's health and their immediate and long-term needs. The nursing assessment of patients on admission to hospital or on attendance at clinics is key to clinical decision-making and to planning patient care that takes account of the individual patients' needs and circumstances. Nurses have responsibility for carrying out the initial and ongoing patient assessments, for initiating interventions that take patients' needs into consideration and for evaluating the effectiveness of these interventions.

The nursing assessment is one component within a larger, multidisciplinary team assessment during which the patient is assessed by different healthcare professionals as part of the care pathway and patient referral process. A multifactorial assessment of the older person for falls, for example, can involve the nurse, doctor, physiotherapist, occupational therapist, optician and other healthcare professionals working in specialist areas of practice such as cardiac assessment. As a member of the multidisciplinary team, the nurse often plays a key role in coordinating the patient assessment and ensuring that appropriate referrals are made and followed up.

The principles of nursing assessment presented in this chapter are in line with the national guidelines from the professional nursing board in Ireland, *An Bord Altranais*, and in the UK the Nursing and Midwifery Council (NMC). The principles need to be read in conjunction with local policies and procedures for the nursing assessment, which are usually set by the hospital or healthcare employer. At ward or unit level, more specific assessment procedures may apply; for example, cerebrovascular or stroke units may include an assessment of swallowing and mood as part of the assessment of a patient newly diagnosed with a cerebrovascular accident – a stroke.

The purpose of nursing assessment

Assessment is the first stage in the nursing process and is key to developing a care plan that is tailored to a patient's individual needs (Figure 1.1).

The purpose of assessment is to achieve the following:

- **Obtain baseline data and track changes.** On admission to hospital or on a first visit to the clinic, it is important to carry out a comprehensive assessment of the patient to establish a set of baseline data against which subsequent assessments can be compared and any changes indicating a deterioration or improvement in the patient's condition tracked.
- **Early recognition of the critically ill or deteriorating patient.** Identifying patients who are 'at risk' is key to initiating a rapid response from the medical emergency or rapid response team. 'Track and Trigger' (e.g. Alert® and other early warning systems) incorporate objective physiological and subjective criteria that can be used to support the nurse's decision about when to call the medical team for help and avert more serious patient emergencies (National Institute for Health and Clinical Excellence [NICE], 2007). If a Track and Trigger system has not been set up in the hospital, a nurse who is concerned about a patient should take urgent action and notify the medical team.
- **Risk assessment.** Assessment is the first step in preventing complications, the aim being to identify patients who are 'at risk' of developing complications associated with their healthcare problem, hospitalisation and reduced mobility. Key areas for risk assessment include pressure ulcers, infection, falls and constipation. Local hospital policy may include risk assessment tools as part of the admission procedure, for example the Braden, Waterlow and Norton scores to identify patients at risk of pressure ulcers and to activate an action plan and interventions to prevent pressure ulcers developing.
- **Screening for health problems.** Nursing assessment provides an ideal opportunity for health promotion and for screening patients for risk factors associated with obesity, cancer, cardiovascular disease, diabetes mellitus and other major Irish and UK health problems. It also provides the opportunity to screen for specific problems such as emotional distress or organisms important in infection control (e.g. methicillin-resistant *Staphylococcus aureus* [MRSA] and vancomycin-resistant *Enterococcus* [VRE]).

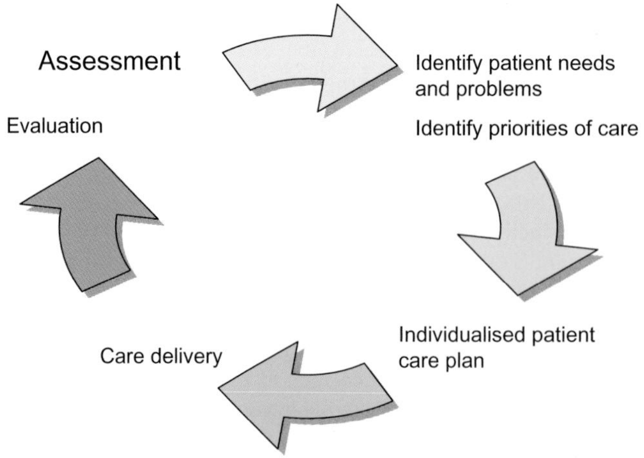

Figure 1.1 Assessment – the first stage in the process of planning patient care.

- **Identify actual and potential problems and prioritise care.** The patient's current problems (actual problems) and problems that could develop in the future (potential problems) need to be identified so that the care plan can be tailored to individual patient needs. Importantly, once the range of patient problems has been identified, care can be prioritised so that major problems are dealt with first.
- **Care planning, tailored to individual patient needs.** The purpose of assessment is not only to determine and document the patient's current condition, but also to provide evidence for the planning and provision of nursing care. Although standardised care plans are available in some units or hospitals, the nursing actions that are required to meet a patient's needs and problems should be tailored to take account of individual patient needs.
- **Discharge planning.** Patient assessment also includes the early identification of patients' needs for forward planning and organising the supports and community services necessary to facilitate a timely discharge from hospital. Recent trends indicate that patients' stay in hospital is shortening, the use of day surgery is increasing, and policies on early discharge and discharge planning are setting the standards for healthcare practice (Capelastegui *et al.* 2008; Saczynski *et al.* 2010; Shepperd *et al.* 2010). Although the reasons for a delay in discharging the patient home from hospital are multifactorial, patient assessment that includes information about the patient's home and social circumstances, family and community supports will help prevent problems arising from a poor knowledge of a patient's home situation or the support available, and will avert delays related to non-medical reasons.

Assessment frameworks

An important principle underpinning the nursing approach to patient assessment is that it is systematic, comprehensive and person-centred. Many of the assessment frameworks used in clinical practice are linked to nursing theories such as the activities of living (Roper *et al.* 2000) or the self-care deficit theory of nursing (Orem 2001), or to other theory including Maslow's (1999) hierarchy of needs.

Nursing models and theories serve as a guide for clinical practice and provide for a structured approach insofar as they map out what areas to include in a patient assessment. The number of new or modified assessment frameworks for nursing practice is ever increasing, but a common feature across different nursing assessments is the inclusion of the core aspects of physical, psychosocial and spiritual assessment within the context of family, community and environment (Figure 1.2). The decision of which assessment framework to use is made by healthcare organisations and nursing management, who then oversee its implementation in their admission procedures and nursing documentation. This is important because it provides a way of assuring a standardised approach to nursing assessment and quality patient care.

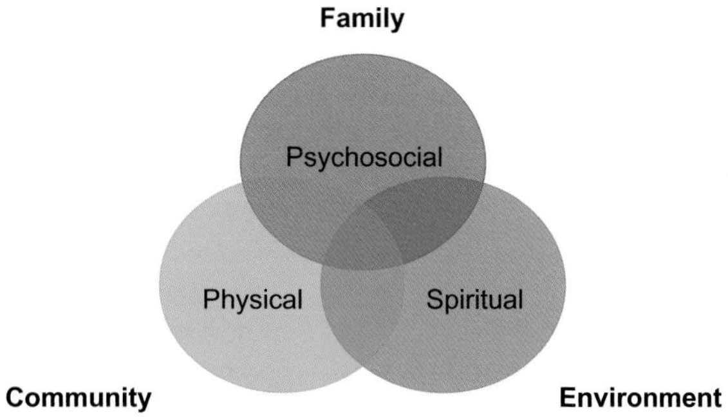

Figure 1.2 Key aspects to include in a patient assessment.

In terms of how this translates into practice and what information is gathered during the nursing assessment, the broad areas to consider include biographical and health data, a systematic review of patient systems and functions, and a social assessment:

- **Biographical and health data.** Obtaining information about the patient's health history is vital for putting the current problem or illness into context (Kaufman 2008).

Assessment of . . .	. . . in relation to the following aspects
The patient's understanding of the reason for admission Biographical and contact details Religion Past medical and surgical history Previous history of healthcare-associated infections, e.g. MRSA, VRE and *Clostridium difficile* Allergies Drugs and medications The patient's knowledge of hospital policy, such as visiting, patients' property and valuables	Identifying significant information that affects current health status and care-planning

- **Patient assessment.** This involves a 'head-to-toe' systematic review of the patient. A review of systems and functions enables the nurse to elicit information about problems and provide vital clues to support a clinical diagnosis or uncover a problem of which the patient is unaware. The depth of the patient assessment will depend on the patient's condition and the urgency of the clinical situation (Tagney 2008).

Assessment of . . .	. . . in relation to the following aspects
Breathing; smoking history Cardiovascular system Communication Diet, nutrition and hydration Elimination Mobility Personal hygiene Skin condition Sleep patterns Sexual health Concerns, anxieties, fears and mood	The key problem as identified by the patient Changes in function Coping strategies in dealing with changes Level of dependence/independence The patient's normal activity, function and behaviour Health beliefs and lifestyle behaviour Preventive health measures including screening and immunisation

- **Social assessment.** Taking a social history enables an early identification of patients' needs and problems that might delay discharge from hospital. Social history-taking is not always considered a priority in acute healthcare services, but it helps nurses to identify the patient's needs so that appropriate referrals can be made to the health and social services and service delivery is coordinated (Atwal 2002).

Assessment of . . .	. . . in relation to the following aspects
Marital status Occupation Whether the patient is living alone or with others, has a carer or is providing care for another person Social networks and supports Housing or accommodation situation Informal support from family, neighbours or voluntary community groups Current community or home services – does the patient have a home help or meals-on-wheels, go to a day centre or receive support from a public health (or community) nurse or other personnel? Access to shops for food, chemist, doctor, dentist, health clinic, bank/post office Access to exercise or sports facilities	Impact of the health problem on work, day-to-day living, lifestyle and family Coping strategies – how the patient currently manages to deal with problem Current supports used by the patient Identification of unmet support service needs

Visit www.wileyfundamentalseries.com/medicalnursing and read Reflective Question 1.1 to think more about this topic.

Methods of assessment

The methods of assessment that are used to gather the information for clinical decision-making include interviewing the patient and obtaining a health history, carrying out a physical examination, making clinical observations and using risk assessment tools.

Interviewing and obtaining a health history

Taking a patient history is an essential part of assessment as an accurate history can provide over 80% of the information required for diagnosis (Epstein *et al.* 2008). Obtaining an accurate history is not just about asking a list of questions, but also requires establishing an effective patient–nurse relationship in which the patient feels that the nurse is interested in understanding their healthcare problems (Elliott 2010). This involves putting patients at their ease, providing as much privacy as possible, ensuring the nurse is familiar with any information already gathered, being sensitive to cultural differences and inviting patients to tell their story (Tagney 2008).

Once the introductions have been completed, obtaining a health history begins with inviting the patient to tell their story and using an open question such as, '*Can you tell me what has brought you here today?*' After an explanation has been given, the nurse moves to asking key and targetted questions to build up a comprehensive picture of the patient's problem: '*How has it affected you? Have you noticed what makes it worse or what helps? Have you noticed any changes in . . . ? How does this compare with previous times you have had this problem?*' More targetted questions are used to focus on eliciting whether there are any associated symptoms so the nurse needs to be familiar with the patterns associated with specific health problems.

Investing in the end of the interview and considering the closing questions is vital to ensuring ongoing continuity in the patient–nurse relationship in future consultations. Ending the interview involves summarising, framing information using the patient's perspective and providing opportunity for the patient to add further information. A closing question such as '*Is there anything else we haven't covered that you would like to discuss?*' enables patients to provide additional information. During the first nurse–patient encounter, some patients may find it difficult to disclose problems and may be unwilling to do so until they know and have established a trusting relationship with the nurse. One helpful way in which the nurse can let the patient know there will be further opportunities to discuss issues is by saying, for example, '*If you think of anything else later on, let me know and we can have a chat then.*'

Physical examination

Physical examination provides objective data and is used to corroborate evidence gathered from the patient interview and clinical observation. Examination involves measurement of the '**vital signs**', including temperature, heart rate, respiratory rate and blood pressure. The patient's **weight** is recorded and, if indicated, the patient's body mass index may also be calculated to determine whether the patient has a normal weight or is under- or overweight. **Urinalysis** using a dipstick reagent strip and a clean sample of fresh urine from the patient is used to screen for abnormal substances such as glucose or protein. Any abnormalities detected in the urinalysis should be followed up by more specific laboratory tests to investigate the cause and perhaps detect a previously undiagnosed condition such as diabetes mellitus. The patient's **skin** condition is examined; in addition to carrying out a pressure ulcer risk assessment, any abnormalities such as the presence of bruises, rashes and peripheral oedema are noted.

Clinical observation

Observation is an integral part of patient assessment as it provides an additional layer of information gathered during the patient–nurse interaction, physical examination and routine ward-based tests. Observation provides a means of gathering vital indicators about the patient's condition and well-being, and this information contributes to the overall evidence supporting clinical decision-making.

During the interaction with the patient, the nurse takes note of non-verbal cues. Indicators of patient anxiety or distress can prompt the nurse to investigate further using gentle questioning or to return for a follow-up visit if the patient is unwilling or not ready to discuss their problems at that time. Observing patients as they walk around the ward, move from chair to bed, get dressed and close buttons or zips can provide important information about their mobility, balance and dexterity. Observing the patient's general appearance includes noting the colour of the face and body and any abnormal signs such as nasal flaring, which can indicate respiratory distress. Abnormal smells or odours such as the odour of ketones on the patient's breath may indicate fasting or diabetic ketoacidosis. Observing the patient's behaviour noting inappropriate responses and actions can indicate neurological, metabolic, endocrine or mental health problems.

Information gathered from observing the patient is used along with that assimilated from the patient interview and physical examination to make sense of the patient's health problem and to support clinical decision-making.

Assessment tools

Nurses can make use of a range of assessment tools and rating scales as part of their assessment of the patient. These provide a standardised approach to assessing specific aspects of the patient's condition that can otherwise be difficult to measure (Table 1.1).

The Glasgow Coma Scale (Teasdale & Jennett 1974), for example, provides a means of assessing a patient who is becoming increasingly drowsy and unresponsive and, importantly, enables nurses to communicate the findings in a way that other healthcare professionals will understand. Using the Glasgow Coma Scale, the patient is assessed on three specific items of (1) best eye-opening, (2) best verbal response, and (3) best motor response. The patient's response on each of these items is converted into a numerical score, with the total score used to determine the level of consciousness.

The Early Warning Score (EWS; McGaughey *et al.* 2007) is an example of another type of tool that not only measures the patient's status, but also identifies an action plan for the healthcare professional

Table 1.1 Examples of assessment tools and rating scales

Assessment aspect	Assessment tools and rating scales
Level of consciousness	Glasgow Coma Scale (Teasdale & Jennett 1974) AVPU (Alert, Voice, Pain, Unresponsive; McNarry & Goldhill 2004)
Acutely ill or patient deteriorating	Alert® (Smith 2003) Manchester Triage Scale (Manchester Triage Group 2006) Early Warning Score (McGaughey *et al.* 2007)
Pressure ulcer risk	Braden scale (Bergstrom *et al.* 1987) Waterlow score (Waterlow 2005) Norton score (Norton *et al.* 1975)
Moving and handling	*Manual Handling Assessments in Hospitals and the Community: An RCN Guide* (Royal College of Nursing 2003)
Falls	*Falls – the Assessment and Prevention of Falls in Older People* (NICE 2004)
Pain	Pain thermometer – numeric rating scale Abbey Pain Scale for patients who are unable to verbalise or articulate their needs (Abbey *et al.* 2004)
Patient distress	National Comprehensive Cancer Network Guidelines *Distress Management*, Version 1.2011 (National Comprehensive Cancer Network 2011)
Bowel elimination	Bristol Stool Form Chart (Lewis & Heaton 1997, © 2000 Norgine Ltd.) Rome III criteria (Longstreth *et al.* 2006) Eton scale for constipation (Kyle *et al.* 2005)

to follow. In the EWS, the physiological parameters are set and used to initiate further interventions. For example, if a patient's temperature exceeds a predetermined level, blood cultures will be taken.

Other assessment tools are used to identify patients at risk, for example, of developing pressure ulcers. These predictive tools help nurses to identify at-risk patients so that interventions can be put in place to prevent pressure ulcers occurring. Pressure ulcer risk assessment tools are, however, only one component of risk assessment. Gould *et al.* (2002) found that tools such as the Braden, Waterlow and Norton scales are not always accurate as they can either over- or underpredict risk. Therefore, pressure ulcer risk assessment tools serve as guides, and the nurse's own clinical judgement should also be taken into consideration.

Patient self-assessment tools are also available whereby patients use a visual analogue scale or brief questionnaire to assess themselves. The pain thermometer is one example – on this, the patient scores how severe the pain is by using a rating scale of 1–10 where 1 is no pain and 10 is the worst pain imaginable. Another example of such a tool is the patient distress self-assessment tool developed by the National Comprehensive Cancer Network (2011) in America. This uses a distress 'thermometer' along with a tick box checklist of practical, family, emotional and physical problems and spiritual or religious concerns encountered with cancer patients.

Rapid assessment of the acutely ill patient

A full patient assessment that includes a detailed review of physical, psychosocial and preventive health needs, a physical examination and routine tests can take several hours to complete. An in-depth assessment requires time and is appropriate for elective, non-emergency cases and for patients on their first visit or admission to the hospital or clinic. Given that nurses also work in acute care situations, however, rapid assessment skills are also important, especially as the early recognition of a deterioration in the critically ill or unstable patient is vital to managing the care of such acutely ill individuals. Depending on how acute or unstable the patient's condition is, some examples of rapid assessment systems are outlined here.

'Track and Trigger'

Delays in recognising patients who are acutely ill on admission to hospital or in detecting clinical deterioration during their hospital stay can result in serious consequences. An analysis of 425 patient deaths that occurred in UK acute hospitals in 2005 showed that 64 deaths were related to a failure to detect and recognise changes in patients' vital signs, a failure to act upon the worsening vital signs or delays in the patient receiving medical attention (National Patient Safety Agency 2007).

To avoid delays in the detection and recognition of acute illness and in starting appropriate interventions, NICE (2007) recommends that a physiological Track and Trigger system is used to monitor all adult patients in acute hospital care settings. NICE recommends that the patient's heart rate, respiratory rate, systolic blood pressure, level of consciousness, oxygen saturation and temperature are monitored and that key changes in these physiological observations are used to trigger a response. The response to a low score involves increasing the frequency of observations and alerting the nurse in charge to changes in the patient's condition. The response to a medium score involves making an urgent call to the patient's primary medical team, and the response to a high score involves making an emergency call to the medical team, which includes a doctor skilled in assessing critically ill patients and in advanced airway management and resuscitation skills. In addition to initiating appropriate interventions, the Track and Trigger system includes information about when to transfer the patient to the critical care area for ongoing care.

Alert®

For use in situations in which a patient is deteriorating, some hospitals have introduced the Alert® system for rapid assessment of the critically ill patient. This acts as a decision-making tool to alert healthcare professionals to patients who are acutely ill, to determine the level of urgency and to know when to call the emergency medical team. The Alert® framework (Smith 2003) is just one example of a rapid and systematic approach to assessment that trains healthcare professionals to rapidly assess a patient whose condition is deteriorating. It follows an ABCDE sequence in which A is **a**irway, B is **b**reathing, C is **c**irculation, D is **d**isability (neurological assessment including assessment of the level of consciousness and/or use of the Glasgow Coma Scale) and E is **exposure** (anything that may contribute to the patient's deterioration).

Cardiopulmonary resuscitation

In emergency, cardiac arrest and life-threatening situations in which the patient is unresponsive, the immediate priorities are to assess the patient for signs of life (Resuscitation Council UK 2010). If the patient shows no signs of life, the nurse calls the resuscitation team and if no carotid pulse is present, starts cardiopulmonary resuscitation. Once these priorities have been addressed, other important assessments can then be made.

Documenting patient assessment and record-keeping

After assessing the patient, it is important that nurses record their findings and so provide documentary evidence about the patient's condition. This written information is vital for providing baseline data and ensuring continuity of patient care. It provides information that other nurses and healthcare professionals can refer to when planning and coordinating patient care. Although patient assessment forms and nursing documentation are set by local hospital policy and procedures, the national professional guidelines for recording nursing practice and patient assessment advise the following:

- An accurate assessment of the person's physical, psychological and social well-being, and, whenever necessary, the views and observations of family members in relation to that assessment' should be included in a patient record. (*An Bord Altranais* 2002, p. 2)
- Evidence in relation to the planning and provision of nursing care should be included as part of a patient record. (*An Bord Altranais* 2002, p. 2)
- Record details of any assessment and reviews undertaken, and provide clear evidence of the arrangements made for future and ongoing care. This should also include details of information given about care and treatment. (NMC 2009, p. 4)

The information gathered from an assessment when the patient is first admitted to hospital or first visits an outpatient clinic needs to be recorded. It provides the evidence to support clinical decisions and a rationale for the individualised patient care plan. Ongoing or continuous patient assessment when monitoring to evaluate changes in a patient's condition in changing circumstances also needs to be recorded, and nursing actions documented. Nursing assessment may also identify patient problems that need to be referred for further assessment by an appropriate healthcare professional such as a physiotherapist, dietitian, social worker, speech therapist or occupational therapist.

The importance of nursing documentation is emphasised by policy-makers and professionals in Ireland (*An Bord Altranais*, 2002), the UK (NMC, 2009) and internationally (Wang *et al.* 2011). However, evidence from a review of quality audits of nursing documentation in actual clinical practice has revealed some deficiencies (Wang *et al.* 2011). Although documentation does not always capture the full extent of what happens in actual nursing practice, Wang *et al.* found several studies that revealed insufficient recording of psychological, social, cultural and spiritual aspects of care. Other deficiencies highlighted by these authors included a lack of documentation of the patient's vital signs, diagnosis leading to hospitalisation, assessment of pressure ulcers and assessment for specific care issues, including older patients with chronic heart failure, the physical characteristics of wounds or patients with pain and cognitive impairment. The implications for practice, therefore, are that if documentation is to serve as a vital communication tool between nurses and other caregivers for the exchange of information gathered at assessment, attention needs to be paid to ensuring there are no gaps in documenting patient assessment.

Conclusion

The nursing assessment of the patient is complex as it involves using different methods to gather information on diverse aspects of patient care across a range of acute and chronic healthcare situations. Nursing assessment generates information that is used to inform nursing actions and interventions. From this information, the patient's problems are identified, further investigations to determine the cause of the problem are selected, and decisions are made about what observations need to be tracked and which referrals to other healthcare professionals are needed.

The pace at which nursing assessment is carried out is determined by the patient's condition and whether it is an emergency, the level of patient distress, how quickly the patient's condition is deteriorating, whether the patient's condition is stable or unstable, and whether the patient is presenting with an acute or chronic illness. The principles of nursing assessment in this chapter are intended to serve as a framework to guide nurses in organising their patient assessment. The key to nursing assessment, however, is to listen to the patient and work towards an understanding the nature of the healthcare problem from the patient's perspective.

Now visit the companion website and test yourself on this chapter:
www.wileyfundamentalseries.com/medicalnursing

References

Abbey, J., Piller, N., DeBellis, A. *et al.* (2004) The Abbey pain scale: a 1-minute numerical indicator for people with end-stage dementia. *International Journal of Palliative Nursing*, **10**(1):6–13.

An Bord Altranais (2002) *Recording Clinical Practice: Guidance to Nurses and Midwives*. Dublin: An Bord Altranais.

Atwal, A. (2002) Nurses' perceptions of discharge planning in acute health care: a case study in one British teaching hospital. *Journal of Advanced Nursing*, **39**(5):450–8.

Bergstrom, N., Braden, B.J., Laguzza, A. & Holma, V. (1987). The Braden Scale for predicting pressure sore risk. *Nursing Research*, **36**(4):205–10.

Capelastegui, A., España, P.P., Quintana, J.M. *et al.* (2008) Declining length of hospital stay for pneumonia and post-discharge outcomes. *American Journal of Medicine*, **121**(10):845–52.

Elliott, N. (2010) 'Mutual intacting': a grounded theory study of clinical judgement practice issues. *Journal of Advanced Nursing*, **66**(12):2711–21.

Epstein, O., Perkin, D., Cookson, J., *et al.* (2008). *Clinical Examination*, 4th ed. Edinburgh: Mosby.

Gould, D., Goldstone, L., Gammon, J., Kelly, D. & Maldwell, A. (2002) Establishing the validity of pressure ulcer risk assessment scales: a novel approach using illustrated patient scenarios. *International Journal of Nursing Studies*, **39**(2):215–28.

Kaufman, G. (2008) Patient assessment: effective consultation and history taking. *Nursing Standard*, **23**(4): 50–6.

Kyle, G., Prynn, P., Oliver, H. & Dunbar, T. (2005) The Eton Scale: a tool for risk assessment for constipation. *Nursing Times*, **101**(18):50–1.

Lewis, S.J., & Heaton, K.W. (1997) Stool form scale as a useful guide to intestinal transit time. *Scandinavian Journal of Gastroenterology*, **32**:920–4.

Longstreth, G., Thompson, W.G., Chey, W., Houghton, L., Mearin, F. & Spiller, R. (2006) Functional bowel disorders. *Gastroenterology*, **130**:1480–91.

McGaughey, J., Alderdice, F., Fowler, R., Kapila, A., Mayhew, A. & Moutray, M. (2007) Outreach and Early Warning Systems (EWS) for the prevention of intensive care admission and death of critically ill patients on general hospital wards. *Cochrane Database of Systematic Reviews*, (3):CD005529.

McNarry, A.F., & Goldhill, D.R. (2004). Simple bedside assessment of level of consciousness: comparison of two simple assessment scales with the Glasgow Coma Scale. *Anaesthesia*, **59**:34–7.

Manchester Triage Group (2006) *Emergency Triage/Manchester Triage Group*, 2nd ed. London: BMJ.

Maslow, A.H. (1999) *Toward a Psychology of Being*. New York: Wiley.

National Comprehensive Cancer Network (2011) *NCCN Clinical Practice Guidelines in Oncology, Distress Management.* Version 1.2011. Retrieved 7th March 2011 from http://www.nccn.org/professionals/physician_gls/pdf/distress.pdf.

National Institute for Clinical Excellence (2004) *Falls: The Assessment and Prevention of Falls in Older People*. Clinical Guideline No. 21. London: NICE.

National Institute for Health and Clinical Excellence (2007) *Acutely Ill Patients in Hospital: Recognition of and Response to Acute Illness in Adults in Hospital*. Clinical Guideline No. 50. London: NICE.

National Patient Safety Agency (2007) *Safer Care for the Acutely Ill Patient: Learning from Serious Incidents*. PSO/5. London: National Patient Safety Agency.

Norton, D., McClaren, R. & Exton-Smith, A. (1975) *An Investigation of Geriatric Nursing Problems in Hospital*. Edinburgh: Churchill Livingstone.

Nursing and Midwifery Council (2009) *Record Keeping: Guidance for Nurses and Midwives*. London: NMC.

Orem, D. (2001) *Nursing: Concepts of Practice*, 6th ed. St Louis: Mosby.

Resuscitation Council (UK) (2010). *Resuscitation Guidelines 2010*. London: Resuscitation Council UK.

Roper, N., Logan, W. & Tiereny, A. (2000) *The Roper-Logan-Tierney Model of Nursing: Based on Activities of Living*. Edinburgh: Churchill Livingstone.

Royal College of Nursing (2003) *Manual Handling Assessments in Hospitals and the Community: An RCN Guide*. London: RCN.

Saczynski, J.S., Lessard, D., Spencer, F.A. *et al.* (2010) Declining length of stay for patients hospitalized with AMI: impact on mortality and readmissions. *American Journal of Medicine*, **123**(11):1007–15.

Shepperd, S., McClaran, J., Phillips, C.O., *et al.* (2010) Discharge planning from hospital to home. *Cochrane Database of Systematic Reviews*, (1):CD000313.

Smith, G. (2003) *ALERT: Acute Life Threatening Events, Treatment and Recognition*. Portsmouth: University of Portsmouth.

Tagney, J. (2008) Skills in taking an accurate cardiac patient history. *British Journal of Cardiac Nursing*, **3**(1):8–13.

Teasdale, G., & Jennett, B. (1974) Assessment of coma and impaired consciousness. A practical scale. *Lancet*, **13**(2), 81–4.

Wang, N., Hailey, D. & Yu, P. (2011) Quality of nursing documentation and approaches to its evaluation: a mixed-method systematic review. *Online Journal of Advanced Nursing* **67**:doi 10.1111/j.1365-2648.2011.05634.

Waterlow, J. (2005). *Pressure Ulcer Prevention Manual*. London: Wound Care Society.

2

Principles of drug administration

Sue Jordan

College of Human and Health Science, Swansea University, Swansea, West Glamorgan, UK

Contents

Introduction 13
Drug formulation 13
How the body handles drugs:
Pharmacokinetics 13
Therapeutics 21
Conclusion 21
References 21
Further reading 23
Glossary 24

Learning outcomes

Having read this chapter, you will be able to:

- Understand how changes in drug formulations affect drug absorption and therapeutic outcome
- Discuss the nursing implications of the pharmacokinetics of oral administration
- Relate principles of drug absorption, distribution and elimination to the management of medications
- Describe the precautions taken to ensure that changes in drug elimination do not adversely affect patients

Fundamentals of Medical-Surgical Nursing: A Systems Approach, First Edition. Edited by Anne-Marie Brady, Catherine McCabe, and Margaret McCann.

Introduction

Medical advances of the latter half of the 20th century produced drugs powerful enough to correct pathophysiological disturbance; however, alterations in physiology may have unintended consequences. It is estimated that twice as many people die from medical errors as from breast cancer, motor vehicle accidents or HIV/AIDS (Kohn *et al.* 1999), and preventable **adverse drug reactions (ADRs)** account for some 3.7% of hospital admissions (Howard *et al.* 2007). Medication administration is increasing in complexity. More physiologically vulnerable patients are sustained by complex regimens, narrowing the margin for error. Without due attention to drug administration and elimination, the amount of drug entering or leaving the body can fluctuate, resulting in either **therapeutic failure** or ADRs.

Drug formulation

The formulation of a medicine refers to its physical and chemical composition. This includes both the specified active ingredients and other chemicals present, the **excipients** or 'packing chemicals', as listed on the product label. The formulation, together with absorption (see the section on 'Absorption'), determines the extent to which the drugs reach their destinations, i.e. their **bioavailability**.

Excipients

Excipients stabilise the active ingredient or modify its release. They may be responsible for ADRs. For example, some medicines contain sodium ions (e.g. some penicillins and warfarin) or potassium ions (e.g. some multivitamin preparations). The sodium content of many antacid indigestion remedies and some proprietary analgesics can be sufficient to precipitate fluid retention and breathlessness in people with incipient heart failure. Aspartame is present in many drugs, for example co-amoxiclav and didanosine; these products should be avoided by people with phenylketonuria. Oral medicines containing sugar promote dental caries (Mentes 2001). Medicines available in 'sugar-free' forms contain sorbitol, which can cause diarrhoea, particularly when administered via **enteral** feeding tubes (Phillips & Nay 2008). Excipients may also be responsible for **hypersensitivity responses**.

Excipients may differ between brands; therefore, the release of the active ingredients, and hence their bioavailability, may be different. Important examples include antiepileptic drugs, lithium preparations, antipsychotic agents, ciclosporin and modified-release formulations. Where a condition, such as epilepsy, is controlled on a certain branded product, changing to another brand or a (cheaper) generic drug may result in a loss of disease control (Chappell 1993).

Visit www.wileyfundamentalseries.com/medicalnursing and read Reflective Question 2.1 to think more about this topic.

Liquids and solids

The physical formulation of a drug affects its rate of absorption. Before being absorbed, tablets must disintegrate and the active ingredients must dissolve. The rate at which this occurs depends on the formulation. For example, drugs will be absorbed more rapidly and completely from liquids than tablets. This can be useful: for example, paracetamol liquid relieves pain more rapidly than tablets, and liquid risperidone is an effective alternative to injections of antipsychotic agents (Currier & Simpson 2001). However, when the formulation of a medicine is changed from tablets to liquid, its bioavailability increases, and ADRs may appear for the first time.

How the body handles drugs: Pharmacokinetics

Pharmacokinetics describes how the body absorbs, distributes and eliminates drugs.

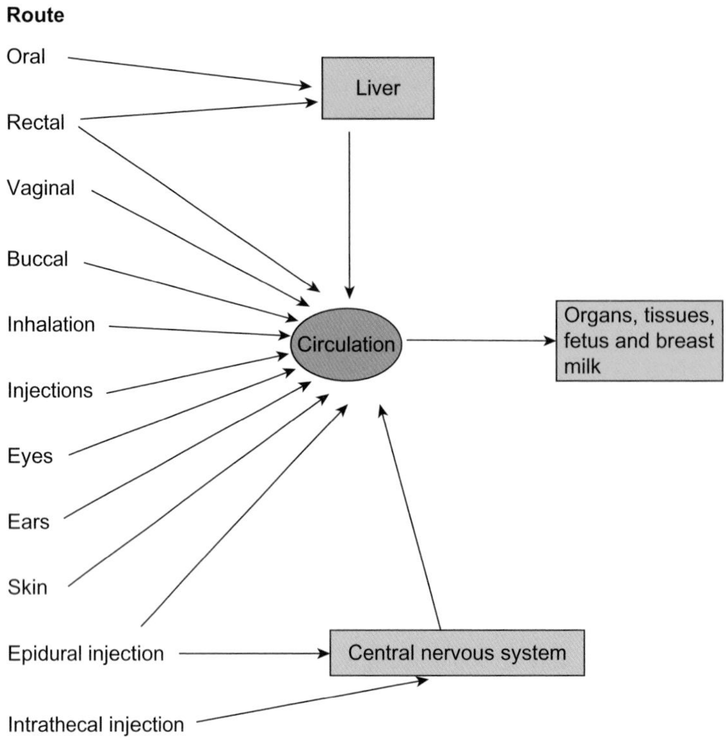

Figure 2.1 Routes of administration. Arrows represent the passage of drugs. Adapted from Jordan (2010) with permission from Palgrave Macmillan.

Absorption

Absorption makes drugs available to the body fluids for distribution, and determines their bioavailability. Regardless of the route of administration, drugs enter the circulation; the rate and extent of absorption are reduced only by topical administration (Figure 2.1). Important barriers to drug absorption and distribution include the gut wall, capillary walls, cell membranes, the blood–brain barrier, the placenta and the blood–milk barrier. Drugs administered orally pass to the liver, where they are metabolised, whereas drugs administered by other routes pass directly into the circulation. Therefore, the latter may be more effective, but they may also cause more severe ADRs. The proportion of drug passing straight into the circulation cannot be predicted with rectal, epidural or spinal administration.

Drug administration

Practitioners avoid touching medicines if at all possible (Railton 2007). Gloves are worn when handling drugs that could be absorbed through skin (e.g. creams, transdermal patches, anticancer drugs and nitrates) or can cause irritation and contact dermatitis (e.g. chlorpromazine) (Smith *et al.* 2008).

Oral administration

Most drugs are given orally, for convenience. All tablets and capsules should be swallowed with a full glass of water with the patient sitting upright and remaining upright for 30 minutes (McKenry *et al.* 2006). This prevents prolonged contact between the drug and the lining of the mouth and oesophagus, which is vulnerable to corrosive substances, particularly bisphosphonates, aspirin, iron and potassium salts. Older adults may find tablets and liquids difficult to swallow and may prefer to take orodispersible preparations with soft food, such as puddings.

Crushing or breaking tablets

Crushing tablets alters their bioavailability, usually by hastening absorption, and this sudden rise in drug concentration can cause ADRs. Breaking, crushing or chewing **enteric-coated** tablets destroys their modified-release mechanisms. If a tablet is crushed or a capsule is opened, fine particles may be released into the air. This may result in:

- absorption through the respiratory tract or skin of the administrator (cytotoxics, hormones, steroids or prostaglandins);
- the growth of resistant microorganisms in non-disposable equipment or in the lungs or skin of the administrator (antibiotics).

Breaking or splitting tablets can cause large dose deviations or weight losses, with important clinical consequences. Splitting devices are used when this cannot be avoided (Verrue *et al.* 2011).

Food

Food and herbs can affect drug bioavailability by binding the drug, increasing gastric acidity, blood and bile flow, delaying gastric emptying, impairing transport across the intestine and altering elimination (Custodio *et al.* 2008; Tarirai *et al.* 2010). Foods, vitamins and herbs can also counteract or augment drug actions.

Optimising drug absorption may require administration on an empty stomach or with food.

Administration on an empty stomach

Some drugs, for example bisphosphonates and tetracyclines, will be not be absorbed at all if given with food. These drugs should be administered 1–2 hours before or 2 hours after a meal.

Food, antacids, bulk-forming laxatives and guar gum may bind to drugs, keeping them within the intestines and to a varying degree decreasing their absorption. Examples include furosemide (frusemide), calcium-channel blockers, erythromycin stearate, tetracyclines and iron preparations.

Drugs whose absorption is decreased by food also have the potential to interact with enteral feeds. If these drugs are administered within 2 hours of an enteral feed, there is a risk that their therapeutic effect will be lost. Where enteral feeds are set to run throughout the day, specialist advice should be sought.

The absorption of some drugs (e.g. iron, ketoconazole, some antifungal or antiviral agents, a few antibiotics and dipyridamole) depends on gastric acidity. Gastric acidity may be too low for drug absorption between meals in older patients and those with HIV/AIDS, or if antacids, **H2-receptor antagonists** (e.g. ranitidine) or proton pump inhibitors (e.g. omeprazole) are co-administered (Lahner *et al.* 2009). Acidity may be increased by vitamin C or Coca-Cola (Schmidt & Dalhoff 2002). A few drugs, such as ampicillin and some forms of erythromycin, are destroyed by gastric acid; others, such as furosemide, metformin, atenolol and pravastatin, are less soluble in acidic environments (Marasanapalle *et al.* 2009). Full absorption is achieved if administration is separated from meals by 2 hours.

Several enzymes and transporters (carrier proteins) are important in the absorption of nutrients and drugs from the small intestine. Some of these are inhibited by grapefruit and orange juice. The extent of this interaction varies between individuals as well as with different batches of juice. When co-administered within 2–4 hours of some drugs (e.g. the antihistamine fexofenadine, l-thyroxine, ciclosporin and atenolol), fruit juices decrease the absorption and effectiveness of the drug (Dresser *et al.* 2002, Bailey 2010).

Protein-containing meals may reduce the absorption of some anti-Parkinson medications (such as co-beneldopa and co-careldopa), worsening the tremor, stiffness and pain, as rated by the patients themselves. Amino acids in the meal may compete with l-dopa for sites on transporters across the blood–brain barrier and the gut (Nyholm *et al.* 2002).

Administration with food

For some drugs, for example nifedipine, a drug–food interaction is beneficial in that it prevents the sudden onset of the drug's action. Co-administration with food may ameliorate nausea or irritation of the gastrointestinal tract, although sometimes at the cost of reduced or delayed absorption, as is seen with carbamazepine, valproate, iron and aspirin.

The type of food may also be important (Custodio *et al.* 2008). For example, tetracyclines are not absorbed in the presence of calcium-containing foods such as dairy products, and digoxin is not absorbed with a high-fibre meal. The fat content of the meal may also be important, either because the drugs dissolve in fat (e.g. isotretinoin) or because fat stimulates bile secretion, which increases drug absorption (e.g. griseofulvin) (Schmidt & Dalhoff 2002).

Many studies on drug–food interactions have been undertaken with unfortified meals. The extra constituents of vitamin- or mineral-enriched foods may bind to some drugs, reducing their absorption (Wallace & Amsden 2002). For example, calcium-fortified orange juice impairs the absorption of fluoroquinolones (Neuhofel *et al.* 2002).

For most drugs, it is important to *maintain a constant relationship between medication and meals*, so that plasma concentrations of the drug do not vary from day to day.

Distribution

Distribution is the movement of drugs around the circulation and into the tissues and fat for storage (Figure 2.2). Distribution is affected by:

- **Plasma protein binding.** Some drugs (including antiepileptics, warfarin and anticancer agents) circulate bound to plasma proteins. When plasma protein levels are low (e.g. with malnutrition, burns or pregnancy, or in neonates), ADRs may occur.
- **Lipid solubility**, that is, whether the drug dissolves in fatty tissues, including the brain
  All drugs acting on the central nervous system are highly lipid soluble. Distribution and storage are affected by adiposity, age and sex. For example, those with generous fat deposits need more nitrous oxide to achieve analgesia for wound dressing and take longer to recover.
- **Transporters embedded in cell membranes** in tissues and organs, for example P-glycoprotein. Transporters regulate drug uptake and efflux, and their action may be accelerated or inhibited by co-administered drugs (Zhang *et al.* 2010). For example, omeprazole delays the elimination of methotrexate, risking its accumulation (Haidar & Jeha 2011).
- **The binding properties of the drug.** Some drugs have unusual binding characteristics. For example, tetracyclines bind to growing bones and teeth and should not be administered to anyone who is growing, pregnant or breast-feeding.

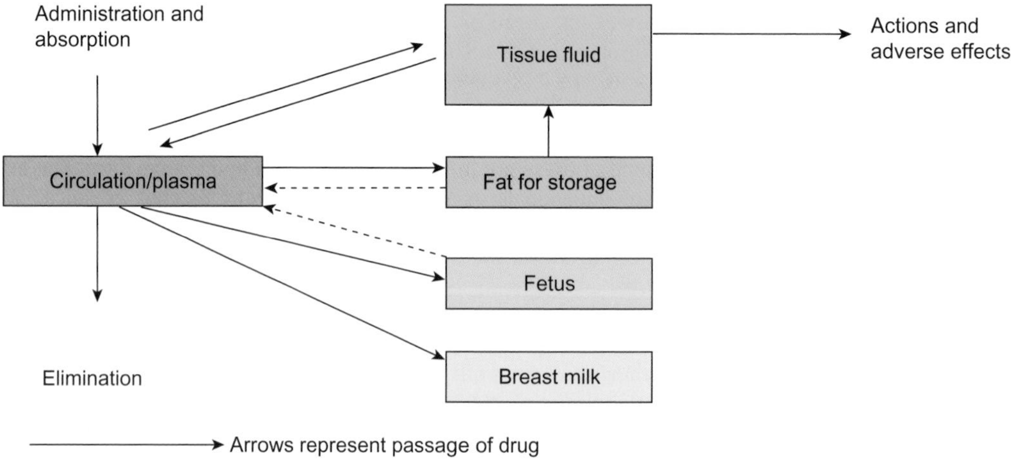

Figure 2.2 Drug distribution and body compartments. Arrows represent the passage of drugs. NB: The return of metabolites from fetus to mother varies between drugs. The fetus and the breast milk are distinct body compartments, which should always be considered when medicines are administered. Adapted from Jordan (2010) with permission from Palgrave Macmillan.

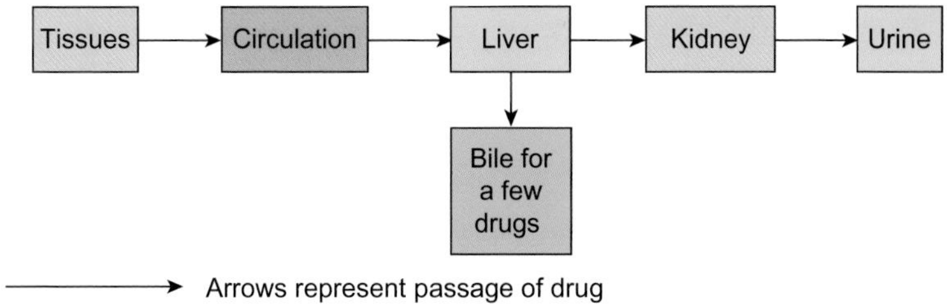

Figure 2.3 Usual routes of drug elimination. Arrows represent the passage of drugs. Adapted from Jordan (2010) with permission from Palgrave Macmillan.

- **Blood flow.** Conditions affecting the circulation, such as heart failure, blood loss or a heart attack, divert blood, and circulating drugs, away from the peripheries and gut and towards the heart, brain and lungs. The reduced circulation to the gut means that drugs administered orally may be poorly absorbed.

Visit www.wileyfundamentalseries.com/medicalnursing and read Reflective Question 2.2 to think more about this topic.

Drug elimination

The route of elimination varies between drugs. A few drugs are eliminated unchanged, whereas others are extensively metabolised (Figure 2.3).

Drug metabolism

Most metabolism occurs in the liver, but the gastrointestinal tract and the central nervous system contain enzymes responsible for the metabolism of some drugs. Metabolic processes allow the body to utilise and detoxify foreign substances. There are no simple tests to assess the liver's capacity to metabolise and eliminate drugs (Perucca *et al.* 2006). Drug metabolism depends on:

- genetic make-up;
- the liver's environment, i.e. the chemicals reaching the liver from the gut and the circulation;
- liver impairment, for example due to malnutrition, cirrhosis or hepatitis;
- the stage in the life cycle.

If metabolism is accelerated, drugs will be removed too rapidly, and signs and symptoms of illness will return. However, if metabolism is inhibited or blocked, the drug will accumulate. Some foods and herbs can interfere with metabolism and increase or decrease the effects of certain drugs, and re-timing the administration of medicines may not prevent these interactions.

Accelerated clearance

The regular ingestion of some foods (barbecued meats, caffeine or alcohol) or drugs (including some antiepileptics, rifampicin, rifabutin, St John's Wort and some antiviral agents) or exposure to tobacco accelerates the action of enzymes in the gut lining and liver. This can increase the rate of elimination of some drugs, for example diazepam, clozapine and oestrogens. Ciclosporin or digoxin may be rendered ineffective by St John's Wort (Fugh-Berman 2000). To accommodate this, the prescriber may increase the dose of medication.

Visit www.wileyfundamentalseries.com/medicalnursing and read Reflective Question 2.3 to think more about this topic.

Reduced clearance

The activity of certain enzymes in the gut lining and liver is inhibited not only by certain drugs, such as ketoconazole, fluoxetine, erythromycin, cimetidine and high doses of alcohol, but also by grapefruit, and possibly by grapefruit and other juices. These reduce the elimination of several drugs, particularly in the elderly: 200–250 mL of grapefruit juice can double the bioavailability of most calcium-channel blockers (except for diltiazem), the effect lasting for some 24 hours (Dresser *et al.* 2000). For other drugs (e.g. dextromethorphan, a cough suppressant), clearance remains low for over 3 days. Further work may expand the list of drugs affected: carbamazepine, warfarin, amphetamines, some statins, most calcium-channel blockers, some antiviral agents, sildenafil and related drugs, zopiclone, benzodiazepines, pimozide, tacrolimus, ciclosporin, amiodarone, sertraline, buspirone, ergotamine (including LSD), some cytotoxics and ranolazine (Kiani & Imam 2007; Seden *et al.* 2010; *British National Formulary* 2011).

Visit www.wileyfundamentalseries.com/medicalnursing and read Reflective Question 2.4 to think more about this topic.

Drug excretion

Most drugs depend on the kidneys for elimination and clearance. However, some drugs such as corticosteroids and oestrogens are excreted via the bile (see Figure 2.3). The kidneys control salt and water balance and eliminate waste products to maintain a stable internal environment for the rest of the body. Two processes are involved: glomerular filtration (in the Bowman's capsules), which is measured by the **glomerular filtration rate (GFR)**, and tubular secretion and reabsorption. Drug excretion may rely on either or both of these processes, depending on the drug involved.

The GFR is usually considered the best overall measure of the kidneys' ability to eliminate drugs in health and disease (Levey *et al.* 1999). For several drugs, prescribers need to know the GFR before initiating therapy. If the GFR is too low, some drugs, such as lithium or metformin, will not be given. For other drugs, a reduced dose will be prescribed at prolonged intervals, as seen with gentamicin.

If the GFR falls, the elimination of most drugs is impaired, causing their accumulation and ADRs. GFR is therefore regularly checked to assess any changes in the patient's ability to eliminate drugs. It is affected by:

- changes in the blood flow to the kidneys, for example with dehydration (including the administration of diuretics, and excess alcohol or caffeine), shock, heart failure and the administration of **non-steroidal anti-inflammatory drugs** (**NSAID**s) or **angiotensin-converting enzyme inhibitors (ACEIs)**;
- renal disorders and the loss of nephrons (e.g. repeated infection, pre-eclampsia, hypertension and long-term prostatic enlargement);
- acute illness, as blood flow and renal function can change rapidly, affecting drug concentrations. A urine output below 30 mL per hour must be reported because renal damage may be occurring and drugs could rapidly accumulate.
- sex, as women have lower GFRs than men. The combined effect of age and gender means that older women have a reduced ability to eliminate drugs, and therefore an increased risk of ADRs;
- the life cycle.

The composition of the urine can affect drug elimination. For example, lithium is excreted more completely if salt intake is high; however, if the sodium concentration decreases, due to reduced salt intake, diarrhoea and vomiting or excessive sweating, lithium is no longer passed into the urine and can accumulate, causing **toxicity**. Some drugs pass more readily into an alkaline urine; therefore, a

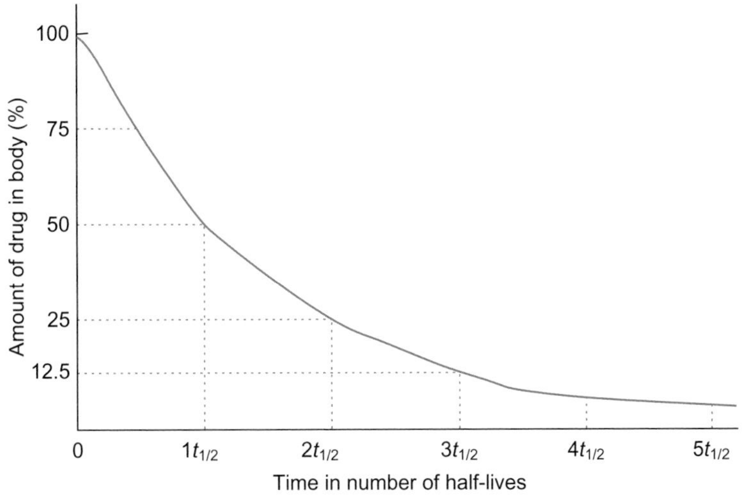

Figure 2.4 Graph to illustrate elimination half-life ($t_{1/2}$) following a single intravenous dose. Most drugs follow this pattern of elimination. During the first half-life, 50% of the drug is eliminated from the body. After three half-lives, 87.5% of the drug has been removed. After 4–5 half-lives, this dose of the drug has effectively disappeared. Adapted from Jordan (2010) with permission from Palgrave Macmillan.

change of diet or the ingestion of antacids may cause the therapeutic failure of lithium, aspirin or aminoglycosides (Wallace & Amsden 2002).

Elimination half-life

The absorption, distribution and elimination of a drug can be measured, and constants such as elimination half-life can be calculated. The elimination half-life for each drug is the time taken for the concentration of the drug in plasma and the amount of drug in the body to fall to half its maximum value (Buxton 2006) (Figure 2.4). The half-life is used to calculate:

- the dose interval;
- the time to eliminate a drug;
- the time taken from an initiation or change of therapy before the concentration of the drug reaches a 'steady state' (Endrenyi 2007; see the section on 'Steady-state concentration').

A drug's half-life depends on its biological properties and the recipient's ability to eliminate it. The duration of action of a drug increases in direct proportion to its half-life. For most drugs, the dose has less impact on the duration of action than the half-life.

To maintain the drug's concentration within the **therapeutic range**, the dosage interval for many drugs is approximately one half-life. Should drug administration intervals be much longer than this, the fluctuations in the drug's concentration in the plasma may lead to therapeutic failure (Buxton 2006).

Fifty percent of a dose will be eliminated one half-life after discontinuation. For example, tetrahydrocannabinol has a half-life of 50 hours, and therefore will be detectable in blood and urine samples for several days after ingestion. In contrast, diamorphine has a half-life of 1.25 ± 0.25 hours and will be cleared from the body in a much shorter time.

Visit www.wileyfundamentalseries.com/medicalnursing and read Reflective Question 2.5 to think more about this topic.

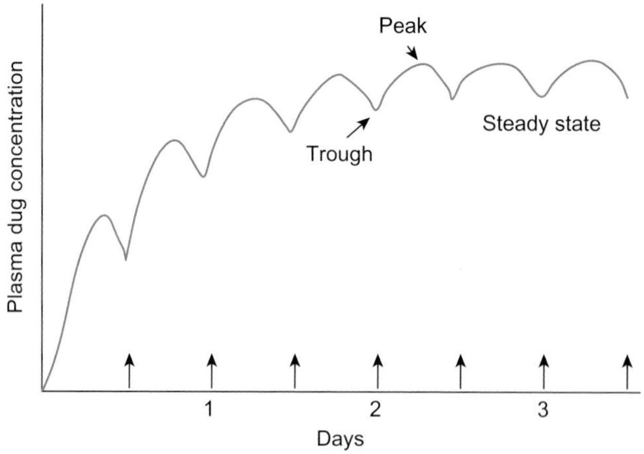

Figure 2.5 Diagram to illustrate the accumulation of a drug with repeated dosing: repeated twice-daily oral dosing of a drug with a half-life of 12 hours. The drug accumulates for 3–5 half-lives and then reaches a steady state in which the amount of drug eliminated equals that taken in. Adapted from Jordan (2010) with permission from Palgrave Macmillan.

Steady-state concentration

Many drugs accumulate with repeated dosing (Figure 2.5). For most drugs at normal doses, repeated administration at regular intervals will result in a relatively constant plasma concentration, or a steady state. At this concentration, the rate of drug elimination is equal to the rate of administration, i.e. what goes in, goes out. The full effects of the drug and dose-related ADRs often do not appear until a steady state has been reached. The time taken to reach a steady state is 4–5 times the drug's elimination half-life (Endrenyi 2007). If the drug's half-life is known, it is possible to predict when dose-related ADRs are most likely to appear for the first time.

Visit www.wileyfundamentalseries.com/medicalnursing and read Reflective Question 2.6 to think more about this topic.

In emergencies, it is not always possible to wait 3–5 half-lives for a therapeutic effect to occur. Therefore a high dose, known as a **loading dose**, will be administered in to achieve a therapeutic concentration rapidly. Loading doses may be administered in acute care, for example if cardiac dysrhythmias are to be treated with digoxin or amiodarone. These doses are individually calculated and not routine; therefore, extra care is needed during administration (National Patient Safety Agency 2010).

For a few drugs, including phenytoin, alcohol, some **selective serotonin-reuptake inhibitors (SSRIs)** and salicylates (including aspirin), elimination does not depend on a single half-life. This is because the enzymes and transporters responsible become 'saturated' and eliminate the drug at a constant rate. Such drugs are more likely to have a prolonged duration of action. For example, adults can eliminate alcohol at a rate of 8–10 g (150–220 mmol) per hour (approximately equivalent to a half pint of beer, a glass of wine or a measure of shorts). Consequently, if 10 pints of beer (or the equivalent) are consumed, high concentrations of alcohol may persist in the body the following day (Masters 2001). This pattern of drug elimination is also observed following overdosage with several drugs, particularly aspirin.

Therapeutics

Not all medicines effectively treat or manage disease. Even if a drug is working on the body's cells, there may be no noticeable response. The clinical response shows considerable individual variation, and doses may need to be adjusted for age, gender, weight, body surface area, pregnancy, kidney function or genetic make-up. Even so, the response is not always predictable, and practitioners must always be alert for idiosyncratic **hypersensitivity or hypersusceptibility reactions**, the most severe of which is **anaphylaxis** (Jordan 2008).

Conclusion

Drug administration is one of the highest-risk aspects of practice. Any failure to consider the details of formulation, distribution and elimination variables, drug interactions or administration schedules may compromise the efficacy of therapeutic regimens and even patient safety.

Now visit the companion website and test yourself on this chapter:
www.wileyfundamentalseries.com/medicalnursing

References

Bailey, D.G. (2010) Fruit juice inhibition of uptake transport: a new type of food-drug interaction. *British Journal of Clinical Pharmacology*, **70**(5):645–55.

British National Formulary (2011) *British National Formulary* 61. London: British Medical Association/Royal Pharmaceutical Society of Great Britain.

Buxton, I. (2006) Pharmacokinetics and pharmacodynamics. In: Brunton, L., Lazo, J. & Parker K. (eds), *Goodman & Gilman's The Pharmacological Basis of Therapeutics*, 11th edn (pp. 1–39). New York: McGraw-Hill.

Chappell, B. (1993) Implications of switching antiepileptic drugs. *Prescriber*, **4**(18):37–8.

Currier, G. & Simpson, G. (2001) Risperidone liquid concentrate and oral lorazepam versus intramuscular haloperidol and intramuscular lorazepam for treatment of psychotic patients. *Journal of Clinical Psychiatry*, **62**(3):153–7.

Custodio, J.M., Wu, C.Y. & Benet, L.Z. (2008) Predicting drug disposition, absorption/elimination/transporter interplay and the role of food on drug absorption. *Advanced Drug Delivery Reviews*, **60**(6):717–33.

Dresser, G. Bailey, D., Leake, B.F. *et al.* (2002) Fruit juices inhibit organic anion transporting polypeptide-mediated drug uptake to decrease the oral availability of fexofenadine. *Clinical Pharmacology and Therapeutics*, **71**(1):11–20.

Dresser, G., Spence, D. & Bailey, D. (2000) Pharmacokinetic-pharmacodynamic consequences and clinical relevance of cytochrome P450 3A4 inhibition. *Clinical Pharmacokinetics*, **3**(1):41–57.

Edwards, I.R. & Aronson, J.K. (2000) Adverse drug reactions: definitions, diagnosis, and management. *Lancet*, **356**:1255–9.

Endrenyi, L. (2007) Pharmacokinetics: principles and clinical applications. In: Kalant, H., Grant, D. & Mitchell, J. (eds), *Principles of Medical Pharmacology*, 7th edn (pp. 50–61). Toronto: Elsevier.

Fairgrieve, S., Jackson, M., Jonas, P. *et al.* (2000) Population based, prospective study of the care of women with epilepsy in pregnancy. *BMJ*, **321**:674–5.

Fugh-Berman, A. (2000) Herb–drug interactions. *Lancet*, **355**: 134–8.

Haidar, C. & Jeha, S. (2011) Drug interactions in childhood cancer. *Lancet Oncology*, **12**(1):92–9.

Howard, R., Avery, A., Slavenburg, S. *et al.* (2007) Which drugs cause preventable admissions to hospital? A systematic review. *British Journal of Clinical Pharmacology*, **63**(2):136–47.

International Conference on Harmonisation (1996) *ICH Harmonised Tripartite Guideline for Good Clinical Practice*. Marlow, Buckinghamshire: Institute of Clinical Research.

Jordan, S. (2008) *The Prescription Drug Guide for Nurses*. Maidenhead: Open University Press/McGraw-Hill.

Jordan, S. (2010) *Pharmacology for Midwives: the Evidence Base for Safe Practice*, 2nd edn. Basingstoke: Palgrave/Macmillan.

Kiani, J. & Imam, S.Z. (2007) Medicinal importance of grapefruit juice and its interaction with various drugs. *Nutrition Journal*, **30**(6):33.

Kohn, L., Corrigan, J. & Donaldson, M. (1999) *To Err Is Human: Building a Safer Health System*. Washington DC: National Academy Press.

Lahner, E., Annibale, B. & Delle Fave, G. (2009) Systematic review: impaired drug absorption related to the co-administration of antisecretory therapy. *Alimentary Pharmacology and Therapeutics*, **29**(12):1219–29.

Levey, A., Bosch, J., Lewis, J., Greene, T., Rogers, N. & Roth, D. (1999) A more accurate method to estimate glomerular filtration rate from serum creatinine: a new prediction equation. *Annals of Internal Medicine*, **130**:461–70.

McKenry, L., Tessier, E. & Hogan, M. (2006) *Mosby's Pharmacology in Nursing*, 22nd edn. St Louis: Elsevier Mosby.

Marasanapalle, V.P., Crison, J.R., Ma J, Li X. & Jasti, B.R. (2009) Investigation of some factors contributing to negative food effects. *Biopharmaceutics and Drug Disposition*, **30**(2):71–80.

Masters, S. (2001) The alcohols. In: Katzung, B. (ed.), *Basic and Clinical Pharmacology*, 8th edn (pp. 382–94). New York: McGraw-Hill.

Mentes, A. (2001) pH changes in dental plaque after using sugar-free paediatric medicine. *Journal of Clinical Paediatric Dentistry*, **25**(4):307–12.

National Patient Safety Agency (2010) *Preventing Fatalities from Loading Doses: Rapid Response Report NPSA/2010/RRR018*. NPSA. Retrieved 31 May 2011 from http://www.nrls.npsa.nhs.uk/patient-safety-data.

Neuhofel, A., Wilton, J., Victory, J.M., Hejmanowsk, L.G. & Amsden, G.W. (2002) Lack of bioequivalence of ciprofloxacin when administered with calcium-fortified orange juice. *Journal of Clinical Pharmacology*, **42**(4):461–6

Nyholm, D., Lennernas, H., Gomes-Trolin, C. & Aquilonius, S.M. (2002) Levodopa pharmacokinetics and motor performance during activities of daily living in patients with Parkinson's disease on individual drug combinations. *Clinical Neuropharmacology*, **25**(2):89–96.

Perucca, E., Berlowitz, D., Birnbaum, A. *et al.* (2006) Pharmacological and clinical aspects of antiepileptic drug use in the elderly. *Epilepsy Research*, **68**(Suppl. 1):S49–63.

Phillips, N.M. & Nay, R.A. (2008) systematic review of nursing administration of medication via enteral tubes in adults. *Journal of Clinical Nursing*, **17**(17):2257–65.

Railton, D. (2007) *Knowledge Set: Medication*. Oxford: Harcourt Education/Heinemann.

Schmidt, L. & Dalhoff, K. (2002) Food–drug interactions. *Drugs*, **62**(10):1481–502.

Seden, K., Dickinson, L., Khoo, S. & Back, D. (2010) Grapefruit–drug interactions. *Drugs*, **70**(18):2373–407.

Smith, S., Duell, D. & Martin, B. (2008) *Clinical Nursing Skills: Basic to Advanced Skills*, 7th edn. Upper Saddle River, NJ: Pearson/Prentice Hall.

Tarirai, C., Viljoen, A.M. & Hamman, J.H. (2010) Herb–drug pharmacokinetic interactions reviewed. *Expert Opinion in Drug Metabolism and Toxicology*, **6**(12):1515–38.

Verrue, C., Mehuys, E., Boussery, K., Remon, J.-P. & Petrovic, M. (2011) Tablet-splitting: a common yet not so innocent practice. *Journal of Advanced Nursing*, **67**(1):26–32.

Wallace, A.W. & Amsden, G.W. (2002) Is it really OK to take this with food? *Journal of Clinical Pharmacology*, **42**(4):437–43.

Zhang, L., Reynolds, K. S., Zhao, P. & Huang, S.-M. (2010) Drug interactions evaluation: an integrated part of risk assessment of therapeutics. *Toxicology and Applied Pharmacology*, **243**: 134–45.

Further reading

British Association for Parenteral and Enteral Nutrition (2004) *Administering Drugs via Enteral Feeding Tubes: A Practical Guide*. London: BAPEN.

Chan, L. (2002) Drug–nutrient interaction in clinical nutrition. *Current Opinion in Clinical Nutrition and Metabolic Care*, **5**(3):327–32.

Chen, N., Aleksa, K., Woodland, C., Rieder, M. & Koren G. (2006) Ontogeny of drug elimination by the human kidney. *Pediatric Nephrology*, **21**(2):160–8.

Clark, A.J. (1933) *The Mode of Action of Drugs on Cells*. London: Edward Arnold.

DeWoskin, R.S. & Thompson C.M. (2008) Renal clearance parameters for PBPK model analysis of early lifestage differences in the disposition of environmental toxicants. *Regulatory Toxicology and Pharmacology*, **51**(1):66–86.

Fairgrieve, S., Jackson, M., Jonas, P. *et al.* (2000) Population based, prospective study of the care of women with epilepsy in pregnancy. *BMJ*, **321**:674–5.

Ginsberg, G., Hattis, D., Sonawane, B. *et al.* (2002) Evaluation of child/adult pharmacokinetic differences from a database derived from the therapeutic drug literature. *Toxicological Sciences*, **66**(2):185–200.

Ginsberg, G., Hattis, D., Russ, A. & Sonawane, B. (2005) Pharmacokinetic and pharmacodynamic factors that can affect sensitivity to neurotoxic sequelae in elderly individuals. *Environmental Health Perspectives*, **113**(9):1243–9.

Harvey, S. & Jordan, S. (2010) Diuretics: implications for nursing practice. *Nursing Standard*, **24**(43):40–9.

Hayes, D., Hendler, C.B., Tscheschlog, B. *et al.* (eds) (2003) *Medication Administration Made Incredibly Easy*. Philadelphia: Springhouse/Lippincott, Williams & Wilkins.

Holmer Pettersson, P., Jakobsson, J. & Owall, A. (2006) Plasma concentrations following repeated rectal or intravenous administration of paracetamol after heart surgery. *Acta Anaesthesiologica Scandinavica*, **50**(6):673–7.

Jentink. J., Dolk. H., Loane, M.A. *et al.* (2010) EUROCAT Antiepileptic Study Working Group. Intrauterine exposure to carbamazepine and specific congenital malformations: systematic review and case-control study. *BMJ*, **2**:c6581.

Jordan, S., Griffiths, H. & Griffith, R. (2003) Continuing professional development: administration of medicines. Part 2. Pharmacology. *Nursing Standard*, **18**(3):45–55.

Morrell, M.J. (2003) Reproductive and metabolic disorders in women with epilepsy.*Epilepsia*, **44**(Suppl. 4): 11–20.

Naysmith, M. & Nicholson, J. (1998) Nasogastric drug administration. *Professional Nurse*, **13**(7): 424–51.

Rang H, Dale M., Ritter J. & Flower R. (2007) *Pharmacology*, 6th edn. Edinburgh: Elsevier/Churchill Livingstone.

Sassarini, J., Clerk, N. & Jordan, S. (2010) Epilepsy in pregnancy In: Jordan, S. (ed.), *Pharmacology for Midwives: The Evidence Base for Safe Practice*, 2nd edn (pp. 361–76). Basingstoke: Palgrave Macmillan.

Thomson F., Naysmith M. & Lindsay A. (2000) Managing drug therapy in patients receiving enteral and parenteral nutrition. *Hospital Pharmacist*, **7**(6):155–64.

Tucker, J. (2007) Rectal and vaginal drug delivery. In: Aulton, M. (ed.), *Aulton's Pharmaceuticals*, 3rd edn (pp. 606–15). Edinburgh: Elsevier.

Wilkinson, G. (2001) Pharmacokinetics. In: Hardman, J., Limbard, L., Molinoff , P., Ruddon, R. & Goodman Gilman, A. (eds.), *Goodman & Gilman's The Pharmacological Basis of Therapeutics*, 10th edn (pp. 3–30). New York: McGraw-Hill.

Glossary

This chapter contains some difficult terminology. Rather than disrupt the text with explanations, we have added a short glossary.

Angiotensin-converting enzyme (ACE) inhibitors	ACEs, e.g. enalapril and lisinopril, are prescribed for hypertension or heart failure (see Jordan 2008)
Adverse drug reactions (ADRs)	ADRs are any untoward and unintended responses in patients or investigational subjects to a medicinal product that is related to any dose administered. Serious ADRs are those that result in death, are life-threatening, necessitate hospitalisation or prolong hospitalisation, result in persistent or significant disability or incapacity, or are congenital anomalies (International Conference on Harmonisation 1996). The term 'side effects' is reserved for dose-related and therapeutically unrelated adverse effects (Edwards & Aronson 2000)
Anaphylaxis	A serious life-threatening hypersensitivity reaction, characterised by low blood pressure, shock and difficulty breathing
Antagonists or blockers	These bind to receptors and block them, preventing the agonist reaching the receptor and activating it. For example, the beta-blockers (propranolol or atenolol, for example) block the actions of the sympathetic nervous system, slow and stabilise the heart rate and induce bronchoconstriction
Bioavailability	A measure of absorption, or the fractional extent to which the drug dose reaches its site of action
Excipient	A vehicle added to a prescription to confer a suitable consistency or form to a pharmaceutical product
Enteral	By way of the gastrointestinal tract
Enteric-coated preparations	A term designating a special coating applied to tablets or capsules that prevents the release and absorption of their contents until they reach the intestine

Glomerular filtration rate (GFR)	GFR is the volume of fluid filtered into the nephrons every minute, i.e. the sum of the volume of filtrate formed each minute in all functioning nephrons. The normal GFR for a standard male (body surface area 1.73 m^2) is 100 mL per minute; the value for a female is 90% of this. A GFR below 60 mL per minute per 1.73 m^2 surface area indicates renal disorder and is associated with an increased risk of cardiovascular disease. GFR is usually calculated from the serum creatinine concentration, and reported as eGFR (estimated eGFR). Where drug doses are finely balanced, at the extremes of body weight or if there are risks of toxicity, other methods of calculating the GFR are used, such as the Cockroft and Gault formula (*BNF* 2011). These calculations require the patient's weight, which should be written on the drug chart
Hypersensitivity/hypersusceptibility response	A response quantitatively greater than is usual for a given dose
Loading dose	A large initial dose of drug given to reach a rapid therapeutic level of the drug
Non-steroidal anti-inflammatory drugs (NSAIDs)	NSAIDs, or 'aspirin-like drugs', share certain therapeutic actions and ADRs. They modify the inflammatory reaction and the associated pain, and reduce fever. NSAIDs include ibuprofen and diclofenac
Selective serotonin reuptake inhibitors (SSRIs)	SSRIs, e.g. fluoxetine and sertraline, are prescribed for the management of depressive illness or obsessive-compulsive disorders
Therapeutic failure	The situation in which treatment does not have the required effect
Therapeutic range	Drug plasma concentrations that will provide therapy but avoid toxicity to the patient. Above the therapeutic range, toxic effects may appear. Below the therapeutic range, the drug does not have the desired effect
Toxicity	The quality of being poisonous

3

Principles of intravenous therapy

Lisa Dougherty

Royal Marsden NHS Foundation Trust, Sutton, Surrey, UK

Contents

Introduction 27
Anatomy and physiology of the veins 27
Overview of vascular access devices 29
Administration of intravenous therapy 30
Principles of infection prevention 35
Maintaining a closed intravenous system 36
Maintaining patency 36
Managing complications 36
Blood transfusion therapy 39
Conclusion 40
References 40
Further reading 43

Learning outcomes

Having read this chapter, you will be able to:

- Understand the anatomy and physiology of the veins
- Describe the types of vascular access device
- Describe the methods for administering intravenous medications
- Understand how to choose the appropriate infusion device
- Describe how to prevent infection in intravenous therapy
- Recognise the signs and symptoms of the related complications

Fundamentals of Medical-Surgical Nursing: A Systems Approach, First Edition. Edited by Anne-Marie Brady, Catherine McCabe, and Margaret McCann.

Introduction

Parenteral therapy is the administration of drugs or fluids by any route other than by mouth or rectum and includes the intravenous and subcutaneous routes (Royal College of Nursing [RCN] 2010). For the purposes of this chapter, it refers to intravenous therapy. Intravenous therapy is now an integral part of the majority of nurses' professional practice and requires both knowledge and skills (RCN 2010).

Anatomy and physiology of the veins

Veins consist of three layers (Figure 3.1):

- The **tunica intima** is a smooth endothelial lining that allows the passage of blood cells. If this becomes damaged, it increases the risk of thrombus formation (Weinstein 2007; Dougherty & Watson 2011). Within the lining are folds of endothelium called valves, which keep the blood moving towards the heart, preventing the backflow of blood. Valves are present in the larger vessels and at points of branching, and are present as bulges in the veins (Weinstein 2007; Collins 2011).
- The **intima media** is the middle layer of the vein wall and is composed of muscular tissue and nerve fibres (vasoconstrictors and vasodilators) that stimulate the vein to contract or relax. The tunica media controls the distension or collapse of the veins (Weinstein 2007; Scales 2008). Stimulation of this layer is by a change in temperature, mechanical or chemical stimulation.
- The **tunica adventitia** is the outer layer and consists of connective tissue that surrounds and supports the vessel (Collins 2011).

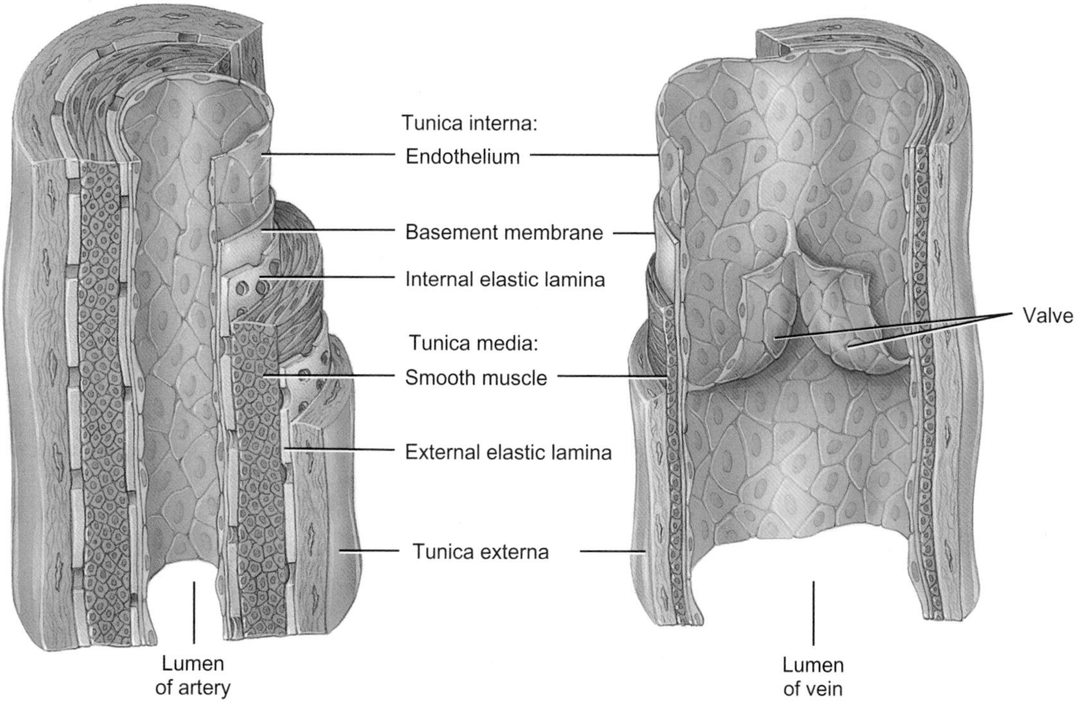

Figure 3.1 Structure of a vein. Reproduced from Nair, M. & Peate, I. (2009) *Fundamentals of Applied Pathophysiology* with kind permission from Wiley Blackwell.

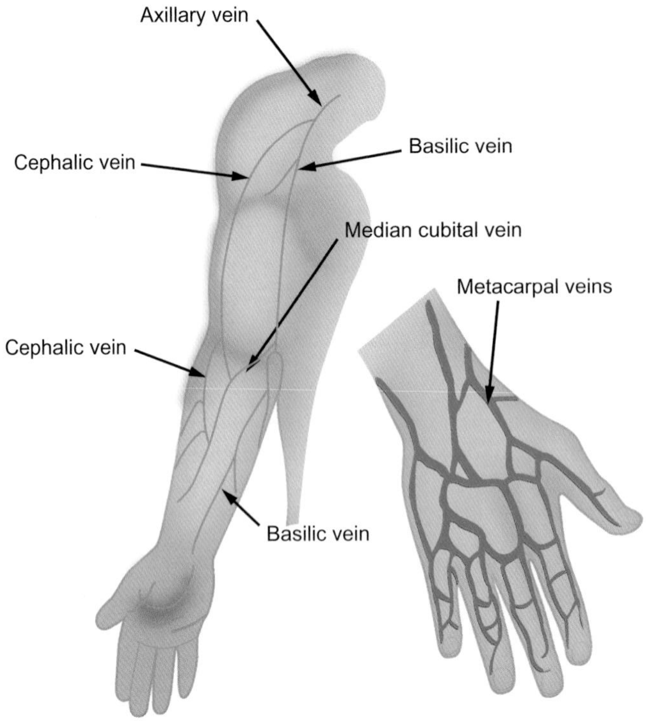

Figure 3.2 Simplified diagram of the right upper limb veins. Reproduced from Hamilton H & Bodenham A (2009) *Central Venous Catheters* with kind permission from Wiley Blackwell.

Veins of the peripheral circulation

The superficial veins of the upper limb are most commonly chosen for cannulation and the insertion of midlines and peripherally inserted central catheters because they are numerous and accessible. There are three main veins (Ernst 2005; Witt 2011; Figure 3.2):

- The **cephalic vein** is a large vein starting at the thumb and extending past the axilla. It is easily accessible but care must be taken to avoid accidental arterial puncture or damage to the radial nerve (Masoorli 2007; Dougherty 2008).
- The **basilic vein** is a large vein on the ulnar side of the forearm; it has numerous valves that can impede the advancement of a cannula, and care must also be taken to avoid accidental puncture of the median nerve and brachial artery (Garza & Becan-McBride 2005).
- The **metacarpal veins** are easily accessible, but use of these veins is contraindicated in the elderly, in whom skin turgor and subcutaneous tissue are diminished (Weinstein 2007; Witt 2011).

Veins of the central venous circulation

A central vein is one near the heart (Chantler 2009). The veins commonly used for central venous catheterisation are the internal jugular, subclavian and femoral veins (Farrow *et al.* 2009; Figure 3.3). The tip of a central venous access device usually ends in the superior vena cava, which descends vertically to the upper part of the right atrium of the heart (Farrow *et al.* 2009).

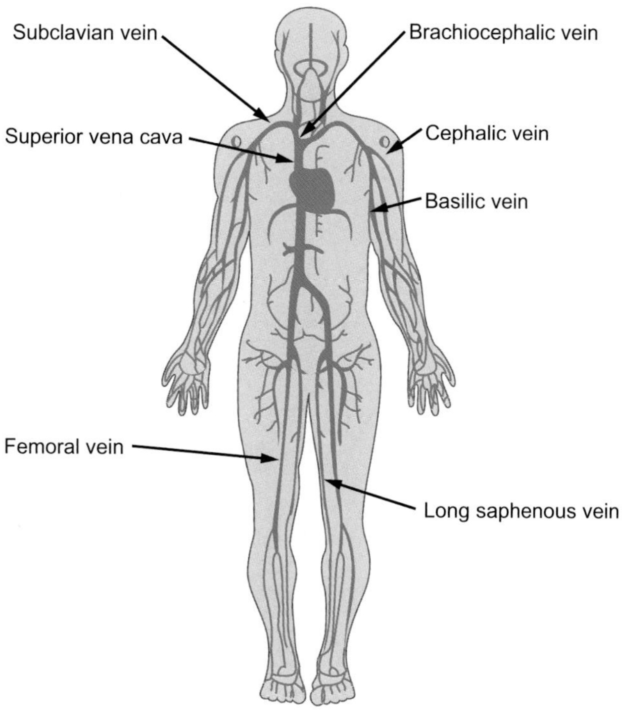

Figure 3.3 Veins used for central venous catheterisation. Reproduced from Hamilton, H. & Bodenham, A. (2009) *Central Venous Catheters* with kind permission from Wiley Blackwell.

Overview of vascular access devices

A vascular access device (VAD) is a device that is inserted into a vein, via the peripheral or central vessels, for either diagnostic (blood sampling or central venous pressure reading) or therapeutic (administration of medications, fluids and/or blood products) purposes (Dougherty & Watson 2011). Most devices (except tunnelled catheters and ports) can be removed by nurses following instruction. However, the insertion of any device is usually carried out by nurses who have received specific training.

Peripheral devices include peripheral cannulas and midline catheters and tend to be used for days (peripheral cannulas) to weeks (midline catheters) (Figure 3.4).

Central venous access devices (Figure 3.5) are placed into the central veins (jugular, subclavian or femoral) and include both short-term devices that stay *in situ* for weeks to long-term access devices that can be in for months or years. Their care can be influenced by their design, and some have valves at the tip or in the hub to prevent blood backflow and resulting occlusions (Dougherty & Watson 2011).

Visit www.wileyfundamentalseries.com/medicalnursing and read Reflective Question 3.1 to think more about this topic.

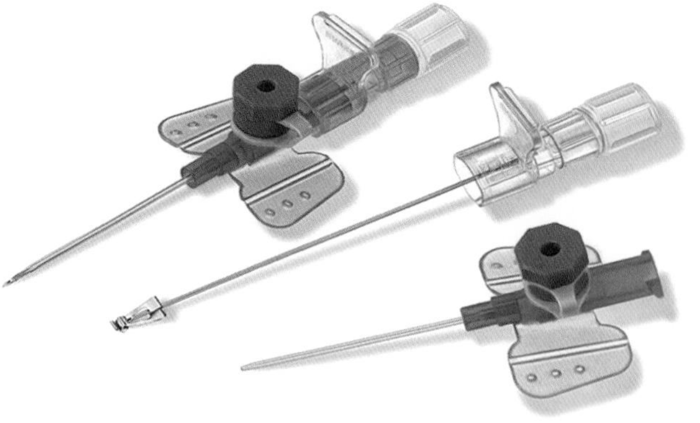

Figure 3.4 Ported cannula (safety). Reproduced from Phillips, S., Collins, M. & Dougherty, L. (2011) *Venepuncture and Cannulation* with kind permission from Wiley Blackwell.

Administration of intravenous therapy

Any nurse administering intravenous drugs must be competent in all aspects of intravenous therapy and act in accordance with the professional nursing body (Box 3.1). Training and assessment should comprise both a theoretical and practical component and include legal and professional issues, fluid balance, pharmacology, drug administration, local and systemic complications, infection control issues, use of equipment and risk management (Hyde 2008; RCN 2010).

Preparation of intravenous therapy

Pre-prepared infusion fluids with additives such as potassium chloride should be used whenever possible. This reduces the risk of extrinsic contamination, which can occur when adding drugs to infusion fluids (Weinstein 2007). Only one addition should be made to each bag of fluid after the compatibility has been ascertained as more additions can increase the risk of incompatibility occurring, leading to, for example, precipitation (Weinstein 2007; Whittington 2008). Drugs should never be added to blood, blood products, i.e. plasma or platelet concentrate mannitol solutions, sodium bicarbonate solution, and so on. Only specially prepared additives should be used with fat emulsions or amino acid preparations (Downie *et al.* 2003).

Potential incompatibility between the drug and diluents, contributing factors such as drug brand, pH, concentration and the effect of light or temperature, and the recommended duration of infusion must be checked prior to preparation. If insufficient information is available, a reference book (e.g. the *British National Formulary* [*BNF*] 2011) or the product data sheet must be consulted (National Patient Safety Association [NPSA] 2007; Whittington 2008).

The additive and fluid must be mixed well to prevent the layering effect that can occur with some drugs and to avoid the risk of administering a bolus injection of the drug (Whittington 2008). Following any additions to the infusion fluid, the container must be inverted a number of times to ensure mixing before the fluid is hung on the infusion stand (NPSA 2007). The infusion container should be labelled clearly after the addition has been made. Infusion bags should not be left hanging for longer than 24 hours. In the case of blood and blood products, this is reduced to 5 hours (McClelland 2007; RCN 2010).

Inspection of fluids, drugs, equipment and their packaging must be undertaken to detect any points at which contamination may have occurred during manufacture and/or transport. This intrinsic contamination may be detected as cloudiness, discoloration or the presence of particles (Weinstein 2007; RCN 2010; *BNF* 2011). If the nurse is unsure about any aspect of the preparation and/or administration of a drug, he or she should not proceed but should consult a senior member of

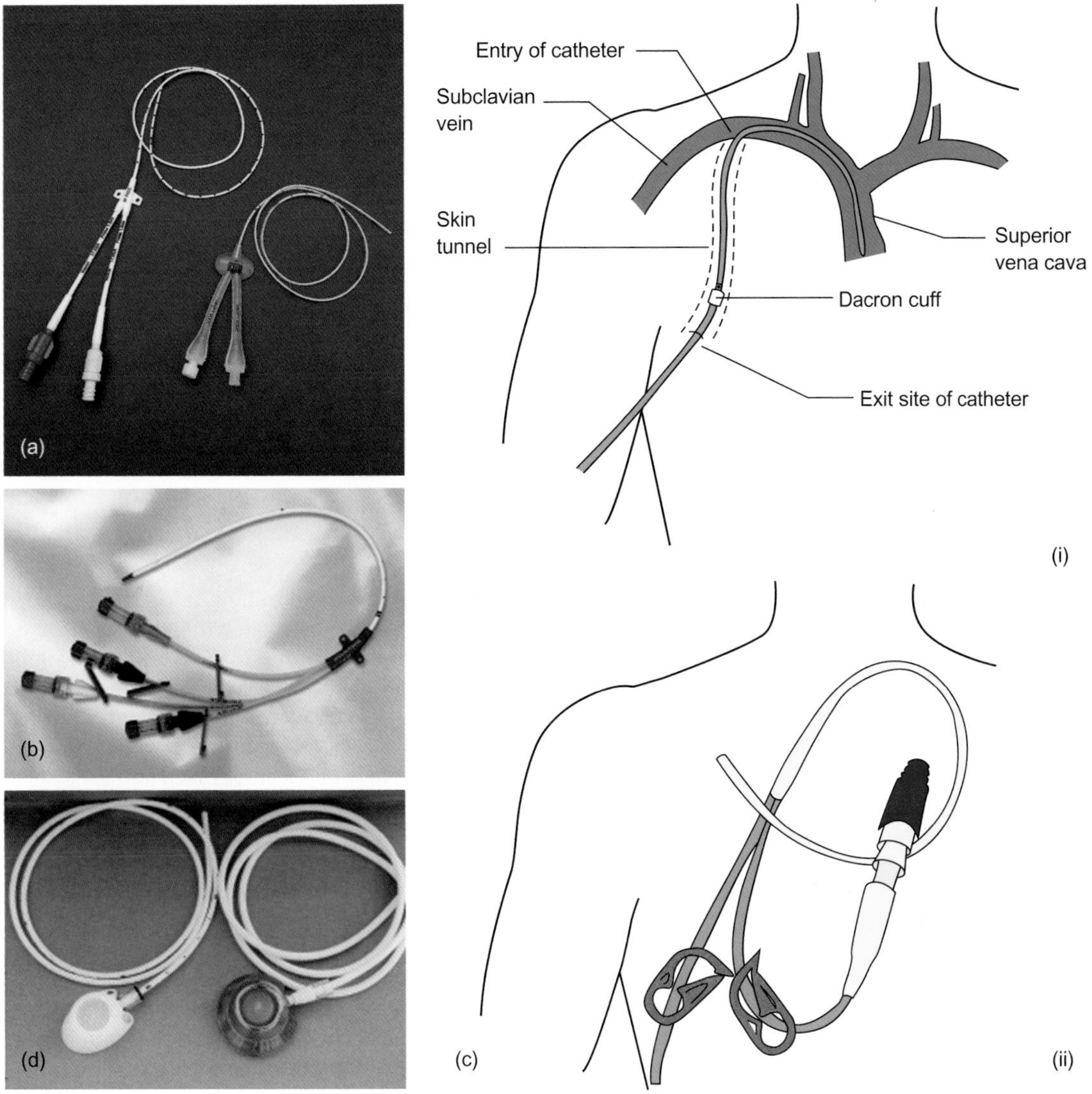

Figure 3.5 (a) Types of peripherally inserted central catheter. (b) Non-tunnelled multilumen central venous catheter. (c) Anatomical positioning of a tunnelled catheter. (d) Implantable ports. Reproduced from Dougherty, L. & Lister, S. (2011) *The Royal Marsden Hospital Manual of Clinical Nursing Procedures* with kind permission from Wiley Blackwell.

staff (Nursing and Midwifery Council 2008). Constant monitoring of the infusion fluid mixture for cloudiness or the presence of particles should occur, as should checking the patient's condition and intravenous site for patency, extravasation or infiltration (Downie *et al.* 2003; Weinstein 2007; Whittington 2008).

Methods of administering intravenous drugs

There are three methods of administering intravenous drugs: continuous infusion, intermittent infusion and direct intermittent injection.

Box 3.1 The nurse's responsibilities in relation to intravenous drug administration (adapted from Dougherty & Watson 2011)

- Knowledge of the therapeutic use of the drug or solution, its normal dosage, side effects, precautions and contraindications
- Checking the drug prescription chart
- Preparation of the drug aseptically and safely, checking the container and drug for faults, using the correct diluent and only preparing it immediately prior to administration
- Identification of the patient and allergy status prior to administration
- Checking and maintaining patency of the VAD
- Inspection of the site of the VAD and managing/reporting complications where appropriate
- Control of the flow rate of infusion and/or speed of injection
- Monitoring the condition of the patient and responding to/reporting changes
- Ensuring accurate, legible and immediate documentation of all drugs administered

Continuous infusion

This is defined as the intravenous delivery of a medication or fluid at a constant rate over a prescribed time period, ranging from several hours to several days, to achieve a controlled therapeutic response (Whittington 2008; Turner & Hankins 2010). It tends to be used when the drugs to be administered needs to be highly diluted or maintenance of steady blood levels of the drug is required (Turner & Hankins 2010). A continuous infusion is often used to replace fluids and rehydrate a patient. Examples of common infusion fluids used are **crystalloids** (solutions that, when placed in a solution, mix and dissolve into the solution and cannot be distinguished from the resultant soluton) such as 0.9% sodium chloride, glucose 5%, Hartmann's solution and sodium bicarbonate, and **colloids** (solutions used to expand the intravascular space, known as plasma expanders) such as albumin, mannitol, gelatins (e.g. Gelofusine) hetastarchs and dextrans (Phillips 2010).

Intermittent infusion

This is the administration of a small-volume infusion, i.e. 25–250 mL, over a period of between 15 minutes and 2 hours (Turner & Hankins 2010; Dougherty & Ansell 2011). This may be given as a specific dose at one time or at repeated intervals (Dougherty & Ansell 2011). An intermittent infusion may be used when a peak plasma level is required, the pharmacology of the drug dictates a specific dilution, the drug will not remain stable for the time required to administer a more dilute volume or the patient is on a restricted intake of fluids (Whittington 2008). Drugs commonly administered as an intermittent infusion include antibiotics. Delivery of the drug by intermittent infusion can be via a 'Y' set or can be piggybacked (via a needle-free injection port) or a burette set with a chamber capacity of 100 or 150 mL, but only if the primary infusion is of a compatible fluid (Turner & Hankins 2010).

Direct intermittent injection

This is also known as an intravenous push or bolus and involves the injection of a drug from a syringe into the injection port of the administration set or directly into a vascular access device (Turner & Hankins 2010; Dougherty & Ansell 2011). They tend to be used when a maximum concentration of the drug is required in the vital organs. A 'bolus' injection may be given rapidly over seconds, as in an emergency, for example adrenaline, where the drug cannot be further diluted for pharmacological or therapeutic reasons or does not require dilution. A controlled 'push' injection is given over a few minutes where a peak blood level is required and cannot be achieved by a small-volume infusion (Turner & Hankins 2010).

Rapid administration could result in toxic levels and an anaphylactic-type reaction. Manufacturers' recommendations for the rate of administration (i.e. millilitres or milligrams per minute) should be adhered to. In the absence of such recommendations, administration should proceed slowly, over 5–10 minutes (Whittington 2008; Dougherty & Ansell 2011). Delivery of the drug by direct injection may be via the cannula through a resealable needleless injection cap, via an extension set or via the injection site of an administration set if the infusion in progress is compatible in order to dilute the drug further and reduce local chemical irritation (Dougherty & Ansell 2011). If the infusion fluid is incompatible with the drug, the administration set may be switched off and a compatible solution may be used as a flush (NPSA 2007).

Principles of administration

If a transparent dressing is not in place, any gauze or occlusive dressing must be removed prior to administration to allow inspection of the device site for any complications such as phlebitis or infiltration (Finlay 2008). Patency of the vein must also be confirmed prior to administration, and the vein's ability to accept an extra flow of fluid or irritant chemical must also be checked using a 10 mL or larger syringe containing 0.9% sodium chloride to prevent damage to the device (Dougherty 2008; RCN 2010). If a number of drugs are being administered, 0.9% sodium chloride must be used to flush the device in between each drug to prevent interactions. In addition, 0.9% sodium chloride should be used at the end of the administration to ensure that all the drug has been delivered. The device should then be flushed to ensure patency is maintained (Dougherty & Ansell 2011).

All details of the prescription and all calculations must be checked carefully in accordance with hospital policy in order to ensure safe preparation and administration of the drug(s). The nurse must have knowledge of the solutions, their effects, their rate of administration, the factors that affect the flow of infusion, the complications that could occur when flow is not controlled and how to select the most appropriate device for accuracy of delivery to best meet the patient's flow control needs (according to age, condition, setting and prescribed therapy) (Weinstein 2007; Dougherty & Ansell 2011).

Infusion devices

An infusion device is designed to accurately deliver measured amounts of fluid or drug over a set period of time, to achieve the desired therapeutic response and to prevent complications (Medicines and Healthcare products Regulatory Authority [MHRA] 2010; Quinn 2008).

Gravity infusion devices

Gravity infusion devices depend entirely on gravity to deliver the infusion. The system consists of an administration set (containing a drip chamber and a roller clamp to control the flow) and is usually measured by counting drops (Dougherty & Ansell 2011). The indications for use are:

- the delivery of fluids without additives;
- that adverse effects are not anticipated and solutions do not need to be infused with absolute precision;
- that the patient's condition does not give cause for concern and complications are not anticipated (Quinn 2008).

Calculation of infusion rates

The flow rate is calculated using a formula that requires the following information: the volume to be infused, the number of hours the infusion is running for and the drop rate of the administration set (which will differ depending on the type of set) (Box 3.2). The number of drops per millilitre is

Box 3.2 Formula for calculation of the drop rate

$$\frac{\text{Volume to be infused}}{\text{Time in hours}} \times \frac{\text{Drop rate}}{60\text{minutes}} = \text{Drops per minute}$$

In this equation, 60 is a factor for the conversion of the number of hours to the number of minutes

dependent on the type of administration set used and the viscosity of the infusion fluid. Increased viscosity causes the size of the drop to increase. For example, crystalloid fluid administered via a solution set is delivered at the rate of 20 drops/mL; the rate of packed red cells given via a blood set will be calculated at 15 drops/mL (Quinn 2008).

Flow rates can be influenced by:

- the composition and viscosity of the fluid (Quinn 2008);
- the height of the container (the recommended height being 1–1.5 m above the infusion site) and any alterations in the patient's position, as these may alter the flow rate and necessitate a change in the speed of the infusion to maintain the appropriate rate of flow (Weinstein 2007; Hadaway 2010);
- the position of the patient – if the infusion is reliant on gravity, patients should be instructed to keep their arm lower than the infusion (Quinn 2008);
- the components of the administration or extension set, for example filters (Hadaway 2010; MHRA 2010);
- the size of the device and the vein, as well as where the device is located – for example, there may be a decrease in flow when a patient bends their arm if a cannula is sited over the elbow joint (Quinn 2008; MHRA 2010);
- whether the patient adjusts the control clamp or changes the height of the container, thereby making flow unreliable. Some pumps have tamper-proof features to minimise the risk of accidental manipulation of the infusion device (Hadaway 2010).

Visit www.wileyfundamentalseries.com/medicalnursing and read Reflective Question 3.2 to think more about this topic.

Volumetric pumps

Volumetric pump devices (Figure 3.6) pump fluid from an infusion bag via an administration set and work by calculating the volume delivered (Quinn 2008). This is achieved when the pump measures the volume displaced in a 'reservoir' (an integral component of the administration set) by a piston or peristaltic action (Hadaway 2010). It is indicated for large-volume infusions, and the rate is set as millilitres per hour (MHRA 2010).

Syringe pumps

These are low-volume, high-accuracy devices designed to infuse small volumes at low flow rates (Quinn 2008). The volume for infusion is limited to the size of the syringe used in the device, usually a 60 mL

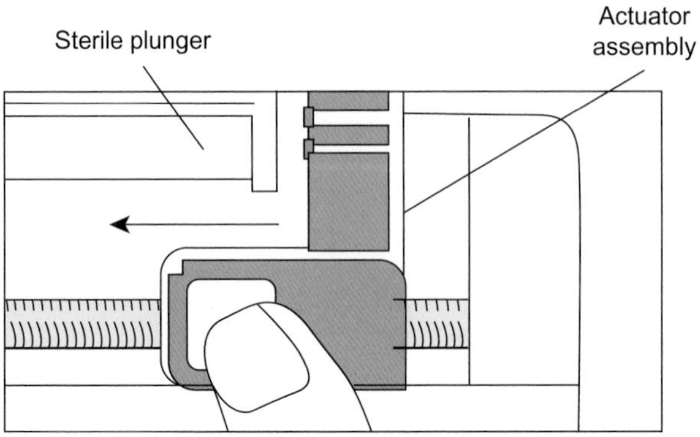

Figure 3.6 Volumetric pump. Reproduced from Dougherty, L. & Lister, S. (2011) *The Royal Marsden Hospital Manual of Clinical Nursing Procedures* with kind permission from Wiley Blackwell.

syringe. The plunger of the syringe is driven forward by the pump at a controlled rate and is calibrated in millilitres per hour (MHRA 2010).

Ambulatory infusion devices

These are infusion devices that pump in the same way as a volumetric or syringe pump, but by nature of their size, they are portable and useful in the ambulatory setting (hospital or home care). Such devices are suitable for patients who have been prescribed continuous infusional treatment for a period of time, for example from 4 days to 6 months, and enables the patients to receive treatment at home (Dougherty & Ansell 2011). Syringe drivers such as Graseby MS24 are set in millimetres per 24 hours, while a McKinley syringe pump is set in millilitres per hour. These devices are often used for symptom management and palliative care (Dickman *et al.* 2007; Quinn 2008).

Care must be taken when setting up a syringe driver as they have been involved in medication errors (Dickman *et al.* 2007; NPSA 2010). All devices must be properly maintained and serviced (MHRA 2010), and staff using an infusion device must receive training prior to using one (Quinn 2008; MHRA 2010).

Principles of infection prevention

An aseptic non-touch technique must be adhered to throughout all intravenous procedures (Rowley 2001). The nurse must employ good hand-washing and drying techniques using a bactericidal soap or a bactericidal alcohol handrub (Pratt et al. 2007; Hart 2008; RCN 2010). It is desirable that a closed system of infusion is maintained wherever possible, with as few connections as is necessary for its purpose (Finlay 2008; Hart 2008). Any extra connections within the administration system increase the risk of infection; three-way taps, for example, have been shown to encourage the growth of microorganisms because they are difficult to clean (Finlay 2008; Hart 2008).

Cleaning of the site

Chlorhexidine 2% in 70% alcohol has been shown to be the most effective agent for skin cleaning around the VAD site prior to insertion and between dressing changes (Maki *et al.* 1991; Department of Health [DH] 2007, 2010; Pratt *et al.* 2007). Solutions should be applied with friction in back and forth strokes for at least 30 seconds and allowed to air dry for 30–60 seconds to ensure disinfection (McGoldrick 2010). The injection sites on administration sets or injection caps should also be cleaned using a 2% chlorhexidine alcohol-based antiseptic prior to use (Pratt *et al.* 2007).

Inspection of the site

The insertion site should be inspected at least once a day for signs of complications such as infiltration, phlebitis or infection, for example redness at the insertion site of the device or pyrexia (RCN 2010), and the site assessed using a scale such as the Visual Infusion Phlebitis score (DH 2010).

Securement and dressings

The aim of a securement device is to secure the device to the skin and prevent movement or dislodgment of the device, which will in turn reduce the risk of mechanical phlebitis and infection (Dougherty & Watson 2011). Types of securement include, tape, sutures and self-adhesive anchoring devices applied to the skin such as StatLocks (Moureau & Iannucci, 2003). Dressings are used to provide a sterile cover to protect the device from contamination. Sterile gauze or a transparent film dressing can be used for peripheral cannulas, but the recommendation for a central venous access device site is a transparent dressing (Pratt *et al.* 2007; DH 2010; RCN 2010). They are moisture permeable, thereby reducing the collection of moisture under the dressing (Casey & Elliott, 2010).

Changing equipment

Administration sets should be changed according to how they are used (intermittent or continuous therapy), the type of device and the type of solution. In order to ensure the set is changed on time, it must be labelled with the date and time of change (NPSA 2007; RCN 2010). If the vascular access device is changed, all the tubing should also be replaced (Pratt *et al.* 2007). All solution administration sets and stopcocks used for continuous infusions should be replaced every 72 hours unless clinically indicated, for example if drug stability (leaching of insulin into the plastic) data indicate otherwise. Intermittent infusion sets should be discarded after each use and not allowed to hang to avoid reuse (Pratt *et al.* 2007; RCN 2010). Administration sets used for lipid emulsions and parenteral nutrition should be changed at the end of the infusion or within 24 hours of initiating the infusion (Pratt *et al.* 2007; RCN 2010). Blood administration sets should be changed at least every 12 hours and after every second unit of blood (McClelland 2007; Pratt *et al.* 2007; RCN 2010).

Maintaining a closed intravenous system

If equipment becomes accidentally disconnected, air embolism or blood loss may occur (Perucca 2010). Needle-free connections provide a more secure connection, and all intravenous equipment, i.e. administration sets, extension sets and injection caps, should have these fittings (Dougherty, 2006). Needle-free systems provide a closed environment, which further reduces the risk of air entry (Dougherty 2006). Before changing the equipment, the nurse should ensure that the catheter or administration set is clamped to prevent the introduction of air into the system (Dougherty & Watson 2011).

Maintaining patency

Patency is defined as the ability to infuse through and aspirate blood from a VAD (Dougherty 2006). It is important at all times for the patency of the device to be maintained. Blockage can result in damage, infection, inconvenience to patients and disruption to drug delivery. Occlusion of the device can be caused by non-thrombotic reasons (formation of precipitation due to inadequate flushing between incompatible medications or mechanical causes, e.g. kinking, tight sutures or pinch-off syndrome) or thrombotic reasons (clot formation when an administration set or electronic infusion device is turned off and left for a prolonged period, or there is inadequate flushing of the device when not in use) (Hadaway 2010; Dougherty & Watson 2011).

Two types of solution are used to maintain patency in VADs; 0.9% sodium chloride, used to flush peripheral cannulas (and some valved central VADs), and heparin, used to flush most central VADs (Goode *et al.* 1991; RCN 2010; Dougherty & Watson 2011). Due to the risk of errors with heparin, its use must be considered carefully (NPSA 2008). Patency can be achieved by using a continuous infusion to 'keep vein open' ('KVO') or by intermittent flushing, using a pulsated (push-pause) flush to create turbulent flow when administering the solution and finishing with positive pressure (Goodwin & Carlson 1993; Cummings-Winfield & Mushami-Kanji 2008). This is accomplished by maintaining pressure on the plunger of the syringe while disconnecting the syringe from the injection cap, which prevents reflux of blood into the tip, reducing the risk of occlusion (Hadaway 2010; Infusion Nursing Society 2011).

Managing complications

Phlebitis

Phlebitis is defined as inflammation of the intima of the vein (Perucca 2010) and is usually associated with pain and tenderness along the cannulated vein, erythema, warmth and streak formation with or without a palpable cord (Mermel *et al.* 2009).There are three main types (Lamb & Dougherty 2008):

- **Mechanical** – related to irritation and damage to a vein by large-gauge cannulas, sited where there is movement, for example the antecubital fossa, not adequately secured or left *in situ* for too long.
- **Chemical** – related to chemical irritation from drugs such as antibiotics and chemotherapy.
- **Bacterial** – when the site become infected due to poor hand-washing or poor aseptic technique.

Prevention includes appropriate device and vein selection and further dilution of drugs, along with regular monitoring of the site (Jackson 1998; Lamb & Dougherty 2008; Morris 2011). The cannula is removed at the early signs of phlebitis, and warm or cold compresses can be applied to the affected site. If bacterial phlebitis is suspected, a swab of the insertion site should be taken and the cannula tip sent to the microbiology laboratory (Lamb & Dougherty 2008).

Visit www.wileyfundamentalseries.com/medicalnursing and read Reflective Question 3.3 to think more about this topic.

Infiltration and extravasation

Infiltration is defined as the leakage into the surrounding tissues of non-vesicant solutions or medications that do not cause tissue necrosis. However, they can result in long-term injury due to local inflammatory reactions or from compression if they are large-volume infiltrates (Doellmann *et al.* 2009; Schulmeister 2009; RCN 2010).

Extravasation is defined as leakage or discharge of solutions into the tissues, although when vesicants (drugs that cause the formation of blisters with subsequent tissue necrosis) leak into the surrounding tissues, immediate action is required if local tissue damage is to be prevented (Figure 3.7) (Polovich *et al.* 2009; Schulmeister 2009).

Some patients are at greater risk, for example children and older adults, those with poor venous access, patients with chronic conditions such as diabetes or cancer and those who are receiving certain medications such as anticoagulants. Signs and symptoms include burning or stinging, swelling or redness at the site. Prevention is by adequate securement of the device to prevent dislodgement, appropriate selection of both vein and device, and knowledgeable and skilled staff inserting and caring for VADs (Dougherty 2010). Close monitoring of the device's insertion site will ensure early recognition. Immediate management is to stop the injection or infusion, remove the peripheral device, elevate the

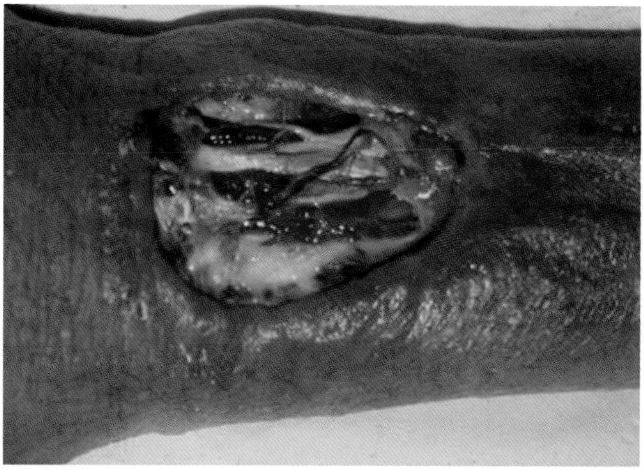

Figure 3.7 Extensive damage following an extravasation of doxorubicin. Reproduced from Dougherty, L. & Lamb, J. (2008) *Intravenous Therapy in Nursing Practice* with kind permission from Wiley Blackwell.

arm and then follow local policy, which may include use of heat or cold packs, injection of an antidote or referral to a plastic surgeon (Dougherty 2010).

Thrombosis

A thrombosis is a clot of blood that can be present at the tip of a catheter or can surround the catheter. Symptoms include complaints of pain in the area, such as the arm or neck, oedema of the neck, chest and upper extremity, periorbital oedema, facial tenderness, tachycardia, shortness of breath and sometimes a cough, signs of a collateral circulation over the chest area, jugular venous distension and discoloration of the limb (Dougherty 2006). Selection of the correct position for catheter tip placement in the superior vena cava and monitoring of catheter function will help in prevention (Mayo 2000). Anticoagulation may be necessary if the patient has had previous thromboembolic events (Bishop 2009). Treatment can be either catheter removal and/or anticoagulation (Gorski *et al.* 2010).

Sepsis

Infection can occur locally at the insertion site or systemically. Signs of local infection include oedema, erythema that may track along the length of the catheter, tenderness and exudate such as pus at the insertion site. Septicaemia is a systemic infection that is usually characterised by pyrexia, flushing, sweating and rigors (the latter occurring particularly when the catheter is flushed) and may be prevented by a good aseptic non-touch technique and use of evidence-based guidelines, for example for a peripheral or central venous catheter care bundle (DH 2007).

If the patient develops symptoms of an infection, swabs of the insertion site along with blood cultures (from the device and peripheral veins) should be taken. Depending on the clinical condition of the patient, it may be necessary to remove the device and administer intravenous antibiotics (Gorski *et al.* 2010). The tip of the cannula or catheter should be sent to microbiology for culture and sensitivity.

Visit www.wileyfundamentalseries.com/medicalnursing and read Reflective Question 3.4 to think more about this topic.

Circulatory overload and dehydration

Circulatory overload can be caused by infusion of fluids of the same tonicity as plasma into the vascular circulation (e.g. sodium chloride 0.9%), large-volume infusions running over multiple days, or rapid fluid infusion into patients with compromised cardiac, liver or renal status (Macklin & Chernecky 2004; Lamb & Dougherty 2008). It can result in left-sided heart failure, circulatory collapse and cardiac arrest (Dougherty & Ansell 2011). Treatment consists of withholding all fluids until excess water and electrolytes have been eliminated by the body and/or diuretics have been administered to promote a rapid diuresis (Weinstein 2007).

Dehydration may be caused by underinfusion. It occurs in patients unable to take sufficient fluids (elderly, unconscious or incontinent patients) or who have excess insensible water loss via the skin and lungs, or occur as a result of certain drugs taken in excess (Weinstein 2007). Treatment involves replacement of the required fluids.

Circulatory overload and dehydration can be related to the rate and volume of the infusion fluids. Prevention includes a thorough assessment of patient before commencing intravenous therapy, close monitoring of the patient, maintaining infusion rates as prescribed and the use of infusion devices where required (Lamb & Dougherty 2008).

Speed shock

Speed shock is a systemic reaction that occurs when a substance foreign to the body is rapidly introduced into the circulation (Weinstein 2007; Perucca 2010). It can occur when intravenous bolus injections or large volumes of fluid are administered too rapidly, resulting in toxic concentrations (Lamb & Dougherty 2008; Perucca 2010). Toxicity may be manifested by an exaggeration of the usual pharmacological actions of the drug or by signs and symptoms specific for that drug or class of drugs. Signs and symptoms include a flushed face, headache, dizziness, chest congestion, tachycardia, hypotension, syncope, shock and cardiovascular collapse (Weinstein 2007; Perucca 2010).

Prevention involves the nurse having knowledge of the drug and the recommended rate of administration (Dougherty & Ansell 2011). When infusing using gravity flow, the solution should be checked to ensure it is flowing freely before adjusting the rate, and it should then be monitored regularly (Perucca 2010). For high-risk medications, an electronic flow control device is recommended (RCN 2010). Although most pumps have an anti-free-flow mechanism, the roller clamp should always be closed prior to removing the set from the pump (MHRA 2010). If speed shock occurs, the infusion must be slowed down or discontinued. Medical staff should be notified immediately and the patient's condition treated as clinically indicated (Perucca 2010).

Blood transfusion therapy

Blood transfusion is the administration of a blood component or plasma-derived product to the patient (Gray *et al.* 2007; Shaw 2011). Any written order for a blood component must be checked to ensure that it is correctly completed and that it contains specific information (Box 3.3).

Prior to the transfusion, the nurse must ensure that the patient has been informed of the proposed transfusion and has had an opportunity to raise any concerns, understands the risks and benefits of the transfusion and has agreed to having the transfusion (Shaw 2011). Pre-transfusion, or baseline, observations including blood pressure, temperature, pulse and respiratory rate must be undertaken, evaluated and documented (RCN 2006).

Venous access needs to be established and, if already in place, checked for patency prior to setting up the transfusion. Blood components may be administered via either peripheral cannulas or a central venous access device, but blood must be transfused through a sterile blood component administration set with an integral mesh filter (170–200 μm) (McClelland 2007). Platelets and plasma components may be administered through a normal blood administration set or a platelet or cryoprecipitate set (McClelland 2007). Gravity or electronic infusion devices may be used for the administration of blood

Box 3.3 Checklist for prescription of blood products (adapted from RCN 2006)

- The patient's core identifiers
- The date (and time if appropriate) the blood component is required
- The type of blood component to be administered
- Any clinical special transfusion requirements, e.g. irradiated or cytomegalovirus-seronegative blood, or a blood warmer
- The volume or number of units to be transfused (giving a precise volume in millilitres for paediatric transfusions)
- The time over which each unit is to be transfused (giving the precise rate or length of time for a specified volume to be transfused if it is a paediatric transfusion)
- Any special instructions, e.g. concomitant drugs required, such as diuretics
- The prescriber's signature

components, but the latter only with an administration set that is designated for the specific infusion device selected (Shaw 2011).

The check at the bedside is the key to ensuring that the right patient receives the right blood, and it is therefore essential that checking is performed thoroughly prior to the transfusion of each component (Oldham *et al.* 2009). On completion of a blood transfusion, the patient's observations should be taken and recorded, as well as details of any reactions to the transfusion. Intravenous fluids prescribed to follow the transfusion should be administered through a new administration set appropriate for that infusion. The traceability documentation confirming the fate of the component should be returned to the laboratory (Shaw 2011).

Conclusion

The administration of intravenous therapy is an everyday aspect of medical and surgical nursing work but is an activity with considerable professional responsibility. Awareness of the risks and potential complications with rigorous application of best practice standards contributes greatly to patient safety.

Now visit the companion website and test yourself on this chapter:
www.wileyfundamentalseries.com/medicalnursing

References

Bishop, E. (2009) Aftercare and management of central venous access devices. In: Hamilton, H. & Bodenham, A. (eds), *Central Venous Catheters* (pp. 221–37).Chichester: Wiley-Blackwell.

British National Formulary (2011) *British National Formulary* 61. London: British Medical Association/Royal Pharmaceutical Society of Great Britain.

Casey, A.L. & Elliott, T.S. (2010) Prevention of central venous catheter-related infection: update. *British Journal of Nursing*, **19**(2):78–82.

Chantler, J. (2009) Applied anatomy of the central veins. In: Hamilton, H. & Bodenham, A. (eds), *Central Venous Catheters* (pp. 14–33). Chichester: Wiley-Blackwell.

Collins, M. (2011) Anatomy and physiology. In: Phillips, S., Collins, M. & Dougherty, L. (eds), *Venepuncture and Cannulation* (pp. 44–67). Oxford: Blackwell Publishing.

Cummings-Winfield, C. & Mushani-Kanji, T. (2008) Restoring patency to central venous access devices. *Clinical Journal of Oncology Nursing*, **12**(6):925–34.

Department of Health (2007) *Saving Lives: Reducing Infection, Delivering Clean and Safe Care. High Impact Intervention No 1 (Central Venous Bundle) and No 2 (Peripheral IV Cannula Care Bundle).* London: DH.

Department of Health (2010) *Peripheral Cannula Care and Central Venous Catheter Care – High Impact Interventions.* Retrieved 22nd June 2011 from http://hcai.dh.gov.uk/whatdoido/high-impact-interventions/.

Dickman, A., Schneider, J. & Varga, J. (2007) *The Syringe Driver: Continuous Subcutaneous Infusions in Palliative Care*, 3rd edn. Oxford: Oxford University Press.

Doellmann, D., Hadaway, L., Bowes-Geddes, L.A. *et al.* (2009) Infiltration and extravasation: update on prevention and management. *Journal of Infusion Nursing*, **32**(4):203–11.

Dougherty, L. (2006) *Central Venous Access Devices: Care and Management*. Oxford: Blackwell Publishing.

Dougherty, L. (2008) Obtaining peripheral vascular access. In: Dougherty, L. & Lamb, J. (eds), *Intravenous Therapy in Nursing Practice*, 2nd edn. Oxford: Blackwell Publishing.

Dougherty, L. (2010) Extravasation: prevention, recognition and management, *Nursing Standard*, **24**(48):48–55.

Dougherty, L. & Ansell, L. (2011) Medicines management. In: Dougherty, L. & Lister, S. (eds), *The Royal Marsden Hospital Manual of Clinical Nursing Procedures*, 8th edn (Chapter 16). Oxford: Wiley-Blackwell.

Dougherty, L. & Watson, J. (2011) Vascular access devices. In: Dougherty, L. & Lister, S. (eds), *The Royal Marsden Hospital Manual of Clinical Nursing Procedures*, 8th edn (Chapter 18). Oxford: Wiley-Blackwell.

Downie, G., MacKenzie, J. & Williams, A. (eds) (2003) Medicine management. In: Downie, G., Mackenzie, J., Willams, A. & Hind, C. (eds), *Pharmacology and Medicines Management for Nurses*, 3rd edn (pp. 49–91). London: Churchill Livingstone.

Ernst, D.J. (2005) *Phlebotomy for Nurses and Nursing Personnel*. West Terre Haute, IN: Quality Books.

Farrow, C., Bodenham, A. & Millo, J. (2009) Cannulation of the jugular veins. In: Hamilton, H. & Bodenham, A. (eds), *Central Venous Catheters* (pp.78–91). Chichester: Wiley-Blackwell.

Finlay, T. (2008) Safe administration of IV therapy. In: Dougherty, L. & Lamb, J. (eds), *Intravenous Therapy in Nursing Practice*, 2nd edn (pp. 143–66). Oxford: Blackwell Publishing.

Garza, D. & Becan-McBride, K. (2005) *Phlebotomy Handbook – Blood Collection Essentials*, 7th edn. Upper Saddle River, NJ: Prentice Hall.

Goode, C.J., Titler, M., Rakel, B. *et al.* (1991) A meta-analysis of effects of heparin flush and saline flush: quality and cost implications. *Nursing Research*, **40**(6):324–30.

Goodwin, M.L. & Carlson, I. (1993) The peripherally inserted central catheter: a retrospective look at three years of insertions. *Journal of Intravenous Nursing*, **16**(2):92–103.

Gorski, L., Perucca, R. & Hunter, M. (2010) Central venous access devices: care, maintenance, and potential problems. In: Alexander, M., Corrigan, A., Gorski, L., Hankins, J. & Perucca, R. (eds), *Infusion Nursing: An Evidence-Based Approach*, 3rd edn (pp. 495–515). St Louis: Saunders Elsevier.

Gray, A., Hearnshaw, K., Izatt, C. *et al.* (2007) Safe transfusion of blood and blood products. *Nursing Standard*, **21**(51):40–7.

Hadaway, L.C. (2010) Anatomy and physiology related to infusion therapy. In: Alexander, M., Corrigan, A., Gorski, L., Hankins, J. & Perucca, R. (eds), *Infusion Nursing: An Evidence-Based Approach*, 3rd edn (pp. 139–77). St Louis: Saunders Elsevier.

Hart, S. (2008) Infection control in IV therapy. In: Dougherty, L. & Lamb, J. (eds), *Intravenous Therapy in Nursing Practice*, 2nd edn (pp. 87–116). Oxford: Blackwell Publishing.

Hyde, L (2008) Legal and professional issues in IV therapy. In: Dougherty, L. & Lamb, J. (eds), *Intravenous Therapy in Nursing Practice*, 2nd edn (pp. 1–22). Oxford: Blackwell Publishing.

Infusion Nursing Society (2011) *Standards for Infusion Therapy*. Norwood, MA: Infusion Nursing Society USA.

Jackson, A. (1998) Infection control – a battle in vein: infusion phlebitis. *Nursing Times*, **94**(4):68, 71.

Lamb, J. & Dougherty, L. (2008) Local and systemic complications of intravenous therapy. In: Dougherty, L. & Lamb, J. (eds), *Intravenous Therapy in Nursing Practice*, 2nd edn (pp. 167–96). Oxford: Blackwell Publishing.

McClelland, B. (2007) *Handbook of Transfusion Medicine*, 3rd edn. London: HMSO.

McGoldrick, M.S. (2010) Infection prevention and control. In: Alexander, M., Corrigan, A., Gorski, L., Hankins, J. & Perucca, R. (eds), *Infusion Nursing: An Evidence-Based Approach*, 3rd edn (pp. 201–27). St Louis: Saunders Elsevier.

Macklin, D. & Chernecky, C.C. (2004) *IV Therapy*. St Louis: Saunders.

Maki, D.G., Ringer, M. &Alvarado, C.J. (1991) Prospective randomised trial of povidone-iodine, alcohol, and chlorhexidine for prevention of infection associated with central venous and arterial catheters. *Lancet*, **338**:339–43.

Masoorli, S. (2007) Nerve injuries related to vascular access insertion and assessment. *Journal of Infusion Nursing*, **30**(6):346–50.

Mayo, D.J. (2000) Catheter-related thrombosis. *Journal of Vascular Access Devices*, **5**(2):10–20.

Medicines and Healthcare products Regulatory Authority (2010) *Device Bulletin Infusion Systems DB2003* (02) v2.0 November. London: MHRA.

Mermel, L.A., Allon, M., Bouza, E. *et al.* (2009) Clinical practice guidelines for the diagnosis and management of intravascular catheter-related infection: 2009 update by the Infectious Diseases Society of America. *Clinical Infectious Diseases*, **49**(1):1–45.

Morris, W. (2011) Complications. In: Phillips, S., Collins, M. & Dougherty, L. (eds), *Venepuncture and Cannulation* (pp. 175–222). Oxford: Blackwell Publishing.

Moureau, N. & Iannucci, A.L. (2003) Catheter securement: trends in performance and complications associated with the use of either traditional methods or adhesive anchor devices. *Journal of Vascular Access Devices*, **8**(1):29–33.

Nursing and Midwifery Council (2008) *The Code: Standards of Conduct, Performance and Ethics for Nurses and Midwives*. London: NMC.

National Patient Safety Association (2007) *Promoting the Safer Use of Injectable Medicines*. Alert 20. London: NPSA.

National Patient Safety Association (2008) *Risks with Intravenous Heparin Flush Solutions*. Safety bulletin. NPSA/2008/RRR002; 24/4/08. London: NPSA.

National Patient Safety Agency (2010) *Safer Ambulatory Syringe Drivers*. NPSA/2010/RRR019, 16/12/10. London: NPSA.

Oldham, J., Sinclair, L. & Hendry, C. (2009) Right patient, right blood, right care: safe transfusion practice. *British Journal of Nursing*, **18**(5):312–20.

Perucca, R. (2010) Peripheral venous access devices. In: Alexander, M., Corrigan, A., Gorski, L., Hankins, J. & Perucca, R. (eds), *Infusion Nursing: An Evidence-Based Approach*, 3rd edn (pp. 456–79). St Louis: Saunders Elsevier.

Phillips, L. (2010) Parenteral fluids. In: Alexander, M., Corrigan, A., Gorski, L., Hankins, J. & Perucca, R. (eds), *Infusion Nursing: An Evidence-Based Approach*, 3rd edn (Chapter 13). St Louis: Saunders Elsevier.

Polovich, M., Whitford, J.M. & Olsen, M. (eds) (2009) *Oncology Nursing Society. Chemotherapy and Biotherapy Guidelines and Recommendations for Practice*, 3rd edn. Pittsburgh, PA: Oncology Nursing Press.

Pratt, R.J., Pellowe, C.M., Wilson, J.A. *et al.* (2007) epic2: National evidence-based guidelines for preventing healthcare-associated infections in NHS hospitals in England. *Journal of Hospital Infection*, **65** (Suppl. 1):S1–64.

Quinn, C. (2008) Intravenous flow control and infusion devices. In: Dougherty, L. & Lamb, J. *Intravenous Therapy in Nursing Practice*, 2nd edn (pp. 197–224). Oxford: Blackwell Publishing.

Royal College of Nursing (2006) *Right Blood, Right Patient, Right Time*. London: RCN.

Royal College of Nursing (2010) *Standards for Infusion Therapy*, 3rd edn. London: RCN.

Rowley, S. (2001) Theory to practice. Aseptic non-touch technique. *Nursing Times*, **97**(7):vi–viii.

Scales, K. (2008) Anatomy and physiology related to intravenous therapy. In: Dougherty, L. & Lamb, J.(eds), *Intravenous Therapy in Nursing Practice*, 2nd edn (pp. 23–48). Oxford: Blackwell Publishing.

Schulmeister, L. (2009) Antineoplastic therapy. In: Alexander, M., Corrigan, A., Gorski, L., Hankins, J. & Perucca, R. (eds), *Infusion Therapy: An Evidence Based Approach* (pp. 366–7). Philadelphia: Saunders Elsevier.

Shaw, C. (2011) Nutrition. In: Dougherty, L. & Lister, S. (eds), *The Royal Marsden Hospital Manual of Clinical Nursing Procedures*, 8th edn (Chapter 24). Oxford: Wiley-Blackwell.

Turner, M.S. & Hankins, J. (2010) Pharmacology. In: Alexander, M., Corrigan, A., Gorski, L., Hankins, J. & Perucca, R. (eds), *Infusion Nursing: An Evidence-based Approach*, 3rd edn (pp. 263–98). St Louis: Saunders Elsevier.

Weinstein, S. (2007) *Plumer's Principles and Practices of Intravenous Therapy*, 8th edn. Philadelphia: Lippincott.

Whittington, Z. (2008) Pharmacological aspects of IV therapy. In: Dougherty, L. & Lamb, J. (eds) *Intravenous Therapy in Nursing Practice*, 2nd edn (pp. 117–46). Oxford: Blackwell Publishing.

Witt, B. (2011) Vein selection. In: Phillips, S., Collins, M. & Dougherty, L. (eds), *Venepuncture and Cannulation* (pp. 91–107). Oxford: Blackwell Publishing.

Further reading

Dougherty, L. (2011) Implanted ports: benefits, challenges and guidance for use. *British Journal of Nursing*, **20**(8):2–19.

European Union (2010) *EU Directive to Prevent Injuries and Infection to Healthcare Workers from Sharp Objects*. Retrieved 22nd June 2011 from http://www.hse.gov.uk/healthservices/needlesticks/eu-directive.htm.

Gabriel, J. (2008) Long-term central venous access. In: Dougherty, L. & Lamb, J. (eds), *Intravenous Therapy in Nursing Practice*, 2nd edn (pp. 321–51). Oxford: Blackwell Publishing.

4

Principles of nutritional care

Carolyn Best and Helen Hitchings

Royal Hampshire County Hospital, Winchester, Hampshire, UK

Contents

Introduction	45
Nutritional screening and assessment	45
Calculating nutritional requirements	47
Dietary guidelines	48
Effect of illness on nutrition	48
Refeeding syndrome	49
Effect of surgery on nutrition	51
Nutritional support	52
Conclusion	56
References	57

Learning outcomes

Having read this chapter, you will be able to:

- Discuss the nursing role in identifying patients at risk of malnutrition in hospital
- Identify the potential complications related to malnutrition
- Recognise how nursing actions can positively affect the patient's experience and nutritional intake
- Understand the role of nursing in managing patients who require nutritional support

Fundamentals of Medical-Surgical Nursing: A Systems Approach, First Edition. Edited by Anne-Marie Brady, Catherine McCabe, and Margaret McCann.

Introduction

A balanced diet should provide sufficient nutrients in the form of the energy, protein, vitamins and minerals that are required to keep an individual healthy. The ongoing absence or relative lack of some or all of these nutrients may lead to malnutrition. During illness, or following surgery, an individual's nutritional requirements may change, and at these times the provision of appropriate levels of nutrition is vital to provide the body with ample nutrients to aid recovery. Nurses are responsible for ensuring that patients within their care receive the appropriate type and level of assistance necessary to ensure that their nutritional requirements are met via the oral, artificial enteral or parenteral routes as appropriate.

Nutritional screening and assessment

Nutritional screening

Nutritional screening is a process used to identify those patients at risk of malnutrition. The National Institute of Clinical Excellence (NICE; 2006) and Department of Health (2007) recommend that all patients should be nutritionally screened on admission to hospital. The responsibility for this tends to lie with nurses as part of their admission assessment.

A basic nutrition screen may include some or all of:

- a review of the patient's normal dietary intake and drug and medical history;
- the patient's weight on admission or, where this is not possible, obtaining a reported weight from the patient, family or carers, or from previous health records;
- height measurements;
- body mass index (BMI):

$$\text{BMI}\,(\text{kg/m}^2) = \frac{\text{weight (kilograms)}}{\text{height (metres)}^2}$$

- a history of any recent weight loss or gain;
- an 'eyeball assessment', i.e. looking at the person for obvious signs of weight loss or malnutrition.

The initial screening acts as a baseline against which to monitor a patient's progress or deterioration. Without this information and an ongoing review, it is difficult to determine how effective any interventions are. The documentation also acts as evidence that nutritional screening has been conducted and which nutritional care plan was implemented. Those patients identified as being at high risk of malnutrition through screening are usually referred to a dietitian for a more thorough nutritional assessment. Some screening tools use the BMI and unplanned weight loss to calculate the overall risk of malnutrition (Box 4.1).

A BMI should not be used in isolation to determine whether someone is at risk of malnutrition as malnutrition can also affect those who are in the normal and overweight categories. A number of screening tools are in use in hospitals, care homes and primary care, one of the most commonly used screening tools being the malnutrition universal screening tool (MUST) developed by the British Association of Parenteral and Enteral Nutrition (BAPEN) (Elia 2003a; the tool can be found at http://www.bapen.org.uk/must_tool.html).

Where a screening tool is not used, nurses should perform a basic nutrition screen by undertaking the actions listed above and using their clinical judgement to calculate the patient's risk of malnutrition. It is important to recognise that the screening process should not be viewed as a one-off event; nutritional screening should be ongoing and repeated weekly for inpatients (NICE 2006). Where the patient is a poor historian or is unconscious, information should be sought from the family or carers. Without the routine use of a screening tool, there is no clear means of checking whether patients' nutritional needs are being met and whether they are at risk of malnutrition.

Box 4.1 BMI

- A person with a BMI of between 20 and 25 kg/m^2 is considered to be in the normal range
- A person with a BMI below 20 kg/m^2 is considered to be at higher risk of malnutrition, particularly if the BMI is below 18.5 kg/m^2
- A BMI greater than 25 kg/m^2 suggests that an individual is overweight

It is important to recognise that these BMI values should be used only as a guide. The BMI gives no indication of body composition or the proportions of fat and lean body tissue. Therefore, some muscular individuals appear to have a higher BMI when they are not actually 'overweight'.

The categories of BMI vary slightly for different population groups, so while a healthy BMI in white individuals is 20–25 kg/m^2, the range for those of Asian, Caribbean, African or Aboriginal origin is 18.5–23 kg/m^2 (World Health Organization 1996). Nevertheless, BMI is still commonly used in clinical practice.

Nursing action plans

When screening has been completed, an appropriate nursing action plan should be implemented without delay. Nursing action plans may include:

- recording the food and fluid intake (usually for up to 3 days);
- ensuring that a high-protein diet is ordered for the patient;
- ensuring that nutritional supplements are offered between meals or to replace a meal;
- recording the weight regularly – at the same time of day, on the same scales (where possible), and in similar clothing to aid consistency in providing accurate weight trends.

Appropriate and timely nutritional intervention following screening can be sufficient to enable many patients to meet their nutritional needs. Where there is little improvement in nutritional intake or the patient requires specialised nutritional advice, referral to another healthcare professional, for example a dietitian or a speech and language therapist, may be necessary.

Referral to a dietitian or speech and language therapist

Referral to a dietitian should be initiated where:

- a high nutritional risk score is present on screening, identifying an increased risk of malnutrition;
- additional or specialist nutrition is required, such as enteral tube feeding or parenteral nutrition;
- a more detailed nutrition assessment is required.

The involvement of a speech and language therapist may be initiated if the patient has swallowing problems with an oral diet or fluids.

Nutritional assessment

A detailed, specific and in-depth appraisal of an individual's nutritional state is usually undertaken by a dietitian following the identification of malnutrition by nutrition screening. An individual's nutritional requirements will vary depending upon their age, gender and mobility, whether acute or chronic illness is present, the stage of that illness and their underlying nutritional state (although this list is not exhaustive). Dietary reference values (Department of Health 1991) provide guidance on nutritional requirements for various groups of individuals but do not take into account medical conditions or factors that may affect a particular individual's nutritional requirements.

It is essential that any person in hospital who is identified as being at risk of malnutrition is monitored regularly and their estimated requirements are adjusted to reflect any change in their clinical condition.

Visit www.wileyfundamentalseries.com/medicalnursing and read Reflective Question 4.1 to think more about this topic.

Nutritional assessment will consider the following:

- **An individual's current nutritional status:** their weight, when they last ate, and what constitutes their normal diet. This will include:
  - evidence of weight loss, as unintentional weight loss, especially if rapid, is a concern in all hospital patients, regardless of their original body weight;
  - asking the patient about their most recent weight. If they cannot be weighed, enquire whether there are any changes in the way clothing or rings fit, or even whether dentures have become looser.
- **The nutritional implications of their medical condition:** for example surgery, intravenous fluids, pyrexia or gastrointestinal losses (through vomiting, diarrhoea and drains):
  - Is the patient dehydrated?
  - Do they have sunken eyes, a dry mouth and fragile papery skin?
  - Are they confused?
  - Is there any evidence of fluid retention (oedema), such as swollen ankles? This may mask weight loss. Accurate fluid balance is essential so that changes in hydration status are not mistaken for changes in actual body weight.
- **The severity and likely duration of their disease or illness:** although this can sometimes be difficult to predict:
  - Are they low in mood? As well as being a sign of poor nutrition, poor mood may also affect appetite.
  - Are they breathless? This will affect the patient's ability to eat, and possibly the ability to obtain and prepare food. It may also be a symptom of anaemia.
  - Is there evidence of pressure ulcers? If present, these will increase the patient's nutritional requirements.
- **The activity level of the individual:** whether they are bed-bound or mobile around the ward.
  - Reduced mobility may be a side effect of malnutrition, but if an individual's mobility was already affected before admission to hospital, they may have been unable to obtain, prepare or eat food for some time at home, compounding the problem.
- **Dietary assessment:** which will focus on an individual's actual intake from food, oral nutritional supplements, enteral feeding or parenteral nutrition. It is sometimes difficult to obtain an accurate history from the individual so intake charts, if completed accurately, can be particularly useful. If individuals are able, it can be useful for them to complete their own.

Calculating nutritional requirements

By estimating an individual's nutritional requirements, the aim of treatment is to:

- meet their specific nutritional requirements;
- ensure that nitrogen (protein) loss is minimised;
- minimise or prevent the risk of weight loss or gain unless this is a desirable outcome;
- ensure that sufficient vitamins and minerals are provided;
- achieve an appropriate level of hydration (fluid balance).

Providing the patient with the appropriate level of nutrition prevents the loss of body fat and protein stores and the ongoing adverse effects associated with malnutrition (Box 4.2). Overfeeding should be avoided in the short term to prevent associated biochemical derangements such as hyperglycaemia, the development of fatty liver and the additional stresses placed on the body. Long-term overfeeding should be avoided to prevent obesity.

Box 4.2 Ongoing adverse effects of malnutrition

- Impaired immune function, placing the individual at increased risk of infections
- Increased risk of tissue breakdown and pressure ulcers
- Muscle wasting and weakness as the body breaks down protein and fats for energy, leading to impaired respiratory and cardiac function
- Delayed wound healing
- Increased risk of postoperative complications
- Apathy and depression
- A general sense of weakness and illness

Dietary guidelines

There are many specific dietary guidelines for different subgroups within both hospital and the community, for example those with coeliac disease, diabetes, short bowel syndrome, etc. Most hospitals will have their own specific dietary information, but additional information can be obtained from other sources (see the online additional resources). Although nurses need to have a basic awareness of the needs of different diets, expert advice will be provided by the dietitian. Nurses should understand the concept of a healthy diet and will need to understand the symbols on menu sheets to be able to advise patients on foods suitable for their specific diet.

Effect of illness on nutrition

Nutrition Screening Week, a national survey facilitated by BAPEN across the UK and the Republic of Ireland in January 2010, highlighted that 1 in 3 patients being admitted to hospital were already in a malnourished state. Once in hospital, 6 out of 10 older people are at risk of becoming malnourished or their situation getting worse (Elia 2003b; Age Concern, 2006). Those who are malnourished often experience a significantly higher incidence of complications during treatment, have longer hospital stays (Elia 2003b; Age Concern, 2006) and have a higher mortality rate than those who are well nourished on admission (Best 2008). Once in hospital, there are numerous reasons why a patient's nutritional intake may be affected.

Medical condition

Due to underlying medical conditions, patients may experience one or a combination of the following problems:

- a deterioration in their ability to swallow safely (dysphagia) due to, for example, a cerebrovascular accident or degenerative neurological disorder;
- uncontrolled pain or discomfort;
- nausea or vomiting;
- infection, resulting in discomfort, confusion and/or reduced appetite;
- increased fluid losses due to diarrhoea or malabsorption;
- being nil by mouth awaiting a swallow assessment or surgical procedure;
- a change in their functional ability to care for themselves, leading to difficulties in:
  - completing a menu;
  - removing wrapping from food containers, opening packaging or removing lids from bottles or cartons;
  - cutting up food;
  - managing a normal-consistency diet;
  - asking for help.

Side effects of medication

Many drugs have unwanted side effects, and if a number of medications are taken simultaneously, the risk of developing side effects increases. Problems experienced may include:

- changes in the taste and smell of food, for example with antibiotics or chemotherapy;
- changes in appetite, for example when taking steroids;
- constipation, for example with opiates;
- diarrhoea, for example with magnesium supplements;
- drowsiness, for example in patients on benzodiazepines;
- dry mouth, for example with tricyclic antidepressants.

Psychological status

A change in psychological status may occur due to the onset of acute illness, infection or dementia and may be exhibited as:

- acute or chronic confusion or memory loss;
- poor comprehension;
- poor motivation to eat;
- an inability to recognise food;
- the inability to eat unaided;
- feeling different from others due to a change in food consistency as a result of, for example, a deterioration in swallowing, requiring purées or a soft diet.

Other issues

Other issues that may affect an individual's ability to eat (Age Concern 2006; Patients Association 2010) include:

- disruption of the patient's mealtimes due to ward rounds, personal care or investigations;
- being off the ward when meals are delivered;
- language difficulties or a lack of understanding of the instructions given;
- poor sight or hearing;
- being unaware of how to order food and what is available outside patients' mealtimes;
- poorly fitting or absent dentures.

Many of these issues can be easily addressed by nursing staff at ward level, improving the patient's experience of meals and reducing the likelihood of them not receiving their appropriate nutrition in a timely manner. Other factors affecting appetite are outlined in Table 4.1.

Refeeding syndrome

Refeeding syndrome occurs when an individual who has received suboptimal levels of nutrition for an extended period of time is given uncontrolled levels of food or nutrition fairly quickly. If not identified or managed carefully, refeeding syndrome puts the patient at increased risk of developing cardiac arrhythmias, respiratory failure, haematological abnormalities, convulsions or even death. Refeeding syndrome can occur in patients who are fed orally, enterally or parenterally. To understand the implications of refeeding syndrome, it is necessary to explore how starvation affects the body.

Process of starvation

As nutritional intake decreases, there is less carbohydrate available for energy, leading to a reduction in insulin concentration and an increase in glucagon levels. When immediate energy stores run low, the body turns to use fat and protein as an alternative source of energy.

Table 4.1 Other problems affecting appetite

Problem	Caused by	Treatment
Constipation	Medication, e.g. opiates Lack of dietary fibre Medical conditions Reduced mobility Insufficient oral food and fluid intake	Adequate hydration Regular aperients
Nausea/vomiting, abdominal distension	Constipation Medical conditions, e.g. poor gastric emptying Side effect of other medications, e.g. antibiotics or chemotherapy	Antiemetics prior to food Constipation – treat as above Offer food that is appetising, well presented and in small portions Offer meals in an unhurried atmosphere Cold food may be tolerated better than hot food, due to a reduced aroma
Poor oral hygiene	Poorly fitting dentures, making eating difficult and possibly leading to mouth ulcers Oral thrush (candida), making eating painful and affecting the taste of food Mouth ulceration, making eating painful Gingivitis – as above	Treatment should be specific to the route of the problem: • New dentures • Antifungal treatment • Vitamin B and C replacement
Other issues including: • Diarrhoea • Uraemia (high blood urea levels due to dehydration or poor kidney function) • Medical conditions, e.g. postoperative ileus • Psychological issues around eating • Increasing age • Dementia		Treatment should include: • Ensuring the patient is adequately hydrated • Providing small appetising meals in an unhurried atmosphere • Providing assistance with eating where appropriate • To stimulate appetite in stable older patients, offering a small amount of alcohol prior to a meal

During this process:

- glycogen stores in the liver are rapidly converted to glucose;
- glucose is synthesised from protein and fat (gluconeogenesis);
- fats from adipose tissue are broken down, releasing large amounts of fatty acids and glycerol, which replace carbohydrate as the major source of energy.

Skeletal and cardiac muscle is also broken down (catabolised), leading to muscle weakness and an overall depletion in electrolytes. Electrolyte levels within cells drop, but blood serum levels may still appear within normal range. When food is reintroduced, the body switches from metabolising fat to metabolising carbohydrate, and changes from catabolism to a stimulation of protein synthesis. To

Box 4.3 Patients at risk of refeeding syndrome (NICE 2006)

There is a risk of refeeding syndrome if the patient has one or more of the following:

- BMI less than 16 kg/m²
- Unintentional weight loss greater than 15% within the last 3–6 months
- Little or no nutritional intake for more than 10 days
- Low levels of potassium, phosphate or magnesium prior to feeding

Or
The patient has two or more of the following:

- BMI less than 18.5 kg/m²
- Unintentional weight loss greater than 10% within the last 3–6 months
- Little or no nutritional intake for more than 5 days
- A history of alcohol abuse or drugs including insulin, chemotherapy, antacids or diuretics

enable this process, insulin levels rise and electrolytes are transferred back into cells, leaving blood serum electrolyte levels low.

Those patients classified as at high risk of developing refeeding syndrome (Box 4.3) should recommence with low levels of protein and energy intake. NICE (2006) recommends starting nutrition at a maximum of 10 kcal/kg per day and increasing levels slowly to meet or exceed full needs within 4–7 days. Blood electrolytes should be monitored, and group B vitamins, including thiamine, and multivitamin/multimineral supplementation should also be prescribed. Providing such low levels of nutrition initially is very likely to result in suboptimal fluid levels, and therefore supplementary intravenous fluids may be required.

Effect of surgery on nutrition

Injury caused by surgery initiates an inflammatory response leading to the release of cytokines, acute-phase proteins and stress hormones (Ljungqvist *et al.* 2006), and this release of mediators into the circulation has a major impact on the body's metabolism (Braga *et al.* 2009). As the patient's metabolic rate changes, so will the body's nutritional requirements. In the initial 24 hours following major surgery, nutritional needs will be reduced while the body copes with the assault, but overall requirements will increase as the body begins the healing process.

Preoperative care

The majority of patients undergoing surgery will continue their normal nutritional intake until 6 hours before surgery and continue to drink clear fluids for up to 2 hours before (Brady *et al.* 2003). Patients should be screened preoperatively and, if malnourished, consideration should be given to perioperative nutritional support to minimise the risks of developing refeeding syndrome (Powell-Tuck *et al.* 2011).

Patients who are in a malnourished state before surgery are at greater risk of complications (see Box 4.2). Therefore it may be appropriate to optimise the patient's nutritional state with artificial nutritional support in the weeks prior to elective surgery. One option is to offer carbohydrate drinks preoperatively with the aim of improving recovery postoperatively. Drinks are usually given 2–3 hours before an operation (Ljungqvist *et al.* 2006). Most enteral feeding companies have their own specialised preoperative nutritional supplement formulation – a clear carbohydrate drink with small levels of electrolytes to aid absorption. These are significantly different from the usual 'oral nutritional supplements' and should not be confused as normal nutritional supplements are not suitable for this purpose.

Postoperative care

Patients undergoing a minor operation will often be able to start eating and drinking fairly quickly following their return to the ward. However, for those patients who were malnourished preoperatively, a more cautious introduction to nutrition may be necessary, using oral supplements or artificial nutrition support continuing until the patient is able to take sufficient nutrition orally. If a patient develops infectious complications after surgery, artificial nutritional support is generally required (Braga *et al.* 2009). The type of nutrition support provided will depend upon the type of surgery the patient has undergone and whether their gastrointestinal tract is functioning and accessible.

Visit www.wileyfundamentalseries.com/medicalnursing and read Reflective Question 4.2 to think more about this topic.

Nutritional support

Nutritional support or artificial nutrition may be given via the oral, enteral or parenteral route and is delivered in various forms. Once the need for nutrition support has been identified, the least invasive method should be used. The least invasive method of providing nutritional support is by supplementing oral intake. Where oral intake fails to meet nutritional needs or is unsafe, the patient may progress to an enteral feeding tube.

Supplementing oral intake

The easiest method of supplementing the diet is to increase the number or size of meals and snacks provided, although larger meals may be off-putting for some patients. Nutritious drinks such as milky coffee, milk or a milkshake between meals may be easier and more acceptable than another meal or snack in individuals with poor appetites (Best 2008). It is essential that patients are provided with an appropriate level of assistance to enable them to eat their meals or snacks.

When the provision of additional food, fortified food or snacks is unsuccessful, the next step is to consider using a nutritional supplement. These supplements tend to come in the form of nutritionally complete liquids provided in a small carton or bottle – for example Fortisip, Ensure, Clinutren and Resource. 'Nutritionally complete' means that if sufficient quantities of the supplement are taken each day, the patient's nutritional requirements for all vitamins and minerals, energy and protein can theoretically be met. They are not, however, nutritionally complete in one bottle or carton.

Supplements commonly come in three types: milkshake, fruit juice style or yogurt style. In addition, some companies offer a savoury, soup-style supplement. When ill or malnourished, some people experience taste changes so be sure to offer your patient a combination of different flavours until they can find what suits them. Offering your patient a variety of different supplements will also help to prevent taste fatigue. There are other powdered supplements that can be made with fresh milk, such as Build-up, Complan, Enshake and Scandishake Mix, which may be more palatable for some people but are not nutritionally complete.

Visit www.wileyfundamentalseries.com/medicalnursing and read Reflective Question 4.3 to think more about this topic.

Nursing responsibility for oral nutrition

Nurses are responsible for ensuring that patients and clients eat the right food at the right time with the right supervision and assistance (Royal College of Nursing 2007). As the nursing role has become increasingly complex, activities such as serving patients' meals in hospital have been devolved to other healthcare professionals, leaving the nursing role in patients' nutritional care ill-defined (Jeffries *et al.* 2011). Even when nurses are not directly involved in delivering meals to patients, they still retain the responsibility for ensuring that patients in their care receive the nutrition that is appropriate to their needs. Simple measures such as are essential to ensure that patients meet their nutritional needs orally (Hospital Caterers Association 2004):

- appointing a mealtime coordinator;
- assessing and documenting the level of assistance that patients require at mealtimes;
- minimising unnecessary interruptions;
- ensuring that staff are available to provide assistance over mealtimes.

Enteral tube feeding

Enteral tube feeding can be provided via a nasogastric tube (NGT), nasojejunal tube, gastrostomy tube or jejunostomy tube.

Nasogastric feeding

Short-term enteral feeding (2–6 weeks) is normally provided through an NGT as this provides a relatively easy means of bypassing the oral cavity while providing direct access to the stomach. Insertion of an NGT can be undertaken at the bedside and generally requires no anaesthetic. Although this is a relatively simple procedure to undertake, there are risks associated with placement of an NGT (Box 4.4). There have been two National Patient Safety Alerts in recent years regarding the placement and checking of NGTs (National Patient Safety Agency [NPSA] 2005, 2011).

A fine-bore NGT should be used as it is more comfortable for the patient and reduces the risk of rhinitis, pharyngitis or oesophageal erosion. It should be radio-opaque throughout its length, so that its position can be monitored on X-ray (if required), and have clear markers to aid measurement during insertion and for bedside checks (NPSA 2011). The NGT is inserted via the nostril, along the nasopharynx, down through the oesophagus and into the stomach (Figure 4.1).

Once the tube has been inserted, its gastric positioning needs to be confirmed, which is usually undertaken using pH indicator strips, gastric placement being confirmed by a pH between 1 and 5.5. Each test result is documented on a chart kept at the patient's bedside (NPSA 2011). X-rays should only be undertaken if gastric placement cannot be confirmed using pH indicator strips and should only be used following initial NGT placement (NPSA 2011).

Gastrostomy tubes

A gastrostomy provides a more permanent means of access to the stomach to enable longer term enteral feeding (>6 weeks). It provides safe access directly into the stomach through the development of a fistula through the abdominal wall. There are four different types of gastrostomy tube (Table 4.2) of which the percutaneous endoscopic gastrostomy (PEG) tube (Figure 4.2) is the most commonly used.

Postpyloric feeding

Postpyloric feeding may be considered for patients in whom gastric feeding is unsafe or problematic, for example patients with gastroparesis, pancreatitis or aspiration pneumonia. The tip of the feeding

Box 4.4 Risks of NGT insertion

Consider the patient history during assessment for:
Previous facial injuries
Facial surgery or polyps
Upper gastrointestinal strictures or disease
Oesophageal varices
Base of skull fractures

Potential risks during the insertion procedure:
Inadvertent placement in the:

- Bronchial tract
- Oesophagus
- Small intestine

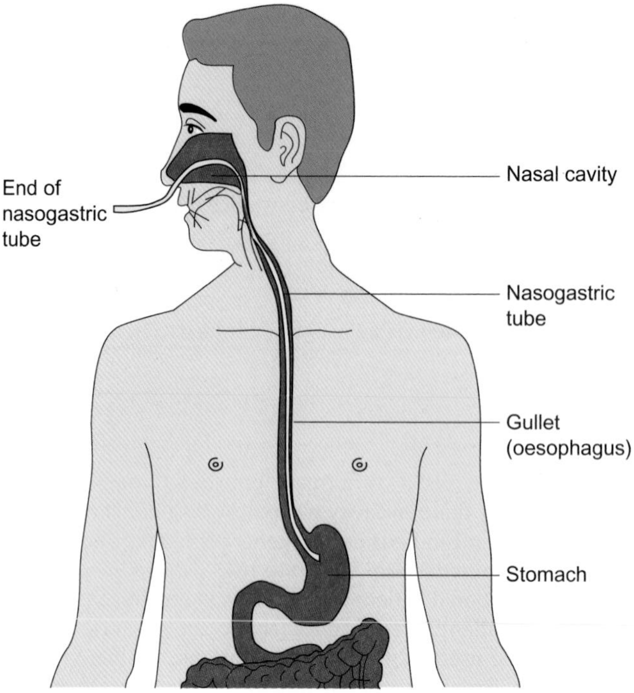

Figure 4.1 NGT insertion.

Table 4.2 Types of gastrostomy tube

Type of gastrostomy tube	Rationale for use
PEG	The most common method of primary gastrostomy insertion
Radiologically inserted gastrostomy or fluoroscopically guided percutaneous gastrostomy	May be the method of choice if endoscopic placement is not available or is inadvisable
Balloon gastrostomy	May be used for primary placement or as a percutaneous replacement where further endoscopic or radiological intervention is to be avoided
Button or low-profile device	Tend to be used in younger adults and children

tube bypasses the stomach and sits in the small intestine. Three types of tube are used for postpyloric feeding (Table 4.3).

Enteral tube feeds

There are many different enteral tube feeds. Some contain fibre, some provide more calories per millilitre than others, and the level of electrolytes may vary between feeds. Feeds are generally presented in sterile ready-to-use containers and can hang for a maximum of 24 hours, after which any remaining feed should be discarded.

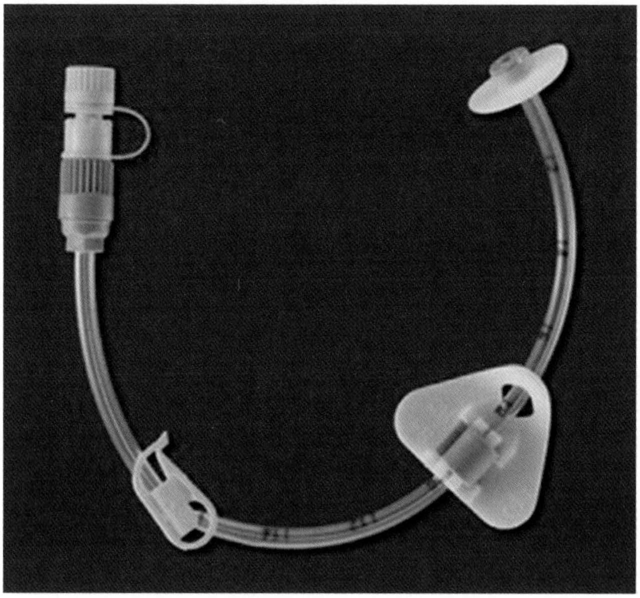

Figure 4.2 PEG tube. Courtesy of Fresenius Kabi.

Table 4.3 Enteral feeding tubes used for postpyloric feeding

Type of tube	Method of placement
Nasojejunal tube	Appears very similar to an NGT. They may be single or dual lumen Dual-lumen tubes have one gastric port for gastric decompression and one jejunal port for feeding They can be placed endoscopically, radiologically or at the bedside by specially trained healthcare professionals Some nasojejunal tubes may be assisted into the small bowel using prokinetic drugs to help stimulate gastric emptying and position the tube correctly
Percutaneous endoscopic gastrojejunostomy	Created following the placement of a PEG tube, a long small-gauge tube is passed through the lumen of the PEG and pulled down into the small intestine
Surgical jejunostomy	Placed directly into the jejunum at laparotomy May be tunnelled and secured using a Dacron cuff or held in place by sutures at the abdomen

Methods of providing enteral feed

A feed can be delivered through an enteral feeding tube in a number of ways:

- continuously via a pump providing a set rate of feed over a specified number of hours;
- intermittent infusion (with or without a pump);
- using a syringe to deliver larger volumes of feed (bolus) at agreed timeslots throughout the day.

The method of administration used will depend upon the patient's medical condition, their ability to tolerate the feed, their nutritional requirements and their preferences.

Patient monitoring

Enteral feed should be stored and administered at room temperature to avoid gastric discomfort associated with the administration of cold feed. The patient should be positioned with the head and shoulders raised to an angle of at least 30° and be monitored closely for any potential side effects (as discussed above) during feeding and for at least an hour on completion of the feed. While nutritional support is being provided, the patient should be monitored to check for:

- changes in weight;
- changes in oral intake;
- fluid balance;
- electrolyte deficiencies;

so that their feeding regimen can be adjusted accordingly.

If a decision is made that nutritional support is no longer required, there is usually a gradual reduction in feed with continued monitoring, to ensure that patients can maintain their nutritional status without support. In the same way that nutritional support is escalated using a step-by-step approach, so it is sensible to reduce it using the same approach.

Parenteral feeding

If feeding into the gastrointestinal tract is not tolerated or the gut is not available, nutritional needs have to be met via the parenteral route. Parenteral nutrition is delivered through a central venous catheter (CVC) with a dedicated lumen. To minimise the risk of infection if central access is only required for the administration of parenteral nutrition, a single-lumen catheter should be used (Pratt *et al.* 2007). However, as parenteral nutrition is often commenced when the patient is acutely ill, a multilumen CVC may be required to provide access for a number of treatments simultaneously. In such cases, one lumen must be reserved solely for the administration of parenteral nutrition and should be labelled clearly to prevent the administration of other therapies or the withdrawal of blood.

Before using parenteral nutrition, micronutrients and trace elements should be added to the feed, and additional electrolytes and nutrients may also be required. Due to the increased infection risks associated with using the central circulation to provide nutrition, parenteral nutrition is used only when all other options of providing nutrition have been explored. The patient receiving parenteral nutrition will require close monitoring of bloods and fluid balance and strict aseptic care of the CVC. Nurses providing care for patients requiring PN will usually require additional local training.

Visit www.wileyfundamentalseries.com/medicalnursing and read Reflective Question 4.4 to think more about this topic.

Conclusion

Many factors affect the nutritional status of a patient coming into hospital, including increasing age, illness, an inability to cope, drug treatment and socioeconomic factors. As the care of health-related problems is increasingly being managed in primary care settings, patients who are admitted to hospital are often acutely ill before admission and may already have some signs of malnutrition. Once in hospital, the risks increase due to episodes where patients are placed on 'nil by mouth' for investigations or procedures required to investigate and treat their illness or disease. In addition, appetite often decreases when a person is ill. Therefore it is not surprising that some patients may leave hospital in a more malnourished state that when they arrived.

Providing an appropriate and timely level of nutritional support is essential to maximise the patient's nutritional status and recovery from illness. The use of a step-by-step approach is often the safest means of progressing – from oral supplementation to parenteral nutrition. However, it is essential to consider the risks that accompany artificial nutritional support as the provision of nutritional care via enteral or parenteral feeding tubes is not without complications. Therefore the balance of risk versus benefit must be considered for each patient before nutritional support is commenced. Nurses play a central role in many of these discussions as they often have a more holistic view of the patient and any family or carers involved. It is essential that nurses are represented within multidisciplinary teams and act as the patient's voice if and when the patient is unable to represent their own view, to ensure that the appropriate level of nutrition is provided by the appropriate route.

Now visit the companion website and test yourself on this chapter:
www.wileyfundamentalseries.com/medicalnursing

References

Age Concern (2006) *Hungry to be Heard: The Scandal of Malnourished Older People in Hospital*. London: Age Concern England.

Best, C. (2008) *Nutrition: A Handbook for Nurses*. Chichester: Wiley Blackwell.

Brady, M., Kinn, S. & Stuart, P. (2003) Preoperative fasting for adults to prevent perioperative complications *Cochrane Database System Review*, (4):CD004423..

Braga, M., Ljungqvist, O., Soeters, P., Fearon, K., Weimann, A. & Bozzetti, F. (2009) ESPEN Guidelines on Parenteral Nutrition: Surgery. *Clinical Nutrition*, **28**:378–86.

Department of Health (1991) *Dietary Reference Values for Food Energy and Nutrients for the United Kingdom*. Report on Health and Social Subjects No. 41. London: HSMO.

Department of Health (2007) *Improving Nutritional Care: A Joint Action Plan from the Department of Health and Nutrition Summit Stakeholders*. London: Department of Health.

Elia, M. (2003a) *Screening for Malnutrition: A Multidisciplinary Responsibility. Development and Use of the 'Malnutrition Universal Screening Tool' ('MUST') for Adults.* Malnutrition Advisory Group (MAG). Redditch, Worcestershire: BAPEN.

Elia, M. (2003b) *The 'MUST' report: nutritional screening of adults: a multidisciplinary responsibility. A report by the Malnutrition Advisory Group of the British Association for Parenteral and Enteral Nutrition*. Redditch, Worcestershire: BAPEN.

Hospital Caterers Association (2004) *Protected Mealtimes Policy*. London: HCA.

Jeffries, D., Johnson, M. & Ravens, J. (2011) Nurturing and nourishing: the nurses' role in nutritional care. *Journal of Clinical Nursing*, **20**(3–4): 317–30.

Ljungqvist, O., Fearon, K. & Little, R.A. (2006) Nutrition in surgery and trauma. In: Gibney, M.J., Elia, M., Ljungvqist, O. & Dowsett, J. (eds), *Clinical Nutrition* (Chapter 19). Oxford: Nutrition Society/Blackwell.

National Institute of Clinical Excellence (2006) *Nutrition Support for Adults. Oral Nutrition Support, Enteral Tube Feeding and Parenteral Nutrition*. Clinical Guideline No. 32. London: NICE.

National Patient Safety Agency (2005) *Reducing the Harm Caused by Misplaced Nasogastric Tubes*. Patient Safety Alert 05. London: NPSA.

National Patient Safety Agency (2011) *Reducing the Harm Caused by Misplaced Nasogastric Feeding Tubes in Adults, Children and Infants*. Patient Safety Alert NPSA/2011/PSA00. London: NPSA.

Patients Association (2010) *Listen to Patients, Speak up for Change*. London: Patients Association.

Powell-Tuck, J. Gosling, P., Lobo, D. *et al.* (2011) *British Consensus Guidelines on Intravenous Fluid Therapy for Adult Surgical Patients*. Redditch, Worcestershire: BAPEN.

Pratt, R.J., Pellowe, C.M., Wilson, J.A. *et al.* (2007) epic2 National Evidence-Based Guidelines for Preventing Healthcare-Associated Infections in NHS Hospitals in England. *Journal of Hospital Infection*, **65S**:S1–64.

Royal College of Nursing (2007) *Nutrition Now*. London: RCN.

World Health Organization (1996) Anthropometric reference data for international use: recommendations from a WHO Expert Committee. *American Journal of Clinical Nutrition*, **64**:650–8.

5

Principles of infection prevention and control

Sile Creedon[1] and Maura Smiddy[2]

[1]*School of Nursing and Midwifery, University College Cork, Cork, Ireland*
[2]*Department of Epidemiology and Public Health, University College Cork, Cork, Ireland*

Contents

Introduction 59
Physiology associated with infection 59
Overview of common microbiology and pathogenic organisms 62
Frequently encountered pathogenic microorganisms 63
Infection control principles 64
Asepsis 66
Decontamination 66
Healthcare waste management 72
Isolation of patients 72
Care bundles 73
Conclusion 76
References 76

Learning outcomes

Having read this chapter, you will be able to:

- Define healthcare-associated infections and differentiate between endogenous and exogenous infections
- Discuss colonisation versus infection
- Describe how infections are transmitted
- Identify frequently encountered pathogenic microorganisms
- Identify techniques used and indications for healthcare workers to engage in hand hygiene
- Describe and discuss standard precautions, including the use of personal protective equipment, decontamination and waste management
- Describe transmission based precautions

Fundamentals of Medical-Surgical Nursing: A Systems Approach, First Edition. Edited by Anne-Marie Brady, Catherine McCabe, and Margaret McCann.

Introduction

The prevention and control of infection is a fundamental element of nursing practice, and all healthcare professionals have the responsibility to adhere to evidence-based guidelines in order to control infection in clinical settings. A healthcare-associated infection is defined as 'a localized or systemic condition that results from an adverse reaction to the presence of an infectious agent(s) or its toxin(s) and . . . that was not present or incubating at the time of admission to the hospital' (Horan *et al.* 2008, p. 1).

Physiology associated with infection

Microorganisms live in continuous interaction with their environment. The main portal of entry for microbes is the skin and mucosal surfaces of the gastrointestinal, respiratory and urogenital tracts (Figure 5.1). Interaction with bacteria leads to colonisation of epithelial surfaces, a coexistence that is usually harmonious and beneficial for the host (commensalism). It leads to the development of a complex open ecosystem formed by the interaction of resident and transiently present microbes.

Resident microbes, usually bacteria, are microorganisms that live permanently on human epithelial cells. They are not harmful and cannot be eliminated unless using a surgical scrub technique. They may also be referred to as '**endogenous**'.

Transient microbes are microorganisms that we acquire when we interact with other humans and our environment. They can be removed by washing or cleaning. They may also be referred to as '**exogenous**'. Under some conditions, the interaction with endogenous microbes can be harmful for the host, and opportunistic infections may occur.

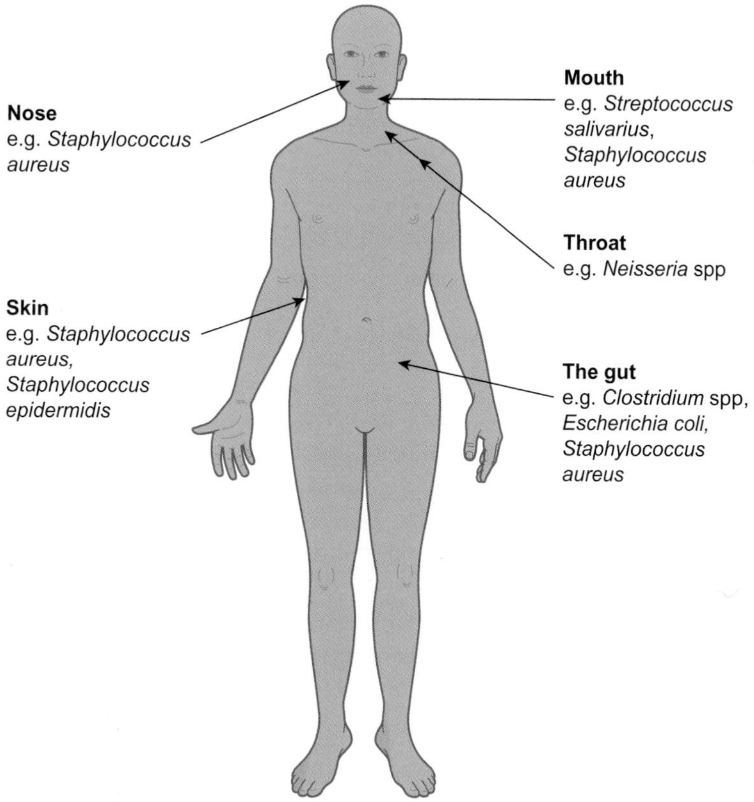

Figure 5.1 Common sites for the presence of commensal bacteria on the human body.

Colonisation versus infection

Colonisation means that a pathogen grows in the host without causing signs or symptoms of illness such as tissue invasion, damage or inflammation. **Infection**, on the other hand, means that the pathogen actually invades the host's tissues and causes signs and symptoms of illness. *Salmonella* (a Gram-negative, rod-shaped bacterium), responsible for food poisoning, is a good example of a pathogenic microorganism. Microorganisms that colonise the human body differ from pathogenic microorganisms in the following ways:

- They rarely cause infection or disease in people who are healthy.
- They may become pathogenic if introduced to another site within the same individual. For example, *Escherichia coli* are normally found in the gastrointestinal tract but may cause a urinary tract infection if introduced into the urinary tract.

It is not possible to differentiate colonisation from infection from a laboratory analysis of clinical specimens alone; the clinical condition of the patient or client must also be considered. Clinically, infection presents as:

- symptoms of pain, pyrexia, dysuria, purulent sputum, the presence of pus and inflammation;
- significant levels of bacteria reported from the laboratory analysis of the specimen, for example a sputum or wound swab;
- other investigations that supports the diagnosis of infection, for example an abnormal chest X-ray or elevated leucocyte (white blood cell) count. The normal range for the leucocyte count is 4300–10,800 cells/mm^3, or 4.3–10.8 $\times 10^9$ cells/L.

Transmission of infection

Microorganisms that cause healthcare associated infections can be acquired in different ways.

Endogenous infections are caused by bacteria present in the person's normal flora because of transmission to sites outside their natural habitat (e.g. the urinary tract), damage to tissue (e.g. wounds) or inappropriate antibiotic therapy that allows overgrowth of the organism (e.g. *Clostridium difficile* or yeast species). For example, Gram-negative bacteria in the digestive tract frequently cause surgical site infections after abdominal surgery or urinary tract infections in patients who have had a urinary catheter inserted.

Exogenous or cross–infections are caused by the transmission of microorganisms from another patient or member of staff. Microorganisms are transmitted between patients:

- through direct contact between patients (via hands, saliva droplets or other body fluids);
- in the air (droplets or dust contaminated by a patient's bacteria);
- via staff engaged in direct patient care (e.g. hands, clothes or nose and throat) who become transient or permanent carriers, subsequently transmitting microorganisms to other patients by direct contact during care;
- via objects contaminated by the patient (including equipment), the staff's hands, visitors or other environmental sources (e.g. water or food).

Endemic or epidemic exogenous environmental infections are caused by the transmission of microorganisms from the healthcare environment. Several types of microorganism survive well in the hospital environment, for example in water, damp areas and occasionally in sterile products or disinfectants (as with *Pseudomonas* sp., *Acinetobacter* sp. and *Mycobacterium* sp.). They can be found:

- in items such as linen, equipment and supplies used in care; good hygiene normally limits the risk of bacteria surviving as most microorganisms require humid or hot conditions and nutrients to survive;
- in food;
- in fine dust and droplet nuclei generated by coughing or speaking (as bacteria smaller than 10 μm in diameter remain in the air for several hours and can be inhaled in the same way as fine dust).

The cycle of infection is such that infection or disease may be transmitted when key elements are present (Box 5.1 and Figure 5.2).

Box 5.1 The cycle of infection (adapted from Health Protection Surveillance Centre 2009)

- **Infectious agent:** an organism that causes disease (e.g. a bacterium, virus, fungus or protozoon)
- **Reservoir or source of infectious agent:** the place where an infectious agent lives and grows (e.g. the gastrointestinal and upper respiratory tracts for the normal flora)
- **Portal of exit:** any body opening that allows the infectious agent to leave (e.g. the mouth, nose, rectum or breaks in the skin)
- **Means of transmission:** how the infectious agent travels from the infected person to another person. The principle routes of transmission are contact (indirect and direct), droplet and airborne. The mode of transmission varies by type of infectious agent, and some may be transmitted by more than one route
- **Portal of entry:** any body opening that allows the infectious agent to enter (e.g. the nose, mouth, eyes, mucous membranes, a surgical or non surgical break in the skin or medical devices such as urethral catheters that bypass the body's natural defences)
- **A susceptible host:** a non-infected person who could get infected. The factors that influence the acquisition and severity of the infection are related to the virulence of the infectious agent and host factors such as extremes of age, underlying disease, treatment for complex diseases, immunosuppression and whether the patient is the recipient of an organ and tissue transplants

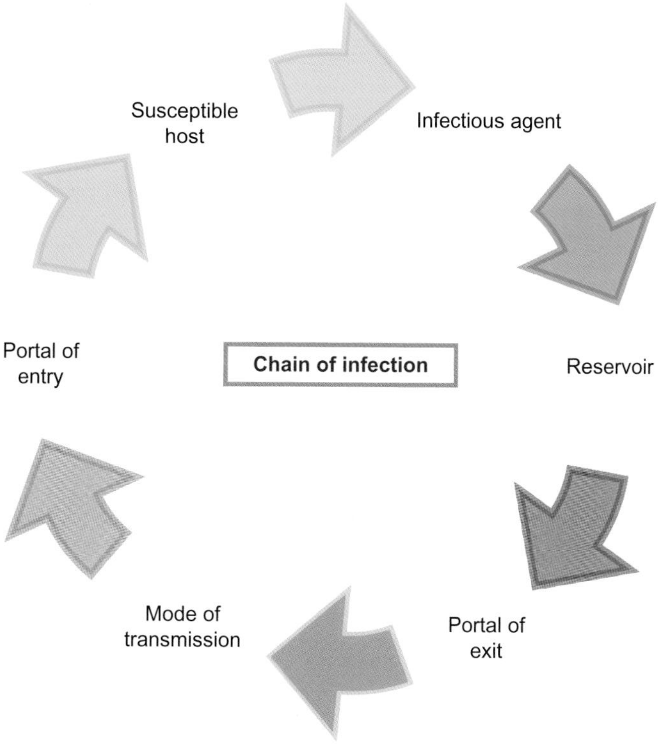

Figure 5.2 The cycle of infection.

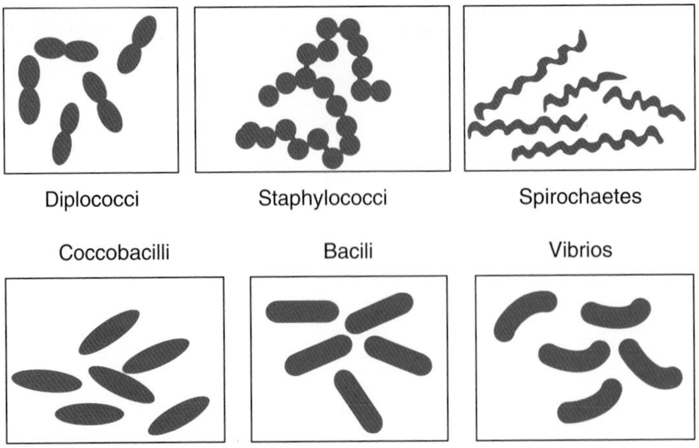

Figure 5.3 Shapes of different bacteria. Reproduced from Nair, M. & Peate, I. (2009) *Fundamentals of Applied Pathophysiology* with kind permission from Wiley Blackwell.

Overview of common microbiology and pathogenic organisms

Bacteria

Bacteria are grouped according to their ability to absorb crystal violet stain (Gram stain) and their shape (morphology). They come in many shapes and sizes (Figure 5.3), for example:

- Gram-positive, e.g. *Staphlococcus aureus*;
- Gram-negative, e.g. *Clostridium difficile*.

Bacteria are colourless and usually invisible to the microscope, and the colourful Gram stain was developed in order to visualise them. If the cell absorbs this violet dye, it will appear blue. These microorganisms are referred to as Gram-positive microorganisms. If they do not absorb the violet dye, they appear red and are called Gram-negative organisms. Bacterial infections may be treated using antibiotics.

Viruses

Viruses are basic life forms composed of a protein coat, called a capsid, that surrounds the genetic material. Viruses contain genetic material that is either DNA or RNA but not both. Viruses are much smaller than other microorganisms and are measured in nanometers ($1\,nm = 1 \times 10^{-9}\,m$). Viruses are too small to be seen with a light microscope so an electron microscope must be used. Viral infections may be treated using antiviral medications.

The most frequently encountered viral infections are:

- herpes simplex type 1 (cold sores);
- herpes zoster (chickenpox or shingles).

Fungi

Fungi are eukaryotic cells (i.e. their contents are enclosed in a membrane) that lack chlorophyll. Thus, they cannot generate energy through photosynthesis, and they require an aerobic environment. Fungi cause a number of diseases in humans that may be categorised as cutaneous or systemic. Fungal infections may be treated using antifungals and may be:

- cutaneous infections such as ringworm;
- systemic fungal infections such as candidiasis.

Frequently encountered pathogenic microorganisms

Multidrug-resistant organisms are now one of the most challenging aspects of the prevention and control of infection. Control of these organisms is best tackled through comprehensive surveillance, appropriate management and antibiotic stewardship programmes (Strategy for the Control of Antimicrobial Resistance in Ireland [SARI] 2005; Coia *et al.* 2006). Precautions and procedures required when caring for patients who acquire these microorganisms are outlined in Table 5.4 later in the chapter.

Methicillin-resistant *Staphylococcus aureus*

Staphylococcus aureus is a Gram-positive aerobic bacterium that is present on the skin of about 30% of the population and is the most common causative organisms of skin infections. Methicillin-resistant *Staphylococcus aureus* (MRSA) is a type of *Staphylococcus aureus* that has become resistant to many of the antibiotics used to treat infections with it. MRSA is spread by touching contact with a patient who is colonised or infected with the organism, through contact with the individual's environment or via contaminated equipment. These patients are cared for using contact isolation precautions.

Glycopeptide-resistant enterococci

Enterococci are Gram-positive anaerobic bacteria that are normal bowel commensals. Glycopeptide-resistant enterococci include enterococci resistant to vancomycin, a glycopeptide antibiotic. These are commonly referred to as vancomycin-resistant enterococci.

Enterococci readily survive in the patient environment and on equipment, especially in toilet areas. Patients with known or suspected infection or colonisation with glycopeptide-resistant enterococci should therefore be cared for using contact isolation precautions.

Other healthcare-associated infections: *Clostridium difficile*

Clostridium difficile or 'C. diff.' is a Gram–negative, spore-forming, rod-shaped bacterium. It is present in the bowel of about 3% of healthy adults and about 66% of infants. It does not usually cause disease in healthy individuals as the natural flora of the gut keep it in check. However, when the gut commensals are compromised due to exposure to antibiotics, *Clostridium difficile* organisms multiply and produce two toxins – A and B – which cause inflammation and diarrhoea.

Clostridium difficile spores can withstand exposure to heat, alcohol and other disinfectants and survive readily in the environment, resulting in a sustained risk to patients. Some patients can be asymptomatic, but they can also develop symptoms of diarrhoea, abdominal cramps, fever and leucocytosis. Patients with severe disease can develop pseudomembranous colitis, which is associated with significant mortality. Risk factors for acquisition of infection include exposure to antibiotics, increased age and associated treatment with antacid medications (Garey *et al.* 2008). *Clostridium difficile* can also be transmitted via the orofaecal route.

The disease is usually self-limiting and treatment is often not required. Patients with known or suspected *Clostridium difficile* infection must be cared for using contact isolation precautions until they have been diarrhoea-free for 48 hours and are producing stools that are normal for that patient.

Infection control principles

Standard precautions

Standard precautions are taken by healthcare workers to protect themselves and patients against exposure to blood and/or body fluid. Implementation of standard precautions minimises the risk of transmission of infectious agents. These precautions are based on the principle that all blood, body fluids, secretions, excretions except sweat, non-intact skin and mucous membranes may contain transmissible infectious agents.

Standard precautions apply to **ALL** patients at **ALL** times regardless of their diagnosis.

Patient placement

Empiric precautions

All patients known or suspected of having an infectious disease should where possible be isolated in a single room using the appropriate precautions to prevent the spread of the infectious condition (Siegel *et al.* 2007). These empiric transmission-based precautions include contact precautions, droplet precautions and airborne precautions; these will be covered in greater detail under 'Isolation of patients'.

Cohort isolation

In some circumstances, it will not be feasible to obtain a single room, in which case patients who are suspected of having the same infectious condition may be cared for in the same room. It is important to remember, even when patients are cared for in a cohort situation, that all aspects of the standard precautions must be adhered to between each patient contact.

Designated ward-specific precautions

In hospitals with a consistent large number of patients with the same infectious condition, for example MRSA, these may be cared for on a specific ward allocated for patients with only that condition.

Patient movement and transfer

The precautions that need to be utilised will depend on the mode of transmission of the infectious agent. Patient movement should be limited to essential purposes to reduce the risk of transmitting the infectious agent to others. All departments and wards involved in the movement of the patient must be informed of the patient's condition prior to transfer; this ensures that the appropriate precautions will be implemented in an efficient and timely manner. Personal protective equipment (PPE), for example gloves, aprons, gowns, masks and face and eye shields, must be worn by the healthcare workers and sometimes the patient. Decontamination of the environment and medical equipment must be carried out after the infectious patient has had contact with it.

Hand hygiene

Hand hygiene is recognised internationally as the most important element in the prevention of infection and as the cornerstone of patient safety (Pratt *et al.* 2001; McFee 2009; World Health Organization [WHO] 2009; D. Pittet, personal communication, 12th January 2012).

- **Social hand hygiene** involves washing the hands with ordinary soap and warm running water for at least 15 seconds, and then drying them with a disposable paper towel. On visibly clean hands,

Table 5.1 The WHO's 5 Moments for Hand Hygiene

	Moment	Rationale – Why?	Rationale – When?
1.	**Before touching a patient**	To protect the patient/client against colonisation and, in some cases, against exogenous infection, by harmful germs carried on your hands	Clean your hands before touching a patient/client when approaching him/her
2.	**Before clean/ aseptic procedure**	To protect the patient/client against infection with harmful germs, including his/her own germs, entering his/her body	Clean your hands immediately before accessing a critical site with infectious risk for the patient (e.g. a mucous membrane, non-intact skin, an invasive medical device)
3.	**After body fluid exposure risk**	To protect you from colonisation or infection with patient's harmful germs and to protect the health-care environment from germ spread	Clean your hands as soon as the task involving an exposure risk to body fluids has ended (and after glove removal)
4.	**After touching a patient**	To protect you from colonisation with patient/client germs and to protect the health-care environment from germ spread	Clean your hands when leaving the patient's side, after having touched the patient/client
5.	**After touching patient surroundings**	To protect you from colonisation with patient/client germs that may be present on surfaces/objects in patient surroundings and to protect the health-care environment against germ spread	Clean your hands after touching any object or furniture when living the patient surroundings, without having touched the patient/client

Reprinted with kind permission from WHO, 2009.

social hand hygiene may be undertaken using an alcohol handrub product, and this will effectively remove transient organisms (SARI 2005).

- **Antiseptic hand hygiene** involves washing the hands with soap and water, or other detergents containing an antiseptic agent (WHO 2009). The aim of an antiseptic handwash or handrub is to remove all transient organisms, and this achieves a higher level of cleanliness than does social hand-washing (SARI 2005).
- **Surgical hand antisepsis** involves an antiseptic handwash or antiseptic handrub performed preoperatively by the surgical team to eliminate transient flora and reduce resident skin flora. Such antiseptics often have persistent antimicrobial activity (WHO 2009).

Table 5.1 and Figure 5.4 outline the golden rules of hand hygiene (WHO 2009).

If exposure to potential spore-forming pathogens, including outbreaks of *Clostridium difficile*, is strongly suspected or proven, hand-washing with soap and water is the preferred means. Hand hygiene is the single most important intervention to prevent transmission of infection and should be a quality standard in all healthcare institutions (Figures 5.5 and 5.6).

PPE for healthcare workers

PPE includes the use of barriers such as gloves, gowns and eye protection, and respiratory protection such as masks, to protect the mucous membranes, airways, skin and clothing from contact with infectious agents (Siegel *et al.* 2007). Items of PPE can be used alone or in combination to protect the wearer

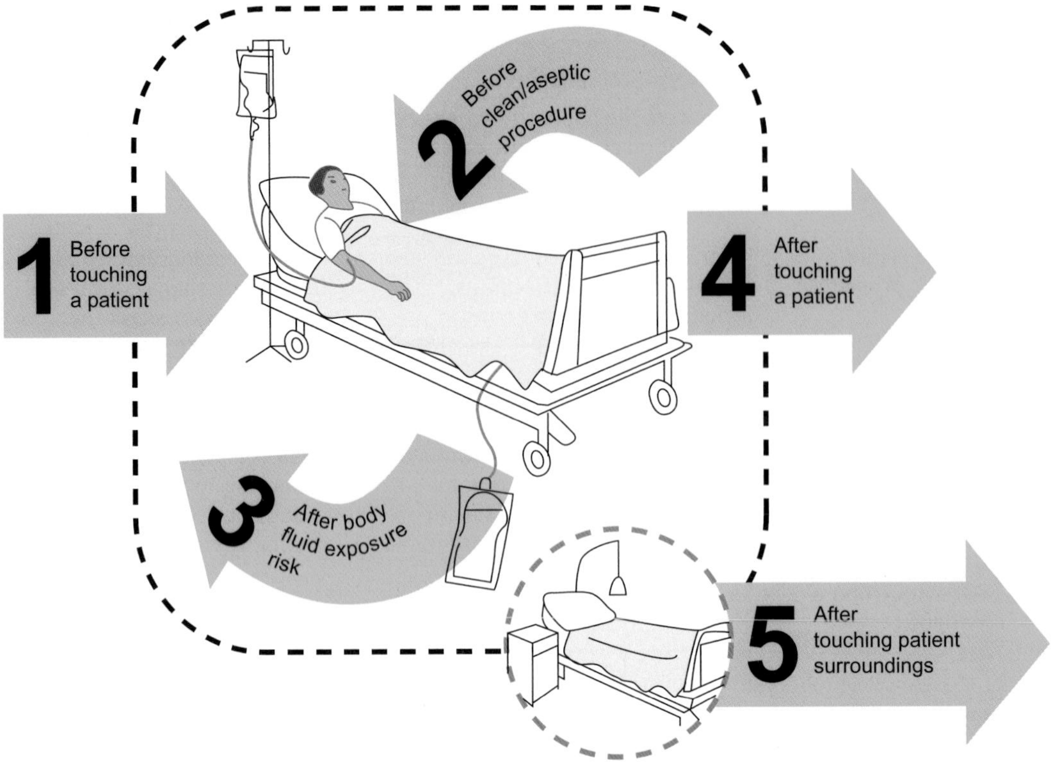

Figure 5.4 The WHO's 5 Moments for Hand Hygiene. Reprinted with kind permission from WHO, 2009.

from the potential risk of transmissible infection. The choice of PPE is dependent on the task to be undertaken and the risk associated with it (Table 5.2).

Asepsis

Aseptic technique refers to the actions that are implemented by the healthcare worker to protect the patient from pathogenic microorganisms during invasive clinical procedures.

Aseptic non-touch technique (ANTT) is a method of applying aseptic technique in a universal manner. The technique focuses on identifying key parts and key sites and taking appropriate measures to prevent the transmission of infection to the patient through hand hygiene, a non-touch technique, the use of aseptic fields and the use of sterilised equipment and equipment that has been decontaminated appropriately to render it aseptic. **Key sites** are open wounds, including insertion and puncture sites. **Key parts** are the parts of the procedure equipment that come into direct or indirect contact with active key parts connected to the patient, any liquid infusion or any key site (Association for Safe Aseptic Practice [ASAP] 2011). ANTT principles are based on both clinical practice and clinical and organisational management (ASAP 2011; Box 5.2).

Decontamination

The healthcare environment should be a clean, safe place for the patient to inhabit and for staff to work in. Microorganisms readily survive in dust and contaminated areas. There are a number of key terms associated cleaning in the health care environment (Box 5.3).

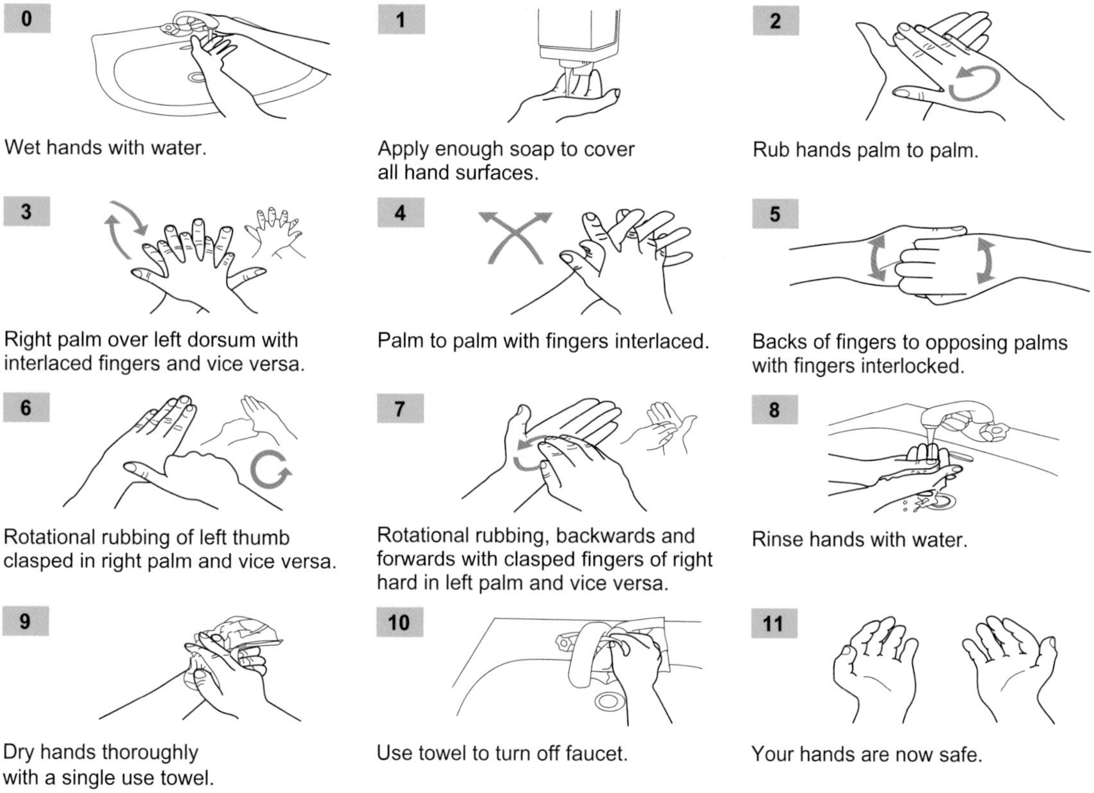
0
Wet hands with water.
1
Apply enough soap to cover all hand surfaces.
2
Rub hands palm to palm.
3
Right palm over left dorsum with interlaced fingers and vice versa.
4
Palm to palm with fingers interlaced.
5
Backs of fingers to opposing palms with fingers interlocked.
6
Rotational rubbing of left thumb clasped in right palm and vice versa.
7
Rotational rubbing, backwards and forwards with clasped fingers of right hard in left palm and vice versa.
8
Rinse hands with water.
9
Dry hands thoroughly with a single use towel.
10
Use towel to turn off faucet.
11
Your hands are now safe.

Figure 5.5 How to handwash. Reprinted with kind permission from WHO, 2009.

Decontamination of the environment

The environment should be free of clutter to facilitate cleaning. The environment should be cleaned with a neutral detergent and water except in circumstances that require additional disinfection, for example spillages of blood and body fluid (Table 5.3), or if there is contamination with specific organisms that require patients to be cared for in isolation using transmission-based precautions. Frequency of cleaning is dependent on the patient's level of hygiene and the degree of environmental contamination. Surfaces that are in close proximity to the patient, such as patient care equipment, commodes, etc. should be cleaned routinely. Disinfection should be carried out when required using a product that has microbial activity against the infectious agent likely to contaminate the patient care environment, for example hypochlorite 1000 ppm or 1:10 dilution, following the manufacturer's instructions.

Visit www.wileyfundamentalseries.com/medicalnursing and read Reflective Question 5.1 to think more about this topic.

Equipment

Non-critical (low-risk) equipment, such as equipment that is not in contact with patients or with intact skin, may be decontaminated with a neutral detergent and water. Equipment must be dried thoroughly after cleaning. Semi-critical/critical (intermediate and high-risk) equipment such as reusable invasive medical devices (scalpels and surgical instruments) and endoscopes require decontamination by disinfection and sterilisation. These items also must be stored and handled in a manner that prevents breaks in or damage to the outer packaging, which would render the device unsuitable for use until reprocessed. Sterile packaged items of equipment must be used prior to the expiry date detailed on the packaging.

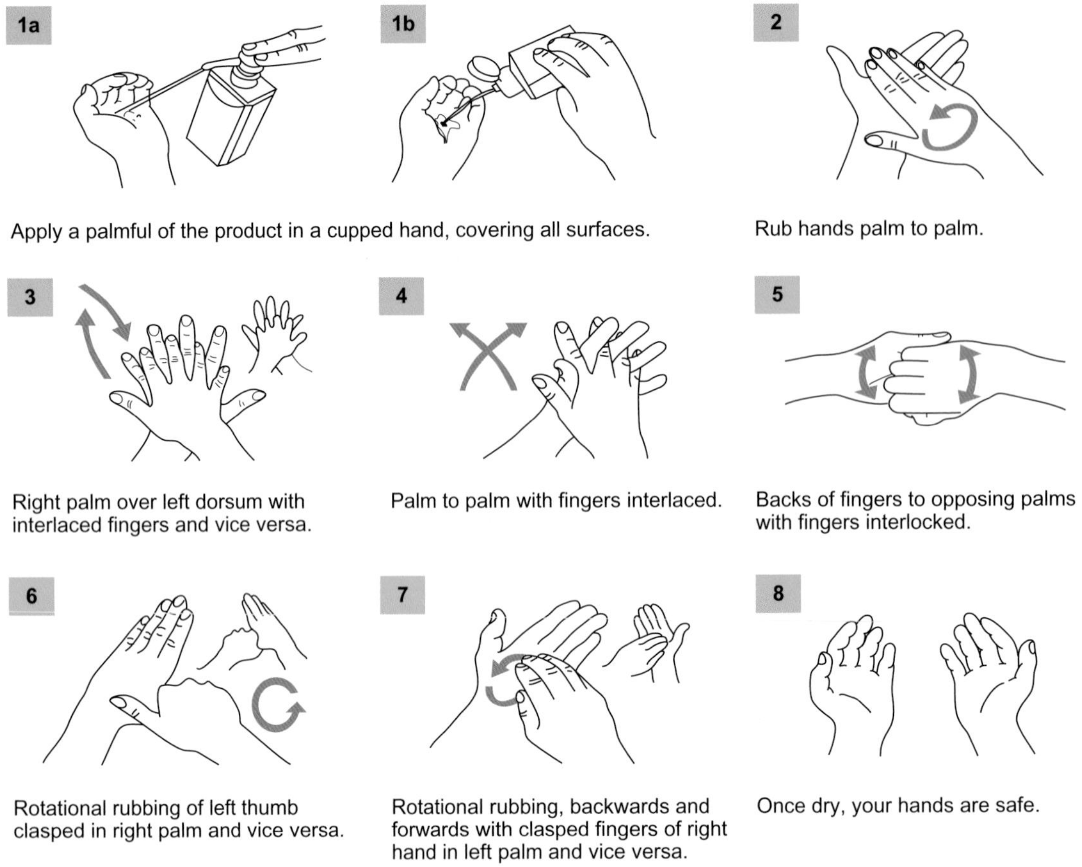
1a
1b
Apply a palmful of the product in a cupped hand, covering all surfaces.
2
Rub hands palm to palm.
3
Right palm over left dorsum with interlaced fingers and vice versa.
4
Palm to palm with fingers interlaced.
5
Backs of fingers to opposing palms with fingers interlocked.
6
Rotational rubbing of left thumb clasped in right palm and vice versa.
7
Rotational rubbing, backwards and forwards with clasped fingers of right hand in left palm and vice versa.
8
Once dry, your hands are safe.

Figure 5.6 How to hand-rub. Reprinted with kind permission from WHO, 2009.

Table 5.2 How to choose your PPE

Type of PPE	Indications for use	Protective effect
Gloves	Anticipating direct contact with blood or body fluids, mucous membranes, non-intact skin and other potentially infectious material Having direct contact with patients who are colonised or infected with pathogens transmitted by the contact route, e.g. multiresistant organisms Handling or touching visibly or potentially contaminated patient care equipment and environmental surfaces (Siegel *et al.* 2007) Indicated prior to sterile procedures (WHO 2009)	Protects the healthcare worker Protects the healthcare worker Protects the healthcare worker Protects the patient
Aprons and gowns	Anticipating direct contact with blood or body fluids, mucous membranes, non-intact skin and other potentially infectious material Having direct contact with patients who are colonised or infected with pathogens transmitted by the contact route, e.g. multiresistant organisms During sterile procedures	Protects the healthcare worker Protects the healthcare worker Protects the patient

Table 5.2 (*Continued*)

Type of PPE	Indications for use	Protective effect
Face protection – masks	Different types of mask are available: standard surgical masks, masks with a fluid shield and masks that provide greater protection to the wearer, such as FFP2 and FFP3 masks. The choice of mask to be worn is dependent on the task being undertaken. Masks are only effective when fitted and worn appropriately	
Face protection masks	Placed on healthcare personnel to protect them from contact with infectious material from patients, e.g. respiratory secretions and sprays of blood or body fluids	Protects the healthcare worker
	Placed on coughing patients to limit the potential dissemination of infectious respiratory secretions from the patient to others (i.e. respiratory hygiene/cough etiquette) (Siegel *et al.* 2007)	Protects the healthcare worker
	There is insufficient evidence to confirm that wearing of a face mask during surgery reduces the risk of surgical site infection (National Collaborating Centre for Women's and Children's Health 2008; Lipp & Edwards 2010)	It is unproven whether there is a protective effect for the patient
Goggles and face shields	The choice of eye protection to be worn depends on the risk to the healthcare worker. Personal glasses are not considered to be sufficient protection against blood and body fluid exposure, and specifically designed goggles or faces shields must be worn. Goggles cover the eye area alone, while face shields that extend from chin to crown ensure greater protection. As with masks, a number of types may be required to ensure individual healthcare needs	Protects the healthcare worker
Respirators	Respirators should not be confused with masks. Respirators are designed to prevent and reduce the risk of transmission of airborne pathogens from an infected patient to others Respirators should also be worn when carrying out aerosol-generating procedures, i.e. intubation, suctioning and bronchoscopy, in patients who are deemed as high risk of transmitting airborne infection, e.g. patients known to or suspected of having multidrug-resistant pulmonary tuberculosis (National Centre for Health and Clinical Excellence 2011) or influenza (Siegel *et al.* 2007) Respirators are only effective when worn correctly, and all staff must be educated regarding how to don and remove the equipment. All staff should be 'fit-tested' to ensure they understand how to put on and wear the equipment correctly. Examples of respirators are FFP2 and FFP3	Protects the healthcare worker

Box 5.2 Points to remember when implementing ANTT

- Always wash the hands effectively
- Always use the no-touch technique
- Take appropriate equipment precautions
- Take steps to protect key parts from contamination at all times

Box 5.3 Definitions (adapted from National Hospital Office 2006)

- **Contamination** – the soiling of inanimate objects with potentially infectious substances. In the clinical situation, this is most likely to be organic matter, but it can also include inorganic substances such as dust. Such contamination maybe transferred via the inanimate object to a susceptible host
- **Decontamination** – a process that removes or destroys contamination and therefore prevents microorganisms reaching a susceptible site in sufficient quantities to cause infection
- **Cleaning** – a process that physically removes contamination but does not necessarily destroy microorganisms. Cleaning is a prerequisite for equipment decontamination to ensure effective disinfection or sterilisation
- **Disinfection** – a process that reduces the number of viable microorganisms but which may not inactivate some bacterial spores
- **Disinfectant** – a chemical agent that is, under defined conditions, capable of disinfection
- **Sterilisation** – a process that renders an object free from viable microorganisms, including viruses and bacterial spores

Table 5.3 Management of blood and body fluid spillage

Ensure spillages are dealt with promptly Organisations should have standardised spillage kits in designated locations			
Before all spillages	**Blood spillage management**	**Body fluid spillage management**	**After all spillages**
Utilise a hazard/spillage sign to ensure the safety of patients, visitors and staff Don PPE: gloves and an apron and required equipment Ensure spillages are dealt with promptly Organisations should have standardised spillage kits in designated locations	Cover the spillage with disinfectant solution/granules Use hypochlorite 10,000 ppm. Leave for the recommended contact time, usually 2–5 minutes Remove spillages using paper towels and place these into a healthcare risk/clinical waste bag Wipe the area with disinfectant solution, ensuring that all traces of blood are removed	Do not use chlorine-based disinfectants directly on acidic solutions, e.g. urine and vomitus Using paper towels, remove the spillage and place the towels into a healthcare risk waste bag Once the fluid has been removed, wipe the area with the disinfectant solution, ensuring that all traces of the fluid are removed	Place all waste into a healthcare risk waste bag Remove gloves and apron Perform hand hygiene Ensure the area is washed with detergent and water to remove all traces of the disinfectant

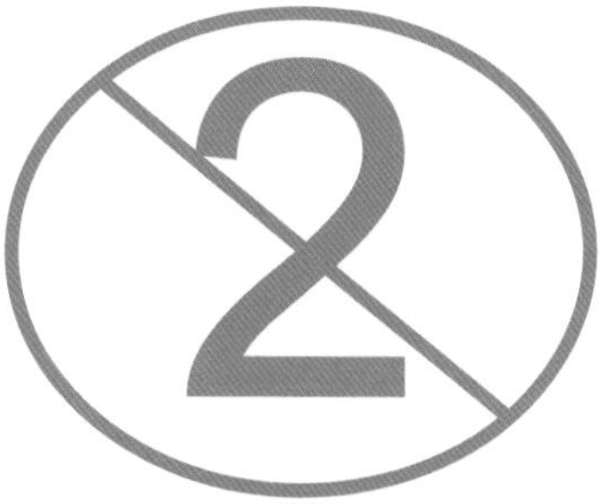

Figure 5.7 'Single use only' sign.

Equipment should be in a good state of repair and non-porous to facilitate decontamination. All equipment should be cleaned according to the manufacturer's instructions. Equipment must be cleaned by a designated person in a standardised manner after each patient use. Equipment must always be cleaned prior to maintenance and should be tagged with a decontamination certificate specifying this. The Medicines and healthcare Products Regulatory Agency advises that a device designated as only for single use must not be reused. It should be used only on an individual patient during a single procedure and then discarded. The 'single use only' sign (Figure 5.7) is present on the packaging of medical devices and equipment.

A medical device that is intended for single patient use, for example nebuliser tubing, means that the device may be used for more than one episode of use on one patient only. The device may be reprocessed between each use as per the manufacturer's instructions.

Visit www.wileyfundamentalseries.com/medicalnursing and read Reflective Questions 5.1 and 5.2 to think more about this topic.

Dishes and eating utensils

Wash utensils after each meal in a dishwasher or using washing-up liquid detergent and hot water. Wear non-sterile household gloves for manual washing. Dry utensils with paper towels or with a freshly laundered tea towel. Launder tea towels after every meal serving or when they are stained.

Uniforms

Uniforms must be changed immediately if they become visibly soiled or contaminated. They must be washed at the hottest temperature suitable for the fabric. Washing uniforms in a 60°C wash for more than 10 minutes removes sufficient microorganisms to render the uniform safe to wear. Uniforms should be changed at the start of each duty (Scottish Government Health Directorate 2008; Department of Health [DH] 2010). To maintain a professional appearance, it is recommended that clinical uniforms should not be worn outside the workplace. Nails should be kept clean, short and unvarnished (Scottish Government Health Directorate 2008; DH 2010).

Laundry and linen

- Laundry should be handled, transported and processed in a manner that prevents transmission of infectious agents to other patients, healthcare workers and the environment.
- Items contaminated with blood and/or body fluid and used laundry from infectious patients should be placed in a water-soluble bag with soluble stitching placed in a laundry bag that identifies the contents as infectious. Sluicing of contaminated linen should never occur.

Healthcare waste management

Healthcare non-risk or domestic waste is disposed of into black or clear bags. This type of waste does not require incineration and can be disposed of at an appropriately licensed landfill site.

Healthcare risk waste or clinical waste can be defined as:

> any waste which consists wholly or partly of human or animal tissue, blood or other body fluids, excretions, drugs or other pharmaceutical products, swabs or dressings, syringes, needles or other sharp instruments, being waste which unless rendered safe may prove hazardous to any person coming into contact with it. (Controlled Waste Regulations, 1992, p. 1)

This waste can be divided into three categories: waste that poses a risk of infection, waste that poses a chemical hazard, and medicines and medicinally contaminated waste that contain pharmaceutically active agents. This waste is disposed of into largely into yellow clinical waste bags and is destroyed by incineration or treated sufficiently to render it safe for landfill; this process is known as alternative technology. 'Sharps' are defined as any item capable of puncturing the skin; these items are disposed of into yellow rigid containers. Potentially offensive material refers to non-infectious human waste such as sanitary towels and continence wear. These items are disposed of into yellow and black striped bags or according to local policy. This type of waste does not require incineration and can be disposed of in an appropriately licensed landfill site.

Sharps waste management

The following principles should always be followed:

- Always dispose of sharps immediately into an appropriate (rigid European Union-marked) container at the point of use.
- The user of the sharp is responsible for its safe disposal.
- Dispose of sharps with the needle pointed away from the handler.
- Sharps containers must be mounted on a wall or using an appropriate device to ensure stability and reduce the risk of spillage.
- Sharps containers must be closed when not in use.
- Sharps containers must be locked when two-thirds full prevent overfilling.

Isolation of patients

Isolation can be defined as placing patients apart from others or alone: 'Patients may be nursed in isolation if they have a disease or condition with the potential to spread or because they are highly susceptible to acquiring infection as a result of an underlying condition or therapy' (Welsh Assembly Government 2004, p. 27). Isolation can have a negative impact on the patient's sense of well-being as patients report feelings of depression and anxiety (Knowles 1993; Gammon 1998; Morgan *et al*. 2009; Abad *et al*. 2010). Provision of information and education of patients regarding the reason for isolation precautions are recommended to reduce negative psychological effects (Abad *et al*. 2010).

When patients require care using isolation precautions due to their susceptibility to infection, this is known as protective isolation. When isolation precautions are implemented due to the presence of a known or suspected infectious disease or condition this is implemented using transmission-based precautions (Siegel *et al*. 2007).

Transmission-based precautions

These are additional precautions used in addition to standard precautions to prevent infection when a patient is known to have or is suspected of having an infectious disease.

Contact precautions

Contact precautions are used to prevent the transmission of epidemiologically significant organisms that are spread by direct or indirect contact, for example multidrug-resistant organisms such as MRSA (Table 5.4).

Droplet precautions

Droplet precautions (Table 5.4) are applied, in addition to standard precautions, to prevent the transmission of infectious agents spread through close respiratory or mucous membrane contact with respiratory droplets (i.e. large-particle droplets bigger than 5 µm in size that are generated by coughing, sneezing or talking). These droplets are propelled a short distance (approximately 1 m) and do not remain suspended in the air. Examples of diseases transmitted by droplets are: mumps, meningitis (*Neisseria meningitidis*), whooping cough (*Bordetella pertussis*) and severe acute respiratory syndrome.

Airborne precautions

Airborne precautions (Table 5.4) are applied, in addition to standard precautions, to prevent the transmission of infectious agents that are transmitted from person to person via the airborne route. Airborne transmission occurs when droplet nuclei or small particles are dispersed into air currents and carried for long distances before being inhaled, thereby causing infection. An isolation room with a mechanical ventilation system is recommended for airborne precautions. Examples of infections for which airborne precautions should be used are infectious pulmonary and laryngeal tuberculosis during sputum-inducing procedures, multidrug-resistant pulmonary tuberculosis, chickenpox (varicella zoster virus), measles (rubeola virus), rubella virus infection (German measles) and viral hemorrhagic fevers (Lassa, Ebola, Marburg and Crimean-Congo viruses).

Isolation signs

Signage for isolation rooms can vary depending on the hospital. Some hospitals use a colour-coded system that denotes the type of precautions. Pictograms can also used, or basic information can be provided, such as instructions to remove white coats and put on gloves and aprons. Some patients may require more than one type of transmission-based precaution depending on their known or suspected condition.

Care bundles

The care bundle involves grouping together key elements of care for procedures and the management of specific diagnoses in order to provide a systematic method for improving and monitoring the delivery of clinical care processes, (Cooke & Holmes 2007). Care bundles are implemented to ensure the implementation of quality evidence-based care and to reduce patients' risk of adverse events, such as healthcare-associated infection. Implementation of care bundles reduces patients' morbidity and mortality (Marwick & Davey 2009; Barochia *et al.* 2010; Rello *et al.*, 2010; Venkatram *et al.* 2010). Care bundles can be developed for almost any intervention or procedure, for example the care of peripheral cannulas and central lines, wound management, urinary catheter management and sepsis management.

Visit www.wileyfundamentalseries.com/medicalnursing and read Reflective Question 5.3 to think more about this topic.

Table 5.4 Transmission-based precautions

Type	Placement	PPE	Hand hygiene	Equipment	Environment	Movement and transfer
Contact precautions	Single room (with an anteroom) when possible If a single room is not available, put the patient in a room with others with the same organism	Gloves and an apron or gown when attending to the patient	As per the WHO's 5 Moments for Hand Hygiene (see Table 5.1 and Figure 5.4)	Each patient should where possible have designated equipment that remains in the isolation area for the duration of the patient's stay In the event of equipment needing to be used for more than one patient, it must be decontaminated appropriately following the manufacturer's instructions between patient uses	The patient zone and the environment around the patient should be cleaned as normal on a daily basis Once the patient has been discharged from hospital, the area needs to be cleaned and disinfected to ensure that no pathogenic organisms survive and pose a risk of infection to the next patient to occupy the area All equipment used to clean an isolation room should be disposed of or decontaminated to ensure that no pathogens are spread in the clinical environment	Limit patient movement Efforts must be made during movement or transfer of the patient to minimise contact between the patient and the environment and other patients The area to which the patient is being transferred must be informed of any additional precautions that will be necessary, and waiting areas should be avoided where possible Staff involved in the transfer of the patient will wear appropriate PPE

Droplet precautions	As per contact precautions	Wear a standard surgical mask when attending to the patient Masks should be donned prior to entering the patient's room and not removed until the healthcare worker has left the room Other PPE may be required as per	As per contact precautions	As per contact precautions	As per contact precautions	As per contact precautions The patient is required to wear a standard surgical mask while out of their room Patients are educated to cover their mouth and nose when coughing using a disposable tissue to reduce transmission of pathogenic microorganisms
Airborne precautions	A negative-pressure room or positive-pressure anteroom with a minimum of six air changes per hour and management of an air-handling unit (CDC 2005; American Institute of Architects 2006). Not all units have this facility therefore the door to the patient's room must remain closed	Staff caring for patients requiring airborne isolation precautions must wear a respirator such as an FFP2 or FFP3 (see Table 5.2) As per droplet precautions	As per contact precautions	As per contact precautions	As per contact precautions	As per contact precautions The patient is required to wear a respirator while out of their room. Patients are educated to cover their mouth and nose when coughing using a disposable tissue to reduce transmission of pathogenic microorganisms

Conclusion

Infection control and prevention is a fundamental responsibility in medical and surgical nursing. This chapter has provided a comprehensive summary of relevant microbiology, pathology and risks associated with the infection in hospitals. An overview of the key principles and standards in the prevention and control of infection has been provided.

Now visit the companion website and test yourself on this chapter:
www.wileyfundamentalseries.com/medicalnursing

References

Abad, C., Fearday, A. & Sadfar, N. (2010) Adverse effects of isolation in hospitalised patients: a systematic review. *Journal of Hospital Infection*, **76**:92–102.

American Institute of Architects (2006) *Guidelines for Design and Construction of Hospital and Health Care Facilities*. Washington, DC: American Institute of Architects Press.

Association for Safe Aseptic Practice (2011) *ANTT Theoretical Framework for Clinical Practice.* Version 2.5. Retrieved 28th December 2011 from http://www.antt.org.uk.

Barochia, A.V., Cui, X., Vitberg, D. *et al.* (2010) Bundled care for septic shock: an analysis of clinical trials. *Critical Care Medicine*, **38**(2):668–78.

Centers for Disease Control (2005) Guidelines for preventing the transmission of *Mycobacterium tuberculosis* in health-care settings. *Morbidity and Mortality Weekly Report*, **54**(RR17):1–141.

Coia, J.E., Duckworth, G.J., Edwards, D.I. *et al.* and the Joint Working Party of the British Society of Antimicrobial Chemotherapy, the Hospital Infection Society and the Infection Control Nurses Association (2006) Guidelines for the control and prevention of methicillin-resistant *Staphylococcus aureus* (MRSA) in healthcare facilities. *Journal of Hospital Infection*, **635**:S1–44.

Cooke, F.J. & Holmes, A.H. (2007) The missing care bundle: antibiotic prescribing in hospitals. *International Journal of Antimicrobial Agents*, **30**:25–9.

Department of Health (2010) *Uniforms and Workwear: Guidance on Uniform and Workwear Policies for NHS Employees*. Retrieved 5th January 2012 from http://www.dh.gov.uk/prod_consum_dh/groups/dh_digitalassets/@dh/@en/@ps/documents/digitalasset/dh_114754.pdf.

Gammon, J. (1998) Analysis of the stressful effects of hospitalisation and source isolation on coping and psychological constructs. *International Journal of Nursing Practice*, **4**:84–96.

Garey, K.W., Sethi, S., Yadav, Y. & DuPont, H.L. (2008) Meta-analysis to assess risk factors for recurrent *Clostridium difficile* infection. *Journal of Hospital Infection*, **70**:298–304.

Health Protection Surveillance Centre (2009) *Standard Precautions*, Version 1.0 28th April. Retrieved 12th January 2012 from http://www.hpsc.ie/hpsc/A-Z/Respiratory/Influenza/SeasonalInfluenza/Infectioncontroladvice/File,3600,en.pdf.

Horan, T., Andrus, M. & Dudeck, M. (2008) CDC/NHSN surveillance definition of healthcare-associated infection and criteria for specific types of infections in the acute care setting. *American Journal of Infection Control*, **36**(5):309–32.

Knowles, H.E. (1993) The experience of infectious patients in isolation. *Nursing Times*, **89**:53–6.

Lipp, A. & Edwards, P. (2010) Disposable surgical facemasks for preventing surgical wound infection in clean surgery. *Cochrane Database of Systematic Reviews* (**1**).

McFee, R.B. (2009) Nosocomial or hospital-acquired infections: an overview. *Disease Monthly*, **55**:422–38.

Marwick, C. & Davey, P. (2009) Care bundles: the holy grail of infectious risk management in hospital? *Current Opinion in Infectious Diseases*, **22**(4):364–9.

Morgan, D.J., Diekema, D.J., Sepkowith, K. & Perencevich, E.N. (2009) Adverse outcomes associated with contact precautions: a review of the literature. *American Journal of Infection Control*, **37**:85–93.

National Collaborating Centre for Women's and Children's Health (2008) *Surgical Site Infection: Prevention and Treatment of Surgical Site Infection*. Commissioned by the National Institute for Health and Clinical Excellence. Dorchester: Royal College of Obstetricians and Gynaecologists Press.

National Hospital Office and Health Service Executive (2006) *Cleaning Manual – Acute Hospitals*. Retrieved 12th January 2012 from http://www.lenus.ie/hse/bitstream/10147/65205/1/NationalCleaningStandardsManual.pdf.

National Institute for Health and Clinical Excellence (2011) *Tuberculosis: Clinical Diagnosis and Management of Tuberculosis, and Measures for its Prevention and Control*. London: NICE.

Pratt, R.J., Pellowe, C., Loveday, H.P. *et al.* (2001) The EPIC project: developing national evidence-based guidelines for preventing healthcare-associated infection. *Journal of Hospital Infection*, **47**(Suppl.):S1–8.

Rello, J., Lode, H., Cornaglia, G. & Masterson, R. (2010) A European care bundle for prevention of ventilator-associated pneumonia. *Intensive Care Medicine*, **36**:773–80.

Scottish Government Health Directorate (2008) *NHS Scotland Dress Code*. Edinburgh: SGHD.

Siegel, J., Rhinehart, E., Jackson, M., Chiarello, L.; Healthcare Infection Control Practices Advisory Committee. *Guideline for Isolation Precautions: Preventing Transmission of Infectious Agents in Healthcare Settings* 2007. Retrieved 20 December 2011 from http://www.cdc.gov/hicpac/pdf/isolation/Isolation2007.pdf.

Strategy for the Control of Antimicrobial Resistance in Ireland (2005) *Guidelines for Hand Hygiene in Irish Healthcare Settings*. Dublin: Health Service Executive, Health Protection Surveillance Centre.

Venkatram, S., Rachmale, S. & Kanna, B. (2010) Study of device use adjusted rates in health care-associated infections after implementation of "bundles" in a closed-model medical intensive care unit. *Journal of Critical Care*, **25**:174.e11–18.

Welsh Assembly Government, Public Health Division (2004) *Healthcare-associated Infections*. A Strategy for Hospitals in Wales. Retrieved 6th January 2012 from http://www.wales.nhs.uk/sites3/documents/379/HAI-strategy.pdf.

World Health Organization (2009) *World Health Organization Guidelines on Hand Hygiene in Healthcare: First Global Patient Safety Challenge, Clean Care Is Safer Care*. Geneva: WHO.

6

Principles of acute care for older people

Louise Daly[1], Debbie Tolson[2] and Anna Ayton[1]

[1]*School of Nursing and Midwifery, Trinity College Dublin, Dublin, Ireland*
[2]*School of Nursing, Midwifery and Community Health, Glasgow Caledonian University, Glasgow, UK*

Contents

Introduction	79
Caring for people in later life	79
Older people in the acute care setting	79
Nursing assessment and the older adult	80
Care of the older person with confusion in the acute care setting	81
Medications and the older person	83
Falls and fall prevention	86
Conclusion	87
References	88

Learning outcomes

Having read this chapter, you will be able to:

- Appreciate the complexity of knowledge underlying the safe care of an older person in an acute hospital in relation to the interplay between the reason for admission, ageing, long-term conditions and the risks inherent in the acute environment
- Describe the principles underpinning dignified and respectful nursing with older people, their families and significant others

Fundamentals of Medical-Surgical Nursing: A Systems Approach, First Edition. Edited by Anne-Marie Brady, Catherine McCabe, and Margaret McCann.

Introduction

Ageing is a life-long experience, influenced by many factors that shape an individual's health and capacity to recover from acute illness or trauma. Population ageing is a global phenomenon. In Europe, the number of persons over 60 years is increasing by more than 2 million per year (European Commission 2010). In light of this demographic growth, it is suggested that 'older adults are now the core business of hospital care' (Mezey *et al.* 2006, p. 2).

Older people have complex health needs arising from the interplay of acute and chronic problems including syndromes specifically associated with later life (Inouye *et al.* 2007). Therefore, it is essential that hospital-based nurses understand the principles of providing safe and effective care for older people. This chapter provides an introduction to nursing the older person within the acute hospital. We begin by exploring caring for people in later life and then focus on some of the key considerations in the acute setting, including assessment, confusion, medications and falls.

Caring for people in later life

Tolson *et al.* (2011) contend that caring for people in later life requires nurses to make connections between gerontological caring values and the continually evolving gerontological practice and acute care evidence base. Not all nurses will become experts in gerontological nursing. However, they should be able to apply the principles of gerontological practice (Kagan 2009). The five foundational principles promoted by the United Nations (UN; 1991) reflect the rights of older people to:

- independent life;
- participation in community life;
- safe care;
- self-fulfilment;
- dignity.

These rights acknowledge a full respect of dignity, beliefs, needs and privacy and the right to make decisions about care that is provided. The way nurses think about practice, including beliefs about what is good practice and how to accommodate an older person's preferences for care, is a major determinant shaping perceptions of care quality. Kelly *et al.* (2005) offer an accessible set of practice values grounded in the views of nurses, older people and family carers. These include a commitment to relationship-centred care in which the individual is central, reciprocity, dignity and respect, and negotiation of care decisions.

Considerations of care with older people in any context must extend to the family and in particular to those who provide direct care or care from a distance. Nolan *et al.* (2007) have long advocated that family carers and, where possible, older people should be viewed as co-experts. Promoting partnerships between the cared-for person, the family and staff has been recognised as a strategy for improving nursing quality (Brown *et al.* 2011). The achievement of a practice culture that is safe, dignified and respectful thus becomes a blend of case knowledge (e.g. the management of conditions such as stroke), patient knowledge (e.g. their functional and cognitive abilities) and person knowledge (e.g. the patient's life history and their meaningful relationships, preferences and aspirations) (Liaschenko & Fisher 1999).

Older people in the acute care setting

An emphasis on primary care means that older people entering acute medical-surgical settings are increasingly likely to present with significant and complex care requirements. An atypical presentation (which can complicate the diagnosis), cognitive impairment and comorbidities resulting in disability and functional effects present particular challenges to those seeking and providing care.

Despite providing benefit, acute hospitals are, however, risky environments for older people (Koch *et al.* 2009). Age-related changes in physiological functioning can result in a narrowed potential for recovery following acute illness. As a result, older patients require swift and effective intervention on admission to the acute setting. In addition, interactions between ageing, the characteristics of the environment and clinical syndromes associated with later life can predispose older persons to negative outcomes of hospitalisation. Specifically, older people are at higher risk of the following when hospitalised (Hickman *et al.* 2007; Eliopolous 2010):

- delirium;
- falls;
- pressure ulcers;
- nutritional decline;
- incontinence;
- functional impairment.

Therefore, the management of acute care for older patients should ideally be guided by appropriate principles. Hickman *et al.* (2007) have identified the following as being particularly beneficial: interdisciplinary team approaches in dedicated care of the older person units or drawing on gerontological expertise; focused assessment to avoid complications; an emphasis on discharge planning; and better communication across the continuum of care.

Skilled nursing care can make 'a huge difference to the outcomes and quality of life for older people' (Nursing and Midwifery Council [NMC] 2009, p.6). The best outcomes are achieved when care goals seek to optimise functional ability and independence in tandem with recovery from the acute problem. When this is not possible, rehabilitation strategies aim to maximise residual abilities and self-care capabilities in those who are becoming increasingly frail. For others, the appropriate course of action is to move towards palliation or end of life care. The older person's stay within an acute hospital is often a relatively brief component of the individual's overall care journey; for some patients, however, a longer stay will be required. Therefore, the delivery of acute care nursing for older people is multifaceted and includes facilitating transitions across the continuum of care.

Nursing assessment and the older adult

Effective nursing assessment is a skilled process that can facilitate good clinical judgements and the planning of suitable care with older people and their families (*An Bord Altranais* 2009). As older persons can present with multiple comorbidities and potentially with cognitive impairment, assessments should be undertaken that take cognisance of the bio-psycho-social effects of ageing and the pathologies and geriatric syndromes of later life. Sound assessment leads to the development of a plan of care with the older person. Where this is not possible, a family member or carer should be involved in the information-gathering process. According to the NMC (2009), effective assessment is about forming a firm relationship with older adults to learn how they want to be cared for, which requires getting to know the person as an individual from their own perspective. This requires the upholding of dignity, respect and the promotion of strengths and psychological growth rather than focusing only on the traditional curative biomedical philosophy commonly prevalent in the acute hospital setting.

Person-centred assessment involves gathering information about the physical, psychological, functional, social, cultural, sexual and spiritual status of the older person (see Chapter 1). Assessment must also take account of the person's life story and circumstances, including (NMC 2009):

- personal and family relationships;
- social circumstances;
- previous occupation, to enhance the life story;
- spiritual and cultural beliefs.

This information contributes to the care plan and is as important as the activities of living, which generally provide the overarching assessment framework (NMC 2009).

The assessment process is ongoing and not usually completed in one sitting. Assessment should be paced to match the needs and abilities of the older adult and the multifaceted nature of problems and functional changes (McConnell 1997). The nurse must be able to probe sensitively and deeply into the person's more covert needs (Nolan & Tolson 2000; Parker *et al.* 2006). However, for those working in

Box 6.1 Examples of actual or potential health problems

- Risk of falls
- Urinary or faecal incontinence
- Nutritional problems including a consideration of oral health
- Difficulties with vision or hearing
- Medication-related issues
- Foot problems requiring a chiropody referral
- Poor social circumstances or unsafe home conditions
- Isolation, depression or mental health difficulties
- Elder abuse
- Cognitive impairment

Box 6.2 Examples of types of assessment tools

- Pressure sore prevention tools
- Pain assessment tools
- Falls risk assessment tools
- Nutritional screening tools
- Tools to assess cognition

particular acute settings such as accident and emergency, where there is limited opportunity in terms of time to build relationships, rapid age-appropriate processes are required to gain insight into a person's needs. Drawing on the principles of assessment, nurses can identify underlying problems that affect health and well-being such as those outlined in Box 6.1.

A range of tools can be used to assist in the overall assessment process (Box 6.2). Where such tools are used, nurses should be educated in their application and interpretation, and the tools should be valid, reliable and age-appropriate (*An Bord Altranais* 2009).

Assessment with older persons involves building relationships and ascertaining strengths and abilities, in addition to identifying the problem(s) that led to hospitalisation. It is important that an interdisciplinary team approach is employed, with the individual being central to the process. Effective communication is vital to ensure that there are no misunderstandings regarding the older person's needs and wishes, and to avoid the patient becoming fatigued by the assessment process. The older person should be involved in the planning and evaluation of his or her care throughout the hospital admission. This requires the sharing of information and explanations to enable an informed choice to be made (NMC 2009). Referrals should be made following consultation with the patient and with respect and support of the person's right to make decisions and accept or decline treatment. Assessment should also involve the older person's family or carer, consistent with the relationship-centred approach to care referred to earlier.

Care of the older person with confusion in the acute care setting

In this section, we will explore dementia and delirium, both of which are frequently encountered (either together or separately) by those caring for older people in the acute setting. It is estimated that 25% of older people who present to the accident and emergency department, and between 20% and 25% of hospital inpatients, have a dementia (Thompson *et al.* 2008). These statistics are significant when it is considered that people with dementia may encounter significant difficulties in acute care settings.

Table 6.1 Common types of dementia

Type	Primary symptoms
Alzheimer's disease	Memory and language impairments and loss of motor skills
Vascular dementia	Memory impairment, behaviour changes and sensory motor deficits, such as limb weakness
Dementia with Lewy bodies	Fluctuations of cognitive impairment, visual hallucinations, frequent falls, and emotional and language impairment

Definition

'Dementia is a syndrome that can be caused by a number of progressive illnesses that affect memory, thinking, behaviour and the ability to perform everyday activities' (Wimo & Prince 2010, p.2).

While there are many forms of dementia (including frontotemporal dementias, dementia associated with Parkinson's disease and alcohol-related dementia), the most common types are listed in Table 6.1.

Often, older people with dementia are admitted to an acute hospital for the evaluation and treatment of an acute medical or surgical problem, and the dementia is coincidental to this. In other cases, an older patient may have an underlying dementia that has not yet been diagnosed, and hospitalisation may be an opportunity to intervene. Quality nursing care involves clinical management of the medical condition along with the maintenance of both cognitive and functional abilities, and promotion of quality of life issues (Thompson *et al*. 2008).

Dementia should be understood as a broad term that refers to a bio-psycho-social condition and not just as a disease located within the brain. It is therefore important to know the person with dementia in the context of their unique life and social history. This information can inform care with the aim of maximising positive outcomes. Unfortunately, studies highlight that it is not unusual for healthcare teams to overlook dementia and focus on physical aspects of acute care (Tolson & Smith 1999; Cowdell 2010). This is concerning as potential problems that can arise for the patient with dementia during admission include:

- distress;
- new incontinence;
- behaviours that are challenging;
- untreated pain;
- inadequate food and fluid intake;
- falls;
- sleep disturbance;
- functional decline.

People with dementia who are admitted to an acute hospital are at increased risk of developing delirium. Older persons who do not have dementia also frequently present with delirium or develop delirium while in hospital.

Definition

'Delirium (sometimes called "acute confusional state") is a common clinical syndrome characterised by disturbed consciousness, cognitive function or perception, which has an acute onset and fluctuating course' (National Institute of Health and Clinical Excellent [NICE] 2010, p. 4).

Box 6.3 Examples of risk factors for delirium

- Dementia
- Infection, particularly urinary tract and respiratory infections
- Dehydration and constipation
- Untreated pain
- Disordered electrolyte balance
- Trauma
- Some medications and polypharmacy
- General anaesthesia
- Environmental change
- Alcohol withdrawal

Delirium is a potentially life-threatening condition and should be regarded as a medical emergency. Three overarching types of delirium that are common are (NICE 2010):

- hyperactive delirium, characterised by agitation, restlessness and potentially aggressiveness;
- hypoactive delirium, characterised by inactivity, withdrawal and sleepiness;
- mixed delirium, fluctuating between hypoactive and hyperactivity.

The first aim of person-centred nursing management is identifying risk factors that may be contributing to the individual's delirium (Box 6.3). However, despite its clinical importance, delirium often remains undetected, and left untreated delirium can lead to significant morbidity and death.

Early identification of any cognitive impairment is fundamental to providing appropriate care for persons with dementia and/or delirium. Nurses should not assume that confusion is normal in later life. Each patient's cognitive functioning should be assessed as a component of the overall assessment process previously described.

The presence of dementia or delirium creates particular challenges for older persons, families/carers and staff in a context focused on acute problems and technological aspects of caring. For example, the unfamiliar hospital environment can be challenging for the individual, and the rapid pace and overstimulation can contribute to the incidence of adverse outcomes (Parker *et al.* 2006; Nolan 2007). As a result, people who have dementia in acute hospitals are extremely vulnerable. Care planning should consequently prioritise partnership working, skilled communication, psychological support and the provision of a safe, supportive and enabling environment (Box 6.4).

One of the most challenging aspects of dementia care frequently encountered by nurses in the acute setting is caring for people who display behaviours that challenge. Cohen-Mansfield's (2000) model suggests that such behaviours are an attempt by the person to communicate or fulfil an unmet need (e.g. pain, boredom or frustration). This model can be used to interpret and address the identified need.

Visit **www.wileyfundamentalseries.com/medicalnursing** and read **Reflective Question 6.1** to think more about this topic.

Medications and the older person

Medicines are frequently a contributing factor in acute admissions for older patients. In later life, the body's response to medications can differ due to age-related physiological changes and result in a greater susceptibility to the effects of drugs (Table 6.2). Older persons are particularly subject to alterations in pharmacokinetics (how medications are absorbed, distributed, metabolised and excreted) and pharmacodynamics (drug effects at target receptors or organs). They are also more likely to take

Box 6.4 Nursing interventions to support older persons with confusion in the acute setting

- Completion of a patient profile to get to know the person
- Minimisation of overstimulation, including appropriate lighting and noise reduction
- Use of a model to interpret and manage behaviour that challenges
- Continuity of care staff
- Supervision of, and where necessary assistance with, activities of living
- Consideration of the patient's placement in the ward setting, e.g. within view of staff
- Risk assessment and safety promotion, e.g. bed safety, ensuring clutter-free spaces, patient identification, etc.
- Environmental modification to ease walking and way-finding, e.g. appropriate signage
- Promotion of orientation, e.g. frequent introductions to people and explanations of nursing interventions
- Working with the family and significant others to ensure that familiarity in terms of routines is maintained as far as is possible
- Facilitation of open family visiting
- Use of appropriate communication strategies and sensory aids
- Liaison with community and primary care professionals

Table 6.2 Examples of age-related physiological changes and impacts on medication

Body system	Age-related alteration	Examples of consequences
Gastrointestinal	Decreased gastric peristalsis and motility, and delayed emptying Decreased gastric blood flow Increased gastric pH	Slower drug absorption
Renal	Reduced blood flow, glomerular filtration and number and efficiency of the nephrons	Affects the rate and level of drug excretion and may result in an accumulation of drugs excreted through the renal system
Circulatory	Decreased cardiac output and circulation Reduction in serum albumin	Increased time needed for drug transportation Potential for increased level of unbound drugs in the blood Competition between multiple protein-binding drugs alters effectiveness
Musculoskeletal	Reduction in skeletal muscle mass	Alterations to drug absorption following intramuscular injection
Hepatic	Reduction in hepatic mass Alterations in enzyme function and liver blood flow	Slower rate of drug metabolism Accumulation of drugs leading to potential toxicity

Data from Galbraith *et al.* (2007), Kee *et al.* (2009) and Miller (2012).

multiple medications (Fulton & Allen 2005). The interactive effects of these can predispose older persons to adverse drug reactions, reduced drug effectiveness and medication errors.

As many medication-related issues are preventable, they are a priority for all nurses caring for older patients. Careful individualised management is required, and care planning should consider the potential impact of age-related physiological changes (National Medicines Information Centre 2010). The nurse is responsible for the safe and effective administration of prescribed medicines, which can be achieved using the principles outlined in Chapter 2 and the nine 'rights' of medication administration (Elliott & Liu 2010):

1. Right patient
2. Right drug
3. Right time
4. Right route
5. Right dose
6. Right documentation
7. Right action
8. Right form
9. Right response.

Due to the higher potential for comorbidities, older patients may be prescribed multiple medications. This can lead to polypharmacy, which can result in negative consequences for the person, including cognitive impairment, falls and malnutrition (Kee *et al.* 2009).

Definition

Polypharmacy is 'the prescription, administration, or use of more medications than are clinically indicated in a given patient' (Charles & Lehman 2010, p. 262).

Polypharmacy may also result in drug–drug or drug–disease interactions, and admission to hospital offers the opportunity to review the safety, efficacy and necessity of the patient's current medications (Miller 2012). The Department of Health (2001) recommends medicine reviews for all older persons, particularly those over 75 and those who have been prescribed four or more medications. As members of the interdisciplinary team, nurses should be knowledgeable about drugs that are commonly prescribed for older persons and how to recognise adverse drug reactions, and should be able to communicate medication-related concerns to prescribers.

Non-adherence to medications is also a concern in older persons, particularly those who take multiple drugs. This occurs where the taking of medications departs from prescribed formats, for example under- or overdosage, incorrect time spans between dosages, self-medication and unfilled prescriptions. According to Reddy (2006/2007), non-adherence can lead to avoidable consequences such as poor health, premature death, hospital admission and health system costs. The factors that contribute to older patients' difficulties with medication regimens include:

- cognitive, sensory or functional difficulties;
- a lack of knowledge or understanding;
- cost;
- unwanted or feared side effects;
- complicated drug regimens;
- the use of herbal remedies;
- using multiple pharmacies or prescribers;
- taking over-the-counter medications.

Nurses need to be able to discuss medication usage with older patients and their families or significant others, and to engage in individualised education on medications in conjunction with the

Box 6.5 Examples of interventions to increase adherence to medication

- Care planning with the older patient, family and/or significant other
- Coordination with the interdisciplinary team
- Multifaceted education on medications in conjunction with the pharmacist using appropriate and age-specific educational materials
- Promoting awareness of side effects, adverse reactions and how to seek advice
- Use of reminders (e.g. written reminders, phone calls or alarms)
- Use of aids (e.g. pill or dossette boxes, blister packaging and medication-dispensing systems)
- Monitoring medication-related behaviour
- Regular medication reviews
- Self-administration of medication programmes
- Discharge planning

pharmacist. There are also a range of practical interventions to promote adherence to medication that can be used, depending on the needs of the patient (Box 6.5).

Visit www.wileyfundamentalseries.com/medicalnursing and read Reflective Question 6.2 to think more about this topic.

Falls and fall prevention

The risk of falling increases with age. One in three adults over 65 years and one in two over 85 years will fall annually (National Steering Group on the Prevention of Falls in Older People and the Prevention and Management of Osteoporosis throughout Life 2008). Older persons who fall are more likely than other age groups to experience fractures, reduced functioning, death, longer hospital stays, decreased well-being and psychological effects including fear of falling.

Definition

A fall is 'a sudden, unintentional change in position causing an individual to land at a lower level, on an object, the floor, or the ground, other than as a consequence of sudden onset of paralysis, epileptic seizure, or overwhelming external force' (National Steering Group on the Prevention of Falls in Older People and the Prevention and Management of Osteoporosis throughout Life 2008, p. 14).

As the risk factors for falls are numerous (Box 6.6), assessment is the basis of the effective prevention and management of falls. However, a sensitive approach is required as older persons may be reluctant to report falls due to embarrassment and fear of threats to their autonomy.

All older persons should be asked if they have fallen in the past year. If the person has fallen, the number, context and nature of the falls and their balance and gait should be assessed (NICE 2004). A fall assessment tool should be completed with all older patients on admission to identify those at risk of falling. Based on the assessment, a referral to a falls specialist or service may need to be arranged. In hospitals, falls most commonly occur during transfers at the bedside and in bathrooms (Johnson *et al*. 2011).

When implementing any aspect of care, the nurse should plan ahead and carefully consider the abilities of the older patient, the care task and any environmental hazards that may pose a risk of falls. There are a range of multifactorial fall prevention interventions that can be used in the hospital setting

Box 6.6 Examples of risk factors for falls

Intrinsic risk factors
Age
History of falling
Elimination difficulties, e.g. incontinence or nocturia
Postural hypotension
Gait and balance disorders
Sensory difficulties, e.g. of hearing and sight
Frailty
Cognitive impairment
Muscle weakness
Cardiac arrhythmias

Extrinsic risk factors
Environmental hazards:
- Poor design
- Poor lighting
- Varifocal spectacles
- Clutter
- Bed/side rails
- Slippery or wet floors
- Footwear and clothing
- Unfamiliar environments

Medication issues:
- Certain medications, e.g. diuretics, antihypertensives and sedatives
- Use of four or more drugs
- Polypharmacy

Box 6.7 Examples of interventions to prevent in-hospital falls

Care planning and intervention:
- Risk assessment using valid and reliable tools
- Involvement of the older person and family or significant others
- Assistance with activities of living
- Interventions to compensate for reduced sensory, cognitive or functional abilities
- Use of policies relating to the use of bed rails and restraints
- Discharge planning to include maintenance of bone health and education for the prevention and management of falls
- Provision of written information

Promotion of a safe environment:
- Assessment and modification of environmental hazards
- Nursing the patient within view of the nurses' station
- Properly fitting clothing and footwear
- Ensuring that beds are at their lowest level and that their brakes are functioning
- Ensuring that the call bell and personal belongings are within reach
- Patient identification and (with permission) the use of fall detector technology, in line with hospital policy
- Staff education and development

for those at risk of falling (Box 6.7). These should be individualised to the needs of older patients and acceptable to them, and should also involve members of the interdisciplinary team working in a planned and coordinated manner.

Conclusion

Although the majority of older people live at home and enjoy good health and an active life, as with all age groups, the need for acute care is always a possibility. For older persons who have one or more chronic conditions and increasing frailty, the likelihood of hospital admission is higher. We believe that all acute care nurses consequently require an age-appropriate value and knowledge base along with the competence to deliver skilled nursing care to older people. This will involve an understanding of the effects caused by the interrelationships between age-related changes, comorbidities and syndromes seen in older age (Inouye *et al.* 2007). To this end, this chapter has provided an overview of the principles underpinning dignified and respectful nursing care for older people, and has explored some of the clinical issues that are a particular priority when caring for older patients in acute care settings.

Now visit the companion website and test yourself on this chapter:
www.wileyfundamentalseries.com/medicalnursing

References

An Bord Altranais (2009) *Professional Guidance for Nurses Working with Older People. An Bord Altranais, Dublin.* Retrieved 13th May 2011 from http://www.nursingboard.ie.

Brown, J., Robb, Y., Lowndes, A., Duffy, K., Tolson, D. & Nolan, M. (2011) Understanding relationships within care. In: Tolson, D., Booth, J. & Schofield, I. (eds), *Evidence Informed Nursing with Older People* (pp. 38–54). Chichester: Wiley Blackwell.

Charles, C. & Lehman, C. (2010) Medications and laboratory values. In: Mauk, K. (ed.), *Gerontological Nursing. Competencies for Care*, 2nd edn (pp. 260–83). Boston: Jones & Bartlett.

Cohen-Mansfield, J. (2000) Use of patient characteristics to determine nonpharmacologic interventions for behavioural and psychological symptoms of dementia. *International Psychogeriatrics*, **12**(1):373–86.

Cowdell, E. (2010) The care of older people with dementia in acute hospitals. *International Journal of Older People Nursing*, **5**(2):83–92.

Department of Health (2001) *Medicines for Older People: Implementing the Medicines-related Aspects of the NSF for Older People*. London: Department of Health.

Eliopolous, C. (2010) *Gerontological Nursing*, 7th edn. Philadelphia: Wolters Kluwer/Lippincott Williams & Wilkins.

Elliott, M. & Liu, Y. (2010) The nine rights of medication administration: an overview. *British Journal of Nursing*, **19**(5):300–5.

European Commission (2010) *Commission Staff Working Document. Demography Report 2010*. Retrieved 27th May 2011 from http://epp.eurostat.ec.europa.eu/portal/page/portal/population/documents/Tab/report.pdf.

Fulton, M. & Allen, E.R. (2005) Polypharmacy in the elderly: a literature review. *Journal of the American Academy of Nurse Practitioners*, **17**(4):123–32.

Galbraith, A., Bullock, S., Manias, E., Hunt, B. & Richards, A. (2007) *Fundamentals of Pharmacology. An Applied Approach for Nursing and Health*, 2nd edn. Harlow: Pearson Education Limited.

Hickman, L., Newton, P., Halcomb, E., Chang, E. & Davidson, P. (2007) Best practice interventions to improve the management of older people in acute care settings: a literature review. *Journal of Advanced Nursing*, **60**(2):113–26.

Inouye, S.K., Studenski, S., Tinetti, M.E. & Kuchel, G. (2007) Geriatric syndromes: clinical, research, and policy implications of a core geriatric concept. *Journal of the American Geriatric Society*, **55**(5):780–91.

Johnson, M., George, A. & Thuy Tran, D. (2011) Analysis of falls incidents: nurse and patient preventive behaviours. *International Journal of Nursing Practice*, **17**(1):60–6.

Kagan, S.H. (2009) Guest Editorial: Boundaries and barriers: redefining older people nursing in the 21st century. *International Journal of Nursing Older People*, **4**(4):240–1.

Kee, J., Hayes, E. & McCuistion, L. (2009) *Pharmacology. A Nursing Process Approach*, 6th edn. St Louis: Saunders Elsevier.

Kelly, T.B., Tolson, D., Schofield, I. & Booth, J. (2005) Describing gerontological nursing: an academic exercise or prerequisite for progress? *Journal of Clinical Nursing* **14**(3a):1–11.

Koch, S., Hunter, P. & Nair, K. (2009) Older people in acute care. In: Nay, R. & Garratt, S. (eds), *Older People Issues and Innovations in Care*, 3rd edn (pp. 153–67). Sydney: Churchill Livingstone Elsevier.

Liaschenko, J. & Fisher, A. (1999) Theorising the knowledge that nurses use in the conduct of their work. *Scholarly Inquiry for Nursing Practice*, **13**(1):29–41.

McConnell, E.S. (1997) Conceptual bases for gerontological nursing practice: models, trends and issues. In: Matteson, M.A. & McConnell, E.S. (eds), *Gerontological Nursing: Concepts and Practice*, 2nd edn. Philadelphia: WB Saunders.

Mezey, M., Quinlan, E., Fairchild, S. & Vezina, M. (2006) Geriatric competencies for RNs in hospital. *Journal for Nurses in Staff Development*, **22**(1):2–10.

Miller, C. (2012) *Nursing for Wellness in Older Adults*, 6th edn. Philadelphia: Wolters Kluwer/Lippincott, Williams & Wilkins.

National Institute for Clinical Excellence (2004) *The Assessment and Prevention of Falls in Older People*. Clinical Guideline No. 21. London: NICE.

National Institute for Health and Clinical Excellence (2010) *Delirium: Diagnosis, Prevention and Management*. Clinical Guideline No. 103. London: NICE.

National Medicines Information Centre (2010) Prescribing in the elderly. *Therapeutics Bulletin*, **16**(3):1–6.

National Steering Group on the Prevention of Falls in Older People and the Prevention and Management of Osteoporosis throughout Life (2008) *Strategy to Prevent Falls and Fractures in Ireland's Ageing Population*. Dublin: Health Services Executive.

Nolan, L. (2007) Caring for older people in the acute setting: a study of nurses' views. *British Journal of Nursing*, **16**(7):419–22.

Nolan, M. & Tolson, D. (2000) Gerontological nursing. 1. Challenges nursing older people in acute care. *British Journal of Nursing*, **9**(1):39–42.

Nolan, M.R., Hanson, E., Grant, G. & Keady, J. (2007) *User Participation in Health and Social Care Research: Voices, Values and Evaluation*. Buckingham: Open University Press.

Nursing and Midwifery Council (2009) *Guidance for the Care of Older People*. London: NMC.

Parker, S.G., Fadayevatan, R. & Lee, S. (2006) Acute hospital care for frail older people. *Age and Ageing*, **35**(6):551–2.

Reddy, B. (2006/2007) Medication review as a route to optimising treatment. *Nurse Prescribing*, **4**(11):464–8.

Thompson, F., Girling, D., Greene, S. & Wai, C. (2008) Care of people with dementia in the general hospital. In: Downs, M. & Bowers, B. (eds), *Excellence in Dementia Care. Research into Practice* (pp. 301–18). Maidenhead: McGraw Hill/Open University Press.

Tolson, D. & Smith, M. (1999) An investigation of the components of best nursing practice in the care of acutely ill hospitalized older patients with coincidental dementia: a multi-method design. *Journal of Advanced Nursing*, **30**(5):1127–36.

Tolson, D., Booth, J. & Schofield, I. (2011) Principles of gerontological nursing. In: Tolson, D., Booth, J. & Schofield, I. (eds), *Evidence Informed Nursing with Older People* (pp. 1–17). Chichester: Wiley Blackwell.

United Nations (1991) *United Nations Principles for Older Persons. Resolution 46/91*. Retrieved 15th November 2011 from http://www.unescap.org/ageing/res/res46-91.htm.

Wimo, A. & Prince, M. (2010) *World Alzheimer Report 2010. The Global Economic Impact of Dementia. Executive Summary*. London: Alzheimer's Disease International.

7 Principles of end of life care

Kevin Connaire

Centre for Continuing Education, St Francis Hospice, Dublin, Ireland

Contents

Introduction	91
The nature of dying	91
Comfort at the end of life	91
Communication at the end of life	96
Ethics and end of life care	99
Conclusion	101
References	101

Learning outcomes

Having read this chapter, you will be able to:

- Describe the nature of death and dying
- Describe the main symptoms in the dying process
- Gain an appreciation of the communication needs of the dying person
- Discuss a variety of methods that may be used when communicating with a dying person
- Appreciate the nature of loss for families of a dying person
- Describe the ethical challenges surrounding the administration of nutrition and hydration to a dying person

Fundamentals of Medical-Surgical Nursing: A Systems Approach, First Edition. Edited by Anne-Marie Brady, Catherine McCabe, and Margaret McCann.

Introduction

Death is an inevitability that each person faces in their lives. It is a part of living that brings with it many challenges, not only for the person who is imminently dying, but also for the family and staff who are caring for the dying person. Many patients who are dying face numerous losses, which may be gradual or acute, depending on the disease trajectory. This is a time of stress not only for the patient who is dying, but also for the patient's family as they come to terms with their impending loss. It is not uncommon for the patient who is dying to feel lonely and isolated, which heightens the need for members of the multidisciplinary to increase their skills of sensitivity to each individual situation. Having an awareness of these situations potentially adds to the quality of care for the patient and the family members.

The nature of dying

The nature of dying may be a sudden event, in which a person has been given no time to prepare for it, or it may have been a long, drawn-out protracted event, spanning a number of weeks or months. Some may consider dying to be a normal life event. For others it may involve suffering, be painful or be peaceful. Each of these are very relevant thoughts on the nature of dying and help us to shape our practices in caring for individuals who are dying and their families.

Over the years, numerous attempts have been made to capture the nature of dying. Glaser and Strauss (1965) suggest that there are four patterns of behaviour relating to awareness of death that occur being the dying person and those people who are close to them. These consist of 'closed awareness', 'suspected awareness', 'mutual pretence' and 'open awareness'. Common responses to impending death and dying have been identified by Kübler-Ross (1969), when she proposed that patients progress through a series of five stages including denial and isolation, anger, bargaining, depression and acceptance. Kübler-Ross suggested that individuals eventually attain the stage of acceptance prior to actually dying.

More recently, Copp (1999), attempted to conceptualise the nature of dying. She regarded the dying process within a 'readiness to die' framework, arguing that people approach dying though various degrees of 'readiness': 'person not ready – body not ready', 'person ready – body not ready', 'person not ready – body ready' and 'person ready – body ready'. In situations where patients have reached the stage of 'person ready – body ready', the dying process usually is less stressful for both patients and families. It is not uncommon for patients to experience a range of emotions and struggles as the end of life approaches. Nursing staff who have an understanding of the nature of dying invariably are more equipped to deal with the range of responses that dying patients may experience in the face of impending death.

Visit www.wileyfundamentalseries.com/medicalnursing and read Reflective Question 7.1 to think more about this topic.

Comfort at the end of life

Providing comfort care at the end of life is a central role of the nurse as part of the multidisciplinary team. Kinder and Ellershaw (2011) highlight the need for ensuring patients' comfort as they progress towards the end of life. Failure to initiate comfort measures and effective symptom management for the disease process can lead to further distress for patients, and for families as they witness their dying relative experiencing ineffective pain and symptom management.

As patients near the end of life, their bodies do not require the level of nutrition and hydration that a normal healthy body needs. In essence, their bodies are 'giving up' and 'shutting down'. The main symptoms that people encounter as they approach their end of life are dyspnoea, a death rattle, terminal restlessness, fatigue, nausea and vomiting, agitation and pain. For the purposes of this chapter, the following sections will provide an overview of the management of dyspnoea, the death rattle and pain.

Dyspnoea

Dyspnoea is a common symptom that occurs as the end of life approaches (Woodroof 2004). It is estimated that approximately 70% of patients with advanced disease who are within the last 6 weeks of life experience dyspnoea (Dudgeon *et al.* 2001). The extent and severity the of dyspnoea are influenced by the underlying condition from which the patient is suffering. It may cause patients distress while also reducing their level of activity (Bausewein *et al.* 2007).

The management of dyspnoea in the dying patient requires a multidisciplinary team approach to care. While a variety of active treatments may be implemented prior to the dying phase, treatment in the dying phase needs to be purely symptomatic. Active intervention and investigative procedures have little value at this stage of the dying process. The most common forms of treatment of dyspnoea in the last days of life are oxygen and pharmacological interventions, together with comfort measures.

Oxygen

Oxygen is generally not an effective method of providing symptom relief for dyspnoea in the dying phase. A trial of oxygen for 30–60 minutes may be provided and assessed for its benefit. If it is established that it is of no benefit, the oxygen should be discontinued and an explanation for the lack of benefit be given to the family. In addition, it is advisable to offer alternative strategies such as pharmacological management, possibly complementary therapy or massage, an open window, a fan and repositioning.

Pharmacological interventions

The most common pharmacological interventions for the management of dyspnoea are opioids and benzodiazepines.

Opioids

The use of opioids is common in the management of dyspnoea in the dying person. Opioids are considered to be the most effective drugs to manage patients suffering from breathlessness at the end of life (Chan *et al.* 2005). Morphine reduces inappropriate and excessive respiratory drive and substantially reduces the ventilatory response to hypoxia and hypercapnia. By slowing respiration, breathing may be made more efficient and the sensation of breathlessness reduced (Watson *et al.* 2006). Opioid use may prolong survival by reducing physical and psychological distress and exhaustion. The early use of opioids also improves quality of life and potentially enables the use of lower doses while tolerance to the respiratory depressant effects develops.

While opioids are available in many formats, the most appropriate method of delivery to the patient who is dying is via a continuous subcutaneous infusion (CSCI), but the preferred opioid may also be administered as 'stat'/'prn' (as required) subcutaneous doses. The priority is the patient's comfort, and all measures should be exhausted immediately and the situation continuously reviewed. Following reviews, pharmacological interventions may need to be altered in order to obtain and maintain maximum comfort for the patient in the dying phase.

For maximum effectiveness of the opioids in the treatment of dyspnoea in the last days of life, they may be administered subcutaneously as a 'prn' dose for the management of dyspnoea, as opposed to being used solely for pain management purposes. The 24-hour dose of opioid in the CSCI may need to be increased if the patient is comfortable and pain is currently not an issue but the patient presents with unresolving breathlessness.

Benzodiazepines

Benzodiazepines are classed as anxiolytic sedatives (Wade *et al*, 2005). They are used to reduce anxiety and restlessness, which are symptoms that often occur in the terminal phase of a person's life and may exacerbate any dyspnoea present. Midazolam 2.5 mg stat (which may be increased to 5 mg depending on the patient's response) is generally the drug of choice and may be administered with a 'prn' dose of opioid for symptomatic relief of dyspnoea. It is familiar practice to have 10 mg or more of midazolam in a CSCI per 24 hours for symptom management at the end of life. Although midazolam may cause increased drowsiness and sedation, this effect may be appropriate to maintain the patient's comfort in the dying phase.

Non-pharmacological management of breathlessness in the patient who is dying

The patient's position in bed is important, especially when the patient is no longer able to maintain independence in terms of positioning and instead requires full nursing care and assistance. The upright position uses gravity to assist in lung expansion and to reduce pressure from the abdomen on the diaphragm. If a patient is able to tolerate sitting in an upright position, this may be effective, but it may be contraindicated by pain. Comfort and management of dyspnoea may be attained through pharmacological measures if the patient is most comfortable in the supine position.

Kravits and Berenson (2010) acknowledge the value of complementary therapy in promoting relaxation and improving dyspnoea in patients who are dying. Opening a window or providing a fan may also be beneficial. In addition, involvement of the physiotherapist in promoting breathing exercises may be of benefit in relieving the severity of breathlessness at the end of life.

Visit **www.wileyfundamentalseries.com/medicalnursing** and read **Reflective Question 7.2** to think more about this topic.

Death rattle

As patients who are dying are unable to clear their upper airway, a condition known as a 'death rattle' frequently occurs within the last 48–72 hours of life (Kass & Ellershaw 2003). It is described by Wilders *et al.* (2009) as the noise that commonly occurs caused by the presence of secretions in the upper airways. Wilders and Menten (2002) suggest that a death rattle occurs in up to 95% of patients who are dying from cancer, but it is not solely confined to cancer patients. The presence of a death rattle is frequently a source of distress and discomfort for family members (Hughes *et al.* 1996).

There are two types of death rattle. Type 1 involves a build-up of secretions mainly from the salivary glands as a result of the absence of the swallowing reflex, while type 2 is caused by a build-up of bronchial secretions. Type 1 usually occurs closer to the time of death, whereas type 2 is more gradual in onset owing to the gradual decline in the patient's ability to cough.

Nursing management

The aim of treatment of a death rattle is to minimise the patient's distress and to support the family members throughout this process. Two key nursing interventions – positioning and suctioning – may provide relief for a death rattle.

Positioning

A change of position may be of assistance in relieving the severity of a death rattle. The extent to which the position is changed will be guided by the patient's response to the changing positions; for example, a change from prone to lateral may not be tolerated well, particularly if the patient is haemodynamically compromised. In addition, Corner and O'Driscoll (1999) suggest that gentle physiotherapy measures may assist with increasing the patient's breathing.

Suctioning

For a type 2 death rattle, the use of oropharyngeal suctioning is not usually recommended as it potentially increases the patient's distress and discomfort. For a type 1 death rattle, gentle suctioning may be effective in relieving the build-up of oropharyngeal secretions, but the extent of suctioning needs to be guided by the patient's response to the suctioning.

Pharmacological management

The pharmacological management of the death rattle at the end of life needs to be initiated as soon as there is evidence of that it is occurring (Lawrey 2005). The use of these drugs does not invariably improve the severity of a death rattle, but rather can prevent it from occurring. Pharmacological management of a death rattle consists mainly of a choice of three anticholinergic drugs: hyoscine butylbromide, hyoscine hydrobromide and glycopyrrolate. It is important to remember that anticholinergic drugs will not be effective in removing the sections already present within the upper airway, instead contributing to the production of additional secretions (Bennett *et al.* 2002; Glare *et al.* 2011).

Hyoscine butylbromide is an anticholinergic agent whose effect relates to an inhibition of parasympathetic activation and a reduction in production of secretions. Hyoscine butylbromide does not cross the blood–brain barrier; therefore drowsiness is not an associated side effect. For the management of a death rattle, 20 mg stat subcutaneously can be effective, with 60–120 mg administered subcutaneously via a CSCI over 24 hours. The administration of higher doses is generally preferable if a patient is dying and has symptoms of increased airway secretions.

Hyoscine hydrobromide acts by inhibiting the muscarinic receptors. It decreases peristalsis and dilates the bronchial muscles. Hyoscine hydrobromide should be used with caution in the management of a death rattle because of its tendency to cause drowsiness as it crosses the blood–brain barrier. It may be administered subcutaneously or in a transdermal form, known as Scopoderm. Common dosages for administration range from 0.2 to 0.5 mg subcutaneously every 4–6 hours, or from 0.1 to 0.2 mg per hour by CSCI (Muller-Busch & Jehser 2009). It is frequently indicated for patients with motor neurone disease or various disorders of the head and neck that present with large amounts of oral secretions and drooling.

Glycopyrrolate is also an anticholinergic agent. It rarely causes sedation or delirium (Twycross & Wilcock 2009). It does not cross the blood–brain barrier, so its advantage in use is that it does not cause the patient to become drowsy. Muller-Busch and Jehser (2009) recommend that doses administered may range from 0.1 to 0.2 mg subcutaneously, or 0.4 mg to 1.2 per day via a CSCI.

The effectiveness of anticholinergic drugs in the management of death rattle remains inconsistent. Evidence suggests that the initiation of anticholinergic drugs before the onset of a death rattle is important for its successful pharmacological management.

> Visit www.wileyfundamentalseries.com/medicalnursing and read Reflective Question 7.3 to think more about this topic.

Pain and pain management in the last 48–72 hours of life

Various symptoms may prevail at the end of life, and pain is generally the symptom that patients and their families most fear. Although pain is a common symptom, it does not affect all individuals in their dying phase. Wells (2000) considers that approximately one-third of patients who are actively receiving treatment for cancer and two-thirds of those with advanced malignant disease experience pain. Pain is an extremely individual symptom and often does not correlate with the diagnosis and treatment. The treatment of pain at the end of life involves an individualised patient-specific plan of care and is highly achievable with the appropriate approach to care at the end of life.

Pain may be attributed to a variety of reasons. A holistic approach to care aims to provide the best possible symptom relief and pain relief for patients with a terminal illness. Death and dying raises many questions about the meaning of life and existence, and often individuals' psychological, social and spiritual distress can be portrayed as physical pain; thus, it is imperative that a holistic approach to pain management is provided. An opportunity to discuss spiritual needs may alleviate the patient's concerns and optimise comfort in the dying phase.

Cancer-related pain may be attributed to a variety of causes, including bone pain, nerve compression or infiltration, soft tissue infiltration from the tumour, visceral pain or lymphoedema. The World Health Organization (1986) recommends the use of a three-step analgesic ladder for the management of cancer pain. Step One includes non-opioids ± adjuvants, Step Two includes weak opioids + non-opioids ± adjuvants, and Step Three comprises strong opioids + non-opioids ± adjuvants. For the purposes of this chapter, guidelines relating to pharmacological pain management in the last 72 hours of life will be provided and will relate to Step Three of the World Health Organization analgesic ladder.

At the end of life, individuals are less responsive and are often in an unconscious state, so medications will need to be administered via the subcutaneous route. A multitude of medications including analgesics, anticholinergics, benzodiazepines and antiemetics may be administered subcutaneously as a 'stat'/'prn' dose or continuously via a CSCI, thus controlling multiple symptoms. Most centres use either a SIMS 'Graseby' or a McKinley syringe driver.

Use of CSCIs in symptom management at the end of life

Drugs are generally more bioavailable after injection than via the oral route. This means that the dose of the drug given by CSCI will be less than the dose previously given orally, generally being approximately half of the oral dose (Twycross & Wilcock 2009).

It is common practice to administer up to four different drugs in the same syringe. If mixing two or more drugs does not result in a physical change, for example discoloration, clouding or crystallisation, they are said to be physically compatible. Information regarding drug compatibility ought to be obtained from compatibility charts or from the pharmacist. Generally, saline or water for injection can be used as a diluent to achieve the desired volume in the syringe for CSCI. Water for injection is always used with cyclizine to avoid incompatibility. If dexamethasone is one of the prescribed drugs, it should be the last drug added to reduce incompatibility.

It is recommended that a Luer-lock syringe with a minimum volume of 20 mL should be used to allow greater dilution; a larger syringe may be required depending on the volume of the drugs prescribed. The rate of delivery is based on the length of fluid or the volume represented in millimetres per unit. With the SIMS Graseby MS16A hourly rate syringe driver, the volume of drugs and diluents will always be 48 mm, regardless of the size of syringe. The rate of the infusion will be at 2 mm per hour over a 24-hour period.

Pain management in the last 72 hours of life

Opioids are generally the analgesic of choice for pain management in the last days of life as they can be delivered effectively and efficiently by CSCI. Non-steroidal anti-inflammatory drugs, for example diclofenac, may be administered by CSCI. Diclofenac must not be mixed with any other drugs. Diclofenac, paracetamol and Paralink may be administered rectally to provide pain relief and also act as an antipyretic.

If a patient has previously been receiving opioids via the oral route, this dose will be converted to the subcutaneous dose (this generally being half the oral dose in 24 hours) for administration in a CSCI. Patients who are opioid-naive will be generally be commenced on low-dose morphine subcutaneously per 24 hours with morphine prescribed 'prn'; the dose may be titrated up if necessary according to unrelieved pain and 'prn' requirements.

Opioids commonly used for 'prn' or CSCI administration

In the last hours and days of life, effective pain management is paramount and requires healthcare professionals to act immediately to optimise comfort during the dying phase. It is normal practice that the 24-hour dose of opioid may need to be increased on a daily basis or even more frequently if the patient's comfort has not been achieved. A 'prn' equivalent opioid must always be prescribed to allow analgesic administration as required if the background opioid dose per 24 hours is not providing adequate analgesic relief.

Morphine is generally the first strong opioid of choice for pain management. An alternative opioid may be used if the patient has undesirable side effects with morphine. In addition, if the patient has acute renal failure, another opioid may be more appropriate. The liver is the principal site of morphine metabolism. It is suggested that it takes between 10 and 20 minutes to achieve peak plasma concentration providing pain relief when morphine is administered subcutaneously (Twycross & Wilcock 2009). The lowest dose of morphine to be administered by CSCI is 2.5–5 mg per 24 hours. Depending on the individual's level of pain and 'prn' analgesic requirements, the commencing dose may be titrated accordingly.

Visit www.wileyfundamentalseries.com/medicalnursing and read Reflective Question 7.4 to think more about this topic.

Communication at the end of life

Visit www.wileyfundamentalseries.com/medicalnursing and read Reflective Question 7.5 to think more about this topic.

Communication with patients as they near their end of life presents many challenges to nurses and other members of the multidisciplinary team: (1) not knowing what to say; (2) being uncomfortable with the questions that they may be asked; (3) being unsure of how much the patient may understand; (4) fear of saying something that might upset the patient; and (5) time limitations. Becker (2010, p. 104) succinctly captured the reasons why professional caregivers may avoid communication with the dying as follows:

Fear of the unknown situation
Fear that our lack of knowledge may cause more problems
Fear of unleashing an emotional reaction
Fear of being blamed
Fear that we may get upset

Patients who are nearing their end of life have invariably progressed through an experience or journeyed through illness. Slevin (2006) highlights the importance of taking into consideration a number of variables that influence the illness experience in terms of responses to the illness. These include 'who is experiencing the illness', 'what is being experienced', 'how the experience is being responded to' and 'when and where' the experience has occurred.

Pollard *et al.* (2002) highlight the importance of good communication skills as being integral to the support of patients and families within a palliative care context. These skills include patient and family support, effectiveness within teamwork, facilitating the transition within the illness trajectory and impacting on treatment outcomes. As patients and families experience a range of emotions related to impending loss and anticipatory grief, it is not uncommon for communications to break down at this sensitive time.

Heaven and Maguire (2003) provide a comprehensive framework within which to address communication issues with individuals approaching the end of life. They highlight that a common cause of communication breakdown, particularly in the provision of end of life care, stems from 'selective attention', 'switching', 'offering advice or reassurance', 'passing the buck' and 'using jargon'. While each of those actions may be unintentional, it is crucial that healthcare professionals are conscious of the manner in which they communicate with dying patients and their families, so that the transition towards dying is made as smooth and as dignified as possible. It must also be kept in mind that patients' families are coming to terms with impending loss and are experiencing a variety of emotions and concerns as they witness their family member's condition deteriorating.

As death approaches, the patient's ability to communicate verbally diminishes. This can be a difficult time for family members as they experience this loss. Despite the absence of this ability to talk, communication with the patient should continue.

It is not uncommon for patients to ask difficult questions towards end of life, such as 'How long have I got?', 'Am I dying?' or 'What will my death be like – will it be painful?' These difficult questions can pose challenges to healthcare professionals as they attempt to answer them in an honest manner. It is also important for them to be answered, balancing hope with honesty and empathy (Clayton *et al.* 2009). In an attempt to facilitate good practice in breaking bad news, Buckman's (1992) Six Step Protocol (Table 7.1) outlines key guidelines in order to break bad news effectively; this, when used as a guide to breaking bad news, helps the nurse to take a sensitive approach to addressing a difficult situation.

Gilbert (2006) has succinctly captured the common concerns for relatives when a family member is approaching the end of life. These include the patient's diminishing fluid and food intake, the patient's distressing symptoms, how the patient will die and how they will recognise it, the effectiveness of medications and whether medications will hasten their relative's death. When addressing the needs of families in care of the dying, it is crucial to clarify the nature of families so that family-centred care can be initiated throughout this time. Farrelly (2009) acknowledges that the terminal illness within

Table 7.1 Six Step Protocol for breaking bad news

Step	Activities/processes
Getting started	Getting the physical context right Where? Who should be there? Starting off
Finding out how much the patient knows	The patient's understanding of the medical condition The style of the patient's statements The emotional content of the patient's statements
Finding out how much the patient wants to know	Phrasing the question First reactions Second thoughts
Sharing the information (aligning and educating)	Decide on your objectives (diagnosis/treatment plan/prognosis/support) Start from the patient's starting point Educating
Responding to the patient's feelings	Identify and acknowledge the patient's reaction
Planning and follow-through	Planning for the future Preparing for the worst and hoping for the best Supporting the patient Making a contract/follow-through 'Are there any (other) questions you'd like to ask me now?'

Data from Buckman, R. (1992) *How to Break Bad News: A Guide for Health Care Professionals*. University of Toronto Press. Toronto.

Table 7.2 The transition of fading away

Redefining	Shifting from 'what used to be' to 'what is now'
Burdening	Extra load in caring for a family member Waiting for the family member to die
Struggling with paradox	Wanting to care and wanting to lead a normal life Giving up and being tired of fighting
Contending with change	Changes in relationships, roles, socialisation and work patterns
Searching for meaning	Looking for meaning in order to help understand what is actually happening during the dying process
Living from day to day	Making the most of today Enjoying the time left with the family member
Preparing for death	Meeting the patient's wishes

family members is one of the most distressing experiences that affect families. There is no doubt that families go through a range of emotions, suffering, anticipatory grief and impending change in the face of the death of a family member.

Caring for the family of a dying patient forms part of person-centred and family-centred care. Families may be profoundly affected by the prospect of an impending death, which, as Kristjanson *et al.* (2003) highlight, can result in changing roles and responsibilities within the family circle. Support for families commences as soon as the patient is admitted to the ward, and its intensity increases as the dying trajectory continues. It is not unusual for family members to react and respond to impending loss in different ways, ranging from anger and denial to bargaining, depression and acceptance, as espoused by Kübler-Ross (1969). While much research has been undertaken that attempts to capture the needs of the families of dying patients, Davies and Steele (2010, p. 614) suggests that families' responses to the impending death of a family member may be described as the 'transition of fading away', which centres around seven key experiences they encounter (Table 7.2).

Visit **www.wileyfundamentalseries.com/medicalnursing** and read **Reflective Question 7.6** to think more about this topic.

As there is no gold standard framework for communicating with families as they face impending loss, Woodroof (2004, p. 27) has provided a framework that may be useful, particularly in situations where the information being delivered concerns a poor prognosis. Strategies include the following:

- Explain the uncertainty in estimating an individual patient's response.
- Give a realistic time range.
- Provide realistic hope – helping the patient to achieve what is important for them.
- Recommend that family relationships and worldly affairs be attended to.
- Be prepared to answer questions about the process of dying.
- Provide ongoing support and counselling.
- Reassure about continuity of care.

By addressing family concerns and issues around end of life care using the above framework, it is likely that family members will feel more included and supported throughout their relative's dying trajectory.

Ethics and end of life care

The provision of health services is achieved by the professionalism of various members of the multidisciplinary team (Thompson *et al.* 2003). Healthcare professionals make decisions within their scope of practice that potentially influence patient care, treatment options and outcomes (Botes 2000). Across the lifespan, healthcare providers are presented with ethical dilemmas and are required to make decisions based on their knowledge and expertise. In addition, there is a duty to act in the best interest of patients (Korner *et al.* 2006). A major dilemma for patients, their families and healthcare providers is to examine and identify the potential benefit versus the potential burden of proposed treatments on each individual patient, particularly at the end of life. Daly (2000) highlights the consensus concerning the general ethical principles that ought to influence decisions surrounding the withholding and withdrawal of treatment.

One of the common ethical issues arising towards end of life concerns the withdrawal or withholding artificial nutrition and hydration: 'There is a lack of consensus in society or among experts as to whether it is physically, psychologically, socially, or ethically appropriate to provide artificial hydration and nutrition to a terminally ill person' (Kedziera & Coyle 2006, p. 239; see also Watson *et al.* 2006). Despite society's increasing understanding of and comfort with end of life decision-making, questions concerning the withholding or withdrawing of nutrition and hydration remain particularly challenging to healthcare professionals and family members (Daly 2000). Nutrition and hydration represent basic survival requirements, but there is a lack of clarity and evidence with regard to the benefits or burdens associated with the administration of nutrition and hydration, particularly as the end of life approaches (Kedziera & Coyle, 2006). Healthcare professionals have a moral responsibility to identify each individual treatment and examine its potential benefit versus potential harm (Daly 2000; Smith & Andrews 2000; O'Brien *et al.* 2001; Maillet *et al.* 2002).

There is extensive evidence that patients who are dying do not respond to the administration of artificial nutrition and hydration in the same manner as patients who have the potential for recovery (Dunlop *et al.* 1995; Smith & Andrews 2000). This natural progression of the dying process frequently pertains to individuals' awareness of dying, which, according to Mak and Clinton (1999), influences individuals in achieving a good death. Patients' realisation of impending death regularly coincides with their awareness of their disease progression related to their disinterest and inability to eat or drink. If there is an option to introduce artificial nutrition, patients' values and wishes ought to be explored and respected as much as possible, upholding the principle of autonomy. This respect for the patient is also an underlying premise of beneficence.

Evidence suggests that the administration of artificial fluids to dying patients causes increased respiratory secretions and fluid overload, which may have distressing consequences for the patient (Daly 2000; Smith & Andrews, 2000). The ethical concern generally in caring for individuals with incurable illness is that fluid replacement therapy may be considered for all patients. The inevitability of death as a result of withholding fluid replacement therapy or nutrition is highlighted by several writers (Dunlop *et al.* 1995; Craig 2008). In opposition to this, Mathes (2001) has acknowledged that there is no evidence that nutritional or fluid support for patients with a terminal illness prolongs life. The issues of justice and patient feeding or hydration are challenging. In end of life care, an individual's inability to eat or drink may indicate a change in their disease progression, indicating the onset of death. Fluid replacement may be administered if warranted, but it is likely the requirement may not be for long.

Ethical decision-making models further corroborate attempts to achieve morally and ethically sound decisions. Examples of developed ethical decision-making models are Purtillo's Six Step Model, the DECIDE model and the Ethical Grid Model (see Thompson *et al.* 2003). According to Thompson *et al.* (2003), the DECIDE model provides a practical method of making prudent value judgements and ethical decisions. The DECIDE model, as described by Thompson *et al.* (2003), constitutes the following process shown in Table 7.3.

In summary, ethical deliberation utilising ethical principles, theories and decision-making process frameworks best assists healthcare professionals to achieve the best possible outcome in controversial issues (Maillet *et al.* 2002). The ethical principles of autonomy, beneficence, nonmaleficence and justice assist healthcare professionals in deciding whether artificial nutrition or hydration is appropriate in the context of individuals with life-limiting illnesses, within palliative care practice. Few issues within

Table 7.3 The DECIDE model

	Process	Action from
D	Define the problem	Firstly the ethical issue needs to be identified. Is the individual involved competent or incompetent? What are the patient's rights? In this case the problem is the issue of withholding or withdrawing nutrition or hydration in a terminally ill individual
E	Ethical review	What principles are relevant to the case? Which principles should be given priority? Is the patient autonomous? Apply beneficence, nonmaleficence to uphold the best possible outcome for the patient. Are the patient's best interests the precedence?
C	Consider the options	What options are available? What is the alternative? What is the potential for beneficial outcomes for this patient? What is the potential for producing distressful side effects in this patient? Have the essential facts about the disease process and the likely outcome of the proposed treatments been explained to the patient and family? What are the patient's goals and values? What is the impact of the proposed treatment on the patient or family members?
I	Investigate outcomes	What are the consequences of the action? Which is the most ethical thing to do? What are the benefits and the burdens of the treatment?
D	Decide on action	Having decided on the best option available, establish a specific plan, act decisively and effectively
E	Evaluate results	Having withdrawn, withheld or initiated a course of action, monitor the results of the decision

Reproduced from Thompson, I.E., Melia, K.M., Boyd, K.M. (2003) *Nursing Ethics*, 4th edn, with kind permission of Elsevier.

healthcare are more complex than those concerning the decision to withhold or withdraw life-prolonging treatment. The difficulties pertaining to the decision of whether to withdraw or withhold artificial nutrition or hydration in patients approaching the end of life are influenced by the patient and their family, together with the ethical and moral values of the healthcare professionals involved. The benefits and burdens of artificial nutrition and hydration ought to be evaluated in terms of short-term and long-term goals, and further ethical deliberation may be required depending on the outcome of these goals.

Visit **www.wileyfundamentalseries.com/medicalnursing** and read **Reflective Question 7.7** to think more about this topic.

Conclusion

End of life care is complex. Death can be a long protracted process that requires a comprehensive range of knowledge, skills and competencies that can address the needs of the dying person and their family members. Understanding the nature of the dying process as presented from a theoretical perspective can assist nurses and care-givers to initiate effective caring interventions so that the quality of life of those patients can be enhanced, particularly as the dying process progresses to ultimate death. The most common symptoms that present at the end of life include dyspnoea, a death rattle and pain. The multidisciplinary team may potentially initiate appropriate interventions so as to facilitate a good death for the dying person.

Communication with the dying person can cause much concern for healthcare professionals, but the use of a sensitive approach can enhance the healthcare professional's skills in addressing sensitive issues. Families experience a range of emotions as they witness their family member dying. The 'transition of fading away' framework provides a comprehensive approach to addressing these concerns. It is not uncommon for family members to express concern with regard to the withdrawal of nutrition and hydration at end of life; using an ethical decision-making framework can assist members of the multidisciplinary team to address this ethical dilemma.

Now visit the companion website and test yourself on this chapter:
www.wileyfundamentalseries.com/medicalnursing

References

Bausewein, C., Farquhar, M., Booth, S., Gysels, M. & Higginson, I. (2007) Measurement of breathless in advanced disease: a systematic review. *Respiratory Medicine*, **101**:399–410.

Becker, R. (2010) *Fundamental Aspects of Palliative Care Nursing*, 2nd edn. London: Quay Books.

Bennett, M,. Lucas, V., Brennan, M., Hughes, A., O'Donnell, V. & Wee, B. (2002) Using anti-muscarine drugs in the management of death rattle: evidence based guidelines for palliative care. *Palliative Medicine*, **16**:369–74.

Botes, A. (2000) A comparison between the ethics of justice and the ethics of care. *Journal of Advanced Nursing*, **32**(5):1071–5.

Buckman, R. (1992) *How To Break Bad News: A Guide for Health Care Professionals*. Toronto: University of Toronto Press.

Chan, K., Tse, D., Sham, M. and Thorsen, A. & Thorsen, A. (2005) Palliative medicine in malignant respiratory diseases. In: Doyle, D., Hanks, G., Cherny, N. & Calman, K. (eds), *Oxford Textbook of Palliative Medicine* (pp. 587–618). Oxford: Oxford University Press.

Clayton, J., Butow, P. & Tattersall, M. (2009) Telling the truth. In: Walsh, D. (ed.), *Palliative Medicine* (pp. 620–4). Philadelphia: Saunders Elsevier.

Copp, G. (1999) *Facing Impending Death: Experiences of Patients and their Nurses*. London: Nursing Times Books.

Corner, J. & O'Driscoll, M. (1999) Development of a breathlessness assessment guide for use in palliative care. *Palliative Medicine*, **13**:375–84.

Craig, G. (2008) Palliative care in overdrive: patients in danger. *American Journal of Hospice and Palliative Medicine*, **25**(2):155–60.

Daly, B.J. (2000) Special challenges of withholding artificial nutrition and hydration. *Journal of Gerontological Nursing*, **26**(9):25–31.

Davies, B. & Steele, R. (2010) Supporting families in palliative care. In: Ferrell, B. & Coyle, N. (eds), *Oxford Textbook of Palliative Nursing* (pp. 587–618). Oxford: Oxford University Press.

Dudgeon, D., Kristjanson, L., Sloan, J., Lertzman, M. & Clement, K. (2001) Dyspnoea in cancer patients: prevalence and associated factors. *Journal of Pain and Symptom Management*, **21**(2):95–102.

Dunlop, R.J., Ellershaw, J.E., Baines, J.M., Sykes, N. & Saunders, C.M. (1995) On withholding nutrition and hydration in the terminally ill: has palliative medicine gone too far? A reply. *Journal of Medical Ethics*, **21**(3):141–3.

Farrelly. M. (2009) Families in distress. In: Walsh, D. (ed.), *Palliative Medicine* (pp. 63–9). Philadelphia: Saunders Elsevier.

Gilbert (2006) The last days of life. In: Cooper, J. (ed.), *Stepping into Palliative Care: Care and Practice* (pp. 148–56). Milton Keynes: Radcliffe Medical Press.

Glare, P., Dickman, A. & Goodman, M. (2011) Symptom control in care of the dying. In: Ellershaw, J. & Wilkinson, S. (eds), *Care of the Dying: A Pathway to Excellence* (pp. 33–61). Oxford: Oxford University Press.

Glaser, B. & Strauss, A. (1965) *Awareness of Dying*. Chicago: Aldine.

Heaven, C. & Maguire, P. (2003). Communication issues. In: Lloyd-Williams, M. (ed.), *Psychosocial Issues in Palliative Care* (pp. 21–47). Oxford: Oxford University Press.

Hughes, A., Wilcock, A. & Corcoran, R. (1996) Management of death rattle. *Journal of Pain and Symptom Management*, **12**(5):271–2.

Kass, R. & Ellershaw, J. (2003) Respiratory tract secretions n the dying patient: a retrospective study. *Journal of Pain and Symptom Management*, **26**:897–902.

Kedziera, P. & Coyle, N. (2006). Hydration, thirst and nutrition. In: Ferrell, B. & Coyle, N. (eds), *Textbook of Palliative Nursing* (pp. 239–48). Oxford: Oxford University Press.

Kinder, C. & Ellershaw, J. &. (2011) How to use the Liverpool Care Pathway for the Dying Patient (LCP). In Ellershaw, J. & Wilkinson, S. (eds), *Care of the Dying: A Pathway to Excellence* (pp. 11–41). Oxford: Oxford University Press.

Korner, U., Bondolfi, A., Buhler, E. *et al.* Ethical and legal aspects of enteral nutrition. *Clinical Nutrition*, **25**:196–202.

Kravits, K. & Berenson, S. (2010) Complementary and alternative therapies and palliative care. In: Ferrell, B. & Coyle, N. (eds), *Oxford Textbook of Palliative Nursing* (pp. 545–65). Oxford: Oxford University Press.

Kristjanson, L., Hudson, P. & Oldhan. L. (2003) Working with families in palliative care. In: O'Connor, M. & Aranda, S. (eds), *Palliative Care Nursing: A Guide to Practice* (pp. 271–83) Milton Keynes: Radcliffe Medical Press.

Kübler-Ross, E. (1969) *On Death and Dying*. New York: Macmillan.

Lawrey, H. (2005) Hyoscine vs glycopyrronium for drying respiratory secretions in dying patients. *British Journal of Community Nursing*, **10**(9);421–6.

Maillet, J.O., Potter, R.L. & Heller, L. (2002) Position of the American Dietetic Association: Ethical and legal issues in nutrition, hydration and feeding. *Journal of the American Dietetic Association*, **102**(5):716–25.

Mak, J.M.H. & Clinton, M. (1999) Promoting a good death: an agenda for outcomes research – a review of the literature. *Nursing Ethics*, **6**(2):97–105.

Mathes, M.M. (2001) Withholding and withdrawing nutrition and hydration by medical means: ethical perspectives. *Medsurg Nursing*, **10**(2):96–9.

Muller-Busch, H. & Jehser, T. (2009) Death rattle. In: Walsh, D. (ed.), *Palliative Medicine* (pp. 956–60). Philadelphia: Saunders Elsevier.

O'Brien, T., McQuillan, R., Tighe, P. & Smullen, H. (2001) *Artificial Hydration in Terminally Ill Patients. A Position Paper by the Irish Association for Palliative Care*. Dublin: Irish Association for Palliative Care.

Pollard, A., Cairns, J. & Rosenthal, M. (2002) Transition in living and dying: defining palliative care. In: Aranda, S. & O'Connor, M. (eds), *Palliative Care Nursing: A Guide to Practice* (pp. 5–20). Melbourne: Ausmed Publications.

Slevin, O. (2006) The experience of illness. In: Cooper, J. (ed.), *Stepping into Palliative Care: Relationships and Responses* (pp. 45–57). Abingdon: Radcliffe Medical Press.

Smith, S.A. & Andrews, M. (2000) Artificial nutrition and hydration at the end of life. *Medsurg Nursing*, **9**(5):233–42.

Thompson, I.E., Melia, K.M. & Boyd, K.M. (2003) *Nursing Ethics*, 4th edn. Edinburgh: Churchill Livingstone.

Twycross, R. & Wilcock, A. (2009). *Symptom Management in Advanced Cancer*. Oxford: Radcliffe Medical Press.

Wade, R., Booth, S. & Wilcock, A. (2005) The management of respiratory symptoms. In: Faull, C., Carter, Y. & Daniels, L. (eds.), *Handbook of Palliative Care* (pp. 160–83). Oxford: Blackwell Publishing.

Watson, M., Lucas, C., Hoy. A. & Back, I. (2006) *Oxford Handbook of Palliative Care*. Oxford University Press: Oxford.

Wells, N. (2000) Pain intensity and pain interference in hospitalised patients with cancer. *Oncology Nursing Forum*, **27**:985–91.

Wilders, H. & Menten, J. (2002) Death rattle: prevalence, prevention and treatment. *Journal of Pain and Symptom Management*, **23**:310–17.

Wilders, H., Dhaenekint, P., Clement, P. *et al.* (2009) Atropine, hyoscine butylbromide, or scopolamine are equally effective for the treatment of death rattle in terminal care. *Journal of Pain and Symptom Management*, **38**(1):124–33.

Woodroof, R. (2004). *Palliative Medicine: Evidence-based Symptomatic and Supportive Care for Patients with Advanced Care*. Oxford: Oxford University Press.

World Health Organization (1986) *Cancer Pain Relief*. Geneva: WHO.

8

Principles of perioperative nursing

Joy O'Neill, Bernie Pennington and Adele Nightingale

Faculty of Health, Edge Hill University, Manchester, UK

Contents

Introduction	105
General issues and anaesthesia	105
Patient safety	107
Anaesthesia	108
Roles of circulating and scrub practitioners	113
Aseptic technique/infection control	113
Accountability	114
Patient positioning	115
Surgical sutures	116
Surgical needles	116
Surgical dressings	116
Surgical drains	116
Surgical instruments	116
Surgical specialities	117
Recovery	117
Postoperative nausea and vomiting	121
Pain management	121
Conclusion	122
References	123

Learning outcomes

Having read this chapter, you will be able to:

- Gain a broad understanding of the knowledge underpinning the skills of a perioperative practitioner
- Demonstrate an understanding of the care delivered to patients in the perioperative environment
- Understand the role of risk management within perioperative care

Fundamentals of Medical-Surgical Nursing: A Systems Approach, First Edition. Edited by Anne-Marie Brady, Catherine McCabe, and Margaret McCann.

Introduction

This chapter on perioperative care has been written for student healthcare professionals who may or may not experience a perioperative placement within their training. It provides basic information regarding the role of the theatre practitioner spanning three areas of perioperative practice (anaesthetics, scrub and recovery) and the delivery of effective patient care. The role of a perioperative practitioner (nurse or operating department practitioner) is multifaceted as it encapsulates clinical care, advocacy, risk management and quality assurance. Maintaining a safe perioperative environment ensures that patients are provided with competent and high-quality care.

General issues and anaesthesia

When patient care involves positive interventions and/or treatments to promote restoration of health, much of perioperative nursing concerns itself with preventing harm during the procedure.

The process of consent is the first in a series of risk assessments that take place during the patient episode. The decision by patients to consent to surgery is in itself a risk assessment. This risk assessment weighs the benefits of treatment against the risks of failure, postoperative infection and potential disability (any loss of function). In order to make this assessment, the surgeon seeking consent will usually indicate what percentage risk exists for that specific procedure while the patient is in his or her care – an example of this being a 15% risk of postoperative infection for a knee arthroscopy. Surgeons are also duty-bound to discuss alternative treatments and their associated risks. The patient will then make a balanced judgement of these and whether proceeding with any given treatment justifies these risks.

Surgery can be very dangerous. Even with modern techniques and advanced simulator training, when one pares surgery down it is largely carried out by human beings and with sharp implements. This takes place at a point when a significant proportion of the body's natural coping mechanisms are modified by anaesthesia, and the body's most important defence against infection (the skin) has been breached. Success is entirely dependent on the skill of the surgeon, anaesthetist and theatre practitioners. These are all human beings, and mistakes can and do occur. Surgery is a risky business.

Before deciding the type of anaesthetic that the anaesthetist will deliver, a number of variables need to be considered:

- the patient's preoperative medical/surgical condition;
- the type and length of surgery;
- postoperative considerations.

Preoperative assessment

The aims of preoperative assessment are to determine whether the patient is fit for anaesthesia, to optimise the patient's condition before anaesthesia and to establish the most suitable anaesthetic technique. Currently, the majority of patients attend for elective operative procedures as 'day case' or 'ambulant surgery', i.e. the patient is admitted and discharged on the same day. This changes the way in which preoperative assessment is undertaken.

In most units, day surgery patients are preoperatively assessed by dedicated preoperative assessment nurses via preoperative clinics, telephone and postal questionnaires, and online forms. Elective surgery patients who have pre-existing or complex medical and/or surgical problems are usually admitted prior to the day of their operation to determine a care plan that will take into consideration their coexisting problems. This assessment may utilise a multidisciplinary approach to patient care. Preoperative information is, however, often limited for emergency patients due to the condition in which they present and the urgency that this creates. The emergency patient may be unconscious, confused or otherwise temporarily incapacitated. Assessment usually follows a trauma assessment protocol, with resuscitation and immediate treatment of life-threatening injuries being the priority.

The anaesthetist will communicate any additional risks to the anaesthetic nurse to ensure that additional drugs and airway management equipment are available and checked prior to anaesthesia.

Table 8.1 Preparation of the anaesthetic area (an indicative rather than exhaustive list)

Sundries/disposables	Electronic equipment	Preparation of the theatre/ anaesthetic room
Tourniquets, skin preparation, cannulas, 'sharps' bins and intravenous dressings Intravenous fluids – crystalloids, colloids and pressure bags should be available Stethoscope	Anaesthetic machine/pipelines and cylinders (airway management equipment is discussed later in this chapter) Gas analyser Non-invasive blood pressure Pulse oximeter Capnograph Means of preventing heat loss and warming the patient Deep vein thrombosis prophylaxis	Temperature (between 21 and 23°C) Humidity between 50% and 70% Lighting Diathermy machine Operating table

Preparation of the environment

Planning and preparation are key to the successful delivery of anaesthetic care. The theatre and anaesthetic room are checked to ensure that the temperature, lighting and humidity are within safe parameters (Table 8.1). Both areas needs to be cleaned in line with hospital policy (based on national guidelines), and all sundry and disposable items should be checked for their availability and integrity.

The anaesthetic machine is one of the most important pieces of equipment that needs to be cleaned, checked and calibrated. This is carried out in accordance with Association of Anaesthetists of Great Britain and Ireland (2010) guidelines and hospital policy (if applicable). Although it is imperative that the anaesthetic machine is checked for functionality, it is equally important to have a secondary means of delivering oxygen and ventilating the patient in the event of machine failure during the operation.

Visit www.wileyfundamentalseries.com/medicalnursing and read Reflective Question 8.1 to think more about this topic.

Scrub and circulating staff also assess perioperative risk prior to surgery – for example, tissue viability is a concern to the perioperative nurse as patients are required to be immobile for the duration of surgery. Positioning of the patient for surgery is primarily to enable access to the site of surgery, with the important secondary concern of protecting the pressure areas. It is therefore highly important that an accurate pressure sore risk assessment takes place prior to and during the operation. Typically, bony prominences will be supported by pressure-dispersing gel pads during surgery. A full-body gel pad may be used between the operating table and the supine patient. This may preclude the use of some commercial warming mattresses (see below), but certain ones do provide some pressure relief as well.

The risk of deep vein thrombosis leading to pulmonary embolus is given similar attention (National Institute for Health and Clinical Excellence [NICE], 2010). Immobile patients are susceptible to the formation of blood clots within the lower legs. Treatment to prevent these forming can be medical (low molecular weight heparins) or mechanical. Mechanical means usually take the form of compression boots that intermittently inflate to compress the calf muscles, resulting in a passive pumping action that reduces the likelihood of venous stasis in that area.

A further risk to the surgical patient is posed by inadvertent hypothermia. An anesthetised patient cannot effectively compensate for heat loss due to drug interference with their autonomic nervous system and because of a reduction in muscle tone that prevents heat generation by shivering. In addition, the patient's 'central heating system', the circulatory system, will have slowed down (as shown by a decreased heart rate and blood pressure on induction of anaesthesia) and may be cooling down due the introduction of intravenous fluids at room temperature.

A patient receiving regional anaesthesia via a spinal or epidural route will have a lesser or greater degree of vasodilation, a mechanism the body effectively uses for losing heat. Patients may also be subject to a rapid infusion of fluids in order to manage a sudden drop in blood pressure (a common side effect of a spinal or epidural anaesthetic). Consequently, before patients have even entered the operating room, they are significantly compromised in terms of maintaining their own body temperature. Studies indicate that hypothermic patients (<35.5°C) take longer to recover from anaesthesia, experience greater pain and are more susceptible to postoperative wound infection. When we consider open abdominal or thoracic surgery and the evaporation of body fluids from within those cavities (insensible heat loss), it is easy to see how a patient may quickly become hypothermic. It is therefore imperative that patients' temperatures are accurately recorded before, during and after surgery. Forced-air warming suits, such as the Bair Hugger (Arizant Inc, MN, USA), and the more conservative approach of additional cotton blankets and foil wrap insulation are options.

Perioperative temperature management can be problematic and in the UK is subject to NICE guidelines (National Institute of Health and Clinical Excellence, 2008). These guidelines advocate regular (half-hourly) monitoring of body temperature and recommend that, for any case taking longer than 30 minutes, active warming methods should be considered. Active warming of the patient includes warming of intravenous fluids and the use of either an electrically powered warming mattress or forced-air warming system.

Patient safety

When admitting the patient to the care of the anaesthetic practitioner, it is important to establish that the correct patient is received, for the correct procedure, and that consent has been obtained in an appropriate manner. The anaesthetic practitioner introduces themself to the patient and confirms the following:

- the patient's name and how they would like to be addressed;
- that the patient has been sufficiently prepared for anaesthesia in terms of fasting;
- surgical site marking;
- that any other information that may impact on the patient's care is articulated.

Intraoperative care plans or integrated care pathways are a means of communicating important information relating to the patient and the episode of care to be undertaken. This is often the first contact that the anaesthetic practitioner will have with the patient. Excellent communication skills are required to establish a rapport with the patient in a very short time in a possibly very stressful situation (Wicker & O'Neill 2010). The care plan must be completed succinctly, accurately and legibly.

One of the biggest risks to patients is the risk of surgery on the wrong site. Reasons for this error are listed in Table 8.2.

Recent work into the causes of wrong-site surgery (National Patient Safety Agency 2005) has led to the adoption of the Surgical Safety Checklist by the World Health Organization (WHO), which is promoting this additional safety measure worldwide (World Health Organization, 2008). The Safe Surgery Checklist ensures that the correct procedure is carried out and incorporates a number of additional risk measures such as an assessment of tissue viability, venous thromboembolism, blood loss,

Table 8.2 Causes of surgery on the wrong site

Reason	Causes
Wrong side listed on the operating list	Error recording the decision in the case notes Error listing the operation
Wrong side/site recorded on the consent form	Error reading the case notes Orientation error Patient not consulted Consent sought by junior staff
Wrong side/site marked on the patient	Error reading the case notes Orientation error Patient not consulted Consent sought by junior staff
Wrong limb prepared	Error reading the case notes Orientation error Error on the operating list Error on the consent form Error in the case notes Tourniquet or skin preparation applied without checks

personnel within the theatre, availability of surgical instrumentation/prostheses and allergy risks. What distinguishes this checklist from the other barriers to error is the adoption of a 'time-out' whereby every member of the theatre team stops what they are doing, and the critical check **immediately prior to surgery** takes place with the full attention of the whole team. The WHO (2008) Surgical Safety Checklist has been demonstrated to dramatically reduce errors where a culture of whole-team involvement is present.

Prior to any intervention, the patient will be attached to the basic monitoring equipment, usually non-invasive blood pressure, oxygen saturation and electrocardiograph. Once baseline observations have been observed and recorded, intravenous access will be sought, and in most cases a fluid regimen commenced.

Visit www.wileyfundamentalseries.com/medicalnursing and read Reflective Question 8.2 to think more about this topic.

Anaesthesia

There are a number of ways in which an anaesthetic can be delivered – as general, regional or local anaesthetic. These types of anaesthetic are all based on the principles of the 'triad of anaesthesia' (Davey & Ince 2000). The triad of anaesthesia offers a balanced technique whereby optimal operating conditions are achieved for the patient, anaesthetist and surgeon (Figure 8.1).

The anaesthetist will have made plans for how to maintain the patient's airway. For most surgical procedures, this will achieved using either a laryngeal mask airway (LMA) or an endotracheal tube (ETT). This decision will be made by taking the patient's anatomical and physiological condition and the length and type of surgery into consideration (Table 8.3).

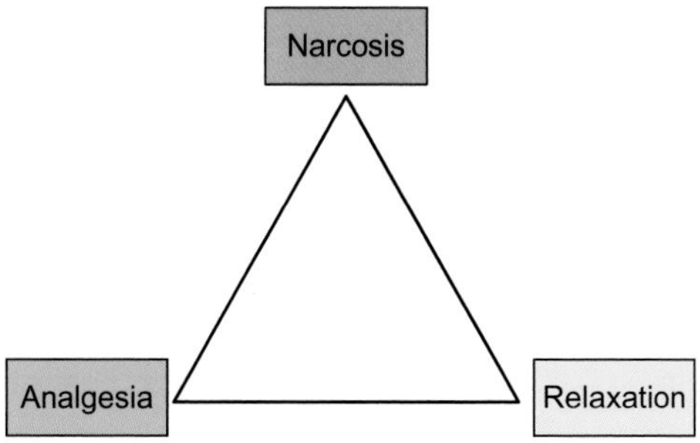

Figure 8.1 The anaesthesia triad.

Table 8.3 Choice of airway maintenance technique

	ETT	LMA
Patient needs	Patients who are known to be at risk of aspiration, i.e. those with: • hiatus hernia • small bowel obstruction • opiate use • pregnancy • a full stomach • trauma/emergency admission Post-arrest – patient may need ventilating Post-surgery requirements – patient may need to be ventilated	Patients who are known to have followed fasting guidelines and do not come into the category for ETT intubation Patients who are free from cardiovascular and respiratory compromise
Surgical needs	Type of surgery, i.e.: • laparoscopic surgery • with patients in particular positions • surgery lasting over 2 hours • surgery in which the surgeon needs to use a muscle relaxant, e.g. laparotomy	Surgery that will take less than 2 hours Surgery in which the patient's position will not interfere with spontaneous breathing or intragastric pressure, i.e. not prone

Endotracheal intubation

Endotracheal intubation is placement of an ETT in the patient's trachea, using a laryngoscope to aid visualisation and assist with placement (Table 8.4).

Laryngeal mask airway

The LMA is used traditionally when a patient is breathing spontaneously, i.e. is not being ventilated. A number of adaptations of the LMA are available, including the i-gel and ProSeal (Gwinnutt 2008). The equipment that is needed for the insertion of an LMA is shown in Table 8.5.

Once all the equipment has been prepared and checked, the anaesthetist will start to preoxygenate the patient. Therefore, if there is a period during which the patient loses consciousness and stops breathing, there will still be a reserve of circulating oxygen available.

Table 8.4 Preparation for endotracheal intubation

Equipment	Rationale
The correctly sized ETT (have one smaller and one larger size available)	Patients are ventilated through an ETT. The tube size needs to be correct to prevent trauma to the trachea and to prevent any leakage of gas from around the cuff
Syringe to inflate the pilot cuff	Required to inflate the cuff
Variety of laryngoscope blades	A laryngoscope is used to aid visualisation of the vocal cords
Lubricating gel (for the ETT)	A water-based gel on the ETT may be necessary in circumstances in which insertion is difficult
Oropharyngeal airways (various sizes)	Prevent the tongue from falling to the back of the pharynx and causing an obstruction
Nasopharyngeal airways (various sizes)	Prevent the tongue from falling to the back of the pharynx and causing an obstruction
Magill forceps	Help with insertion of the ETT between the vocal cords
Bougie (gum elastic or single-use disposable)	Used to railroad an ETT when the view at laryngoscopy is suboptimal
Stylette	Inserted inside an ETT before insertion to change the shape of the tube

Table 8.5 Preparation for insertion of an LMA

Equipment	Rationale
A suitably sized LMA	To prevent any trauma to the soft tissue and teeth To minimise leakage around the cuff
Lubricating gel	A water-based gel on the ETT may be necessary in circumstances where insertion is difficult
Syringe for inflating the cuff	Required to inflate the cuff

Having preoxygenated the patient, a combination of drugs will be administered. Patients are rendered unconscious by the administration of an induction agent delivered intravenously or by the inhalation of an anaesthetic vapour (gas induction). Prior to the induction agent being administered, the anaesthetist will often (apart from with rapid sequence induction or if a difficult airway is anticipated) give an opiate, usually fentanyl. This is to prevent the normal sympathetic response to laryngoscopy, i.e. the patient's response to a painful stimulus.

Laryngoscopy

A laryngoscope is used to aid with visualisation of the vocal cords to allow direct placement of the ETT. This process is known as intubation. The laryngoscope is traditionally a left-handed instrument and has an atomically shaped blade. It is inserted down the right-hand side of the tongue, displacing it to the left. Once the epiglottis has been elevated, the vocal cords should be in view and the ETT is passed between them.

The role of anaesthetic nurse is to provide assistance to the anaesthetist. In order to provide skilled assistance, the nurse must possess an in-depth knowledge and understanding of anaesthesia to anticipate the needs of both the anaesthetist and the patient.

The third element of the triad – analgesia – is required to prevent the patient's sympathetic nervous system responding to the painful stimulus. This is often overcome by administering opioid analgesia on induction. However, the amount of drug and the speed at which it is metabolised may not be adequate to prevent a response to surgical stimuli. The use of intravenous paracetamol is on the increase, and this is often given in the anaesthetic room on induction. An opiate is routinely administered in theatre, whether this be incremental doses of morphine or a continuous infusion of remifentanil. Remifentanil is administered by continuous infusion as part of the total intravenous anaesthesia technique, whereby a continuous infusion of propofol is delivered via a syringe pump in tandem with the remifentanil.

The anaesthetist (or patient or surgeon) may decide against the use of a general anaesthetic. There may be a number of reasons for this including:

- patient choice;
- the patient's medical family history (e.g. a history of malignant hyperpyrexia or suxamethonium apnoea);
- physiological conditions;
- known problems with a difficult airway.

Alternative techniques include regional anaesthesia. This technique will use one of the following:

- a spinal anaesthetic;
- an epidural anaesthetic;
- combined epidural and spinal anaesthesia.

Although spinal and epidural anaesthetics have their differences (Table 8.6), they also have a number of similarities, including:

- the position of the patient:
    - sitting – the anaesthetic practitioner will need a stool (without wheels) for the patient to rest their feet on;
    - lateral – the anaesthetic practitioner must consider whether help is required to hold the patient in position;
- preparation of the patient:
    - basic monitoring;
    - intravenous access with infusion of a crystalloid (or colloid if necessary);
    - a means of delivering oxygen via a face mask (or nasal specs/sponge);
    - location of the anatomical points;
    - aseptic cleaning of the spinal area identified;
- preparation of equipment ¬– using an aseptic non-touch technique (ANTT);
- preparation of the anaesthetic practitioner – again;
- with the anaesthetic practitioner using an aseptic technique with a mask, gown and gloves.

Visit **www.wileyfundamentalseries.com/medicalnursing** and read **Reflective Question 8.3** to think more about this topic.

If patients are non-ambulant, this poses significant health and safety risks to both themselves and the theatre personnel. This risk has been reduced over the last decade or so, with the trend towards ambulatory (day case) surgery enabling a shift towards more patients receiving treatment on specialist operating trolleys, thus reducing the need for staff to employ manual handling techniques. Even for

Table 8.6 Spinal and epidural anaesthesia

Property	Spinal	Epidural
Anatomical differences	Inserted below L3/4 or L4/5	Most commonly performed in the lumbar region
	Inserted through the dura mater into the subarachnoid space	Sits in the epidural space
Type of needle	Uses a small-gauge needle, usually 25G or 27G, either a Whitacre or Sprotte type	Tuohy needle (16–18G)
	Has an introducer and a stylette to aid insertion	Uses a loss-of-resistance syringe filled with either air or saline
Drugs used	Heavy bupivacaine (8% glucose), which makes it a hyperbaric solution	Bupivacaine 0.25–0.75%
Type of surgery	Lower limb or lower abdominal surgery, e.g. lower segment caesarean section	Often used as postoperative pain relief in surgery involving the upper or lower gastrointestinal tract, e.g. oesophagectomy
Onset of anaesthesia	Rapid onset	Slow onset: 20–30 minutes
Duration of anaesthesia	Lasts 2–2.5 hours	Can be set up as a continuous infusion

those patients not requiring a transfer from trolley to table, however, positioning for optimal surgical access may be required. Most of the risk posed here is to theatre personnel, and predictably this risk is higher where the risk is unforeseen, for example with the presentation of a morbidly obese patient. The minimum number of theatre personnel required to move or position an adult patient is four, based on European Manual Handling directives indicating that male staff should move a maximum load of 25 kg and female staff a 15 kg maximum. Careless positioning of the surgical patient can cause considerable harm. Even the most basic surgical position – supine – carries risks. Risks can, however, be reduced by positioning the patient as far as possible in alignment and by continuous monitoring of at-risk areas.

Assessment of infection risk takes into account the site of the surgery (e.g. bowel), existing bacterial activity and the tissue that will be breached (bone infection, for example, being very difficult to manage). Contact infection is managed by the creation of a 'sterile field'. This is discussed in the next section. An additional infection risk may be present via reusable equipment that has been inadequately disinfected. Examples of this are operating tables, suction units and diathermy machines – particularly where staff members handle diathermy pedals that are in regular contact with the floor. Gel pads and operating table supports can also have similar contact with a soiled theatre floor and must be disinfected carefully between patients.

Electrosurgical units, audiovisual stacker systems, suction units, anaesthetic machines, warming units and light source equipment all present the risk of trailing cables. This risk is usually managed via ceiling-mounted booms or pods containing electrical and gas supply socket systems.

Where specimens are taken for pathology examination, a risk of misdiagnosis exists. The biggest risk is error in labelling specimens. This should not occur if labelling takes place in real time, checking takes place and the specimen is despatched as soon as documentation has been completed.

Box 8.1 Roles of the scrub and circulating practitioners

Role and responsibilities of the scrub practitioner

Checks prior to commencement of the operating list:
- Cleanliness of the theatre environment
- Temperature and humidity levels, and efficient air-conditioning, taking the appropriate action if necessary to adjust the levels

Preparation of instrument sets and accessories:
- Swabs
- Needles
- Extra instruments
- Accessories (e.g. sutures and dressings)

Scrubbing-up procedure: wash hands and arms, don sterile gown and gloves
Preparation of instrument trolley and Mayo stand
Passing instruments to the surgeon
Anticipation of the surgeon's needs
Maintenance of the sterile field
Swab, needle and instrument checks
Handling and passing of instruments
Specimens
Documentation (electronic and hard copy)
Cleaning between surgical procedures and at the end of the operating list

Role and responsibilities of the circulating practitioner

Checks prior to commencement of the operating list:
- Cleanliness of theatre environment
- Temperature and humidity levels, and efficient air-conditioning, taking the appropriate action if necessary to adjust the levels

Assisting the scrub practitioner in the preparation of the instrument sets, accessories, swabs, needles and instruments
Preparation of sterile surgical gowns and gloves
Tying donned sterile gowns
Opening instrument sets
Passing accessories to the scrub practitioner
Maintenance of the sterile field
Swab, needle and instrument checks with the scrub practitioner
Anticipation of the scrub practitioner's needs
Safe practice in placing specimens into appropriately sized specimen containers (with the correct medium)
Documentation (electronic and hard copy)
Cleaning between surgical procedures and at the end of the operating list

The soiled theatre floor presents multiple risks that include the spread of infection via carelessly discarded equipment coming into contact with used irrigation, skin preparation and bodily fluids (usually blood). There is also a slip hazard relating to these items. Management of these risks involves mopping between cases, but this poses an additional slip risk as it takes place at a time when multiple staff are preparing the operating room for the next case. Good and timely communication is essential in this instance.

Roles of circulating and scrub practitioners

The scrub team consists of the scrub and circulating practitioners and the surgical team [surgeon and assistant surgeon(s)]. The roles of the scrub and circulating practitioners are outlined in Box 8.1.

Aseptic technique/infection control

Theatre practitioners undertake three methods of hand-washing: social hand-washing, aseptic technique and the surgical scrub. Social hand-washing is used when washing the hands before preparing food, after ablutions and before and after clinical procedures. Aseptic technique is a method of maintaining asepsis and helps to protect healthcare staff and patients from health-acquired infections. The ANTT has now superseded the aseptic hand-wash and includes a seven-stage hand-wash that ensures effective hand-cleansing. This was introduced by the Department of Health in 2003 as part of a strategy to reduce infections and their subsequent cost to the National Health Service (Rowley *et al.* 2010).

The surgical scrub is an extension of the aseptic hand-wash. This procedure helps to eliminate transient flora and reduce the resident skin flora as the scrub cleansing solutions have antimicrobial properties (World Health Organization 2009). Scrub practitioners and the surgical team should follow their theatre policy for their scrubbing procedure.

All types of hand-washing and the use of personal protective equipment (PPE) can reduce the risk of hospital-acquired infection and surgical site infections. PPE includes theatre clothing (top and trousers, or theatre dress), face masks, face masks with a visor or goggles, aprons, gloves (sterile or disposable) and theatre shoes. These should be worn appropriately and disposed of in line with theatre policy. The use of PPE is assessed on an individual basis for each patient and their medical condition and surgical procedure.

Practitioners clean the equipment and operating table to ensure that they are clean and free from dust. Damp dusting is the cleaning of flat surfaces (e.g. trolley tops, work surfaces and anaesthetic machines) to remove dust from the perioperative environment prior to the start of the operating list (Gruendemann & Mangum 2001).

Ventilation, temperature and humidity levels are checked each morning by the scrub and circulating practitioners before the start of the operating list. Normal levels of temperature ('22°C–24°C') and humidity levels (50–60%) inhibit bacterial growth and limit the risk of infection for the patient (Gilmour 2005).

Accountability

After checking the operating list, the scrub and circulating practitioners ensure that all necessary instruments and accessories are available for each surgical procedure. Preparation following basic principles and good communication between members of the theatre team are the key to effective clinical practice, safe patient care and a lack of delay in the operating list.

The circulating practitioner opens the instrument set using an aseptic technique, and the scrub practitioner opens and prepares the instruments for the surgical procedure. The scrub and circulating practitioners check the swabs, needles and individual instruments for all instrument sets against the instrument checklist. Any missing or faulty instrument is identified on the checklist. The quantities of swabs, needles and accessories are noted on a white board to highlight the number of each used in the surgical procedure and for checking purposes when the wound is opened and before it is closed to ensure nothing has been left in the wound at the end of the surgical procedure. The surgeon is told when a correct check has been confirmed.

Surgical swabs are manufactured from gauze and have an X-ray-detectable thread within them to enable easy detection should the swab count be incorrect. Differently size swabs, packed in sets of five, are used during surgery and are chosen by the scrub practitioner according to the particular surgical procedure. The insertion of a swab into the wound or body cavity is documented on a white board to ensure it is accounted for during swab checks.

The swab, needle and instrument checks are undertaken to ensure that no item has been left in the surgical wound. A retained swab or instrument is a potential source of infection and can interfere with the correct anatomy of the wound area, leading to bleeding, loss of function or pain (Wicker & Nightingale 2010).

In the event of a missing item, the sterile scrub practitioner should check the sterile drapes and instrument trolley. The surgeon will check the wound, and the theatre team will check the swabs and accessories given out during the procedure, the waste and linen bags and the theatre environment. If the missing item cannot be located, an X-ray will be taken to establish whether the item is still inside the patient. The surgeon will then remove it, and the scrub practitioner will once again check that everything has been correctly accounted for. If the item is not found, the scrub practitioner will document this in the patient's notes and the theatre register, while the surgeon will document it in the patient's notes. This constitutes a critical incident, and incident reporting is then triggered.

It is of paramount importance to complete all documentation accurately at the end of the surgical procedure. It is the responsibility of the scrub practitioner to ensure that the correct information has been written (in black ink and legibly) on the operating list, patient care plan, operation register, specimen container and histology request form. The same rigour must apply to documentation held electronically on the electronic patient system.

The sterile field

The area around the operating table and the patient covered in sterile surgical drapes is known as the sterile field. Only members of the scrub team can enter this area. Maintaining the sterile field is of paramount importance to prevent exposing the patient to a risk of infection. The scrub and circulating practitioners have to follow their duty of care and acknowledge if they break the sterile field. For example, circulating personnel who are not wearing sterile gowns and gloves could accidentally touch the sterile drapes and possibly cause contamination.

All members of the surgical scrub team will undertake a surgical hand-scrub and put on sterile gloves before they enter the sterile field and before preparation of the surgical instruments and accessories. Theatre policies, including scrubbing-up times and the use of surgical cleansing solutions and sterile gloves, should be followed for these procedures.

The circulating practitioner provides the scrub practitioner with the surgical gown and sterile gloves prior to the scrubbing-up procedure, thus maintaining sterility.

Patient positioning

The theatre team, of which the circulating practitioner is a member, transfers the patient from the patient trolley or bed onto the operating table. They position the patient in the correct position for the surgery (Table 8.7). The anaesthetist coordinates the transfer to ensure that the patient's airway is maintained.

Table 8.7 Surgical positions

Position	Description	Surgical speciality
Supine	Patients are placed flat on their back Also used for the transfer of patients from the patient theatre trolley to the operating table, and the operating table to the patient trolley or bed	All surgical specialities
Trendelenburg	The patient is supine with a head-down tilt	Gynaecology The contents of the abdominal cavity fall under gravity towards the diaphragm, making the organs more accessible to the surgeon
Reverse Trendelenburg	The patient lies supine with a head-up tilt	Head and neck and ear, nose and throat surgery
Lateral	The patient is positioned on the left or right side	General, vascular, urology, plastic, orthopaedic, trauma and thoracic
Lithotomy	The patient lies supine with the legs raised and the feet placed in stirrups The lower end of the operating table is removed	Gynaecology, urology and lower bowel surgical procedures
Prone	The patient lies on his or her front	General, urology, orthopaedic

Data from Smith (2005).

Table 8.8 Surgical sutures

Type	Example
Absorbable	
Natural or synthetic Short-term wound support Decomposes; degrades as the wound heals Used on internal tissues Also for subcutaneous suturing of skin	Vicryl Dexon PDS
Non-absorbable	
Resists the body's attempt to dissolve it May be removed after the surface incision has healed Used for suturing fat, muscle and skin	Linen Ethilon Prolene Silk

Surgical sutures

Each type of suture material is coded by a standard colour for easy identification (Table 8.8). The information on the front of each suture identifies the type and length of the suture material, the date of manufacture, the expiry date, the type of needle and its sterility status.

Surgical needles

Surgical needles are identified by their shape and size. Surgical needles vary in size, shape (straight, curved or J-shaped) and type so the practitioner can choose the relevant needle and suture for the surgical incision.

As an alternative to suturing the skin, surgeons can use skin staples to close the wound. These are applied using a skin closure unit that works in a similar way to a paper stapler.

Surgical dressings

The scrub practitioner should be aware of the issues of wound healing and choose the appropriate dressing for the surgical wound. The surgical dressing acts as a physical barrier between the wound and any microorganisms and sources of infection, and also protects the delicate healing tissue. There are many different dressings, each of which has its own properties (Table 8.9).

Surgical drains

Surgical drains – either passive or active (Table 8.10) – are used by the surgeon to remove fluid (blood or serum) from the surgical wound. The surgeon secures the drain tubing with surgical sutures. Dressings are placed around the tubing to help prevent contamination from the wound dressing.

Surgical instruments

The surgeon uses surgical instruments to dissect, resect or alter tissues during the surgical procedure. They should only be used for their intended purpose (Table 8.11).

Table 8.9 Type of surgical dressing

Type of surgical dressing	Example
Passive – a traditional dressing that provides cover over the wound	Gauze and tulle
Interactive – a polymeric film that is mostly transparent, permeable to water vapour and oxygen, and non-permeable to bacteria	Hydrogels and foam dressings
Bioactive – a dressing that delivers substances active in wound healing, such as hydrocolloids and alginates, and collagens	Tegasorb

Table 8.10 Surgical drains

Type of surgical drain	Example
Passive	
The drain involves a piece of tubing (soft latex, PVC, corrugated plastic or rubber) that carries the fluid from the wound site into a bag The bag prevents contamination of the wound and surrounding skin by microorganisms	Corrugated Robinson Penrose
Active	Medinorm
These involve a closed suction drain that prevents contamination of the wound The negative pressure creates a suction and drains the fluid via a tube into the container (concertina drain, expelled bulb or re-evacuated bottle)	

Surgical specialities

The variety of different surgical specialities undertaken in the theatre environment can vary between theatre departments. Within each speciality, elective (planned) and emergency minor, intermediate and major surgical procedures are undertaken (Table 8.12).

Recovery

Following surgery, all patients are admitted to a recovery area – the post-anaesthetic care unit (PACU) – where they will be cared for in the immediate postoperative period. Practitioners working in the PACU will deliver one-to-one patient care. They will receive a comprehensive handover from the anaesthetist that should include:

- the patient's name;
- the operation or procedure that has been undertaken;
- the type of anaesthetic delivered – spinal, epidural or general anaesthetic;
- the intraoperative management in terms of airway management, observations (vital signs recordings), positioning, warming devices, prophylaxis for deep vein thrombosis, and the drugs and fluids administered;

Table 8.11 Surgical instrumentation

Instrument	Action
Sponge-holding forceps	To hold a swab used in prepping the patient or swabbing a wound
Scalpel/blade	To make an incision
Tissue forceps – with teeth at the end of the forceps	To hold or grasp soft issue
Artery forceps – curved or straight	To clamp or dissect arteries or veins, and to hold small swabs (pledgets)
Dissecting forceps ● Non-toothed (internal tissues) ● Toothed (external tissues – skin or muscle)	To hold tissue when the surgeon is suturing or dissecting it
Dissecting scissors – curved	To dissect tissue
Scissors – curved or straight	To cut tissue or sutures
Needle holder Lightweight needle holder for vascular surgery	To hold and support the suture needle
Retractor (hand-held or self-retaining)	To retract tissue
Towel clip Tapes	To hold surgical drapes in place
Diathermy – monopolar or bipolar	To coagulate, fulgurate and cut tissue
Suction	To remove blood, debris or fluid

- information relating to immediate post-surgery care, for example surgical drains and wound care;
- post-anaesthesia instructions for PACU;
- postoperative instructions for the ward.

It is the responsibility of the recovery practitioner to ask the anaesthetist to stay with their patient until the recovery practitioner is confident of safely and effectively continuing the patient's care.

While obtaining the handover, the practitioner will be observing the patient's airway and recording their vital signs every 5 minutes for 20–30 minutes (Table 8.13).

The PACU documentation will often integrate an early warning score (EWS). This is a tool that is used throughout ward areas in many hospitals as an alert system for deteriorating patients. The rationale behind it is to encourage early recognition of the deteriorating patient and, if necessary, to initiate treatment to prevent further deterioration. The scoring system is numerical, aiming for a score of below 3 for a recovering patient. As Table 8.14 shows, different parameters are given a different numerical value, with the extremes of parameters having the highest scores. The numerical values for the different parameters are added together to determine the EWS, which should then be used in conjunction with the referral guidelines (Rees 2003; Avard *et al.* 2011). A score of 3 for any single parameter or a total score of 3 is a trigger for action (Health Service Executive 2011).

However, in PACU, a high number of patients will initially trigger an alert just by the nature of having undergone an anaesthetic. This should be taken into consideration, and a number of PACUs now have a modified early warning system (MEWS) for use in the immediate postoperative phase (Subbe *et al.* 2001).

Table 8.12 Surgical specialties

Speciality	Surgery – medical system, condition or diseases	Examples of surgical procedures within the identified surgical speciality
General surgery – open and laparoscopic surgery	Digestive system Thyroid gland	Appendicectomy Thyroidectomy Laparoscopic cholecystectomy
Vascular surgery	Circulatory system	Embolectomy Repair of aortic aneurysm
Gynaecological – open and laparoscopic surgery	Female reproductive system	Dilation and curettage Hysterectomy Laparoscopic sterilisation
Urology – laparoscopic and open surgery	Urinary tract Prostrate gland (male patients)	Cystoscopy Transurethral resection of the prostrate
Plastic surgery	Medical conditions and diseases of the limb and breast Reconstructive surgery	Removal of a breast lump Mastectomy
Otolaryngology (ear, nose and throat)	Ear, nose and throat	Adenoidectomy Submucous resection of the nasal septum Mastoidectomy
Maxillofacial and oral surgery	Head, neck and dental specialities Reconstructive surgery	Removal of wisdom teeth
Ophthalmology	Components of the eye and surrounding tissues	Lens implantation for cataract Squint correction
Orthopaedic surgery	Preservation, restoration and repair of the bones, ligaments and muscles	Arthroscopy Total knee surgery
Trauma surgery	Emergency surgery for fractures	Reduction of fractures of the wrist, humerus, tibia and fibula
Cardiac surgery	Circulatory and cardiovascular systems	Open heart surgery Coronary heart bypass
Bariatric surgery	Surgery to reduce obesity	Gastric bypass Gastric banding Gastric balloon

Table 8.13 Basic observations in recovery

Monitoring	Considerations
Airway	Is the airway patent? What type of airway is *in situ*? If patients are maintaining their own airway, is the oxygen delivery device appropriate? Is the oxygen flowing at an appropriate volume or percentage to meet the patient's needs?
Breathing (respiratory rate) (see the text for more information on the early warning score)	Is the patient breathing spontaneously? What is the respiratory rate? What is the depth of breathing – is it shallow or deep? Are the patient's chest movements symmetrical?
Blood pressure (see the text for more information on the early warning score)	Is the blood pressure within normal parameters for this patient? What was the intraoperative blood pressure? What was the preoperative baseline blood pressure? What is the patient's capillary refill time?
Oxygen saturation	Are the oxygen saturation levels within acceptable parameters? Look at the patient's colour Does the patient look adequately oxygenated?
ECG (heart rate and rhythm) (see the text for more information on the early warning score)	What is the patient's heart rate? (<40 beats per minute = an early warning score of 2; 41–50 beats per minute = a score of 1) Is it within normal parameters? Is the patient or bradycardic (<50 beats per minute) or tachycardic (>100 beats per minute)?
Pain score	A variety of pain scores are available; an example is a score of 0–3 with 0 = no pain, 1 = mild pain, 2 = moderate pain, and 3 = severe pain Has an analgesic regimen been prescribed?
Nausea and vomiting	Does the patient feel nauseated or have they vomited? What type of surgery have they had? Have antiemetics been prescribed?
Temperature	Is the patient too cold or too warm? Are they shivering or sweating?
Sedation score (conscious level)	An example of a scoring system for conscious level is the AVPU, where patients are categorised as A = alert, V = responds to voice, P = responds to pain, or U = unconscious
Urine output in catheterised patients (see the text for more information on the early warning score)	See the hospital's policy As an example, urine output can be monitored in millilitres over a 4-hour period, with >160 mL being an average

Table 8.14 An example of physiological parameters used in EWS systems

EWS	3	2	1	0	1	2	3
Respiratory rate (breaths per minute)	<8			9–20	21–30	31–35	≥36
Heart rate (beats per minute)	<40		41–50	51–91	91–110	111–130	>130
Temperature (°C)	<34	34.1–35	35.1–36	36.1–37.9	38–38.5	≥38.6	
Oxygen saturation (%)	<84	85–89	90–92	≥93			
Urine output during 4 hours	<80 mL	81–119 mL		120–800 mL	>800 mL		
Or							
Urine output during 24 hours	<480 mL	480–719 mL		720–4800 mL	>4800 mL		

Postoperative nausea and vomiting

Active vomiting can have a detrimental effect on the patient not only in terms of its being an unpleasant experience, but also because the physical strain can cause damage to sutured incision sites, surgical flaps and anastomosis sites. Any patient may suffer from postoperative nausea and vomiting (PONV), but there are certain factors that may increase its risk, for example:

- surgical interventions;
- factors related to the patient;
- the type of anaesthesia;
- drugs that are known to induce nausea and vomiting, for example opiates;
- the physiological condition of the patient in PACU.

The physiology of vomiting is relatively complex, but having an understanding of how it works enables treatment plans to be formulated. Antiemetic regimens will involve more than one group of drugs as this offers the ability for each drug group to target a specific site of action.

Pain management

Pain management is often addressed and planned prior to surgery so that pain is managed proactively rather reactively once the patient is out of theatre. However, patients do not always respond to pain in the same way, so pain management regimens are dependent on using effective communication skills to elicit information on how much pain patients are suffering and what type of pain it is. It is important to obtain a detailed handover to establish whether the patient has had an analgesic in theatre and if so what type, for example an opiate, non-steroidal anti-inflammatory drug or paracetamol.

Not all pain experienced in recovery can be attributed to surgery; other factors contributing to pain – headaches, bladder distension, pain from positioning, etc. – may need to be considered. It is important to assess the nature and cause of any pain, and a number of tools have been devised to establish severity of pain, including visual and verbal pain scales. As with any drugs that are administered to a patient, there are a number of issues to consider, including what analgesic drugs are available, the pharmacology of these drugs, their indications and contraindications, and also their interactions.

Patients who have been administered opioids will need to be closely monitored for a longer period of time in recovery as opioids can have a number of adverse effects, including respiratory depression and nausea and vomiting.

Any drugs administered in the recovery area should be documented in the patient's recovery care plan. Details required include the drug administered, the dose of the drug, the route by which it was delivered and the time at which it was delivered This record will then be signed by the person who administered the drug.

Specific criteria from PACU are often utilised in recovery and should be met prior to the patient returning to the ward.. These criteria are variable and are adapted for individual recovery areas, often depending on the types of patient and the surgical procedures undertaken. They offers guidance (Association of Anaesthetists of Great Britain and Ireland, 2001) on the minimum safe requirements for vital signs, including:

- conscious level;
- oxygen saturation levels and respiratory rate;
- blood pressure;
- heart rate;
- temperature;
- pain and PONV scores;
- urine output in catheterised patients.

To complete the patients' journey through the theatre department, a comprehensive and succinct handover to the ward staff is necessary. This is carried out verbally as well as being documented in the patient's notes. It will include all vital signs, any infusions (epidurals, intravenous lines, etc.) and information relating to the dressings, drains and irrigation systems used intraoperatively.

Conclusion

The role of the nurse working in the operating theatre is multifaceted, including patient assessment before, during and after surgery, advocacy, risk management and quality assurance. Providing an efficient and safe environment for patients and staff requires that members of the multidisciplinary team work and communicate collaboratively. It also requires the use of clearly defined and documented local, national and/or international policies by all those involved in providing this service.

Now visit the companion website and test yourself on this chapter:
www.wileyfundamentalseries.com/medicalnursing

References

Association of Anaesthetists of Great Britain and Ireland (2001) *Immediate Post Anaesthetic Care*. London: AAGBI.

Association of Anaesthetists of Great Britain and Ireland (2010) *AAGBI Safety Guideline. Management of Severe Local Anaesthetic Toxicity*. London: AAGBI.

Avard, B., McKay, H., Slater, N., Lamberth, P., Daveson, K. & Mitchell, I. (2011) *Training Manual for the National Early Warning Score and associated Education Programme*. Dublin: Health Service Executive.

Davey, A. & Ince, C.S. (2000) *Fundamentals of Operating Theatre Practice*. Cambridge: Cambridge University Press.

Gilmour, D. (2005) Infection control principles. Cited in: Woodhead, K. & Wicker, P. (eds) *A Textbook of Perioperative Care* (p. 89). Edinburgh: Elsevier Churchill Livingstone.

Gruendemann, B. & Mangum, S.S. (2001) *Infection Prevention in Surgical Settings*. St Louis: WB Saunders.

Gwinnutt, C. (2008) *Clinical Anaesthesia*, 3rd edn. Oxford: Wiley & Sons.

Health Service Executive (HSE) (2011) *Training Manual for the National Early Warning Score and associated Education Programme*. Retrieved 22nd May 2013 from http://www.hse.ie/eng/about/Who/clinical/natclinprog/acutemedicineprogramme/earlywarningscore/compass.pdf.

National Institute for Health and Clinical Excellence (2010) *CG92 Venous Thromboembolism – Reducing the Risk: Full Guideline. Clinical Guideline No. 92*. Retrieved 20th May 2013 from http://guidance.nice.org.uk/CG92/Guidance/pdf/English.

National Institute for Health and Clinical Excellence (2008) *Perioperative Hypothermia (Inadvertent): Full Guideline. Clinical Guideline No. 65*. Retrieved 20th May 2013 from http://guidance.nice.org.uk/CG65/Guidance/pdf/English.

National Patient Safety Agency (2005) *Annual Report and Accounts*. London: The Stationery Office.

Rees, J.E. (2003) *Early Warning Scores*. Update in *Anaesthesia* 17(10). Retrieved 6th November 2011 from http://www.nda.ox.ac.

Rowley, S., Clare, S., Macqueen, S. & Molyneux, P. (2010) ANTTV2: an updated practice framework for aseptic technique. *British Journal of Nursing*, **19**(5):s5–10.

Smith, C.(2005) Care of the patient undergoing surgery. Cited in Woodhead, K. & Wicker, P. (eds), *A Textbook of Perioperative Care* (pp. 161–80). Edinburgh: Churchill Livingstone.

Subbe, C.P., Kruger, M., Rutherford, P. & Gemmel, L. (2001) *Validation of Modified Early Warning Scores in Medical Admissions*. Retrieved 6th November 2011 from http://www.qjmed.oxfordjournals.org.

Wicker, P. & Nightingale, A. (2010) Patient care during surgery. Cited in Wicker, P. & O'Neill, J. (eds), *Care of the Perioperative Patient* (pp. 339–78). Oxford: Wiley Blackwell.

Wicker, P. & O'Neill, J. (2010) *Care of the Perioperative Patient*, 2nd edn. Oxford: Wiley Blackwell.

World Health Organization (2009) *Guidelines for Hand Hygiene in Health Care*. Retrieved 20th May 2013from http://whqlibdoc.who.int/publications/2009/9789241597906_eng.pdf.

World Health Organization (2008) *WHO surgical safety checklist and implementation manual* Retrieved 20th May 2013 from http://who.int/patientsafety/safesurgery/ss_checklist/en/.

9 Principles of high-dependency nursing

Tina Day

Florence Nightingale School of Nursing and Midwifery, King's College London, London, UK

Contents

Introduction 125
The high-dependency environment 125
Current policy in high-dependency care 125
Technological developments in high-dependency care 126
The role of the nurse as a member of the high-dependency team 126
Nursing assessment and monitoring of the highly dependent patient 127
Respiratory assessment, monitoring and intervention 128
Cardiovascular assessment, monitoring and intervention 132
Neurological assessment, monitoring and intervention 135
Conclusion 138
References 138

Learning outcomes

Having read this chapter, you will be able to:

- Understand the role and function of high-dependency care in the UK
- Recognise early signs of deterioration and identify appropriate nursing interventions
- Demonstrate an understanding of how to assess a patient's respiratory, cardiovascular and neurological status
- Discuss interventions for a compromised respiratory, cardiovascular and neurological status

Fundamentals of Medical-Surgical Nursing: A Systems Approach, First Edition. Edited by Anne-Marie Brady, Catherine McCabe, and Margaret McCann.

Introduction

Critical care is essential and costs the National Health Service (NHS) over £700 million per year (Department of Health 2010). In August 2010, there were around 3463 adult critical care beds across the UK. This included both intensive care and high-dependency beds (Department of Health 2010) and represented a 56% increase in the number of open and staffed beds since data collection commenced in 2000. It is also well recognised that the cost of critical care has continued to increase. The cost of a patient occupying a high-dependency bed is six times that of a ward bed.

The high-dependency environment

Critical care includes both intensive care unit (ICU) and high-dependency unit (HDU) provision, along with services such as operating theatres and recovery areas, and some parts of emergency care. ICU provides care for patients with multiple organ failure or requiring advanced respiratory support, and HDU provides care for patients no longer needing the support of ICU who are not well enough to be nursed on a general ward (Department of Health 2000). Examples of patients requiring HDU care include postoperative patients and patients requiring single-organ support, such as non-invasive ventilation or haemodynamic monitoring. HDU is frequently used as a 'step down' from ICU or a 'step up' from the ward (Sheppard & Wright 2007).

Current policy in high-dependency care

Key policy documents that underpin current policy and practice include *Comprehensive Critical Care* (Department of Health 2000), *The Nursing Contribution to Comprehensive Critical Care* (Department of Health 2001) and *Beyond Comprehensive Critical Care* (Department of Health 2005). The first two documents made recommendations on nurse to patient ratios, patient dependency, and recruitment and retention strategies. Recommendations were also made about ward staff having HDU skills and competencies, and targets were set. On the basis of this, programmes such as ALERT (Acute Life Threatening Events – Recognition and Treatment), CCrISP (Care of the Critically Ill Surgical Patient) and the Modified Early Warning Score (MEWS) were introduced (White and Garrioch 2002; Smith & Poplett 2002; Health Service Executive 2011). Recommendations were also made that critical care provision should be available to all patients 24 hours a day and, if necessary, the ICU consultant should be involved in care outside the ICU (Department of Health 2000; Creed & Spiers 2010).

The nurse to patient ratio for an HDU is recommended to be 1:2 (Garfield *et al.* 2000), compared with 1:1 in ICU (Intensive Care Society 1997). The document *Comprehensive Critical Care* classified levels of care for the critically ill patient (Box 9.1).

Box 9.1 Classification of critically ill patients (data from Department of Health 2000)

- Level 0 – Patients whose needs can be met through normal ward care in an acute hospital
- Level 1 – Patients at risk of their condition deteriorating, or those recently relocated from higher levels of care whose needs can be met on an acute ward with additional advice and support from the critical care team
- Level 2 – Patients requiring more detailed observation or intervention, including support for a single failing organ system, or postoperative care, and those stepping down from higher levels of care
- Level 3 – Patients requiring advanced respiratory support alone or basic respiratory support together with the support of at least two other organ systems. This includes all patients with complex conditions requiring support for multiorgan failure

Box 9.2 Monitoring equipment for HDUs

- Invasive and non-invasive blood pressure monitoring
- Central venous pressure monitoring
- Pulse oximeters
- Arterial blood gas monitoring
- ECG/cardiac monitoring
- Temperature monitoring
- Cardiac pacing boxes
- Resuscitation equipment
- Ventilation facilities (continuous positive airway pressure/bilevel positive airway pressure)
- Syringe drivers
- Patient-controlled analgesia
- Access to services such as theatres, X-ray and pathology
- Portable monitors for patient transfer

The National Institute for Health and Clinical Excellence (NICE) (2007) guidelines on the care of the acutely ill adult make evidence-based recommendations on the recognition and management of acute illness in the hospital setting. NICE (2007) also endorsed the National Critical Care Outreach Forum's (2003; National Outreach Forum and Critical Care Stakeholders Forum 2007) recommendation for a physiological 'Track and Trigger' system. Track and Trigger scores are sometimes referred to as early warning scores, modified early warning scores or even patient at-risk scores. In the UK, a national NHS score (NEWS) is currently being developed and is undergoing a period of consultation (Prytheron *et al.* 2010). In Ireland, the MEWS system is being introduced into all hospitals (Health and Safety Executive 2011).

Technological developments in high-dependency care

The key elements of high-dependency care are a nurse–patient ratio that allows close observation of patients, monitoring of equipment, an appropriate skill mix and competency base, and constant access to suitably qualified medical and therapy staff (Box 9.2). There are also environmental factors to consider, such as building regulations, bed space, electrical sockets, piped gases and suction, and washing facilities, along with air-conditioning, lighting and acoustics (Sheppard & Wright 2007). Computer systems are now commonplace in HDU.

The aim of technology is to reduce the risk of errors. It can, however, also be seen as imposing, intrusive (Akmerud *et al.* 2008) and difficult to get to grips with. In their study, Akmerud *et al.* (2008) found that, in spite of being constantly observed and monitored, patients did not feel as though they were thought of as individual people; they felt like an object or diagnosis. It is therefore important that patient care does not become dehumanised or invisible as a result of technology as this can impact on the provision of care (Barnard 2004).

The role of the nurse as a member of the high-dependency team

Nurses are normally required to undertake additional postqualification education in high-dependency care (Bassett & Makin 2003). High-dependency and foundation courses have been developed in order to prepare nurses who are new to HDU, and a system of preceptorship is in place. The nursing skill mix in HDU is normally based on a 1:2 nurse–patient ratio, with a nurse in charge and often a healthcare assistant or support worker.

The interdisciplinary team in HDU will consist of medical practitioners, nurses and other allied health professional staff. The medical team will be consultant led, but this person can be a physician (or 'intensivist'), an anaesthetist or a specialist consultant. Medical practitioners are also required to undertake additional postqualification education (Bassett & Makin 2003). Physiotherapists routinely see patients in HDU, but referrals are made to speech and language therapy, occupational therapy and psychological services as required. The pharmacist and microbiologist complete the team.

Nursing assessment and monitoring of the highly dependent patient

It is recognised that the longer patients are in hospital before admission to critical care, the higher their mortality (Goldhill & McNarry 2004). Cardiac arrest on a general ward is neither a sudden nor an unpredictable event and, in most cases, is not caused by a primary cardiac event (Nolan *et al.* 2005). Early recognition and treatment of the signs of impending deterioration may prevent cardiac arrest (Smith 2003).

The 'ABCDE' framework for assessing the sick deteriorating patient is now widely adopted. This framework, adapted from the ALERT course (Smith 2003), has been recommended by the Resuscitation Council (UK) (Resuscitation Council 2006) and can be used when assessing and treating any acutely ill, critically ill or deteriorating patient (Jevon 2010). A systematic approach based on **a**irway, **b**reathing, **c**irculation, **d**isability and **e**xposure ('ABCDE') should thus be used to assess and treat the patient (Jevon 2010).

Airway

The patient who is awake and talking will have a patent airway. Signs of partial airway obstruction include diminished air entry (Jevon & Ewens 2007). This can be accompanied by noises such as gurgling, suggesting the presence of liquid in the mouth or upper airway, snoring, when the tongue obstructs the pharynx, or crowing which occurs during laryngeal spasm (Resuscitation Council 2006). An expiratory wheeze can be the result of airway collapse during expiration, which occurs in asthma. In complete airway obstruction, no breath sounds will be heard.

Emergency management of an upper airway obstruction includes simple manoeuvres such as the head tilt and chin lift (Resuscitation Council 2006), suction (Day 2007; Day *et al.* 2009) and airway adjuncts such as an oropharyngeal or nasopharyngeal airways. Endotracheal intubation may also be required. The patient should also be nursed in the recovery position and be given high-flow oxygen (Resuscitation Council 2006).

Breathing

Signs of respiratory distress include tachypnoea, sweating, the use of accessory muscles and abdominal breathing (Jevon & Ewens 2007; Jevon 2010). There is evidence from empirical work (McQuillan *et al.* 1998; Smith 2003) that a fast respiratory rate is one of the first indicators of deterioration. Assessment of breathing will be discussed in more detail later in this chapter.

Emergency management of breathing disorders includes early recognition and assessment, diagnosis and the administration of high-flow oxygen therapy, with a target peripheral oxygen saturation level (SpO_2) of above 94% (Resuscitation Council 2006). In cases of severe chronic lung disease and other risk factors for hypercapnia, the same target $SpO_2$of 94% should be aimed for until arterial blood gas (ABG) results are available.

Circulation

The patient should be observed for colour, capillary refill, heart rate, rhythm and blood pressure (Kisiel & Perkins 2006; Jevon & Ewens 2007). The patient's temperature should also be assessed, along with the urine output. Assessment of circulation is also discussed in more detail later in this chapter.

The emergency management of circulatory disorders includes establishing intravenous access, administration of fluids and control of bleeding. Patients requiring large ongoing volumes of fluid should not be considered stable even if their vital signs appear normal (National Patient Safety Agency 2007).

Disability

Disability refers to an evaluation of the central nervous system (Jevon & Ewens 2007). A full Glasgow Coma Scale (GCS) assessment can be used in cases of head injury or other neurological conditions. This will be discussed more fully later in this chapter. However, a quicker method, the AVPU framework, can be used (Smith 2003):

- A – **A**lert
- V – Responds to **v**oice
- P – Responds to **p**ain
- U – **U**nresponsive.

Along with a central nervous system assessment, hypoglycaemia must be excluded so a blood glucose level will need to be recorded. Normal blood glucose levels are 3.9–6.2 mmol/L (Bersten *et al.* 2004).

In cases of altered consciousness, emergency management is required to maintain a patent airway. The patient should be placed in the recovery position and given high-concentration oxygen therapy. Endotracheal intubation may also be required, and intravenous dextrose will need to be given if the blood glucose level is less than 3 mmol/L (Woodward & Mestecky 2011).

Exposure

Exposure refers to a complete examination of the patient. This is the end of the initial assessment and treatment period. The environment is also considered here, and a decision will be made on whether to transfer to transfer the patient to a higher level of care.

Respiratory assessment, monitoring and intervention

Respiratory problems are a major cause of acute illness and are one of the leading causes of admission to HDU (Moore & Woodrow 2009). A thorough systematic respiratory assessment is therefore vital (Considine 2005).

The assessment should ideally be undertaken in a private, quiet and warm environment with adequate lighting, but this is often difficult to achieve in a busy HDU. Consideration must also be given patient preparation, including positioning (Simpson 2006). According to Bickley and Szilagyi (2008), the best position to assess the patient is the sitting position, enabling access to both the anterior and the posterior thorax.

History-taking

When undertaking an assessment in any practice setting, an accurate patient history is essential (Epstein *et al.* 2003). These details should be clearly documented in the patient's notes and important issues noted such as the history of the presenting condition, the present health status (i.e. cough, shortness of breath or chest pain), the past medical history, the smoking history, environmental exposure, family history and recent foreign travel (Jarvis 2004).

Primary data

Airway patency

A key aspect of the nurse's role in HDU is maintaining airway patency (Moore & Woodrow 2009). It is unlikely that the patient will be intubated, but there could be a tracheotomy *in situ*. In any patient with an artificial airway, periodic suction should always be applied (Day 2007; Jevon & Ewens 2007). The high-dependency nurse should be familiar with this skill (Day 2007; Day *et al.* 2002, 2009).

Inspection

A respiratory assessment should follow a systematic approach (Epstein *et al.* 2003). This includes using the skills of inspection, palpation, percussion and auscultation to obtain primary data.

Inspection will determine the patient's respiratory rate, depth of breathing and breathing pattern, taking account of any potential variations in relation to age or pre-existing medical conditions, such as acute and chronic lung or cardiac disease (Simpson 2006; Day 2007). A normal respiratory rate is approximately 12–16 breaths per minute (Hinchcliff *et al.* 1996). However, an increased respiratory rate may be seen in the presence of disorder. Similarly, a fall in respiratory rate is also a sign of deterioration (Jevon 2010). This can be a result of medication, including opiates, hypothermia, head injury or central nervous system depression (Adam & Osborne 2005). There is evidence from the literature that respiratory rates have in the past been poorly monitored (Jevon 2010). However, this has improved with the introduction of early warning scores (Creed & Spiers 2010).

The thorax should be assessed for symmetry of movement and use of the accessory muscles (Epstein *et al.* 2003). The skin will also be observed for colour, evidence of sweating and scars. Cyanosis is a blue discoloration as a result of hypoxaemia. Central cyanosis is assessed by observing the lips, although in non-white individuals this is an unreliable indicator; hence, the tongue and mucous membranes inside the mouth will be observed instead (Giuliano & Higgins, 2005). Cyanosis is a late sign of hypoxaemia (Jevon & Ewens 2007).

Palpation

Palpation is a sophisticated skill used to obtain data through the use of touch, with the hands employed to compare both sides of the chest (Epstein *et al.* 2003). This is not routinely performed by the high-dependency nurse and is an advanced assessment skill.

Percussion

Percussion of the chest involves tapping one object against another in order for the chest wall and its underlying structures to move (Simpson 2006) so that sounds are produced. This is also an advanced assessment skill.

Auscultation

Chest auscultation is a fundamental aspect of the respiratory assessment as it provides critical information relating to the condition of the lungs (Epstein *et al.* 2003). Auscultation involves listening to breath sounds transmitted through the thorax with a stethoscope (Middleton & Middleton 2002). The diaphragm of the stethoscope is normally used to listen for breath sounds, whereas the bell is used for low-frequency sounds such as heart sounds. A systematic approach should be taken, comparing left with right during both inspiration and expiration (Simpson 2006).

Secondary data

A number of further or secondary investigations can be used to support findings from the primary data. These include pulse oximetry, ABG analysis and chest radiography (Coombs & Morse 2002).

Pulse oximetry

The pulse oximeter is an essential diagnostic and monitoring tool, and is a simple, non-invasive method of assessing oxygenation (Jevon & Ewens 2007). The level of oxygenation is expressed as a percentage or SpO_2.

Table 9.1 Normal ABG parameters

Parameter	Normal values	Interpretation
pH	7.35–7.45	Assesses overall acid–base status of blood. Small changes can be life-threatening
$PaCO_2$	4.5–6.0 kPa	Measures partial pressure of carbon dioxide in the blood. Reflects respiratory control of acid–base balance
PaO_2	12–15 kPa	Measures partial pressure of oxygen in the blood. A low PaO_2 indicates hypoxaemia
HCO_3^-	22–26 mmol/L	Measures bicarbonate levels in the blood. Reflects metabolic control of acid–base balance
Base excess	−2 to +2	Reflects the quantity of acid or base required to restore the blood pH to 7.4. Negative values reflect acidosis, positive values alkalosis

Crown copyright.

The main function of the pulse oximeter is the early detection of hypoxaemia, as cyanosis is a very late sign and is not normally visible until the oxygen saturation falls below 75%. The normal oxygen saturation level is above 95%, although patients with chronic lung disease may have a lower baseline level due to changes in chemoreceptor activity. Pulse oximeters have an important role in HDU and are part of ongoing respiratory assessment and monitoring (Hatfield & Tronson 2009). However, their effects can be limited because, to obtain accurate results, the patient must have an adequate haemoglobin level. Poor peripheral or vascular perfusion will also lead to errors as oximeters require pulsatile blood flow to calculate oxygenation (Jevon & Ewens 2007). Excessive movement from shivering and nail polish or acrylic nails can also lead to erroneous results.

ABG analysis

ABG analysis is the 'gold standard' for assessing and evaluating gas exchange and acid–base balance (Hess & Medoff 1999; Table 9.1). ABG results provide essential information about the patient's respiratory function and metabolic state (Simpson 2004; Allen 2005). Most patients will have an indwelling arterial line in place, which will give continual access to arterial blood for sampling and analysis. Alternatively, ABG samples can be taken from an arterial 'stab', normally from the radial artery (Woodrow 2004).

Evaluation of ABG results is an essential skill for the high-dependency nurse, as these are normally used to titrate parameters such as ventilation settings or oxygen therapy, and for extubation purposes.

Chest X-ray

A chest X-ray can provide a useful picture of any underlying pathology and evaluate the severity of disease. Important information can also be obtained about local or diffuse respiratory problems, such as local consolidation due to an infection or a tumour, or shadowing due to pulmonary oedema (Epstein *et al.* 2003). Chest X-rays also illustrate the position of the diaphragm, the size of the thoracic cavity and lung function. Portable facilities for taking X-rays are available in the HDU as the patient may not be stable enough to be moved to the X-ray department.

Visit www.wileyfundamentalseries.com/medicalnursing and read Reflective Question 9.1 to think more about this topic.

Respiratory interventions

Oxygen therapy

Highly dependent patients are likely to require oxygen therapy throughout their stay in HDU. Indications for oxygen therapy are based on an evaluation of the patient's ABG results and clinical condition (Moore 2007). It should not be forgotten that oxygen is a drug and must be prescribed. However, although there are guidelines from NICE (2004) for long-term oxygen therapy and from the British Thoracic Society (2008) for patients with chronic lung disease, no such guidelines exist for this group of patients.

Oxygen delivery systems are classed as either low-flow or high-flow systems (Pierce 2007). Low-flow systems, such as nasal cannulas and simple face masks, are also referred to as variable performance systems, and the oxygen concentration delivered is dependent upon respiratory rate and tidal volume. Such systems are unlikely to benefit the patient in HDU. High-flow systems are sufficient to meet the patient's oxygen and ventilation requirements as they have a fixed performance and can deliver higher concentrations of oxygen. These include the Venturi mask (Pierce 2007), which can deliver a fraction of inspired oxygen (FiO_2) of up to 0.6 (or 60%). Alternatively, the non-rebreather mask and bag can be used to deliver even higher oxygen concentrations. The British Thoracic Society (2008) stipulates that the non-rebreather bag (using 10–15 L of oxygen) should be used for all patients with trauma, sepsis, shock or other critical illness.

Non-invasive ventilation

If high-flow oxygen is not sufficient for the patient's oxygen requirements, non-invasive ventilation may be required.

Continuous positive airway pressure ventilation

Continuous positive airway pressure (CPAP) is used for patients with type I respiratory (oxygenation) failure. CPAP improves oxygenation by preventing alveolar collapse and increasing the surface area (i.e. functional residual capacity) available for oxygenation and gas exchange (Bassett & Makin 2003; Moore & Woodrow 2009). With CPAP, pressures are constant throughout the period of inspiration and expiration, and this is delivered non-invasively in HDU by a high-flow generator and administered via a face mask (Figure 9.1). However, CPAP may be poorly tolerated, and problems with mask fitting, leakages and pressure sores have been reported (Kannan 1999).

More recently, alternative methods of delivering nasal CPAP using products such as Vapotherm (Vapotherm Inc., Stevensville, MD, USA) and the Nasal Pillows Mask (Fisher Paykel Healthcare Ltd., Irvine, CA, USA) have been developed. These products maintain a low level of CPAP by delivering high-flow humidified nasal oxygen (Moore 2007). There is anecdotal evidence that these products are more comfortable and may be better tolerated.

Non-invasive positive-pressure ventilation

Non-invasive positive-pressure ventilation (NIPPV) is used for patients with type II respiratory (ventilation) failure. With NIPPV, two alternating pressures are set: a higher one on inspiration and a lower one on expiration (Moore & Woodrow 2009). This allows an increase in tidal volume and thus reduces carbon dioxide retention. This therapy is often referred to as bilevel non-invasive ventilation (Moore & Woodrow 2009).

Masks should be accurately fitted for both CPAP and NIPPV so that leaks are avoided (Kannan 1999). Psychological support is also paramount as the patient can feel claustrophobic and isolated, and will require time to adjust to the therapy. Some studies report a high failure of non-invasive ventilation

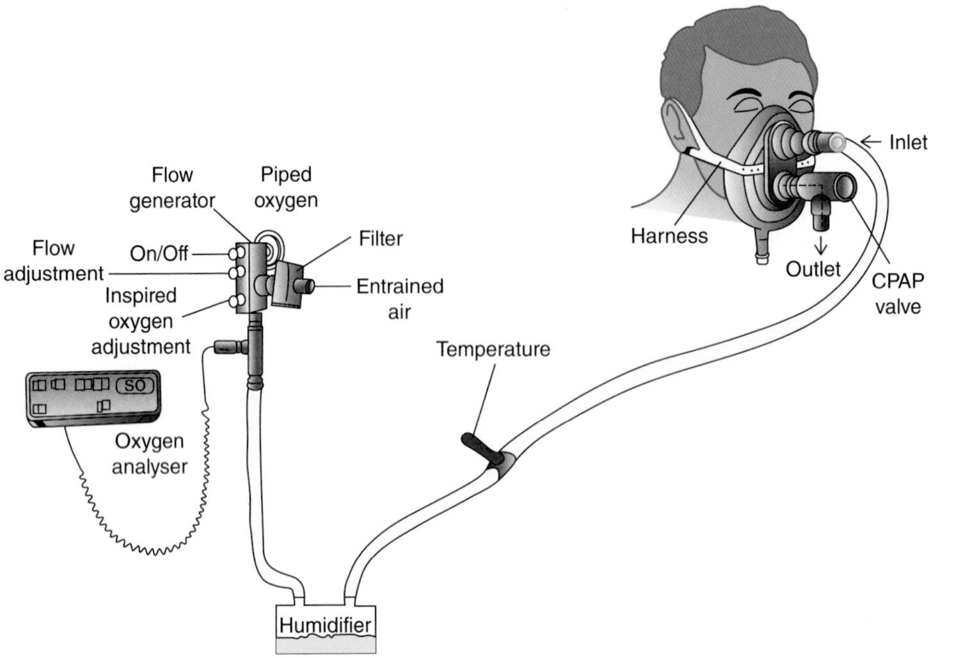

Figure 9.1 CPAP circuit.

(Squadrone *et al.* 2004; Telfer *et al.* 2007) from either refusal of therapy or ineffective treatment. In the event of deterioration, the patient may require transfer to ICU, intubation and ventilation.

Cardiovascular assessment, monitoring and intervention

Alterations in the patient's cardiovascular status are also key indicators of deterioration (Resuscitation Council 2006). Cardiovascular problems can occur as a primary cause of acute illness or as a result of other disorders that compromise cardiac function (Moore & Woodrow 2009).

History-taking

When undertaking a cardiovascular assessment, an accurate patient history is important (Epstein *et al.* 2003). Any history of hypertension, dysrhythmias, circulatory disorders or chest pain should be clearly noted (Epstein *et al.* 2003; Jarvis 2004) along with behavioural issues such smoking or alcohol consumption.

Primary data

Inspection

Alterations in mental status, such as confusion, agitation or lethargy, can be a sign of reduced cerebral perfusion (Robson & Newell 2005). The patient's colour should also be observed and limb perfusion noted. Pale, mottled or cyanosed limbs are indicative of decreased perfusion and increased capillary refill (Jevon & Ewens 2007).

Palpation

Heart rate

In HDU, patients are normally attached to cardiac monitors on which the heart rate is displayed on a beat-by-beat basis. However, the radial pulse should also be recorded manually (Epstein *et al.* 2003). Manual readings will provide information about the regularity of the pulse and its strength and volume, and conditions such as atrial fibrillation may go undetected when pulse readings are taken from automated blood pressure monitors (Moore & Woodrow 2009). A normal heart rate is 72 beats per minute, although this can range from 60 to 100. Heart rates can increase in response to haemorrhage, low blood pressure or sepsis.

Capillary refill

Capillary refill time reflects perfusion (Epstein *et al.* 2003). Pressure should be applied to a finger nail for 5 seconds and then released (Resuscitation Council 2006). Normal capillary refill occurs when colour returns to the nail bed in less than 2 seconds (Gwinnutt 2006). A slow capillary refill suggest poor perfusion. This could indicate reduced cardiac output, vasoconstriction, hypothermia and the influence of factors such as smoking or anaemia.

Percussion

Percussion of the chest involves tapping one object against another in order for the chest wall and underlying structures to move (Simpson 2006) and cause a sound. In this situation, it is used to estimate heart size. This is an advanced assessment skill that is not normally performed by the high-dependency nurse.

Auscultation

Blood pressure refers to the pressure on the artery wall when the heart is either contracting (ventricular systole) or in the relaxation phase (ventricular diastole). A systolic blood pressure below 100 mmHg can trigger early warning scores. There are many causes of hypotension that can affect the highly dependent patient, including haemorrhage, hypovolaemia, sepsis and shock (Dellinger *et al.* 2008).

A more useful indicator of blood flow and organ perfusion is the mean arterial blood pressure (MAP; Garretson 2005). This can be helpful in determining the effectiveness of perfusion to vital organs such as the brain and kidney (Jevon & Ewens 2007). An MAP of greater than 65 mmHg is cited as the minimum perfusion pressure required, although higher pressures of 70 or 80 mmHg are desirable in hypertensive patients (Moore & Woodrow 2009).

Secondary data

Central venous pressure

Central venous pressure (CVP) monitoring is commonplace in HDU. CVP lines are normally placed in either the internal jugular or subclavian vein (Adam & Osborne 2005). The CVP measurement is the pressure of blood returning to the right side of the heart, reflecting the blood volume, vascular tone and heart function (Moore & Woodrow 2009). This value equals the right ventricular end-diastolic (filling) pressure. Normal CVP measurements are 5–10 mmHg from the mid-axilla or 0–5 mmHg from the sternal notch (Henderson 1997).

CVP monitoring allows an assessment of blood volume and cardiac function (Clarke & Ketchell 2011). Other indications include rapid fluid resuscitation, drug administration, parenteral nutrition or the placement of a pacing or pulmonary artery catheter.

A low CVP is indicative of hypovolaemia caused by haemorrhage, fluid loss or poor venous return (Moore & Woodrow 2009). A high CVP can be seen in patients with cardiac failure, hypervolaemia or fluid overload. In health, right-sided pressures reflect stroke volume and ventricular filling, which is normally the same on both sides of the heart. However, in the acutely or critically ill patient, right-sided function may not necessarily reflect left-sided function, and alternative approaches to haemodynamic monitoring may be required (Jevon & Ewens 2007).

Temperature

Core body temperature normally ranges between 35 and 37°C. A temperature of above 37.5°C is defined as a pyrexia and one below 35°C as hypothermia (Marieb 2008). Alterations in temperature are highly significant as pyrexia will increase oxygen consumption (by shifting the oxygen dissociation curve to the right) and hypothermia will reduce oxygen consumption (by shifting the oxygen dissociation curve to the left) (Woodrow 2006). Maintaining temperature within normal parameters is therefore a priority.

Urine output

Other signs of low cardiac output include a poor urinary output (Smith 2003). A compromised cardiovascular system will have an effect on renal perfusion as vasoconstriction will occur. Urine output is therefore an indirect assessment of cardiac output (Jevon & Ewens 2007). It is generally accepted that a urine output of greater than 0.5 mL/kg per hour suggests adequate renal perfusion. A fall in urine output can be an indication of hypovolaemia due to reduced renal perfusion, and if the output is less than 500 mL per day, the kidneys are unable to excrete nitrogenous waste, resulting in urea and electrolyte imbalance and metabolic acidosis (Gwinnutt 2006).

Cardiac rhythm

The highly dependent patient may have developed cardiac dysrhythmias as a result of cardiac disease or in response to other conditions or treatments (Moore & Woodrow 2009). The high-dependency nurse should be familiar with normal sinus rhythm and be able to assess other common dysrhythmias such as tachycardias and bradycardias, atrial fibrillation, ectopics, heart blocks and life-threatening rhythms such as ventricular fibrillation, ventricular tachycardia and asystole (Hatchett & Thompson 2007).

Cardiovascular interventions

Fluid replacement therapy

Patients with cardiovascular compromise may require fluid replacement therapy during their stay in HDU. In hypovolaemic shock, there is inadequate tissue perfusion, and fluid replacement therapy will be required. Although some compensation can occur in the early stages of blood loss, fluid losses of greater than 750 mL are likely to result in physiological changes (McLuckie 2003).

Woodrow (2006) argues that the early detection, prevention and treatment of blood loss is the key to treatment. However, this is also likely to be influenced by the choice of fluids. Restoring the MAP to 70 mmHg is recommended. However, there is much debate over whether colloids or crystalloids should be used (Alderson *et al*. 2004; Table 9.2). Cochrane reviews have generally found no evidence

Table 9.2 Colloids and crystalloids

Colloid	Rationale	Crystalloid	Rationale
Blood	Increases intravascular volume Expensive, risk of reaction	0.9% saline	Expands extracellular fluid compartment
Albumen	Increases intravascular volume Expensive, risk of reaction	5% dextrose	Water moves across intracellular and extracellular compartments
Synthetic products gelatins, starches	Increase intravascular volume Inexpensive, variable lifespan	Dextrose saline	Provides additional electrolytes

to support one as being superior to the other (Alderson *et al.* 2004), although their use may be influenced by cost and availability. As crystalloids move more rapidly across the intravascular and interstitial space, greater volumes are required to achieve the same effect. Colloids remain in the intravascular compartment for longer so smaller volumes are required.

Inotropic support

Drugs to support cardiac function are frequently required in HDU. Patients with cardiogenic shock, cardiac failure or sepsis may require infusions of inotropes to sustain an adequate cardiac output and MAP (McLuckie 2003). Inotropes are drugs that increase cardiac contractility and cardiac output, and agents such as adrenaline, noradrenaline and dobutamine are commonly used to support the patient's blood pressure in HDU (Trim & Roe 2004). These would not be used outside the critical care environment, and the patient requires close observation and monitoring.

Neurological assessment, monitoring and intervention

The patient admitted to HDU may arrive as a consequence of direct or indirect neurological problems. Although patients may be transferred to specialist units, the high-dependency nurse must be able to undertake a comprehensive neurological assessment and facilitate early intervention (Moore & Woodrow 2009; Woodward & Mestecky 2011). Alterations in conscious levels are commonplace in critical care and can either occur suddenly or develop over hours or days (Jevon & Ewens 2007).

History-taking

When undertaking a neurological assessment, an accurate patient history is important (Epstein *et al.* 2003). Any history of changes in mood or behaviour, head injury or seizures should be clearly noted, along with behavioural issues such tiredness, lethargy, altered cognition, hallucinations or motor impairment (Moore & Woodrow 2009).

Primary data

Inspection

The first sign of neurological impairment is often a change in behaviour (Woodward & Mestecky 2011). The high-dependency nurse should be aware of any subtle changes in mood or behaviour and act promptly (Moore & Woodrow 2009).

The AVPU method of assessment, described earlier in the chapter, has now been widely adopted as an easy guide when undertaking an **initial** neurological assessment (Kelly *et al.* 2004). 'Alert' is normal. If the patient is not 'Alert', an assessment must be undertaken. The patient should be asked a question such as 'Hello, are you all right?' If this instigates a verbal response or the patient opens their eyes and looks at the assessor, they are assessed as having responded to 'Voice'. In the event of a lack of response, and taking into account problems such as dysphagia or inability to speak, painful stimuli can be applied (Kelly *et al.* 2004). If the patient does not respond to 'Pain', a diagnosis of 'Unconscious' is made (Smith 2003) and a full neurological assessment must be undertaken. Both Moore and Woodrow (2009) and Woodward and Mestecky (2011) argue that although AVPU is a useful method of assessment, it is not sensitive enough to differentiate between new and pre-existing impairment, nor is it evidence based. It is therefore only relevant to guide early warning scores (Jevon & Ewens 2007).

The GCS

The GCS is the gold standard for assessing consciousness (Woodward & Mestecky 2011). The scale has three sections: eye opening, verbal response and motor response.

Eye-opening

Eye-opening is a measure of arousal; however, this does not necessarily mean that the patient is aware (Woodward & Mestecky 2011). This is always measured first because without it cognition cannot occur (Jevon & Ewens 2007). The maximum score of 4 indicates spontaneous eye-opening, without verbal prompting; a score of 3 indicates eyes open to speech; a score of 2 is to painful stimuli; and the lowest score of 1 is given when there is no response (Jevon & Ewens 2007).

Verbal response

Assessing verbal response is a measurement of awareness or cognition, as speech is a higher level function (Woodward & Mestecky 2011). When assessing verbal response, questions are asked about orientation in time, place and person. The maximum score of 5 indicates complete orientation, whereas a score of 4 means the patient is confused. Lower scores of 3 and 2 indicate inappropriate words and incomprehensible sounds, respectively. The lowest score of 1 is given when there is no verbal response.

Motor response

In assessing motor function, the patient will be asked to obey a simple command such as 'Stick out your tongue'. This will also assess cognition (Woodward & Mestecky 2011). The maximum score of 6 indicates fully obeying commands. If the patient is unable to obey commands, the response to a painful stimulus is assessed. Pain is best applied by the trapezius pinch. The sternal rub and suborbital ridge pressure should not be used as they can cause bruising (Woodward & Mestecky 2011). A score of 5 is given for localising to pain (an appropriate response), 4 for withdrawal to pain and 3 for normal flexion to pain. A score of 2 indicates abnormal flexion, which is often incorrectly identified by nurses (Heron *et al.* 2001), and a score of 1 indicates no response to pain.

The GCS is a useful tool and has been widely tested for validity and reliability (Cavanagh & Gordon 2002; Gill *et al.* 2004). However, as Moore and Woodrow (2009) argue, it does not take into account neurological deficit. If the patient has a hemiparesis, both sides need to be assessed. Scores should be monitored over time and findings interpreted out of the total score of 15. A score of 14 would not normally be a cause for concern, but 13 indicates mild impairment, 9–12 moderate impairment and less than 8 serious impairment, requiring endotracheal intubation for airway protection (Moore & Woodrow 2009).

Pupillary reaction

Pupillary reaction assesses oculomotor cranial nerve function, and compression of this nerve will cause dilated pupils (Fairley 2005). Although not part of the GCS, it is an essential component of the assessment. Abnormalities are associated with brainstem problems. Pupils should be assessed relative to each other and to pre-existing medical conditions such as cataracts or previous eye surgery (Woodward & Mestecky 2011). Medication should also be taken into account.

Pupils should first be inspected to observe whether they are equal in size and an appropriate size for the time of day or amount of light. Their size should be measured. The pupillary reaction should then be assessed by shining a light, such as a pen torch, across each eye, from the outer aspect towards the pupil (Waterhouse 2005). The reaction should be noted. This would be recorded as a brisk (normal) response, a slow (sluggish) response or a lack of response. The consensual reaction should also be assessed by repeating these actions and observing the reaction of the **other** eye (Waterhouse 2005).

Neurological interventions

Sedation

The highly dependent patient may be receiving sedation, the purpose of which is to promote comfort, help the patient to sleep with minimal disturbance, reduce anxiety and facilitate nursing and medical interventions (Gwinnutt 2006). The ideal level of sedation produces a calm and relaxed patient who complies with interventions. However, the effects of over- or undersedation are widely recognised (Gwinnutt 2006).

The most commonly used sedative agents are propofol and midazolam (Gwinnutt 2006). Patients receiving these drugs should be assessed using an appropriate sedation scoring tool on a regular basis. Outdated tools such as the Ramsey Scale (Ramsey *et al.* 1974) can still have a place in HDU, but more recent tools such as the Richmond Agitation Sedation Scale (Sessler *et al.* 2002) are more appropriate for ICU.

The other issue to consider in HDU is the risk of delirium. Up to 80% of patients experience delirium at some stage during their stay (Page & Ely 2011). Many factors contribute to delirium, including lack of sleep, surgical procedures, drugs and age. Tools such as the CAM ICU can be useful for assessing delirium (Page & Ely 2011), and although it may be difficult to prevent, recognising and treating delirium is essential.

Pain control

Pain is assessed under 'Disability' during the ABCDE assessment or when calculating an early warning score (Jevon 2010). Many pain assessment tools exist, but in reality a scale of 0–3 is commonly used whereby three reflects the most severe pain imaginable and zero reflects no pain. This can then be used to guide the analgesic ladder advocated by the World Health Organization (1996). On the first step of the ladder, mild pain, drugs such as paracetamol or non-steroidal anti-inflammatory drugs are administered. The second step, moderate pain, involves the use of weak opioids such as dihydrocodeine or codeine, in conjunction with non-opioids. With the final step, severe pain, strong opioids such as morphine or diamorphine are administered (World Health Organization 1996).

Analgesia can be administered by the intravenous, subcutaneous or oral route in HDU. Patient-controlled analgesia is also used, enabling patients to control their pain themselves within set parameters (applied by a preset dose lock-out). However, although there are documented benefits, there is also evidence that these systems are difficult to use (Mackintosh 2007). An alternative approach for the postoperative patient is epidural analgesia. However, epidurals can cause problems such as hypotension, weakness and numbness, and can even be misplaced (Moore & Woodrow 2009). The high-dependency nurse must therefore be vigilant and follow strict hospital protocols for managing epidurals.

Visit www.wileyfundamentalseries.com/medicalnursing and read Reflective Question 9.2 to think more about this topic.

Conclusion

Caring for the highly dependent patient can be both challenging and rewarding. Not only does it provide the nurse with the opportunity to deliver high standards of person-centred care for an unstable, deteriorating or recovering patient, but there are tremendous learning opportunities as well. The patient is also normally awake and conscious, which makes communication much easier than in an ICU environment. Providing psychological support for patients and their families during this stressful period is a fundamental aspect of care. This chapter has discussed the role and function of high-dependency care in the UK. The importance of a thorough systematic respiratory, cardiovascular and neurological assessment has also been discussed, along with some of the key nursing interventions in HDU.

Now visit the companion website and test yourself on this chapter:
www.wileyfundamentalseries.com/medicalnursing

References

Adam, S. & Osborne, S. (2005) *Critical Care Nursing: Science and Practice*, 2nd edn. Oxford: Oxford University Press.

Akmerud, S., Alapack, R., Fridlund, B. & Ekeberg, M. (2008) Beleaguered by technology: care in technologically intense environments. *Nursing Philosophy*, **9**(2):55–61.

Alderson, P., Bunn, A., Li Wan Po, L., Li, L., Roberts, I. & Schierhout, G. (2004) Human albumen solution for resuscitation and volume expansion in critically ill patients. *Cochrane Database of Systematic Reviews*, (4):CD001208.

Allen, K. (2005) Four step method of interpreting arterial blood gas analysis. *Nursing Times*, **101**(1):42–45.

Barnard, A. (2004) Philosophy of technology in nursing. In: Reed, P., Shearer, N. & Nicholl, L. (eds), *Perspectives on Nursing Theory* (pp. 613–15). Philadelphia: Lippincott.

Bassett, C. & Makin, L. (2003) *Caring for the Seriously Ill Patient*. London: Arnold.

Bersten, A., Soni, N. & Oh, T.E. (2004) *Oh's Intensive Care Manual*, 5th edn. Oxford: Butterworth-Heinemann.

Bickley, L. & Szilagyi, P. (2008) *Bate's Guide to Physical Examination*. New York: Lippincott.

British Thoracic Society (2008) BTS guideline for emergency oxygen use in adults. *Thorax*, **63**(Suppl. VI):1–68.

Cavanagh, S. & Gordon, V. (2002) Grading scales used in the management of aneurismal subarachnoid haemorrhage: a critical review. *Journal of Neuroscience Nursing*, **34**(6):288–95.

Clarke, D. & Ketchell, A. (2011) *Nursing the Acutely Ill Adult*. Basingstoke: Macmillan.

Considine, J. (2005) The role of nurses in preventing adverse events related to respiratory dysfunction: literature review. *Journal of Advanced Nursing*, **49**(6):624–33.

Coombs, M. & Morse, S. (2002) Physical assessment skills: a developing dimension of clinical nursing practice. *Intensive and Critical Care Nursing*, **18**(4):200–10.

Creed, F. & Spiers, C. (2010) *Care of the Acutely Ill Adult: An Essential Guide for Nurses*. Oxford: Oxford University Press.

Day, T.L. (2007) Respiratory assessment in the recovery unit: essential skills for the perioperative practitioner. *Journal of Advanced Peri-operative Practice*, **3**(2):41–9.

Day, T.L., Farnell, S. & Wilson-Barnett, J. (2002) Suctioning: a review of current research recommendations. *Intensive and Critical Care Nursing*, **18**(2):79–89.

Day, T.L., Iles, N. & Griffiths, P. (2009) Effect of performance feedback on tracheal suctioning knowledge and skills: randomised control trial. *Journal of Advanced Nursing*, **65**(7):1423–31.

Dellinger, R.P., Levy, M.M., Carlet, J.M. *et al.* (2008) Surviving Sepsis Campaign: international guidelines for management of severe sepsis and septic shock. *Intensive Care Medicine,* **34**(1):17–60.

Department of Health (2000) *Comprehensive Critical Care: A Review of Adult Critical Care Services*. London: DH.

Department of Health (2001) *The Nursing Contribution to Comprehensive Critical Care*. London: DH.

Department of Health (2005) *Beyond Comprehensive Critical Care: A Report from the Stakeholder Forum*. London: DH.

Department of Health (2010) *Emergency Activity and Critical Care Capacity. Monthly SitReps2010/11*. Retrieved 4th June 2013 from http://collections.europarchive.org/tna/20101125105919/, http://dh.gov.uk/en/Publicationsandstatistics/Statistics/Performancedataandstatistics/EmergencyActivityandCriticalCareCapacity/index.htm.

Epstein, O., Perkin, G., de Bono, D. & Cookson, J. (2003) *Clinical Examination*, 3rd edn. London: Mosby.

Fairley, D. (2005) Using a coma scale to assess patient consciousness levels. *Nursing Times*, **101**(25):38–47.

Garfield, M., Jeffrey, R. & Ridley, S. (2000) An assessment of staffing level required for a high dependency unit. *Anaesthesia*, **55**(2):137–43.

Garretson, S. (2005) Haemodynamic monitoring: arterial catheters. *Nursing Standard*, **19**(31):55–63.

Goldhill, D. & McNarry, A. (2004) The longer patients are in hospital before intensive care admission the higher their mortality. *Intensive Care Medicine*, **30**:1908–13.

Gill, M., Reiley, D. & Green, S. (2004) Inter-rater reliability of Glasgow Coma Scale scores in the emergency department. *Annals of Emergency Medicine*, **43**(2):215–23.

Giuiliano, K. & Higgins, T. (2005) New-generation pulse oximetry in the care of critically ill patients. *American Journal of Critical Care*, **14**(1):26–39.

Gwinnutt, C. (2006) *Clinical Anaesthesia*, 2nd edn. Oxford: Blackwell Publishing.

Hatchett, R. & Thompson, R. (2007) *Cardiac Nursing; A Comprehensive Guide*. London: Churchill Livingstone.

Hatfield, A. & Tronson, M. (2009) *The Complete Recovery Room Book*, 4th edn. Oxford: Oxford University Press.

Health Service Executive (2011) *Training Manual for the National Early Warning Score and Associated Education Programme*. HSE, Dublin. Retrieved 5th June 2013 from http://www.hse.ie/eng/about/Who/clinical/natclinprog/acutemedicineprogramme/earlywarningscore/compasstrainingmanual.pdf.

Henderson, N. (1997) Central venous lines. *Nursing Standard*, **11**(42):49–56.

Heron, R., Davie, A., Gillies, R. *et al.* (2001) Inter-rater reliability of the Glasgow Coma Scale scoring among nurses in sub-specialities of critical care. *Australian Critical Care*, **14**(3):100–5.

Hess, D. & Medoff, P. (1999) Respiratory monitoring. *Current Opinions in Critical Care*, **5**:52–60.

Hinchcliff, S., Montague, S. & Watson, R. (1996) *Physiology for Nursing Practice*, 2nd edn. London: Baillière Tindall.
Intensive Care Society (1997) *Standards for Intensive Care*. London: ICS.
Jarvis, C. (2004) *Physical Examination and Health Assessment*, 4th edn. Philadelphia: Saunders.
Jevon, P. (2010) ABCDE: the assessment of the critically ill patient. *British Journal of Cardiac Nursing*, **5**(6):268–72
Jevon, P. & Ewens, B. (2007) *Monitoring the Critically Ill Patient*, 2nd edn. Oxford: Blackwell Publishing.
Kannan, S. (1999) Practical issues in non-invasive positive pressure ventilation. *Care of the Critically Ill*, **15**(3):76–9.
Kelly, C., Upex, A. & Bateman, D. (2004) Comparison of conscious level assessment in the poisoned patient using the alert/verbal/painful/unresponsive scale and the Glasgow Coma Scale. *Annals of Emergency Medicine*, **44**(2):108–13.
Kisiel, M. & Perkins, C. (2006) Nursing observations: knowledge to help prevent critical illness. *British Journal of Nursing*, **15**(19):1052–6.
Mackintosh, C. (2007) Assessment and management of patients with post-operative pain. *Nursing Standard*, **22**(5):49–55.

McLuckie, A. (2003) Shock: an overview. In: Bersten, A., Soni, N. & Oh, T.E. (eds), *Oh's Intensive Care Manual*, 5th edn (pp. 71–77). Philadelphia: Butterworth-Heinemann.
McQuillan, P., Pilkington, S. & Allan, A. (1998) Confidential enquiry into quality of care before admission to intensive care. *British Medical Journal*, **316**:1853–8.
Marieb, E. (2008) *Human Anatomy and Physiology*, 7th edn. San Francisco: Pearson/Benjamin Cummings.
Middleton, S. & Middleton, P.G. (2002) Assessment and investigations of patient perceptions. In: Prior, J.A. & Prasad, S.A. (eds), *Physiotherapy for Respiratory Care and Cardiac Problems*, 3rd edn (pp. 1–20). London: Churchill Livingstone.
Moore T. (2007) Respiratory assessment in adults. *Nursing Standard*, **21**(49):48–56.
National Critical Care Outreach Forum (2003) *Critical Care Outreach: Progress in Developing Services, Best Practice Guidelines*. London: Department of Health.
Moore, T. & Woodrow, P. (2009) *High Dependency Nursing Care: Observation, Intervention and Support for Level 2 Patients*, 2nd edn. London: Routledge.
National Institute for Health and Clinical Excellence (2004) *Chronic Obstructive Pulmonary Disease: Management of Chronic Obstructive Pulmonary Disease in Adults and Children in Primary and Secondary Care*. London: NICE.
National Institute for Health and Clinical Excellence (2007) *Acutely Ill Patients in Hospital: Recognition of and Response to Acute Illness in Adults in Hospital*. London: NICE.
National Outreach Forum and Critical Care Stakeholders Forum (2007) *Critical Care Outreach Services: Indicators of Service Achievement and Good Practice*. London: Department of Health.
National Patient Safety Agency (2007) *Recognising and Responding Appropriately to Early Signs of Deterioration in Hospitalized Patients*. London: NPSA.
Nolan, J., Deakin, C., Soar, J. *et al*. (2005) European Resuscitation Council Guidelines for Resuscitation 2005: Section 4, Adult Advanced Life Support. *Resuscitation*, **675**:S39–86.
Page, V. & Ely, E. (2011) *Delirium in Critical Care*. Cambridge: Cambridge University Press.
Pierce, L. (2007) *Management of the Mechanically Ventilated Patient*, 2nd edn. St Louis: Elsevier.
Prytheron, D., Smith, G., Schmidt, P. & Featherstone, P. (2010) ViEWS – towards a national early warning score for detecting adult in patient deterioration. *Resuscitation*, **81**(8):932–7.
Ramsey, M., Savage, T. & Simpson, B. (1974) Controlled sedation with alphaxalone and alphadolone. *British Medical Journal*, **2**:656–9.
Resuscitation Council (UK) (2006) *Advanced Life Support*, 5th edn. London: Resuscitation Council (UK).
Robson, W. & Newell, J. (2005) Assessing, treating and managing patients with sepsis. *Nursing Standard*, **19**(50):56–64.
Sessler, C.N., Gosnell, M., Grap, M. *et al*. (2002) The Richmond Agitation-Sedation Scale: validity and reliability in adult intensive care unit patients. *American Journal of Respiratory and Critical Care Medicine*, **166**:1338–44.
Sheppard, M. & Wright, M. (2007) *Principles and Practice of High Dependency Nursing*, 2nd edn. London: Baillière Tindall.
Simpson, H. (2004) Interpretation of arterial blood gases: a clinical guide for nurses. *British Journal of Nursing*, **13**(3):522–9.
Simpson, H. (2006) Respiratory assessment. *British Journal of Nursing*, **15**(9):484–8.
Smith, G. (2003) *ALERT Acute Life Threatening Events – Recognition and Treatment*, 2nd edn. Portsmouth: University of Portsmouth.
Smith, G. & Poplett, N. (2002) Knowledge of aspects of acute care in trainee doctors. *Postgraduate Medical Journal*, **78**:335–8.

Squadrone, E., Frigerio, P., Fogliati, C. *et al*. (2004) Noninvasive vs invasive ventilation in COPD patients with severe acute respiratory failure deemed to require ventilatory assistance. *Intensive Care Medicine*, **30**(7):1303–10.

Telfer, M., Lewin, A. & Jenkins, P. (2007) Assisted ventilation in acute exacerbations of chronic obstructive pulmonary disease. *Journal of the Royal College of Physicians of Edinburgh*, **37**(1):44–8.

Trim, J. & Roe, J. (2004) Practical considerations in the administration of intravenous vasoactive drugs in the critical care setting: the double pumping or piggyback technique-part one. *Intensive and Critical Care Nursing*, **20**:153–60.

Waterhouse, C. (2005) The Glasgow Coma Scale and other neurological observations. *Nursing Standard*, **19**(33):56–64.

White, R. & Garrioch, M. (2002) Time to train all doctors to look after seriously ill patients-CCRiSP and IMPACT. *Scottish Medical Journal*, **47**:127.

Woodrow, P. (2004) Arterial blood gas analysis. *Nursing Standard*, **18**(21):45–52, 54–5.

Woodrow P. (2006) *Intensive Care Nursing: A Framework for Practice*. New York: Routledge.

Woodward, S. & Mestecky, A.M. (2011) *Neuroscience Nursing: Evidence Based Practice*. Chichester: Wiley Blackwell.

World Health Organization (1996) *Cancer Pain Relief*, 2nd edn. Geneva: WHO.

10

Principles of emergency nursing

Valerie Small[1], Gabrielle Dunne[1] and Catherine McCabe[2]

[1]*Emergency Department, St James's Hospital, Dublin, Ireland*
[2]*School of Nursing and Midwifery, Trinity College Dublin, Dublin, Ireland*

Contents

Introduction 143
Historical context of emergency nursing 143
Triage 143
Common surgical emergencies 144
Common medical emergencies 145
Patient assessment in the ED 145
Advanced life support 146
Assessment and stabilisation of emergency trauma conditions 146
Minor trauma 148
Burns 148
Head injuries 151
Assessment and stabilisation of adverse behavioural presentations 152
Care of the critically ill and dying patient in the ED 152
Conclusion 153
References 153

Learning outcomes

Having read this chapter, you will be able to understand:

- The nurse's role as a member of the emergency care team
- The principles of triage
- The principles of advanced life support
- The assessment and stabilisation of emergency medical, surgical or trauma conditions
- The assessment and stabilisation of adverse behavioural presentations
- The care of the critically ill and dying patient in the emergency department

Fundamentals of Medical-Surgical Nursing: A Systems Approach, First Edition. Edited by Anne-Marie Brady, Catherine McCabe, and Margaret McCann.

Introduction

This chapter presents an overview of the role of the healthcare team in emergency care, rapid assessment and the very broad and diverse nature of the types of medical, surgical, social and behavioural conditions that are treated in emergency departments (EDs). Nursing students' experience in EDs is often very limited, but through the use of scenarios this chapter provides an insight into the challenging, dynamic and rewarding aspects of working in an ED.

During your clinical placement in the ED, become familiar with the resuscitation area and how it is prepared for trauma patients. Ask your mentor or preceptor to demonstrate the systematic initial assessment and management of the trauma patient in a simulated clinical situation (although during trauma care training the sequence is presented in a longitudinal process of events, whereas in the actual clinical situation many of these activities occur simultaneously). Finally, observe the assessment, stabilisation and management (including the log roll) of major trauma patients during your placement.

Historical context of emergency nursing

Much like the emergency service itself, emergency nursing has developed over time from the 'casualty departments' of the old voluntary hospitals and workhouses in the UK and Ireland. The term 'casualty' came from the word 'casual', denoting the type of activity of the early departments where patients could access care by 'casually' attending an outpatient department. Despite the introduction of the term 'accident and emergency department' in the UK nearly 50 years ago by the Standing Medical Advisory Committee in the Platt Report (Platt 1962), the term 'casualty' still persists today (Jones 2008).

As with emergency medicine, emergency nursing is a relatively young specialist area of practice: the first Accident and Emergency Forum (now the RCN Emergency Care Association) was established in 1972, and the first accident and emergency course was developed in the UK in 1975. In the years from the casualty service of the 1960s to today's modern emergency care services, the nurse has always been an essential and influential member of the multidisciplinary team. Nurses have pioneered the developments in emergency nursing education (Specialist Certificate, Higher Diploma level), nurse triage, trauma nursing, bereavement care and advanced nurse practitioner services. Despite the challenges, it is emergency nurses who continue to contribute to the debate on how, when and where emergency care should be provided (Jones 2008). Emergency nursing is therefore dynamic, complex and progressive; it is about providing an immediate nursing response to meet the full spectrum of human care (Jones 2008).

Triage

The term comes from the French verb *trier*, meaning to sort or select (Merriam-Webster's Advanced Learner's English Dictionary 2008). Triage originated in the First World War from French medics treating the battlefield wounded at the aid stations behind the front line. It has developed into a system of clinical risk management used internationally in ED departments to prioritise patients' needs (Mackway Jones *et al.* 2006).

A number of triage frameworks now exist, for example the Canadian Triage and Acuity Scale (Bullard *et al.* 2008) and the Australasian Triage Scale (Commonwealth Department of Health and Family Services 1997), but it is the Manchester Triage System that is primarily used throughout Great Britain and Ireland (Mackway-Jones *et al.* 2006). The Manchester Triage System is used to prioritise patients into categories of acuity, which range from life-threatening to non-urgent. The triage category is based on a physical assessment of the patient and accurate history-taking. The signs and symptoms that discriminate between the triage categories are termed 'discriminators' and have been classified (Mackway-Jones *et al.* 2006) into six key factors:

- Life threat
- Haemorrhage
- Pain

Table 10.1 UK triage scale

Category/colour	Name	Maximum target time (minutes) to first contact with the treating clinician
1	Immediate	0
2	Very urgent	10
3	Urgent	60
4	Standard	120
5	Non-urgent	240

Reproduced from Mackway-Jones 2003 with kind permission of Wiley-Blackwell.

- Conscious level
- Temperature
- Acuteness.

Table 10.1 outlines the categories and colour codings of clinical urgency and the maximum target time in minutes to the first contact with the treating clinician. Triage is a brief, face-to-face encounter and not a consultation, should occur within 15 minutes of the patient's arrival or registration and should normally require less than 5 minutes' contact (College of Emergency Medicine *et al*. 2011). Nurse triage should only be undertaken by an experienced registered nurse in emergency care who has received specific training.

The process of triage is based on five steps:

1. Identify the problem.
2. Gather and analyse information related to the solution.
3. Evaluate all the alternatives and select one for implementation.
4. Implement the selected alternative.
5. Monitor the implementation and evaluate the outcomes.

The Manchester Triage Group has produced a list of presentational flow charts for practically all conditions presenting to the ED. These flow charts provide a framework by which the most appropriate clinical priority can be determined. They are too numerous to include in this book but are recommended as an excellent learning resource for students and qualified nurses.

Common surgical emergencies

Surgical emergencies are numerous and varied, and commonly include conditions such as:

- neurological emergencies including skull fractures and head injuries;
- cardiovascular emergencies such as abdominal or thoracic aortic aneurysms;
- respiratory emergencies including traumatic chest injuries, for example flail chest, haemothorax or rib/sternal fractures;
- gastrointestinal emergencies including appendicitis, cholecystitis, abdominal trauma, pilonidal abscess, intestinal obstruction and perforated peptic ulcer;
- genitourinary emergencies such as Bartholin's cyst/abscess and trauma to the bladder or genital area;
- maxillofacial emergencies, for example fractures and/or dislocation of the facial and mandibular bones;

- musculoskeletal injuries, generally due to trauma and including fractures and/or dislocations of the upper and lower limbs, spine, pelvis and neck. Other musculoskeletal injuries include blast injuries and gunshot wounds.

Assessment for all patients presenting to the ED with abdominal pain includes:

- an 'ABCDE' assessment (more details on this assessment are provided later in this chapter and also in Chapter 9);
- urinalysis and culture and sensitivity;
- blood tests (which may include a full blood count, urea and electrolytes and possibly liver function tests);
- an abdominal X ray;
- an ultrasound scan;
- a computed tomography (CT) scan;
- a magnetic resonance imaging scan.

Visit www.wileyfundamentalseries.com/medicalnursing and read Reflective Question 10.1 to think more about this topic.

Common medical emergencies

Medical emergencies are numerous and varied, as can be seen from the following list:

- neurological emergencies including cerebrovascular accidents, meningitis, encephalitis, seizures and altered consciousness;
- cardiovascular emergencies comprising chest pain, unstable angina, myocardial infarction, left ventricular failure, cardiogenic shock or anaphylaxis, and deep venous thrombosis;
- respiratory emergencies such as acute exacerbation of asthma and heart failure, along with conditions such as pneumonia, pulmonary embolism and spontaneous pneumothorax;
- gastrointestinal emergencies, for example epigastric pain, peptic ulcer disease, pancreatitis, alcoholic liver disease, inflammatory bowel disease and gastroenteritis;
- genitourinary emergencies including urinary tract infection, pyelonephritis, retention of urine, renal colic, sexually transmitted infections and priapism;
- endocrine and metabolic emergencies such as hypoglycaemia, diabetic ketoacidosis, hypo- or hyperkalaemia/natraemia, thyrotoxic crisis and hypothyroidism;
- clotting disorders such as haemophilia and sickle cell disease, which are the most common haematological emergencies;
- skin emergencies, for example burns, rashes, urticaria and leg ulcers;
- ENT emergencies including epistaxis, peritonsillar abscesses, tonsillitis and earache;
- other medical emergencies, such as poisoning and drug/alcohol misuse.

Patient assessment in the ED

The management of patients presenting to the ED can be challenging due to the diverse and often complex nature of surgical, medical, traumatic injuries and behavioural and social conditions. The emergency nurse is often the first healthcare professional to assess the patient presenting with an acute surgical condition, so it is essential that nursing assessment is rapid, focused, accurate and continuous. The formulation of an accurate working diagnosis and timely appropriate management is essential in order to reduce overall morbidity and mortality (Small 2008). This requires good communication skills, a knowledge of anatomy, physiology and mechanisms of trauma, proficient assessment skills, critical thinking skills and common sense (Steinmann 2010).

The principles of advanced life support (ALS) are used to assess all patients presenting to the ED. The primary and secondary assessment processes described here can be applied to any emergency

Box 10.1 Primary assessment

A **A**irway (ensure cervical spine support for trauma patients) – patient colour, is the airway open?, is the patient distressed?
B **B**reathing – rate, pattern, effort, sounds, chest movement, oxygen saturation
C **C**irculation – patient colour, pulse rate, rhythm and strength, blood pressure, capillary refill time, blood loss, urine output
D **D**isability – neurological assessment using AVPU (**a**lert, responds to **v**oice, **p**ain, **u**nresponsive), pupil reaction, blood sugar
E **E**xposure – remove clothing to assess for rashes, wounds and thrombosis

Box 10.2 The FGHHI mnemonic

F **F**ull set of vital signs – temperature, pulse, respiratory rate, blood pressure, oxygen saturation, weight
G **G**ive comfort measures – reassurance, dignity, comfort
H **H**istory – past medical history, details related to the present condition, medications, allergies, last intake of food/fluids
H **H**ead-to-toe assessment – including the head, face, neck, chest, abdomen, pelvis and extremities
I **I**nspect the posterior surfaces – bleeding, puncture wounds, oedema, bruising

admission and should be complete within 5 minutes. **Primary assessment** is conducted to identify potentially life-threatening situations and prioritise care. This is done using the ABCDE mnemonic (Resuscitation Council 2010; East 2010; Box 10.1).

Secondary assessment includes a review of ABCDE and continues with the FGHI aspect of the mnemonic (Steinmann 2010; Box 10.2).

A detailed history is taken either following this assessment or concurrently, depending on the condition of the patient.

Advanced life support

ALS is a generic term to describe resuscitation efforts that include a set of life-saving protocols and skills that extend basic life support to further support the circulation and provide an open airway and adequate ventilation. Emergency medical care for sustaining life may include defibrillation, airway management, drugs and medications (Mosby 2009).

ALS may commence in the pre-hospital setting before the patient arrives at the ED. Pre-hospital emergency care refers to any medical care or intervention that a seriously ill or injured person receives from trained personnel before being taken to hospital. In Ireland and the UK, this practice is guided by the Pre-Hospital Emergency Care Council (2008) and the Joint Royal Colleges Ambulance Liaison Committee (2006). ALS guidelines in the UK are produced by the Resuscitation Council (UK) (2010) (Figure 10.1) and the Irish Heart Foundation (which uses the American Heart Association guidelines [2010]: http://circ.ahajournals.org/content/102/suppl_1/I-136) in Ireland).

Assessment and stabilisation of emergency trauma conditions

The majority of people who experience major trauma are under the age of 45 years, and it is the second main cause of death in developed countries (Blank-Reid & Reid 2010). Trauma causes more than 5 million deaths per year (Krug *et al.* 2000).

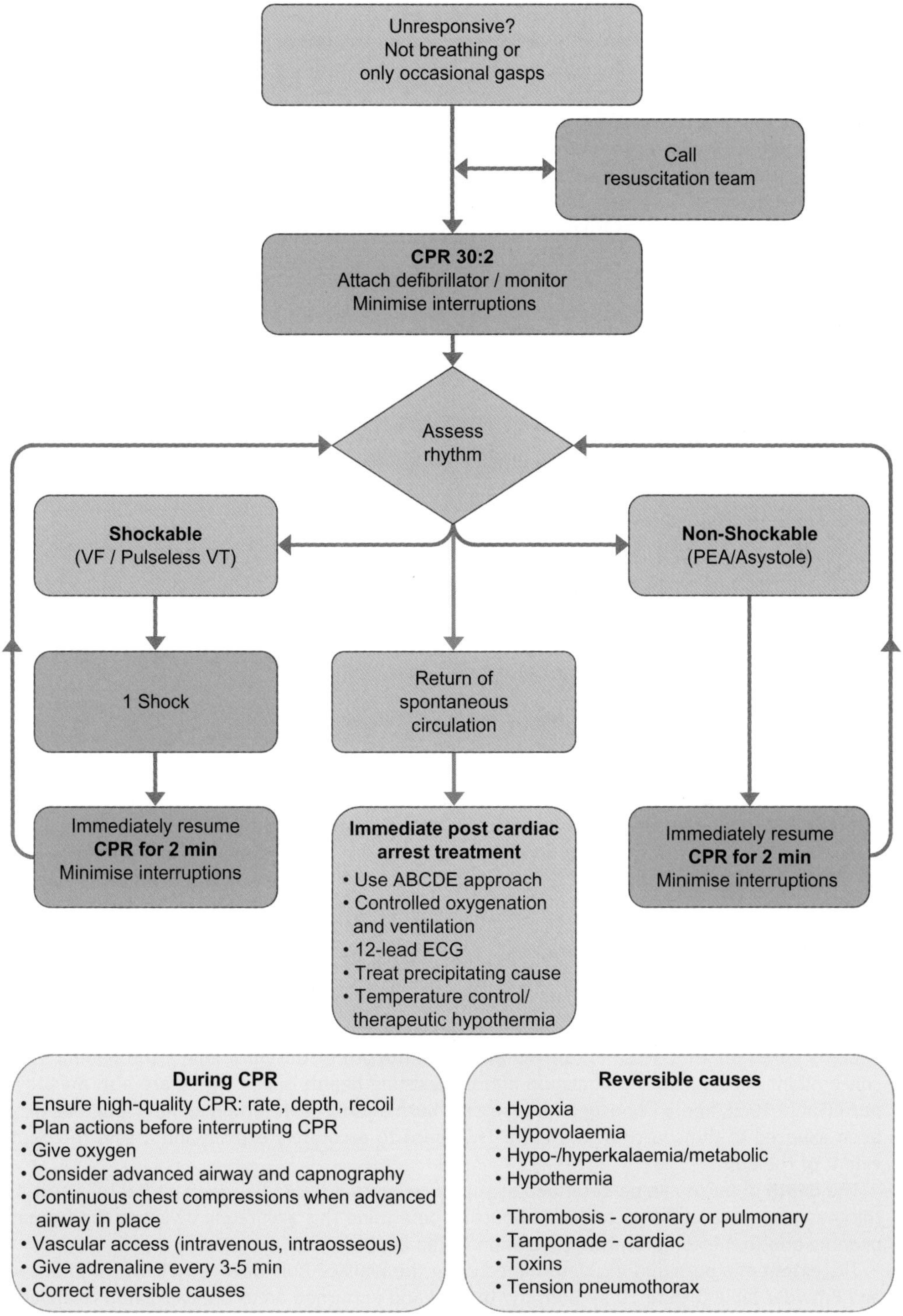

Figure 10.1 ALS guidelines. CPR, cardiopulmonary resuscitation; PEA, pulseless electrical activity; VF, ventricular fibrillation; VT, ventricular tachycardia. Reproduced with kind permission of the Resuscitation Council UK.

The treatment of the seriously injured patient requires a rapid assessment and early intervention with life-saving therapy. Patients are assessed and their treatment priorities established based on the cause and mechanism of their injuries, their vital signs and a primary assessment. The Advanced Trauma Life Support (ATLS) method was developed by the American College of Surgeons and provides a framework for the care of the trauma patient. The hallmark of the ATLS programme is a systematic, concise approach to early care in the 'golden hour' after the injury has been sustained, and is characterised by the need for rapid assessment and resuscitation, which are its fundamental principles (American College of Surgeons 2004). A similar programme, the Advanced Trauma Nursing Course, exists for nurses. The process is known as the 'initial assessment' and includes:

- preparation;
- triage;
- a primary survey (ABCDE);
- resuscitation;
- adjuncts to the primary survey and resuscitation;
- a secondary survey (FGHHI);
- adjuncts to the secondary survey;
- continued post-resuscitation monitoring and re-evaluation;
- definitive care.

Visit **www.wileyfundamentalseries.com/medicalnursing** and read **Reflective Question 10.2** to think more about this topic.

Minor trauma

Some injuries are described as non-life- or limb-threatening, self-limiting injuries (Dawood & Holt 2008). A 'minor injury' as defined generally means a sprain, abrasion, laceration or whiplash-associated disorder. These injuries are caused by torn, stretched or damaged fibres in the muscles, ligaments, tendons or blood vessels, or by damage to tissue. The first aid treatment is an application of ice for 15–20 minutes per hour during the first few hours, which reduces pain and prevents swelling and inflammation.

Burns

People present to the ED with burns that can be classified as minor or major. The severity of the burn injury is based on an assessment of the extent and depth of the burn injury, the patient's age, any concomitant injuries, smoke inhalation and pre-existing health issues. There are also many types of burn (Table 10.2), and a key aspect of assessing burn injuries is determining how long the victim has been exposed to the source of the burn. This helps to accurately explain and assess the depth and extent of the burn.

The **depth** of burns can be described as superficial partial thickness, deep partial thickness and full thickness, but it can take up to 48–72 hours to determine this accurately owing to the formation of oedema and to the compromised circulation (Wraa 2010).

The **extent** of a burn injury is determined using the Wallace Rule of Nines (Figure 10.2) or the Lund and Browder table (Figure 10.3). Both the burned and unburned areas are calculated to ensure accuracy. The exception to the use of these charts is with electrical burns, where the percentage of body surface area is not used to describe the extent of the burn – in these cases, the injury is described anatomically.

Due to the loss of skin in burns, the emergency care of a burn injury focuses on the prevention of infection, on hypovolaemia and on maintaining a normal body temperature. Assessment includes the following steps:

Table 10.2 Aetiology of burns

Types of burn	Mechanism of injury
Electrical	As electricity passes through the body, it meets resistance from the tissue. The smaller the area of contact , the more intense the heat and damage
Chemical	Alkaline substances cause more damage than acids
Frostbite	This is caused by vasoconstriction of the peripheral blood vessels. Intra- and extracellular fluids freeze, forming crystals that damage the tissues
Thermal	Flame, flash, steam, liquid and contact burns

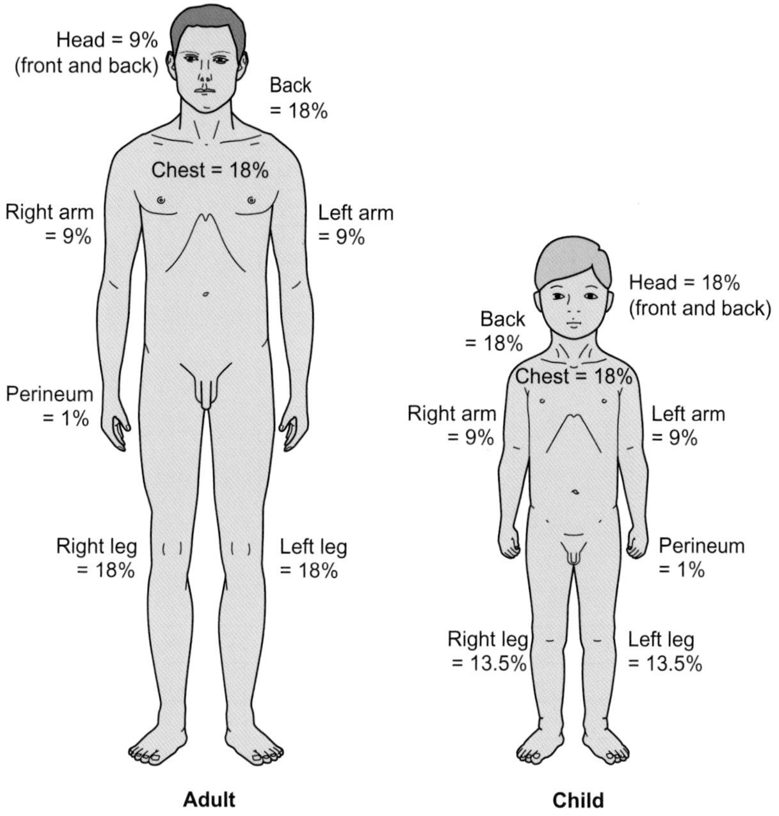

Figure 10.2 Wallace Rule of Nines. Reproduced from Hettiarachty (2004) *ABC of Burns*, with kind permission of Wiley Blackwell.

- Trauma survey – ABCDEF and assess the size and depth of the burn
- History:
  - Time of injury
  - Type of flame, scald or smoke
  - Medical history
- Reassure the patient and family:
  - What is happening now
  - What the plan is over the next 24–48 hours
  - What their level of understanding is.

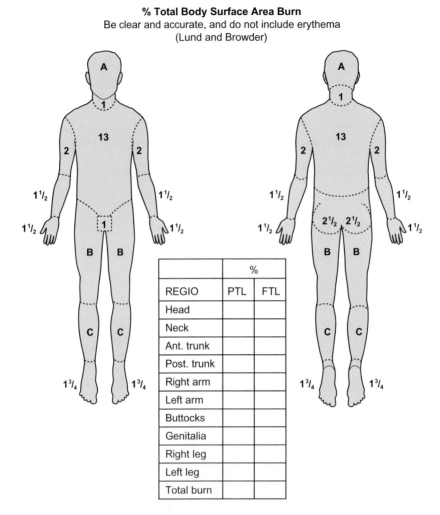

% Total Body Surface Area Burn
Be clear and accurate, and do not include erythema
(Lund and Browder)

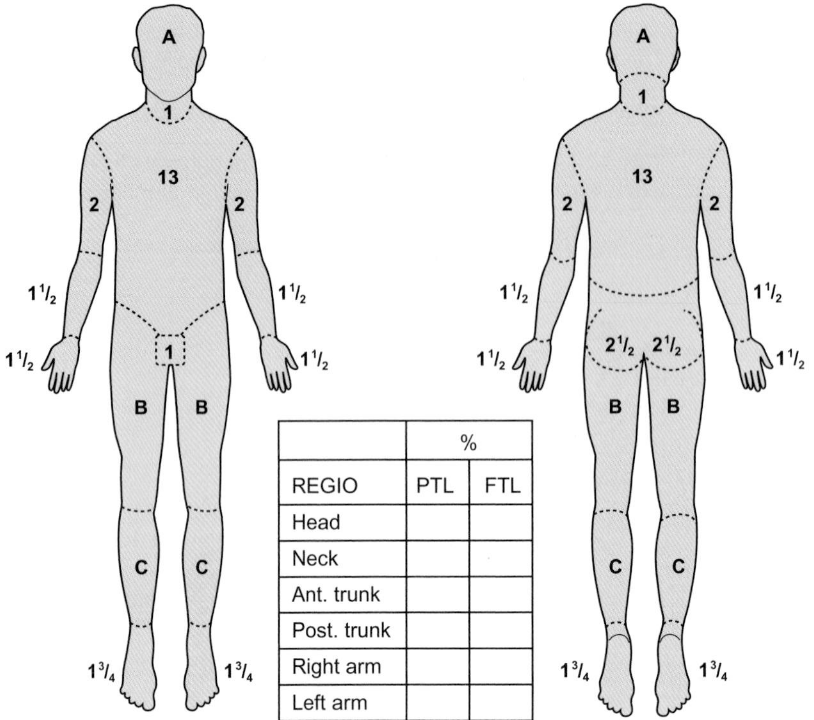

	%	
REGIO	PTL	FTL
Head		
Neck		
Ant. trunk		
Post. trunk		
Right arm		
Left arm		
Buttocks		
Genitalia		
Right leg		
Left leg		
Total burn		

AREA	Age 0	1	5	10	15	Adult
A = $\frac{1}{2}$ of head	$9\frac{1}{2}$	$8\frac{1}{2}$	$6\frac{1}{2}$	$5\frac{1}{2}$	$4\frac{1}{2}$	$3\frac{1}{2}$
B = $\frac{1}{2}$ of one thigh	$2\frac{3}{4}$	$3\frac{1}{4}$	4	$4\frac{1}{2}$	$4\frac{1}{2}$	$4\frac{3}{4}$
C = $\frac{1}{2}$ of one lower leg	$2\frac{1}{2}$	$2\frac{1}{2}$	$2\frac{3}{4}$	3	$3\frac{1}{4}$	$3\frac{1}{2}$

Figure 10.3 Lund and Browder chart. Reproduced from Hettiarachty (2004) *ABC of Burns*, with kind permission of Wiley Blackwell.

If the burn injury is classified as major (more than 20% of the victim's total body surface area being affected), the following are the key points of care in stabilising the patient (Wraa 2010):

- Two large-bore intravenous lines and a central venous catheter should be inserted.
- Take baseline blood samples.
- Insert a urinary catheter.
- Calculate the required fluid replacement from the time of the burn and not from the patient's arrival in the ED – use 2–4 mL × the percentage of the total body surface area burnt × the patient's weight (kg).

- Administer all fluids through a fluid warmer.
- Administer pain relief – short-acting narcotics.
- Dress the wound – clingfilm is ideal for transferring the patient to a burns unit as it does not stick, it protects the wound and it prevents further heat and fluid loss.

Minor burns can be treated with silver sulfadiazine cream (Flamazine) and a dry, secure dressing. In the case of burns to the hands or fingers, Flamazine is applied and the hand is placed in a burn bag (clear plastic) to facilitate movement of the fingers. Dressings should be reviewed after 24 hours.

Head injuries

The National Institute for Health and Clinical Excellence (2007) defines a head injury as any trauma to the head other than shallow injuries on the surface of the face. The Glasgow Coma Scale (GCS; Figure 10.4) (see also Chapter 9) provides an objective, standardised and easily interpreted tool for neurological assessment. The GCS allows healthcare professionals to assess how severely a person's brain has been damaged following a head injury. It scores people on:

- verbal responses (whether they can make any noise);
- physical reflexes (whether they can move);
- how easily they can open their eyes.

The highest possible score is 15, which means that the person knows where they are and can speak and move as instructed. The lowest possible score is 3, meaning that the body is in a deep coma (a sleep-like state in which the body is unconscious for a long period of time). Depending on the score, head injuries are classed as:

- minor – a score of 13 or more;
- moderate – a score of 9–12;
- severe – a score of 8 or less.

Neurological Observation Chart

Glasgow Coma Scale	Eye opening	Open spontaneously (4)	•																(C) = Eyes closed due to swelling
		Open to speech (3)		•	•														
		Open to pain (2)				•	•												
		Closed (1)						•	•	•									
	Verbal response	Orientated (5)																	(T) = intubated
		Confused (4)	•	•	•														
		Inappropriate words (3)				•	•												
		Incomprehensible sounds (2)						•	•										
		No verbal response (1)								•									
		Obeys commands (6)	•	•															
	Motor response	Localises to pain (5)			•														Record best arm response
		Flexion withdrawal (4)				•	•												
		Abnormal flexion (3)						•											
		Extension to pain (2)							•										
		No movement (1)								•									
		Total (out of 15)	14	13	12	9	9	6	5	3									

Figure 10.4 Glasgow Coma Scale. Reproduced from Woodward & Mestecky (2011) Neuroscience nursing: Evidence Based Practice with kind permission of Wiley Blackwell.

With a GCS score of 13–15, any changes in the patient's condition should be monitored closely. Extra vigilance on the part of nursing staff is required with patients who have taken alcohol and/or drugs, which may mask subtle changes. All ED clinicians involved in assessing patients with head injuries should be able to assess the presence and absence of risk factors and the need for CT imaging (National Institute for Health and Clinical Excellence 2007).

Nursing assessment and examination should follow a set or systematic pattern regardless of how severe or trivial an injury may appear. The assessing clinician should establish the history, perform an examination and refer the patient for radiology as appropriate.

Follow-up on discharge

Most minor head injuries do not require treatment. However, the individual should be monitored for 48 hours to check for any changes in their condition, and should be discharged, with a head injury advice sheet, to the care of a responsible adult.

Assessment and stabilisation of adverse behavioural presentations

Behavioural disturbances and aggression in the ED is an increasing problem confronting ED staff every day. The majority of attacks on healthcare workers in general occur in the ED. Patients may self-refer or be referred to the ED by concerned family members or other health professionals, such as GPs or community mental health teams, or may be transported by police or paramedics in an aroused and agitated state for assessment, management and the ruling out of an organic cause for their behaviour. It is the responsibility of the emergency nursing and medical staff to assess and manage these patients properly, without biases, and with the same thoroughness that every patient who presents to ED for treatment is afforded. The risk of violence, i.e. behaviour that involves either a threat of physical or psychological harm to one's self or to others, is considered to be a critical predictor of urgency in mental health triage (Sands 2007).

Patients with behavioural disturbance can challenge clinicians, the nursing and allied staff, and some can even be a challenge to the whole ED, which includes other patients and their relatives. These patients have a high morbidity and mortality rate, and carry a higher medicolegal risk from their behaviour, from injuries they may have obtained or from the underlying organic illness that is causing their adverse behaviour. Emergency nurses and clinicians have a duty of care to these patients to provide assessment and treatment. The challenge is to carry out this duty of care while minimising the risks to the patient, staff and others in ED.

Patients presenting to the ED who are aggressive or hostile towards staff could be displaying behavior that is symptomatic of a number of conditions, including:

- head injury;
- substance abuse and intoxication;
- underlying mental illness;
- hypoxia;
- hypoglycaemia;
- infection – meningitis, encephalitis or sepsis;
- hyperthermia or hypothermia;
- seizures – post-ictally or status epilepticus;
- vascular: stroke or subarachnoid haemorrhage.

Care of the critically ill and dying patient in the ED

Critically ill patients are defined as those patients who are at high risk of actual or potential life-threatening health problems. A critically ill patient is one who has an immediate requirement for any form of organ support (intubation, ventilation or inotropes), or is likely to suffer acute cardiac, respiratory or neurological deterioration requiring such support. The more critically ill the patient is, the more likely he or she is to be highly vulnerable, unstable and complex, thereby requiring intense and vigilant nursing care (American Association of Critical Care Nurses 2008).

Family-witnessed resuscitation is one way of supporting and helping families during a critical or life-threatening event. The family become part of the team by providing support to the patient, which can in turn relieve the sense of helplessness often felt by family members, and enhance communication (Kingsnorth-Hinrichs 2010).

Autopsy remains a very important tool to establish the cause of death in patients dying in ED. The concordance between the ante mortem presumed cause of death recorded in the patient's notes and the real cause is often poor (Vanbrabant *et al.* 2004).

Conclusion

During a clinical placement nursing students will experience or witness the emergency care of patients with a wide variety of acute and possibly life-threatening trauma injuries, acute medical/surgical and behavioural conditions. They will gain an understanding of the role of the nurse in the emergency care team, and observe or participate in the skills of triage, rapid assessment, resuscitation, care of the dying/dead patient and support of family and friends.

Visit **www.wileyfundamentalseries.com/medicalnursing** and read **Reflective Question 10.3** to think more about this topic.

Now visit the companion website and test yourself on this chapter:
www.wileyfundamentalseries.com/medicalnursing

References

American Association of Critical Care Nurses (2008) *Scope and Standards for Acute and Critical Nursing Practice AACN Critical Care Publication, CA*. Retrieved 4th June 2013 from http://www.aacn.org/wd/practice/docs/130300-standards_for_acute_and_critical_care_nursing.pdf.

American College of Surgeons (2004) *Advanced Trauma Life Support*, 7th edn. Chicago: American College of Surgeons.

American Heart Association (2010) *Guidelines for CPR & ECC*. Dallas: American Heart Association.

Blank-Reid, C. & Reid, P.C. (2010) Family presence during resuscitation In: Kunz Howard, P. & Steinmann, R.A. (eds), *Sheehy's Emergency Nursing Principles and Practice*, 6th edn. St Louis: Mosby.

Bullard, M.D., Unger, B., Spence, J., Grafstein, E. & the Canadian Triage and Acuity Scale National Working Group (2008) Revisions to the Canadian Emergency Department Triage. *Canadian Journal of Emergency Medicine*, **10**(2):136–42.

College of Emergency Medicine, Emergency Nurse Consultant Association, Faculty of Emergency Nursing, Royal College of Nursing (2011) *Triage Position Statement*. Retrieved 4th June 2013 from www.collemergencymed.ac.uk/code/document.asp?ID=5898.

Commonwealth Department of Health and Family Services (1997) *The Australian National Triage Scale: A User Manual*. Melbourne: Australian Government Publishing Service.

Dawood, M. & Holt, L. (2008) Skeletal injuries. In Dolan, B. & Holt, L. (eds), *Accident and Emergency Nursing: Theory into Practice*, 2nd edn (pp. 79–122). London: Elsevier.

East, J. (2010) Acute emergency situations. In: Creed, F. & Spiers, C. (eds), *Care of the Acutely Ill Adult: An Essential Guide for Nurses* (pp. 385–425). New York: Oxford University Press.

Joint Royal Colleges Ambulance Liaison Committee (2006) *UK Ambulance Service Clinical Practice Guidelines*. Retrieved 9th July 2012 from http://www2.warwick.ac.uk/fac/med/research/hsri/emergencycare/prehospitalcare/jrcalcstakeholderwebsite/guidelines.

Jones, G. (2008) Nursing in emergency care. In: Dolan, B. & Holt, L. (eds), *Accident and Emergency Nursing: Theory into Practice*, 2nd edn (pp. 1–16). London: Elsevier.

Kingsnorth-Hinrichs, J. (2010) Family presence during resuscitation. In: Kunz Howard, P. & Steinmann R.A. (eds), *Sheehy's Emergency Nursing Principles and Practice*, 6th edn (pp. 148–54). St Louis: Mosby.

Krug, E.G., Sharma, G.K. & Lozano, R. (2000) The global burden of injuries. *American Journal of Public Health*, **90**:523–6.

Mackway-Jones, K., Marsden, J. & Windle, J. (2006) *Emergency Triage: Manchester Triage Group*, 2nd edn. Oxford: Blackwell Publishing.

Mosby (2009) *Mosby's Medical Dictionary*. St. Louis, Elsevier.

National Institute for Health and Clinical Excellence (2007) *Head Injury: Assessment in the Emergency Department*. NICE Guideline No. 56. London: NICE.

Platt, R. (1962) Platt Report. *British Medical Journal*, **2**(5263):1341–2.

Pre-Hospital Emergency Care Council (2008) *A View of Pre-Hospital Emergency Care in Ireland*. Naas: PHECC.

Resuscitation Council (UK) (2010) *Resuscitation Guidelines*. London: Resuscitation Council.

Sands, N. (2007) An ABC approach to assessing the risk of violence at triage. *Australasian Emergency Nursing Journal*, **10**(3):107–9.

Small, V. (2008) Surgical emergencies. In: Dolan, B. & Holt, L. (eds), *Accident and Emergency Nursing: Theory into Practice*, 2nd edn. London: Elsevier.

Steinmann, R.A. (2010) Patient Assessment In: Kunz Howard, P. & Steinmann R.A. (eds), *Sheehy's Emergency Nursing Principles and Practice*, 6th edn (pp. 73–82). St Louis: Mosby.

Vanbrabant, P., Dhondt, E. & Sabbe, M. (2004) What do we know about patients dying in the emergency department? *Resuscitation*, **60**(2):163–70.

Wraa, C. (2010) Burns. In: Kunz Howard, P. & Steinmann R.A. (eds), *Sheehy's Emergency Nursing Principles and Practice*, 6th edn (pp. 340–54). St Louis: Mosby.

Part 2

Adult Medical and Surgical Nursing

Chapter 11	Nursing care of conditions related to the skin	156
Chapter 12	Nursing care of conditions related to the respiratory system	176
Chapter 13	Nursing care of conditions related to the circulatory system	210
Chapter 14	Nursing care of conditions related to the digestive system	240
Chapter 15	Nursing care of conditions related to the urinary system	262
Chapter 16	Nursing care of conditions related to the endocrine system	298
Chapter 17	Nursing care of conditions related to the neurological system	326
Chapter 18	Nursing care of conditions related to the immune system	364
Chapter 19	Nursing care of conditions related to haematological disorders	386
Chapter 20	Nursing care of conditions related to the musculoskeletal system	422
Chapter 21	Nursing care of conditions related to the ear, nose, throat and eye	448
Chapter 22	Nursing care of conditions related to reproductive health	478

11

Nursing care of conditions related to the skin

Zena Moore[1] and Julie Jordan O'Brien[2]

[1]*Faculty of Nursing and Midwifery, Royal College of Surgeons in Ireland, Dublin, Ireland*
[2]*Beaumont Hospital, Dublin, Ireland*

Contents

Introduction	157
The structure and function of the skin	157
Maintaining normal tissue integrity	158
Skin assessment	158
Treatments	160
Common skin diseases	161
Wound healing	165
Wound assessment	167
Wound management	168
Surgical wounds	169
Pressure ulcers	170
Conclusion	172
References	173

Learning outcomes

Having read this chapter, you will be able to:

- Understand and describe the structure and function of the skin
- Understand and describe the pathophysiology of wound healing
- Understand the key components in the assessment of patients with altered tissue integrity
- Understand and describe the most commonly encountered dermatological disorders
- Describe the importance of wound assessment in determining nursing priorities for managing patients with wounds
- Understand the key factors in preventing and managing wounds

Fundamentals of Medical-Surgical Nursing: A Systems Approach, First Edition. Edited by Anne-Marie Brady, Catherine McCabe, and Margaret McCann.

Introduction

This chapter provides an overview of the anatomy, physiology and related disorders of the skin. The nursing assessment, diagnosis and management of skin disorders are also outlined. Case scenarios relating to skin disorders are provided to enhance learning through reflection and discussion.

The structure and function of the skin

The skin is the largest organ of the body and has five main functions: protection, sensation, storage, absorption and heat regulation. The skin is composed of two distinct parts – a superficial layer, the epidermis, and a deeper layer, the dermis (Figure 11.1). The epidermis provides a physical barrier and tissue strength. It is avascular with four separate layers: the stratum corneum (horny layer), stratum granulosum (granular cell layer), stratum spinosum (prickle cell layer) and stratum basale (basal cell layer). The thickness of the epidermis differs across the body, with the soles of the feet and the palms of the hands displaying the thickest layers. The epidermis has a high cell turnover, with surface cells continuously rubbing off and regenerating (Martin 1997).

The dermis is made up of connective tissue, composed of fibroblasts, dermal dendrocytes, mast cells, lymphocytes and macrophages, and blood vessels and lymphatics (Tortora & Derrickson 2011). It provides tissue strength and helps to dissipate external pressure (Bridel-Nixon 1997). Subcutaneous

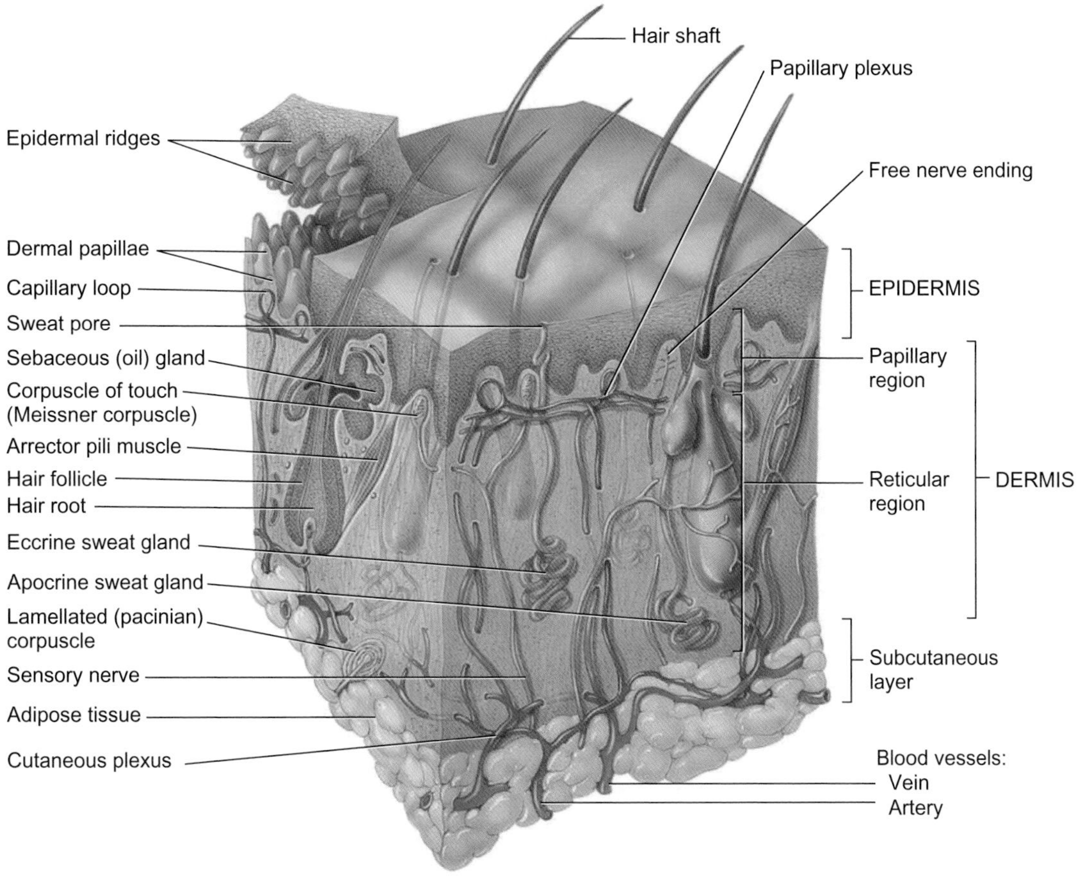

Figure 11.1 Sectional view of skin and subcutaneous layer. Reproduced from Tortora G.J., Derrickson, B. (2011) *Principles of Anatomy and Physiology*, with kind permission of Wiley Blackwell.

tissue lies beneath the dermis. It is made up of loose connective tissue and fat, which provides padding and protection of the bony prominences As the individual ages, the elasticity and resilience of the skin is reduced (Waller & Maibach 2005).

Maintaining normal tissue integrity

A sufficient supply of oxygen and nutrients, the removal of the waste products of cell respiration, and proliferation are essential to maintain healthy tissue. Central to this function are the circulatory and lymphatic systems. The circulatory system is responsible for the delivery of oxygen and nutrients to the tissue and the removal of carbon dioxide and waste products following cell metabolism. The lymphatic system is akin to a drainage system, removing surplus fluid and protein from the tissue spaces (Reddy 1990). It also transports waste products from the cells to the circulatory system, as the wall of the lymph capillary is more permeable than the blood capillaries, so substances can diffuse more readily into the lymphatic system (Reddy 1990).

Waste products, such as carbon dioxide and other by-products of cell respiration and activity, diffuse from the cells into the interstitial fluid and from there diffuse into the capillaries for elimination by the body in sweat or in urine.

Skin assessment

A structured and systematic approach to skin assessment is essential and should be part of the day-to-day care of all patients (Holloway & Jones 2005). It is important to identify any existing skin problems, as well as assess potential risk factors that may influence the integrity of the skin. Skin disorders are by nature visible, so use of the eyes, ears, touch and smell, together with a detailed clinical history, is essential for undertaking a comprehensive examination of the skin (Johannsen 2005).

Setting and equipment

The room should be warm and bright, and have fluorescent lighting to determine changes in the skin. An observant eye, a sensitive touch, a flexible metric ruler, a small torch and a magnifying glass should be available. The patient should wear a disposable gown, leaving their underwear on, so that all areas can be examined; covering the patient with a drape when possible will ensure comfort and dignity (Cole & Gray-Miceli 2002).

The patient's history

The following information (Cole & Gray-Miceli 2002) should be collected:

- Demographic information: name, address, contact telephone numbers, age, gender, ethnicity, marital status, occupation, education and religion.
- At the start, the patient's own words regarding their condition. The nurse gains a sense of direction about which triage questions to ask, for example, 'When did the rash start?' An allergic reaction may involve swelling of the tongue, which would require prompt reaction to prevent anaphylaxis.
- From the 'OLD CARTS' mnemonic, the **o**nset, **l**ocation, **d**uration, **c**haracteristics, **a**ssociated symptoms, **r**elieving factors, **t**iming and **s**everity of the condition.
- The medications and treatments tried.
- The past medical history.
- The family history.
- The patient's social habits – alcohol, tobacco, recreational drugs, diet, exercise, exposure to toxins and sun, and sexual habits.
- Travel – any domestic and international travel in the past year.

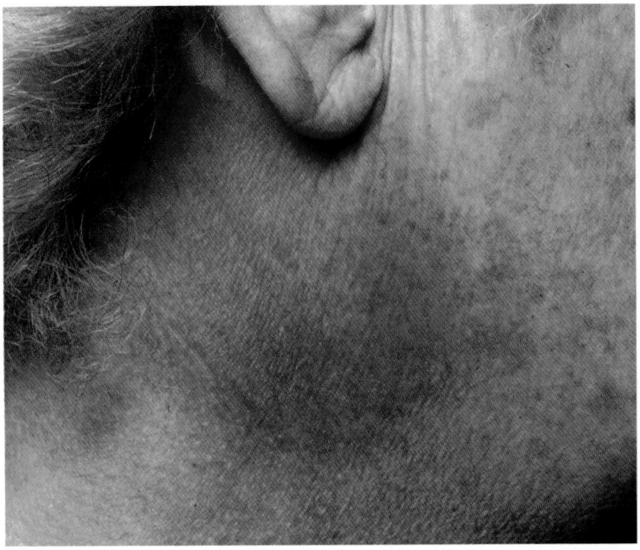

Figure 11.2 Erythema. Reproduced from Buxton, P.K. & Morris-Jones, J. (2009) *ABC of Dermatology*, with kind permission of Wiley Blackwell.

- The patient's occupation – as this may relate to contact dermatitis.
- Their hobbies.
- The skin care routine usually followed – hygiene, the use of soaps, oils and home remedies, and sun exposure.
- Hair and nail care – when assessing the hair, note the texture, colour, brittleness, hair loss and presence of parasites; when assessing the nails, note the length, colour, symmetry, thickness and hygiene, as well as deformities, pitting and splinter haemorrhages.
- Then document the findings including illustrations, photos and body stickers where relevant.

Physical examination

Start at the head and work down over the whole body. Note the condition of mucous membranes of the eyelids, nose and mouth. Pay careful attention to the folds of skin in contact with one another. Check the skin for colour, texture, temperature, moisture, erythema (redness), integrity, sensation and lesions (Figure 11.2). If lesions are found, it is important to record their distribution, arrangement and morphology. Note the site and distribution of the lesions and the shape of any rash. Note other features such as itching, burning, scaling or blisters, whether the lesions are raised (papular) or flat (macular), ulcerated or pigmented, and whether the edges of the lesions are well defined. Note any association with blood vessels, such as telangiectasias, and any odour. Also observe the lesions for plaques, crusts, scabs, wheals, bullae, pustules, cysts or vesicles (Cole & Gray-Miceli 2002).

Diagnosis

This is made in conjunction with the patient's history, a physical examination and the results of specific investigations. In conjunction with what healthcare practitioners can see and what they can palpate with their hands, numerous diagnostic tools offer key information in making a diagnosis (Lawton 2001).

Investigations

A variety of investigations can be employed (Ashton & Leppard 2005):

- **Skin scrapings** of scaly rashes can be sent for mycology examination to out rule fungal infections and prevent the wrong treatment being given. A sample can be taken over an area of itching that is not responding to treatment.
- **Bacterial swabs** can be taken over exuding areas and sent for culture and sensitivity to treat local infections.
- **Doppler ultrasonography** of venous and arterial blood flow is important in order to treat varicose eczema and venous leg ulcers.
- **Patch testing** can be useful to ascertain allergens that may cause allergic contact dermatitis.
- **Punch biopsy** is used to diagnose cancerous cells such as malignant melanomas or pigmented basal cell carcinomas.

Treatments

The following guidelines (Hess 2000) on managing skin complaints are useful during treatment:

- The skin should be assessed at least daily.
- Skin cleansing should be carried out at frequent intervals with pH-balanced cleansers, moisturisers and barrier creams to aid skin integrity
- Care should be taken when washing the skin to avoid excessive rubbing and massage.
- Hygiene needs should be promptly attended to if incontinence is present.
- Extremes of temperature that may cause drying of the skin or excessive moisture should be avoided.
- When repositioning patients, be careful to avoid shearing and friction forces.

Emollients

Emollients are important not only in the treatment of dry skin, but also in the maintenance of healthy skin integrity (Aycliffe 2007). For patients with repetitive skin disorders such as chronic eczema, the regular application of emollients can help to reduce complications. Emollients are mildly anti-inflammatory and should be used regularly by children with atopic eczema for washing and moisturising.

The choice of emollient will depend on the severity of the dryness and the patient's preference, as this will have a significant impact on concordance with treatment (Cork 2006). Emollients include unperfumed wash products, for example bath additives, soap substitutes, skin cleansers and topical preparations such as creams, ointments and lotions (Watkins 2008). Small applications frequently applied are recommended, rather than large amounts in one go; the emollient should be applied in downward strokes in the direction the hair falls to avoid folliculitis (National Collaborating Centre for Women's and Children's Health 2007).

Topical steroids

Topical steroids are prescribed according to their potency and must be applied sparingly to the skin. The choice of potency will depend on the severity of the problem (Ference & Last 2009). Steroids should not be stopped abruptly but tapered off slowly, as otherwise rebound dermatitis/eczema may result (Kartal Durmazlar *et al.* 2009). The dosage should be measured using fingertip units (FTUs), one FTU being the distance from the tip of the adult index finger to the finger's first crease. One FTU equates to a dose of approximately 500 mg and should be enough to cover an area twice the size of an adult flat hand.

Common skin diseases

The psychological impact of wounds, rashes and lesions should never be underestimated. If patients understand their skin disorder and its contributing factors, they will be reassured and are more likely to comply with treatments and skin care regimens (Watkins 2008).

Rashes

Rashes can be endogenous or exogenous. Endogenous rashes are rashes that arise internally, for example atopic eczema or a drug rash triggered by an internal reaction. They are commonly seen all over the body and trunk. Exogenous rashes are rashes that usually arise from an outside source, for example infestations or infections. These rashes may affect only one area of the body (Ashton & Leppard 2005).

Eczema

Eczema is one of the most common skin disorders, with 60% of cases occurring during infancy. Around 2% of adults have chronic severe eczema, which has a severely negative impact on their quality of life (Boyle *et al.* 2009).

Aetiology

There are many causes of eczema, which can be either endogenous or exogenous, or both. Endogenous eczema is related to internal factors and includes atopic eczema, discoid eczema and varicose eczema. Exogenous eczema is related to extrinsic factors and is mediated by the antibody immunoglobulin E. The reaction is triggered by an external stimulus or allergen causing irritant eczema and allergic contact eczema (Greener 2009).

Signs and symptoms

Eczema is an inflammatory disorder characterised by itching, redness, exudation and vesiculation during the acute phase. In the chronic phase, there is also redness and some degree of exudate, but scaling may also be present (Greener 2009).

Treatment

Emollients and topical steroids are the first-line treatments for mild to moderate eczema. Emollients reduce itching and irritation, rehydrate the skin, protect the skin from drying out and may reduce the need for topical steroids. Patients with moderate to severe eczema, and those who do not respond adequately, may require ultraviolet therapy or systemic therapies (Schram *et al.* 2011).

Visit **www.wileyfundamentalseries.com/medicalnursing** and read **Reflective Question 11.1** to think more about this topic.

Psoriasis

Psoriasis is a common chronic inflammatory skin condition that occurs as a result of complex interactions between genetic, environmental and immunological factors. Psoriasis affects 1–3% of population in the UK, with a late onset at average age 33 years. It is common in both males and females, although some studies have shown that up to age 20 it is more common in women. Psoriasis can be genetic but may develop due to environmental reasons, stress or infection. Lifestyle choices such as smoking and alcohol can worsen the condition, although sun exposure can be beneficial for some individuals (Murphy & Reich 2011).

Aetiology

The plaques that are present in psoriasis arise as a result of the hyperproliferation of epidermal cells, which leads to thickening of the skin as a result of the skin trying to replace itself too quickly. The capillaries become dilated, and the white blood cells infiltrate the cells. This stimulates the T cells to release chemokines and cytokines, which cause the keratinocyte hyperproliferation. This results in erythema,

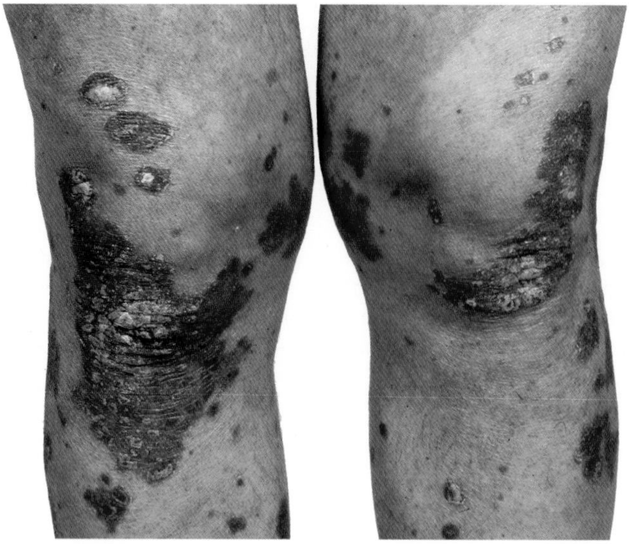

Figure 11.3 Psoriasis. Reproduced from Buxton, P.K. & Morris-Jones, J. (2009) *ABC of Dermatology*, with kind permission of Wiley Blackwell.

inflammation and a scaly appearance of the skin (Griffiths & Barker 2007). Green (2011) describes many types of psoriasis, including:

- chronic plaque psoriasis, which affects the head/hairline, back, abdomen, knees and elbows;
- flexural (inverse) psoriasis, which affects the knees and axillae;
- guttate psoriasis, with widespread coverage;
- erythrodermic psoriasis, affecting 90% of the total body surface;
- pustular psoriasis;
- palmar–plantar psoriasis;
- facial psoriasis;
- scalp psoriasis.

Signs and symptoms

Psoriasis is characterised by dry, scaly, silvery plaques usually over the elbows and knees (Figure 11.3), but it can occur all over the body Psoriasis can be associated with arthritis and nail diseases such as pitting and leuconychia (white patches). Some patients experience psychological distress, depression and low self-esteem due to the physical appearance of their skin (Green 2011).

Treatment

The nurse, alongside the medical team, can produce a care plan suitable for each individual, taking into account their lifestyle and the psychological impact of their psoriasis on them. Treatments can vary and include both topical and systemic therapies. Emollients are the most important part of a skin care regimen to hydrate the dry skin. It is important that patients understand that psoriasis is not contagious nor is it curable, but phototherapy and systemic drugs can help to reduce outbreaks. The use of corticosteroids is not recommended as the psoriasis tends to return as soon as the steroids are stopped. Vitamin A and D in combination with topical tar-based creams can help, although they can stain the clothes (Murphy & Reich 2011).

Acne

Acne is the most common skin condition worldwide, mainly affecting teenagers and young adults. It tends to be more severe in males than females owing to androgens, which produce more sebum secretions in males (Buxton & Morris-Jones 2009).

Aetiology

Acne is caused by increased sebum production, blockage of the follicles, inflammation and altered shedding of the outer layers of the skin. All of these factors arise due to the overproduction of androgens by the adrenal glands (Lavers & Courtenay 2011). It is important to rule out other causes of acne, such as rosacea and folliculitis. Photographs and sebum testing may identify whether oily skin and overproduction of sebum is a problem. For women, it is important to investigate whether hormonal imbalance is a causative factor (Roebuck 2006).

Signs and symptoms

Acne can range from mild to severe. In the mild form, there are no inflammatory lesions and scarring is unlikely. Severe acne, however, involves pustules on the face, back and underarms, and scarring is highly likely.

Treatment

A key concern in the treatment of acne is to lessen the duration and severity of the disease, reducing the risk of scarring and thereby enhancing the individual's psychosocial welfare. Both topical and systemic therapies are used, such as antibiotics, anti-inflammatory agents and hormonal therapies. Other treatments include laser therapy and chemical peels. The patient should be also educated on personal hygiene, diet and the use of cosmetics and toiletries that will not exacerbate the condition (Lavers & Courtenay 2011).

Rosacea

Rosacea is a life-long disorder affecting mainly light-skinned women aged between 30 and 50 years, and affects over 13 million people worldwide (Barton 2008).

Aetiology

The aetiology of rosacea is not fully understood. It is, however, postulated that there is skin thickening, enlargement of the follicles and raised irregularities of the skin as a result of the overproduction of the profibrotic mediator factor XIII (Dahl 2001). *Demodex* mites have been linked to the production of inflammation and pustules (Dahl 2001). Environmental, genetic and psychosocial factors have been linked to the development of rosacea and may also play a role in exacerbating the symptoms (Barton 2008).

Signs and symptoms

Individuals with rosacea present with facial flushing and inflammation, oedema and telangiectasias in the area of the nose. They may also develop papules, pustules and chronic inflammation (Barton 2008).

Treatment

There is no cure for rosacea, but the symptoms may be well controlled. Topical treatments include antibiotics and anti-inflammatory agents. Laser therapy is also a useful addition to reduce the redness and the appearance of the blood vessels (Wolf 2005). Patient education and support is important to help individuals manage their symptoms, avoid exacerbating factors and generally enhance their quality of life (Barton 2008).

Visit www.wileyfundamentalseries.com/medicalnursing and read Reflective Question 11.2 to think more about this topic.

Skin infections

Any break in the continuity of the skin will provide organisms with a portal for entry. Infection will develop depending on the immune status of the patient and the virulence of the organism. Infections in the skin can range from mild to severe and may be caused by, fungi, bacteria or viruses:

- **Folliculitis** is an infection of the hair follicle most often caused by *Staphylococcus aureus*. The bacteria proliferate, resulting in erythema and the development of pustules pierced by hair follicles (Trent *et al*. 2001).

- **Cellulitis** is a common skin infection most often caused by *Staphylococcus aureus* or *Streptococcus pyogenes*. It manifests itself as inflammation of the subcutaneous tissues, which may result in blistering (Trent *et al.* 2001). Symptoms include inflammation, swelling, pain, redness and possibly a high temperature and general malaise.
- **Candidiasis** is a fungal infection located in the skin folds that is caused by *Candida albicans*. The fungi proliferate in a moist environment, causing maceration and altered skin integrity (Aly *et al.* 2001).
- **Herpes zoster** (shingles) is a viral rash that consists of macules and papules and develops into vesicular lesions. The rash may take 2–4 weeks to heal.

Treatment

The treatment of skin infections depends on the diagnosis of the specific causative factor. Treatments include both topical and systemic antibiotics, anti-inflammatory agents and analgesia. The use of local cleansing and wound therapies may also be considered (Aly *et al.* 2001; Trent *et al.* 2001; Laube & Farrell 2002).

Skin infestations

Infestations are highly contagious and cause skin irritation and pruritis (Watkins 2010). Scratching the itchy areas usually exacerbates the condition. Common infestations include fleas, bed bugs, lice, ticks and scabies, which result in pruritis, erythema and swelling, all of which are very uncomfortable for the patient (Watkins 2010).

Treatment

Management includes topical pesticide preparations, anti-inflammatory agents, antihistamines and antibiotics if required. Patients should be advised not to scratch and to attend to hygiene needs regularly using an antiseptic soap. Domestic cleaning is also required, paying attention to clothing, bed linen and carpets (Watkins 2010).

Bullous pemphigoid

Bullous pemphigoid is an autoimmune disorder characterised by blistering and most often affecting the elderly. Immunoglobulin G autoantibodies are deposited in the epidermal basement membrane. This gives rise to the formation of bullae (thin-walled blisters larger than 5 mm in diameter that are filled with fluid), which may occur anywhere on the body (Langan *et al.* 2008; Figure 11.4). Diagnosis

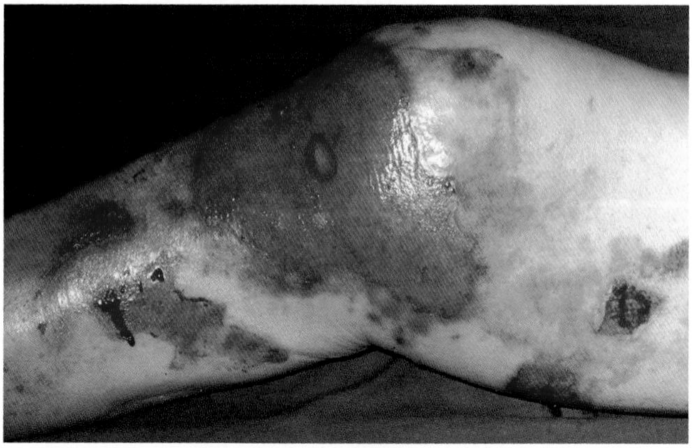

Figure 11.4 Bullous pemphigoid causing erosion. Reproduced from Buxton, P.K. & Morris-Jones, J. (2009) *ABC of Dermatology*, with kind permission of Wiley Blackwell.

is made by immunofluorescence of a sample of the outer area of the blister. A biopsy may also be used to clarify the presence of immunoglobulin G. A blood test may identify a raised eosinophil level (Southwell *et al.* 2009).

Treatment

Treatment of this condition usually involves systemic steroid therapy (Southwell *et al.* 2009). Patients should be educated in order to enhance their ability to live with the condition, and it is important to stress that this is not a contagious condition.

Malignant and non-malignant tumours

Skin cancer is the most commonly diagnosed cancer in the UK, and its incidence is rising annually. However, the majority of skin cancers are not malignant. Early detection enhances the likelihood of successful treatment. Benign lesions include basal cell papillomas, skin tags, dermatofibromas, spider angiomas, blue naevi and port-wine naevi, and pyogenic granulomas. Malignant lesions include squamous cell carcinomas, malignant melanomas and basal cell carcinomas (Freak 2005).

Diagnosis

Diagnosis is made by histopathologic examination of a biopsy specimen of the lesion as this is considered to be the gold standard for diagnosis (Freak 2005).

Treatment

No specific treatment is required for many of the benign lesions, but observation is important to detect changes in the lesions. For malignant lesions, treatment may include surgical excision, cryosurgery, radiotherapy and photodynamic therapy, depending on the nature and severity of the lesion. Observation of lesions is important here too, specifically noting changes in size, shape, colour, bleeding or crusting (Freak 2005).

Wound healing

Wound healing is a normal response to injury and is initiated when the skin's integrity has been interrupted. It occurs as a result of a finely balanced sequence of events. Each stage of healing is regulated by stimulators and inhibitors known as growth factors (e.g. cytokines and matrix metalloproteinases) produced naturally by the body (Tarnuzzer & Schultz 1996).

Early inflammation

The disruption in the integrity of the skin initially causes haemorrhage. This is quickly followed by haemostasis, which occurs in a three-step process: blood vessel contraction, formation of a platelet plug and coagulation (Hart 2002). When vessels are damaged, agents are released that encourage the adhesion of platelets to each and to the vessel wall. Platelets, in turn, release activated contents that cause further adhesion. This platelet plug is sufficient to arrest minor haemorrhage.

However, in cases of more severe haemorrhage, both the intrinsic and extrinsic pathways activate the coagulation pathway in which prothrombin is converted to thrombin. In the last stage of the clotting process, the enzyme thrombin speeds up the conversion of fibrinogen to fibrin, a protein that forms a fibrous network to trap blood cells and platelets in the formation of a clot (Hart 2002).

In order to allow for advancement of wound healing, the clot must be dissolved by a process called fibrinolysis. This is necessary for ease of cell migration and to prevent complete occlusion of the blood vessels, which would further impair perfusion. Both intrinsic and extrinsic activators activate fibrinolysis. Clot dissolution is tightly controlled by the presence of plasma inhibitors, which prevent premature breakdown of the haemostatic mechanism (Hart 2002).

In addition, injured cells release histamine and pain mediators, which increase vascular permeability. This gives rise to the cardinal signs of inflammation: pain, redness, heat and swelling.

Late inflammation

Alpha granules of platelets contain growth factors that diffuse from the wound into the surrounding tissues, thereby stimulating the influx of inflammatory cells (neutrophils and macrophages) into the wounded area; these are primarily involved in phagocytosis and debridement. Macrophages are also a rich source of biological cell regulators that initiate the progression of wound healing (Hart 2002). The debridement of damaged extracellular matrix (ECM) components is necessary to allow the movement of cells into the wounded area. This is facilitated by the release of proteinases by the neutrophils and macrophages, which degrade and remove the damaged ECM and secrete additional growth factors. This process is balanced by the production of inhibitors such as TIMP-1, which limit inappropriate damage to healthy tissues. Both an excessive and a poor inflammatory response are detrimental to wound healing (Trengrove *et al.* 2000).

Production of granulation tissue

Part of the secretory activity of macrophages involves the release of fibroblast growth factor, which is necessary for replacing lost or dead tissue. During this stage of wound healing, fibroblasts are activated and undergo proliferative and synthetic activity in the production of large amounts of fibronectin, later synthesising other proteins (Cherry *et al.* 2000).

Granulation tissue is so called because of its pink granular appearance, rather like cobblestones. It is composed of mesenchymal and non-mesenchymal cells embedded in a loose ECM. The ECM is a stable complex of macromolecules that underlies the epithelial cells and surrounds the connective tissue cells (Juhasz *et al.* 1993). The role of the ECM is to provide tissue with support and act as a centre for cell differentiation and repair. It is composed of large insoluble proteins produced by fibroblasts, and soluble proteins produced by keratinocytes. Fibrous proteins (collagen and elastin) and adhesive proteins (fibronectin and laminin) are the two main classes of matrix protein (Hart 2002). Collagen is rapidly synthesised by fibroblasts following injury, its function being to provide structural integrity and tensile strength (Kumar 2004). The synthesis and degradation of ECM proteins is critical for healing and is regulated by degradative enzymes called proteases (Juhasz *et al.* 1993).

Angiogenesis

Following injury, hypoxia acts as a major stimulus for angiogenesis, which is necessary for new blood formation and restoration of blood flow to the injured area (Cherry *et al.* 2000). Vascular proliferation starts 48–72 hours after injury and lasts for several days. New vessels originate as capillaries from existing small vessels at the wound edge and then develop into new blood vessels.

Epithelialisation

The purpose of this stage of healing is to reconstruct the barrier protection of the skin. It begins a few hours after injury from residual epidermal appendages and ingrowth from the lateral margins of the wound. Uninjured epithelial cells at the wound edges divide to provide new cells. These marginal cells leapfrog across the provisional matrix and stop when the cells meet. When the process is complete, the epithelial cells re-establish normal cell-to-cell and cell-to-basement-membrane supporting structures (Cherry *et al.* 2000).

Contraction

During the proliferative phase of repair, wounds heal by contraction. Myofibroblasts migrate into the wound 2–3 days after injury; these have features similar to fibroblasts and smooth muscle cells. The contractile activity of the fibroblasts and myofibroblasts causes the inward movement of the injured tissue. This in turn reduces the size of the wound and therefore has a positive effect on wound healing time (Cherry *et al.* 2000).

Remodelling

Remodelling is the final phase of wound repair and involves the synthesis and degradation of collagen to increase the tensile strength of the area. This occurs about 3 weeks post-injury and lasts for anything up to 2 years. Gradually, over time, the wound increases its strength, but it will only ever reach 80% of its original strength (Krishnamoorthy *et al.* 2001).

Wound assessment

The process of assessment involves collecting the patient's medical, surgical and social history, current lifestyle information and history of the wound, in order to plan subsequent treatment (Gray *et al.* 2010).

Location

Simple identification of the specific area of the body affected is useful information for all those caring for the patient. Importantly, the location of the wound can also influence the healing outcome and is a point to consider when selecting treatments (Gray *et al.* 2010).

Size

The size of the wound should be measured, and the area calculated and recorded in the patient's notes. A variety of methods are available for measuring the wound, such as photography, digital planimetery, tracing, ruler measurement, mouldings and volumetric calculations. Monitoring the wound area will show whether the wound healing is static, deteriorating or progressing (Gray *et al.* 2010).

Stage of the wound and depth of tissue involved

Assessing the depth of damage will give an indication of the severity of the problem and the likely risk of complications, such as osteomyelitis and deep infection. The European Pressure Ulcer Advisory Panel and the National Pressure Ulcer Advisory Panel (EPUAP/NPUAP, 2009), has developed a common international definition and classification system for pressure ulcers. The system includes four categories or stages:

- Category/stage I: non-blanchable erythema
- Category/stage II: partial thickness
- Category/stage III: full-thickness skin loss
- Category/stage IV: full-thickness tissue.

Two additional categories or stages identified in the USA have also been included:

- Unstageable/unclassified: full-thickness skin or tissue loss
- Suspected deep tissue injury: Depth of damage is unknown.

The International Working Group on the Diabetic Foot has also developed a classification system for the describing the extent of tissue damage in diabetic foot ulcers (Schaper 2004):

- Grade 1 is a superficial full-thickness ulcer, not penetrating any structure deeper than the dermis.
- Grade 2 is a deep ulcer, penetrating below the dermis to the subcutaneous structures and involving fascia, muscle or tendon.
- Grade 3 involves all subsequent layers of the foot, including bone and/or joint (exposed bone or probing to bone).

Wound edges and wound bed

Assessing the colour of the wound bed and wound edges can help to indicate the physiological processes occurring within the wound. Black necrotic tissue is evidence of devitalised tissue. Slough is yellow or white in appearance and adheres firmly to the wound bed. As mentioned above, granulating tissue is so named because of its granular appearance. It should be pale, moist and salmon pink in colour, and its presence suggests normal wound healing (Fletcher 2007). Conversely, a wound that is beefy red and bleeds easily is generally agreed to be unhealthy (Cutting *et al.* 2005). During assessment, the types and percentages of the different tissues within the wound bed should be documented.

Nature of wound drainage

An estimation of the nature and amount of wound fluid will help in judging the progression of wound healing and also enable the practitioner to make an appropriate wound dressing selection. The amount, colour and viscosity of the wound exudate should be recorded, along with a description of whether it is bloody, serosanguineous, serous or purulent (Gray *et al.* 2010). Some dressings may have an effect on the amount and type of fluid produced. Simple methods for assessment include questioning the patient, staff or carers regarding the wear time achieved with particular dressings (Benbow & Stevens 2010). This can be assisted by examination of the previous dressing, clothing, footwear and bed linen, as any staining might indicate excessive wound exudate (Gray *et al.* 2010).

Odour

The presence of malodour of the wound is often a very distressing experience for the patient. The nature and severity of any malodour should be recorded as this may provide an indication of wound deterioration.

Amount of pain or discomfort

Using a validated pain assessment tool, the nature and severity of the pain and any exacerbating factors should be recorded. Furthermore, this assessment should be repeated in order to enable an evaluation of the outcomes of care delivery. Pain associated with wounds results not only from underlying pathology, but also often from dressing choices and dressing techniques (Kammerlander & Eberlein 2002). The location, frequency, associating factors, impact on daily living and effectiveness of treatments need to be included in this assessment in order to develop a more effective programme of management.

Wound management

When wounds are kept moist, they have been shown to heal more rapidly, with a faster rate of epithelialisation, than when they are left to dry out. Many wound care products are based on this concept, for example hydrogels, hydrocolloids, foams, alginates and hydrofibres or hydropolymers, which donate fluid to the wound or absorb excess exudate from the wound, thereby maintaining a moist wound–dressing interface (Moore 2006).

The decision to use a topical antimicrobial agent should be based on the assessment of both the patient and the wound. The use of newer formulation topical antimicrobials, particularly silver- and iodine-containing products, is increasingly being recommended as one component of the management of wounds with a problematic or increasing bacterial burden. If the wound is deemed suitable, a number of antimicrobial choices are available, for example silver, iodine, chlorhexidine, polyhexamethylene biguanide and acetic acid. Furthermore, older products such as honey are re-emerging onto the market, with an increasing research interest into their use being seen. In current clinical practice, however, it is more common for clinicians to use either silver- or iodine-based products as a first line of treatment (Moore & Romanelli 2006).

It is prudent to point out that the uncontrolled use of antimicrobial products is not recommended. Indeed, learning from our experiences with antibiotic resistance, the unnecessary use of topical antimicrobial agents may result in the development of bacterial resistance (Moore & Romanelli 2006).

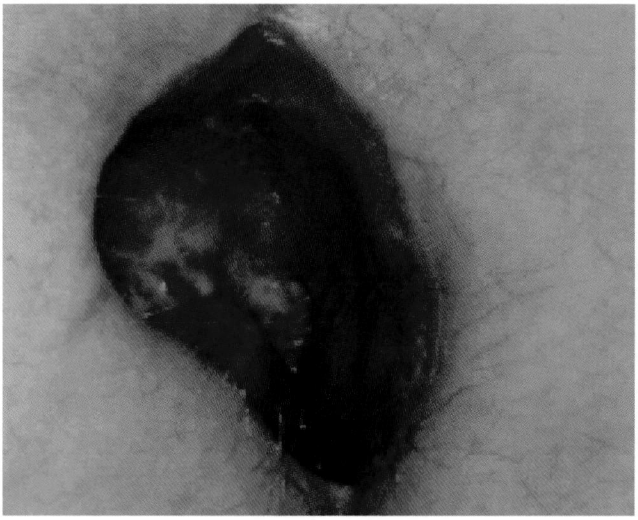

Figure 11.5 Surgical wound healing by secondary intention. Courtesy of Dr Zena Moore.

Surgical wounds

Surgical site infection is estimated to be one of the leading causes of hospital-acquired infection, accounting for 17% of all nosocomial infections (Klevens *et al.* 2007). With the increasing use of ambulatory care, up to 84% of infections are diagnosed after patients have been discharged from hospital, increasing the burden on community services. The mean length of extended hospital stay attributable to surgical site infection is 9.8 days, at an average cost per day of €325/£277 (Gottrup *et al.* 2005).

Methods of closure of surgical wounds

Surgical wounds may heal by primary intention, in which the edges are drawn together with sutures, staples or clips. Alternatively, the wound may be left open to heal by secondary intention, where the wound bed fills with granulation tissue to replace the tissue that has been lost (Gottrup *et al.* 2005; Figure 11.5). Wounds may also heal from a skin graft or tissue flap depending on the amount of tissue loss.

A skin graft involves the surgical removal of a piece of skin from one area of the body for transplantation to another area of the body. The rationale for conducting a skin graft is to rapidly restore tissue integrity, enhance cosmesis, reduce the risk of contracture formation and restore the body's protection from bacterial invasion (Black & Black 2007). There are several different types of graft:

- **Split-thickness**: this includes the epidermis and variable amounts of dermis.
- **Full-thickness**: this includes the epidermis and all the dermis.
- **Composite graft**: this involves small grafts containing skin and underlying cartilage or other tissue (Black & Black 2007).

Survival of the skin graft is dependent on an adequate blood supply, so care should be taken to avoid the development of oedema or infection (Black & Black 2007).

Where there is a large amount of tissue loss, the formation of a flap may be required to cover the defect. A tissue flap is similar to a skin graft except that the amount of tissue transferred is greater and includes skin and underlying structures such as fat, blood vessels and muscle. The original blood vessels either remain attached to the donor area, or are moved and grafted onto the recipient area. Flaps may be classified as either free flaps (with the donor tissue completely removed from the donor site) or local flaps (Black & Black 2007). Local flaps are further divided according to:

- **the anatomic structures involved**: skin, fasciocutaneous tissue (epidermis, dermis and subcutaneous tissue supported by the underlying structures) or myocutaneous tissue (skin, subcutaneous tissue, fascia and muscle);
- **the methods used to move the flap**: advancement (tissue advanced into the defect), rotation (with the flap rotated into the defect) or transposition (the flap being moved across normal skin);
- **the methods used for maintaining perfusion**: random flaps including dermal and subdermal vessels, or axial flaps including an artery.

Successful wound healing outcomes for patients undergoing flap formations is dependent on maintaining an adequate blood supply, facilitating effective wound drainage, avoiding the adverse effects of shearing forces and preventing infection.

Principles of wound management

The key principles of management of surgical wounds are:

- maintenance of the blood supply;
- avoidance of oedema or any build-up of fluid within the wound;
- prevention of infection;
- prevention of wound breakdown or dehiscence;
- restoration of tissue integrity;
- enhancement of quality of life and pain management.

The choice of treatment depends on the method of closure adopted, the presence or absence of infection, the amount of tissue loss (whether it is a cavity or shallow wound), the amount of exudate, the condition of the wound bed and the stage of wound healing (Moore & Cowman 2007).

For wounds healing by primary intention, the wound should be covered with a simple non-adherent, absorbent dressing (Heal *et al*. 2006). The patient may shower after 24–48 hours; the dressing should be removed either before or during the shower and replaced with a clean dressing afterwards (Heal *et al*. 2006). For wounds healing by secondary intention, a variety of dressings and topical agents are available. The wound may be cleansed with potable water or normal saline (Joanna Briggs Institute 2008).

Visit **www.wileyfundamentalseries.com/medicalnursing** and read **Reflective Question 11.3** to think more about this topic.

Pressure ulcers

Up to 23% of all hospital inpatients have a pressure ulcer, most of which occur during hospitalisation for an acute episode of illness/injury (European Pressure Ulcer Advisory Panel 2002). The impact of pressure ulcers on the individual is profound, affecting all domains of the activities of living. The costs associated with the prevention and management of pressure ulcers are also considerable, with one of the main cost drivers being nursing time (Posnett & Franks 2008).

A pressure ulcer can be defined as 'localized injury to the skin and/or underlying tissue usually over a bony prominence, as a result of pressure, or pressure in combination with shear (EUPAP/NPUAP 2009; p. 9; Figure 11.6).

The impact of external mechanical forces on tissue viability

Pathologically, the development of pressure ulcers is a complex process. Impaired perfusion of the loaded area contributes to pressure ulcer development; however, this mechanism alone does not adequately explain the entire process (Stekelenburg *et al*. 2008).

It is estimated that four mechanisms acting within three functional units lead to the development of pressure ulcers (Stekelenburg *et al*. 2008). The three functional units are the capillaries, the interstitial spaces and the cells. The mechanisms involved are local ischaemia, reperfusion injury, impaired interstitial fluid flow and lymphatic drainage, and sustained deformity of the cells. Fundamentally, however, none of this is relevant unless an individual is exposed to prolonged, unrelieved external mechanical loading.

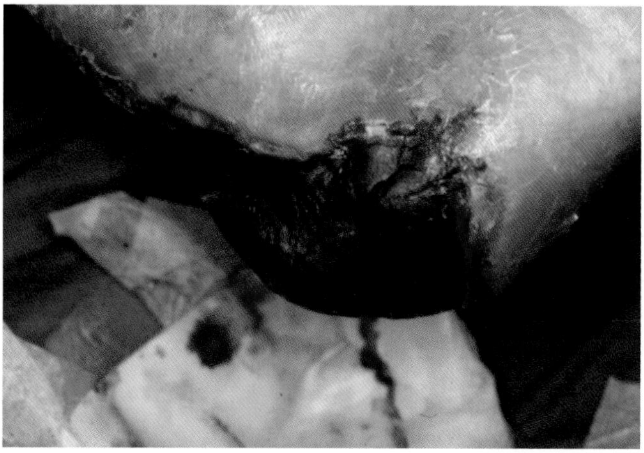

Figure 11.6 A grade 4 pressure ulcer. Courtesy of Dr Zena Moore.

Risk assessment

There are over 100 factors pertaining to the individual that have been suggested to contribute to altering the person's ability to withstand the adverse effects of pressure and shearing forces. However, a number of key factors are considered of primary importance (Moore & Cowman 2008):

- Immobility is important as individuals will be exposed to prolonged external mechanical forces only if they are unable to reposition themselves to relieve the pressure.
- Older individuals are more susceptible due to the likelihood that there will be multiple comorbidities and changes in tissue integrity synonymous with the ageing process.
- Nutritional status is important, as it influences collagen deposition and synthesis, which is needed for tissue strength. Poor nutrition also leads to increased muscle wasting and soft tissue loss, increasing the prominence of bony points.

Pressure ulcer prevention

Repositioning

Repositioning is one of a number of key ways in which nurses and care staff can prevent pressure ulcers among those who cannot reposition themselves (Moore & Cowman 2009). The 30° position is recommended as the most appropriate for the patient, as less pressure will be applied to the bony prominences and therefore the blood supply to the weight-bearing area is not completely occluded.

Support surfaces

A wide variety of support surfaces are currently available for use as part of a pressure ulcer prevention and management programme. Surfaces may be static, and are commonly composed of foam or gel, or alternately can be air-filled (McInnes *et al.* 2008). Static surfaces work on the principle that pressure reduction will be achieved if the pressure between the patient and the mattress is spread over the widest possible area. Alternating air overlays or mattresses operate by periodically removing pressure from varying anatomical sites of the body by the cyclical inflation and deflation of cells within the mattress (McInnes *et al.* 2008). Extra care is needed when caring for patients at risk of pressure ulcers, and a repositioning regimen should be initiated along with use of the support system (EPUAP/NPUAP 2009).

It must be remembered that those patients who require pressure relief or redistribution while in bed are also at risk of pressure ulcer development while sitting out of bed (EPUAP/NPUAP 2009).

Therefore, similar protection should be offered. This can be in the form of a pressure-redistributing cushion, which should be selected based on the patient's individual needs. The patient should not be exposed to prolonged periods of sitting out as this also increases the risk of pressure ulcer development. Furthermore, it contributes to fatigue and may have a negative impact on rehabilitation.

Nutrition

The role of nutrition in the prevention and management of pressure ulcers cannot be overstated (Stratton *et al.* 2005). The EPUAP/NPUAP (2009) pressure ulcer prevention and management guidelines offer very specific advice pertaining to nutrition. These guidelines recommend that all patients should have a regular assessment of their nutritional status, which should include weight measurement, skin assessment and recording of fluid and food intake. For those at risk of nutritional impairment, advice should be sought from the multidisciplinary nutritional team.

Skin care

The EPUAP/NPUAP (2009) guidelines recommend that skin emollients be used to hydrate dry skin as dry skin does not have the same protective function as intact skin and increases the individual's risk of pressure ulceration. The skin should also be protected, using a barrier product, from the damaging effects of excess moisture. In the presence of excess moisture, the mechanical properties of the stratum corneum are altered, thereby reducing the individual's resistance to pressure and shearing forces.

Information on burn injuries to the skin can be found in Chapter 10.

Visit www.wileyfundamentalseries.com/medicalnursing and read Reflective Question 11.4 to think more about this topic.

Conclusion

The skin is the largest organ in the body and provides the key functions of protection, heat regulation, absorption, sensation and storage. Due to the diverse nature, aetiology and variety of skin disorders encountered, assessment, diagnosis and management requires a systematic, rigorous and holistic approach. The patient's history and lifestyle, and a physical examination, are the main factors in diagnosing and effectively managing skin conditions. Fundamental aspects of nursing management are ensuring patient dignity, warmth, comfort and effective management of symptoms including pain, skin irritation and exudates. Common conditions include eczema, psoriasis, acne, rosacea, infection, infestation and tumours.

Now visit the companion website and test yourself on this chapter:
www.wileyfundamentalseries.com/medicalnursing

References

Aly, R., Forney, R. & Bayles, C. (2001) Treatments for common superficial fungal infections. *Dermatology Nursing*, **13**:91–4, 98–101.

Ashton, R. & Leppard, B. (2005) Introduction to dermatological diagnosis. In: Ashton, R. & Leppard, B. (eds), *Differential Diagnosis in Dermatology*, 5th edn (pp. 1–20). Oxford: Radcliffe Medical Press.

Aycliffe, V. (2007) Contact dermatitis and the effect of fragrance allergy. *Dermatological Nursing*, **6**:10–16.

Barton, M. (2008) Rosacea management – why it matters: nursing implications and patient education. *Dermatology Nursing*, **20**:10–14.

Benbow, M. & Stevens, J. (2010) Exudate, infection and patient quality of life. *British Journal of Nursing*, **19**:S30, S32–6.

Black, J. & Black, S. (2007) The role of surgery in wound healing. In: Bryant, R.A. & Nix, D. (eds), *Acute and Chronic Wounds: Current Management Concepts*, 3rd edn (pp. 461–70). St Louis: Mosby Elsevier.

Boyle, R., Bath-Hextall, F., Leonardi-Bee, J., Murrell, D. & Tang, M. (2009) Probiotics for the treatment of eczema: a systematic review. *Clinical and Experimental Allergy*, **39**:1117–27.

Bridel-Nixon, J. (1997) Pressure sores. In: Morison, M., Moffatt, C., Bridel-Nixon, J. & Bale, S. (eds), *Nursing Management of Chronic Wounds* (pp. 153–75). London: Mosby.

Buxton, P. & Morris-Jones, R. (2009) Acne and rosacea. In: Buxton, P. & Morris-Jones, R. (eds), *ABC of Dermatology*, 5th edn (pp. 84–91). Oxford: Wiley Blackwell.

Cherry, G., Hughes, M., Fergusson, M. & Leaper, D. (2000) Wound healing. In: Morris, P. & Wood, W. (eds), *Oxford Textbook of Surgery* (pp. 131–62). Oxford: Oxford University Press.

Cole, J. & Gray-Miceli, D. (2002) The necessary elements of a dermatologic history and physical evaluation. *Dermatology Nursing*, **14**:377–83.

Cork, M. (2006) Improving the treatment of atopic eczema through an understanding of gene–environment interactions. *Exchange: National Eczema Society Journal*, **131**:7–13.

Cutting K, White R, Mahoney P, Harding K (2005) Clinical identification of wound infection: a Delphi approach. In: *European Wound Management Association (EWMA). Position Document: Identifying Criteria for Wound Infection* (pp. 14–16). London: MEP.

Dahl, M. (2001) Pathogenesis of rosacea. *Advances in Dermatology*, **17**:29–45.

European Pressure Ulcer Advisory Panel (2002) Summary report on the prevalence of pressure ulcers. *EPUAP Review*, **4**:49–57.

European Pressure Ulcer Advisory Panel and National Pressure Ulcer Advisory Panel (2009) *Prevention and Treatment of Pressure Ulcers: Quick Reference Guide*. Washington, DC: National Pressure Ulcer Advisory Panel.

Ference, J. & Last, A. (2009) Choosing topical corticosteroids. *American Family Physician*, **79**:135–40.

Fletcher, J. (2007) *Dressings: Cutting and Application Guide. World Wide Wounds*. Retrieved 6th June 2013 from http://www.worldwidewounds.com/2007/may/Fletcher/Fletcher-Dressings-Cutting-Guide.html.

Freak, J. (2005) Identification of skin cancers. 1. Benign and premalignant lesions. *British Journal of Community Nursing*, **10**:8–12.

Gottrup, F., Melling, A. & Hollander, D. (2005) *An Overview of Surgical Site Infections: Aetiology, Incidence and Risk Factors. World Wide Wounds, 2005* Retrieved 6th June 2013 from http://www.worldwidewounds.com/2005/september/Gottrup/Surgical-Site-Infections-Overview.html.

Gray, D., White, R., Cooper, P. & Kingsley, A. (2010) Applied wound management and using the wound healing continuum in practice. *Wound Essentials*, **5**:131–9.

Green, L. (2011) An overview and update of psoriasis. *Nursing Standard*, **25**:47–55.

Greener M. (2009) Eczema: what lies beneath? *Nurse Prescribing*, **7**(10):438–43.

Griffiths, C. & Barker, J. (2007) Pathogenesis and clinical features of psoriasis. *Lancet*, **370**:263–71.

Hart, J. (2002) Inflammation: its role in the healing of acute wounds. *Journal of Wound Care*, **7**(6):205–9.

Heal, C., Buettner, P., Raasch, B. *et al.* (2006) Can sutures get wet? Prospective randomised controlled trial of wound management in general practice. *British Medical Journal*, **332**:1053–6.

Hess, C. (2000) Skin care basics. *Advances in Skin and Wound Care*, **13**:127–8.

Holloway, S. & Jones, V. (2005) The importance of skin care and assessment. *British Journal of Nursing*, **14**(22):1172–6.

Joanna Briggs Institute (2008) Solutions, techniques and pressure in wound cleansing. *Nursing Standard*, **22**:35–9.

Johannsen, L. (2005) Skin assessment. *Dermatological Nursing*, **17**(2):165–6.

Juhasz, I., Murphy, G., Yan, H., Herlyn, M. & Albelda, S. (1993) Regulation of extracellular matrix proteins and integrin cell substratum adhesion receptors on epithelium during cutaneous human would healing. *American Journal of Pathology*, **143**:1458–69.

Kammerlander, G. & Eberlein, T. (2002) Nurses' views about pain and trauma at dressing changes: a central European perspective. *Journal of Wound Care*, **11**:76–9.

Kartal Durmazlar, S., Eskioglu, F., Oktay, B. & Eren, C. (2009) Current threats and problems in the topical use of steroids?: review. *Turkiye Klinikleri Journal of Medical Sciences*, **29**:194–201.

Klevens, R.M., Edwards, J., Richards, C. *et al.* (2007) Estimating health care-associated infections and deaths in U.S. hospitals, 2002. *Public Health Reports*, **122**:160–6.

Krishnamoorthy, L., Morris, H.L. & Harding, K.G. (2001) A dynamic regulator: the role of growth factors in tissue repair. *Journal of Wound Care*, **10**:99–101.

Kumar, R. (2004) The dynamics of acute inflammation. *Journal of Theoretical Biology*, **230**:145–55.

Langan, S., Smeeth, L., Hubbard, R., Fleming, K., Smith, C. & West, J. (2008) Bullous pemphigoid and pemphigus vulgaris – incidence and mortality in the UK a population based cohort study. *British Medical Journal*, **337**:a180.

Laube, S. & Farrell, M. (2002). Bacterial skin infection in the elderly: diagnosis and treatment. *Drugs and Aging*, **19**(5):331–42.

Lavers, I. & Courtenay, M. (2011) A practical approach to the treatment of acne vulgaris. *Nursing Standard*, **25**:55–64.

Lawton, S. (2001) Assessing the patient with a skin condition. *Journal of Tissue Viability*, **11**:113–15.

McInnes, E., Cullum, N.A., Bell-Syer, S.E.M., Dumville, J.C. & Jammali-Blasi, A. (2008) Support surfaces for pressure ulcer prevention. *Cochrane Database of Systematic Reviews*, (4):CD001735.

Martin, P. (1997) Wound healing – aiming for perfect skin regeneration. *Science*, **276**:75–81.

Moore Z (2006) Current issues in wound management. *Irish Pharmacy Journal*, 25–9.

Moore, Z. & Cowman, S. (2007) Assessment and management of surgical wounds. *Enhancing Clinical Practice*, September:5–7.

Moore, Z.E.H. & Cowman, S. (2008) Risk assessment tools for the prevention of pressure ulcers. *Cochrane Database of Systematic Reviews* (16):CD006471.

Moore, Z.E.H. & Cowman, S. (2009): Repositioning for treating pressure ulcers. *Cochrane Database of Systematic Reviews* (2):CD006898.

Moore, Z. & Romanelli, M. (2006) Topical management of infected grade 3 and 4 pressure ulcers. In: European Wound Management Association Position Document, *Management of Wound Infection* (pp. 11–13). London: MEP.

Murphy, G. & Reich, K. (2011) In touch with psoriasis: topical treatments and current guidelines. *Journal of the European Academy of Dermatology and Venereology*, **25**:3–8.

National Collaborating Centre for Women's and Children's Health (UK) (2007) *Atopic Eczema in Children: Management of Atopic Eczema in Children from Birth up to the Age of 12 Years*. NICE Clinical Guideline No. 57. London: RCOG Press. Retrieved 6th June 2013 from http://www.ncbi.nlm.nih.gov/books/NBK49373/.

Posnett, J. & Franks, P.J. (2008) The burden of chronic wounds in the UK. *Nursing Times*, **104**:44–5.

Reddy, N.P. (1990) Mechanical stress effects on lymph and fluid flows. In: Bader, D.L. (ed.), *Pressure Sores: Clinical Practice and Scientific Approach* (pp. 203–20). London: Macmillan.

Roebuck, H. (2006) Acne: intervene early. *Nurse Practitioner*, **31**:24–43.

Schaper, N. (2004) Diabetic foot ulcer classification system for research purposes: a progress report on criteria for including patients in research studies. *Diabetes Metabolism Research and Reviews*, **20**:S90–5.

Schram, M., Roekevisch, E., Leeflang, M., Bos, J., Schmitt, J. & Spuls, P. (2011) A randomized trial of methotrexate versus azathioprine for severe atopic eczema. *Journal of Allergy and Clinical Immunology*, **128**(2):353–9.

Southwell, B., Riaz, F. & Khachemoune, A. (2009) Bullous pemphigoid: a short review. *Dermatology Nursing*, **21**:322–6.

Stekelenburg, A., Gawlitta, D., Bader, D.L. & Oomens, C.W. (2008) Deep tissue injury: how deep is our understanding? *Archives of Physical Medical Rehabilitation*, **89**:1410–13.

Stratton, R.J., Ek, A.C., Engfer, M. *et al.* (2005) Enteral nutrition in prevention and treatment of pressure ulcers: a systematic review and meta-analysis. *Ageing Research Reviews*, **4**:422–50.

Tarnuzzer, R.W. & Schultz, G.S. (1996) Biochemical analysis of acute and chronic wound environments. *Wound Repair and Regeneration*, **4**:321–5.

Tortora, G.J. & Derrickson, B. (2011) *Principles of Anatomy & Physiology; Organization, Support and Movement, and Control Systems of the Human Body*. Hoboken, NJ: John Wiley & Sons.

Trengrove, N., Bielefeldt-Ohmann, H. & Stacey, M. (2000) Mitogenic activity and cytokine levels in non–healing and healing chronic leg ulcers. *Wound Repair and Regeneration*, **8**:13–25.

Trent, J., Federman, D. & Kirsner, R. (2001) Common bacterial skin infections. *Ostomy Wound Management*, **47**:30–4.

Waller, J.M. & Maibach, H.I. (2005) Age and skin structure and function, a quantitative approach (I) blood flow, pH, thickness, and ultrasound echogenicity. *Skin Research and Technology*, **11**:221–35.

Watkins, J. (2010) Pruritis. 4. Infestations. *Practice Nursing*, **21**:247–52.

Watkins, P. (2008) Using emollients to restore and maintain skin integrity. *Nursing Standard*, **22**:51–7.

Wolf, J. (2005) Present and future rosacea therapy. *Cutis* **75**(3 Suppl):4–7; discussion 33–6.

12

Nursing care of conditions related to the respiratory system

Anne Marie Corroon[1] and Geralyn Hynes[2]

[1]*School of Nursing and Midwifery, Trinity College Dublin, Dublin, Ireland*
[2]*Faculty of Nursing and Midwifery, Royal College of Surgeons in Ireland, Dublin, Ireland*

Contents

Introduction	177
Anatomy and physiology	177
Nursing care and assessment of symptoms	183
Respiratory function testing	188
Respiratory interventions	190
Management of specific conditions	193
Conclusion	208
References	208

Learning outcomes

Having read this chapter, you will be able to understand:

- The pathophysiology of the respiratory system
- Important respiratory conditions in adult nursing
- Nursing assessment, planning and management for these respiratory conditions
- The importance of interdisciplinary and integrated approaches to respiratory care

Fundamentals of Medical-Surgical Nursing: A Systems Approach, First Edition. Edited by Anne-Marie Brady, Catherine McCabe, and Margaret McCann.

Introduction

Chronic respiratory illnesses are often associated with a negative impact on quality of life in terms of physical function, anxiety, depression and social isolation. Nurses are well placed to address the complex care needs required to enhance the quality of life of these patients.

This chapter provides an overview of respiratory conditions that dominate hospital care, including respiratory infections such as pneumonia and tuberculosis (TB), respiratory diseases that affect the airways (such as asthma, chronic obstructive airway disease, respiratory failure and bronchiectasis), cystic fibrosis (CF) and lung cancer. The anatomy and physiology of the respiratory system is presented first, followed by an outline of symptoms, diagnosis, treatment and nursing management.

Anatomy and physiology

Function of the respiratory system

The function of the respiratory tract is to exchange gases and assist in regulating blood pH and maintaining acid–base balance.

Respiratory tract

The respiratory tract consists of the nose and pharynx, the larynx, the trachea and two lungs (Figure 12.1). The lungs are covered by the parietal and visceral pleura, and contain bronchi, bronchioles and alveoli. Each lung is subdivided into lobes (Figure 12.2). The pulmonary vascular system facilitates gas exchange in the alveoli.

Mechanics of respiration

Respiration consists of a cycle of inspiration, expiration and rest, through which gas exchange occurs (Figure 12.3).

Control of respiration

Respiration is controlled by a complex set of processes involving an interplay between the cerebral cortex, the respiratory centre, chemoreceptors, proprioceptors and stretch receptors (Figure 12.4). Rate, rhythm, depth and effort all change to meet the demands of the body and maintain normal levels of PaO_2 (the partial pressure of oxygen in the blood; 12–14 kPa), $PaCO_2$ (the partial pressure of carbon dioxide in the blood, which reflects respiratory control of the acid–base balance; 4.6–6.0 kPa) and pH (7.35–7.45) (Woodrow 2004). The following are involved in the control of respiration:

- **Respiratory centre.** Respiration is controlled by the medulla oblongata and the pons in the brainstem.
- **Chemoreceptors.** These monitor the levels of CO_2, O_2 and hydrogen ions (H^+). Hypercapnia (too high a level of CO_2) causes an increase in the level of H^+ and causes hyperventilation, thus increasing the level of O_2 and decreasing CO_2:

$$\uparrow CO_2 \leftrightarrow \uparrow H^+ (\downarrow pH) \leftrightarrow \text{Hyperventilation} \leftrightarrow \uparrow O_2 \text{ and } \downarrow CO_2$$

In contrast, hypocapnia (too low a level of CO_2) causes H^+ levels to fall, which increases pH, but does not cause a change in respiration:

$$\downarrow CO_2 \leftrightarrow \downarrow H^+ (\uparrow pH)$$

Hypoxaemia (too low a level of O_2) initially stimulates breathing, although not as powerfully as hypercapnia. However, extreme hypoxaemia can cause respiratory depression.

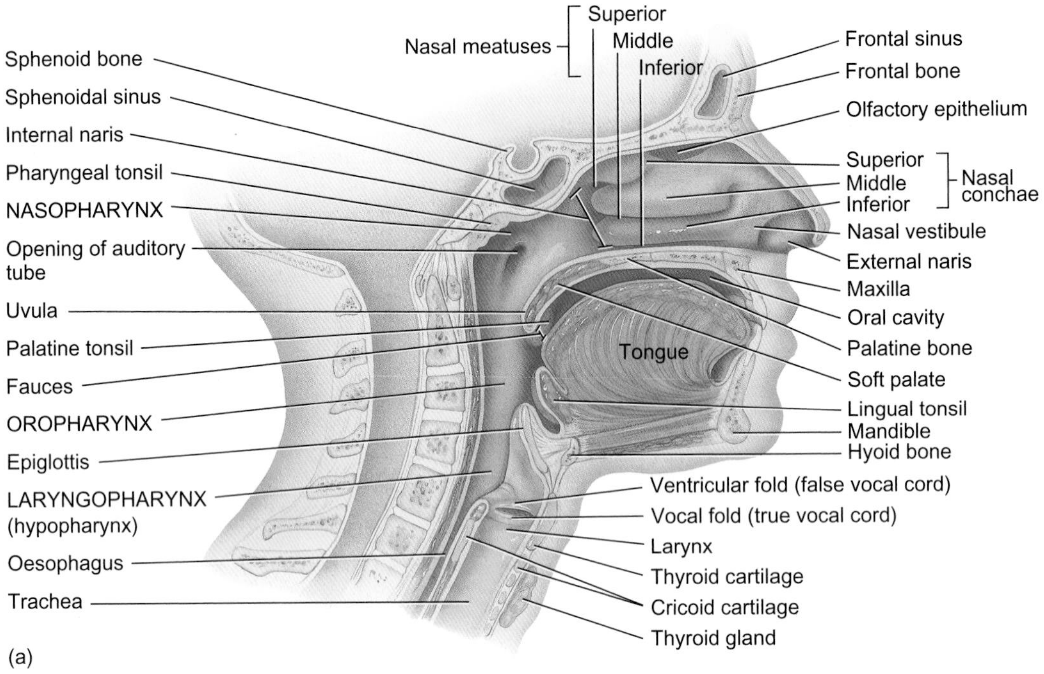

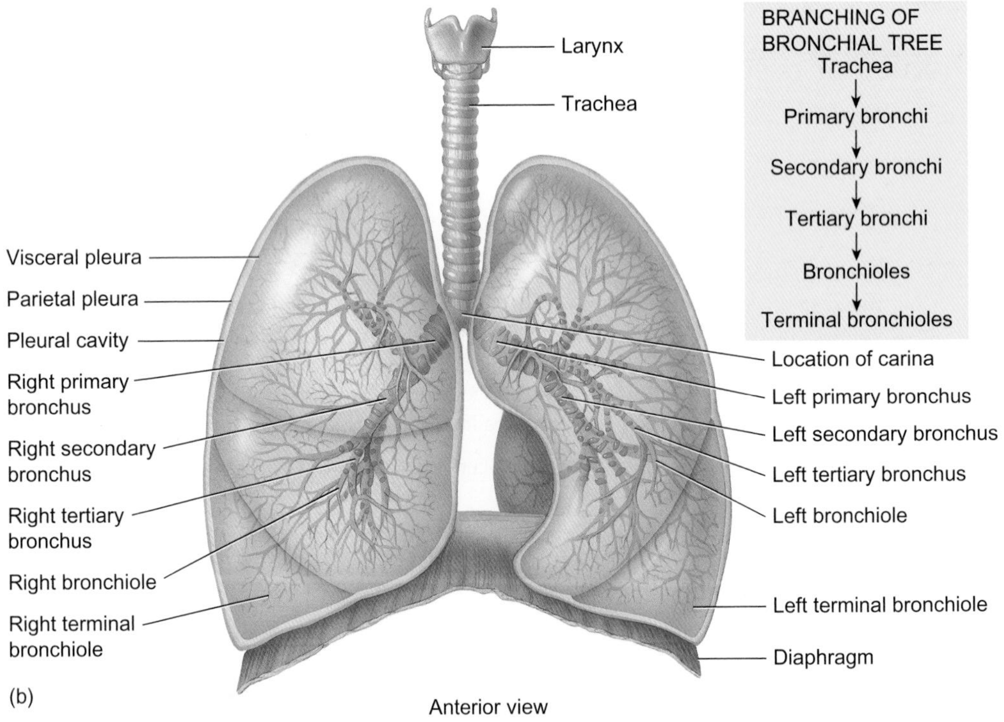

Figure 12.1 (a) The upper respiratory tract. (b) The lower respiratory tract. Reproduced from Tortora, G.J., Derrickson, B. (2011) *Principles of Anatomy and Physiology*, with kind permission of Wiley Blackwell.

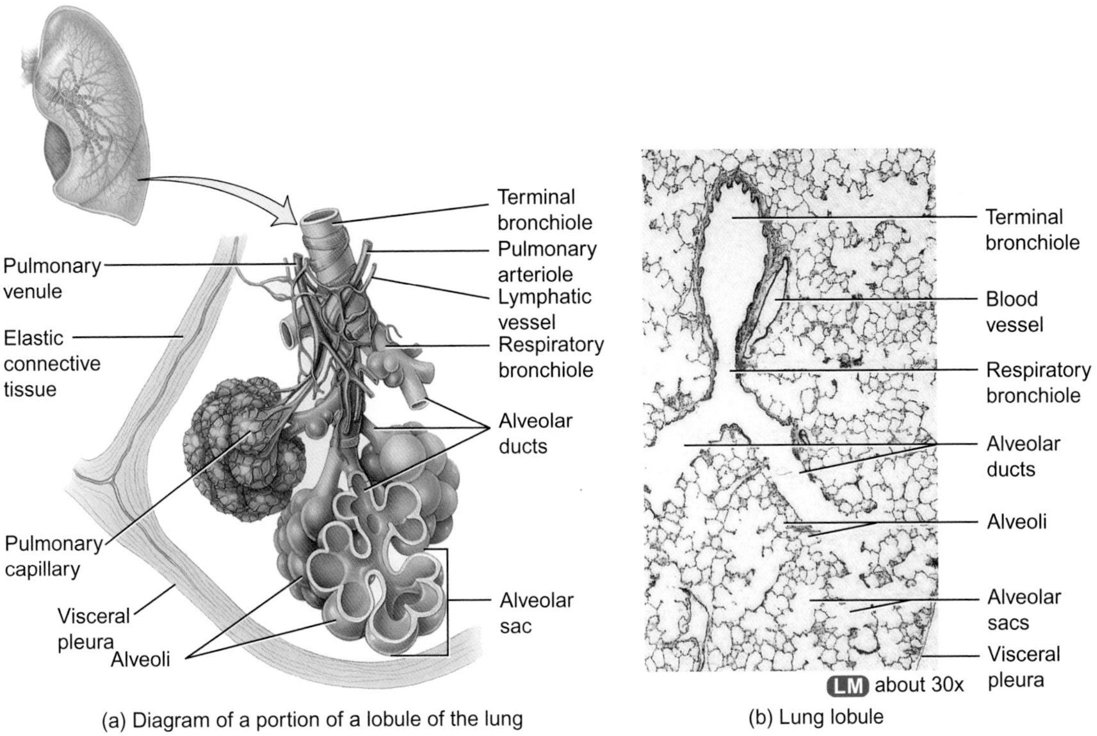

Figure 12.2 Microscopic anatomy of a lung. Reproduced from Tortora, G.J., Derrickson, B. (2011) *Principles of Anatomy and Physiology*, with kind permission of Wiley Blackwell.

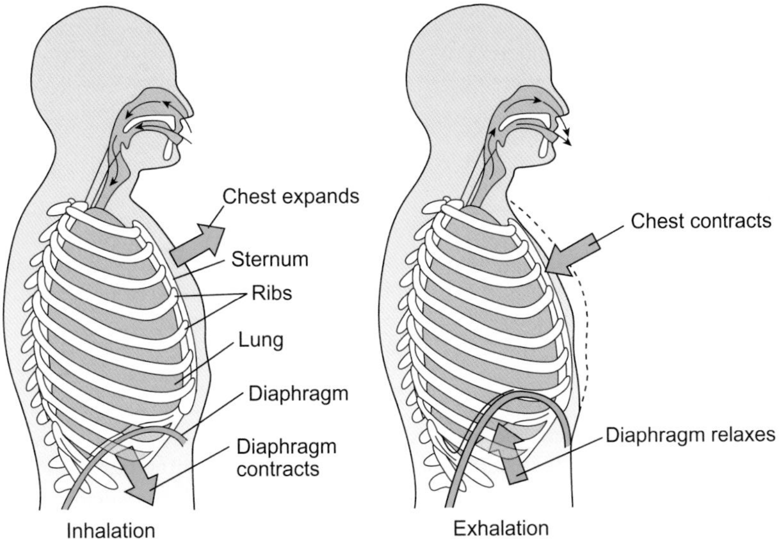

Figure 12.3 Mechanics of respiration. Reproduced from Peate, I., Nair, M. (2011) *Fundamentals of Anatomy and Physiology*, with kind permission of Wiley Blackwell.

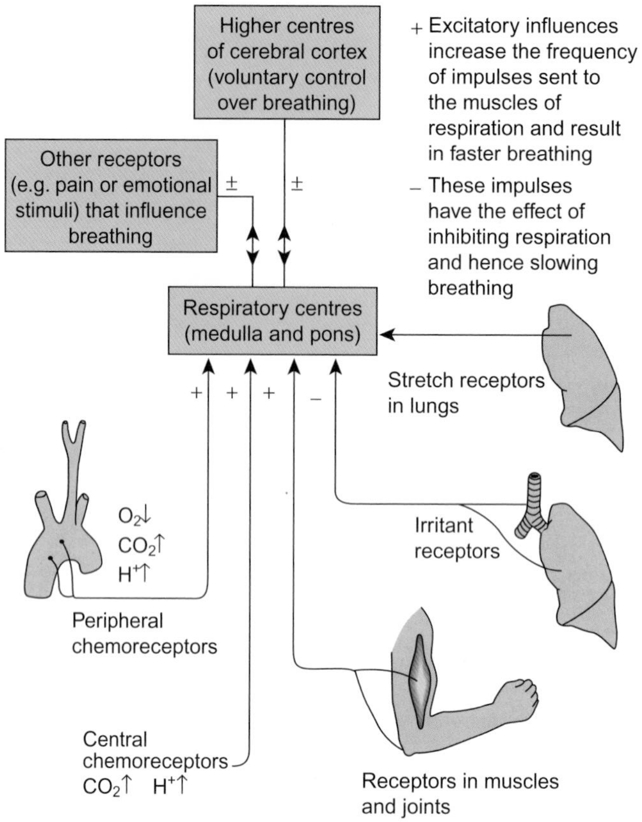

Figure 12.4 Factors influencing the rate and depth of breathing. Reproduced from Dougherty, L. & Lister, S. (2011) *The Royal Marsden Hospital Manual of Clinical Nursing Procedures*, with kind permission from Wiley Blackwell.

- **Stretch receptors** and the inflation reflex. Stretch receptors in the bronchi and bronchioles cause breathing to stop when they are overstretched, leading to expiration.
- **Proprioceptors.** Stimulation of proprioceptors in the muscles and joints increases the rate and depth of breathing.

Gas exchange

In the alveoli, oxygen from the atmosphere is taken up into the pulmonary capillaries to meet the tissues' needs, while carbon dioxide, a waste product of metabolism, is excreted by expiration (Figure 12.5).

Transport of oxygen

Oxygen is almost entirely transported bound to haemoglobin in the blood (98.5%), with 1.5% dissolved in the plasma (Figure 12.5). At rest, only 25% of the oxygen is used by the tissues (Tortora & Derrickson, 2011).

Transport of carbon dioxide

Carbon dioxide is carried in the blood in three forms: approximately 70% as bicarbonate ions (HCO_3^-), approximately 23% as carbamino compounds, and about 7% as dissolved carbon dioxide (Figure 12.6).

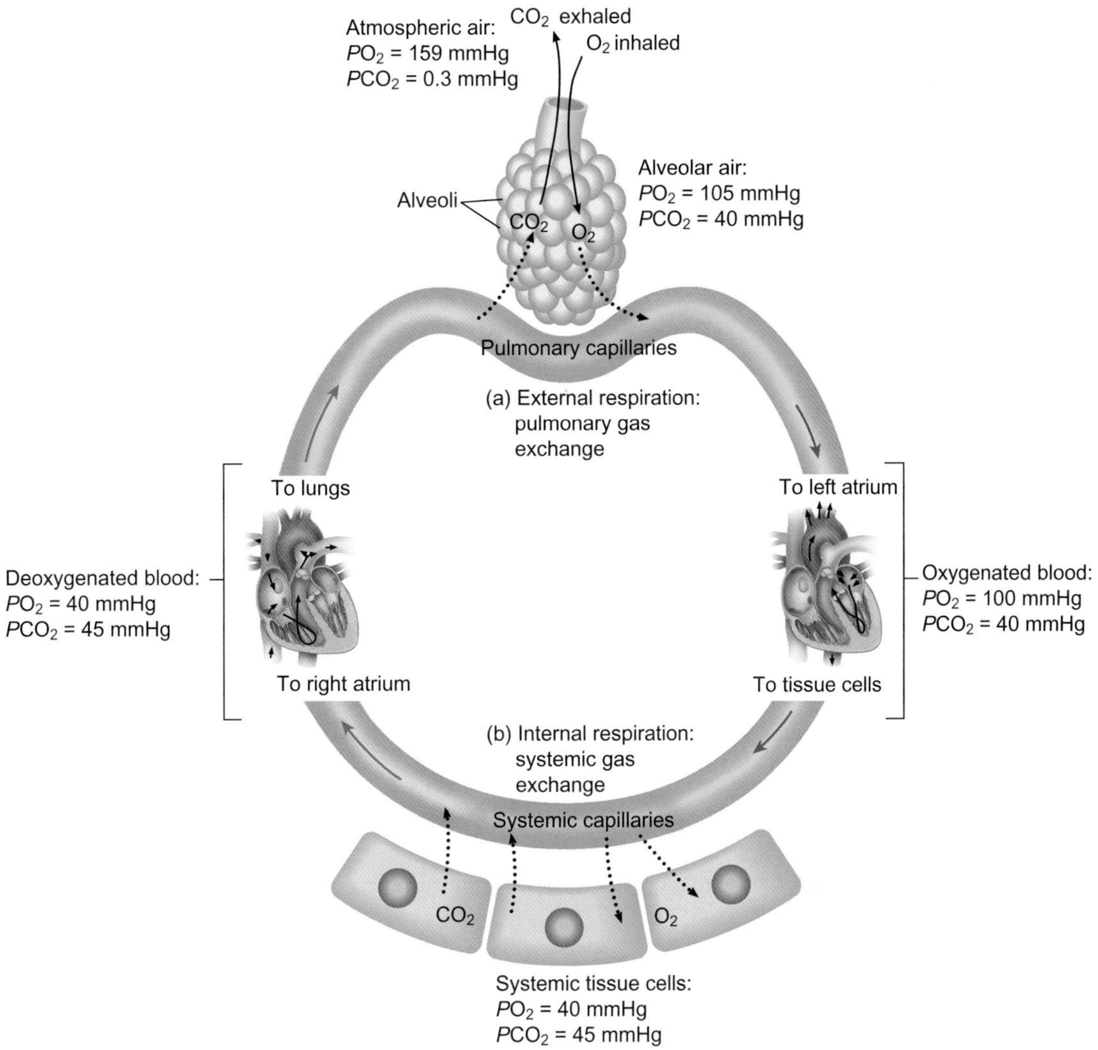

Figure 12.5 Gas exchange. Reproduced from Tortora, G.J., Derrickson, B. (2011) *Principles of Anatomy and Physiology*, with kind permission of Wiley Blackwell.

Regulation of pH

The respiratory system contributes to acid–base balance via the regulation of pH or H^+ associated with the transport of carbon dioxide. Carbon dioxide diffuses into the red cells in the blood and binds with water to form a weak acid, carbonic acid (H_2CO_3), which in turn dissociates into H^+ and HCO_3^-:

$$CO_2 + H_2O \leftrightarrow H_2CO_3 \leftrightarrow H^+ + HCO_3^-$$

$$\text{Carbon dioxide} + \text{Water} \leftrightarrow \text{Carbonic acid} \leftrightarrow \text{Hydrogen ion} + \text{Bicarbonate ion}$$

The free H^+ is buffered by binding with haemoglobin, thereby changing its structure and releasing oxygen to the tissues. Similarly, the build-up of lactic acid during exercise causes a release of oxygen to the tissues.

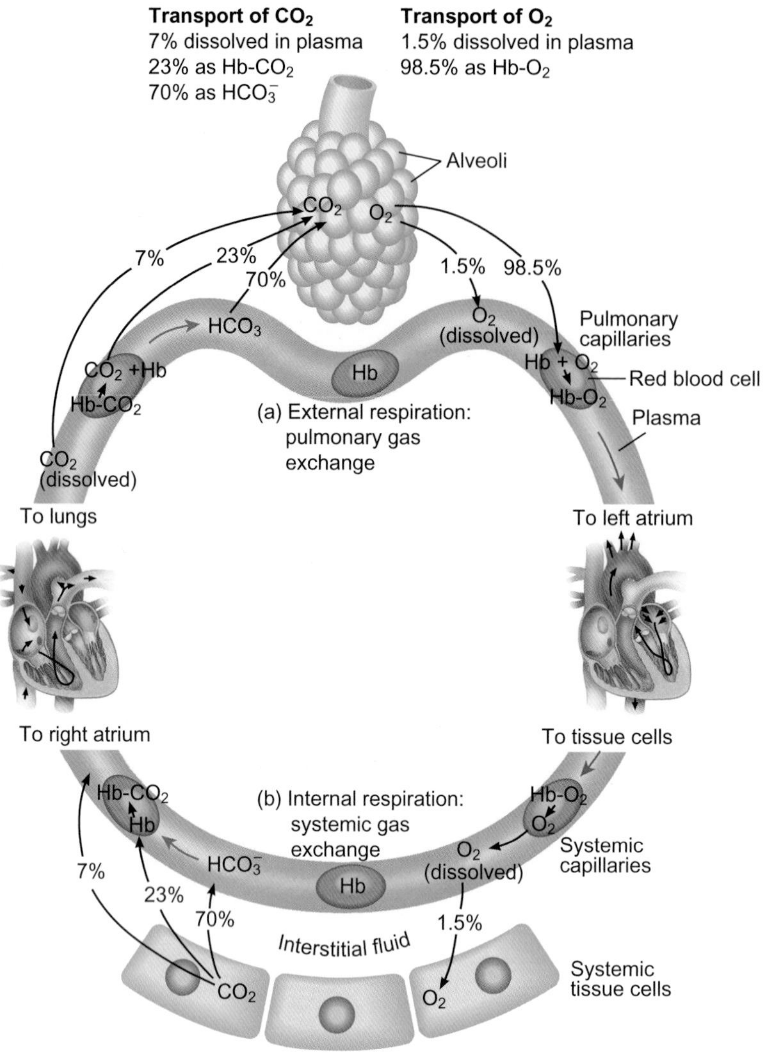

Figure 12.6 Transport of oxygen and carbon dioxide in the blood. Reproduced from Tortora, G.J., Derrickson, B. (2011) *Principles of Anatomy and Physiology*, with kind permission of Wiley Blackwell.

Arterial blood gases

Arterial blood gases (ABGs) indicate the level of functioning of the lungs. Normal ABG measures are presented in Table 12.1.

Ventilation, perfusion and V/Q ratio

Ventilation (V) refers to the flow of air throughout the lungs; whereas perfusion (Q) refers to the flow of blood in the pulmonary capillaries. In ideal circumstances, the two are matched, and their relationship is expressed as the V/Q ratio. V/Q imbalance occurs when there is inadequate ventilation and/or perfusion (Figure 12.7). V/Q imbalance can result in shunting, in which the blood is not oxygenated and remains high in carbon dioxide. The imbalance may be the result of one or a combination of different factors (Box 12.1).

Table 12.1 Normal ABG values

ABG parameter	Normal
pH	7.35–7.45
PaO_2	12–14 kPa
$PaCO_2$	4.6–6.0 kPa
SaO_2	>95%

SaO_2, arterial oxygen saturation.

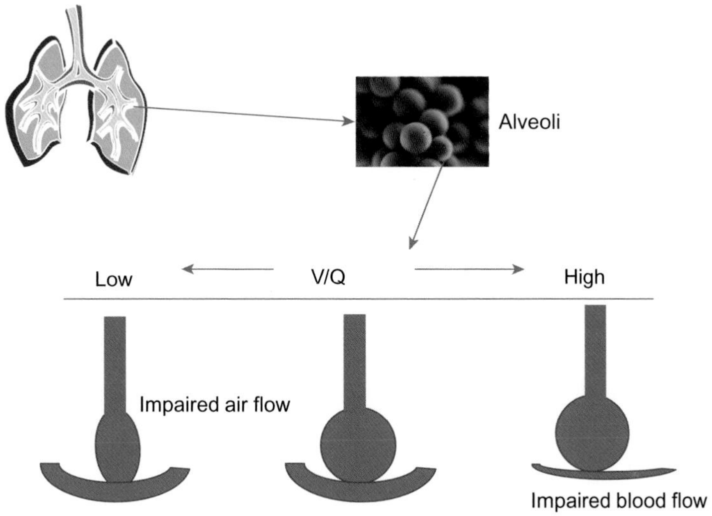

Figure 12.7 V/Q ratio.

Box 12.1 Causes of V/Q imbalance

Inadequate ventilation
Airway blockages
Low compliance
Increased airway resistance
Pulmonary oedema
Atelectasis (collapse of an area of lung tissue that has not ventilated by normal breathing)

Inadequate perfusion
Increased alveolar pressure
Increased pulmonary artery pressure
Gravity
Pulmonary embolism

Nursing care and assessment of symptoms

The nursing assessment of a patient in relation to respiration is an essential aspect of nursing care. Abnormal breathing patterns are not synonymous with respiratory disorders; they can present in cardiac disease, diabetes, head injury, anaemia and muscular and neurological disorders as well. Initial assessment involves identifying health problems and the impact of these on the patient's function and well-being. Similarly, respiratory interventions are not restricted to respiratory conditions and are a necessary part of nursing every acutely ill patient.

Nurse–patient relationship: a partnership in care

Due to the chronicity and adverse effect on health and well-being of most respiratory disorders, building a therapeutic and long-lasting relationship with the patient and the family/carer is critical and must start on the patient's initial contact with the service. A partnership approach to care is fundamental. Support from the nurse enhances patients' ability to self-manage their conditions. The nurse needs to be friendly, accessible and able to explain conditions and management in clear terms, avoiding jargon, while demonstrating empathy and excellent verbal and non-verbal communication skills (Robinson & Scullion 2009). Care needs to be taken to ensure that patients and carers are educated and that all resources and supports are in place to maximise self-care. Regular assessment of patients' inhaler technique if applicable and their understanding of medications and self-management strategies for symptom control is imperative (Conway 2007).

Respiratory assessment

The following information should be collected:

- History – general health and the development of symptoms, along with the patient's social history
- Weight loss or gain
- Night sweats
- Fevers
- Reflux
- Oedema
- Anxiety and/or depression
- Colour of the skin, fingernails, lips, etc.
- Level of consciousness
- Respiratory rate, effort and sounds
- Ability to talk and the use of accessory muscles
- Cough
- Physiological measures of respiratory function.

Respiratory rate, effort and quality, depth and rhythm of breathing should be assessed in conjunction with observing the patient's colour and chest movement (Table 12.2).

Dyspnoea/breathlessness

Dyspnoea, or difficulty breathing, is common to many respiratory disorders. Nursing assessment should include the questions shown in Box 12.2, which will provide a comprehensive outline of the patient's condition.

Cough

The presence, nature and trigger (acute or chronic) of a cough should be assessed (Table 12.3). Cough can be characterised as paroxysmal, barking, hacking, harsh or hoarse, and also be classified as effective or ineffective, and dry or productive.

Haemoptysis

Haemoptysis refers to coughing up blood or bloody sputum. It is associated with lung cancer, pneumonia, abnormalities of the pulmonary blood vessels, pulmonary embolism, TB, bronchiectasis, epistaxis, forceful coughing and cardiac disease. It may also occur as a result of anticoagulant use. The amount produced is assessed using terms such as 'teaspoon', 'tablespoon' and 'cup'.

Table 12.2 General respiratory assessment

Focus	Observe	Normal adult values	Abnormalities	Indications
Respiration	Quality, rate	Rate: 12–18 per minute	Bradypnoea <10 breaths per minute	Head injury Narcotic overdose
			Tachypnoea	Following exertion Pneumonia Diabetic ketoacidosis Pyrexia – rate of breathing increases by 7 breaths per minute for every 10°C rise in the patient's temperature
			Apnoea	Respiratory arrest
	Depth		Shallow or deep	Hyperventilation Hypoventilation (hypercapnia)
	Rhythm	Regular rhythm	Cluster breathing – normal breathing interspersed with apnoeic pauses	Neurological disorders
			Cheyne–Stokes – the rate changes with increasing periods of apnoea	End of life
	Effort		Unable to complete a sentence Use of accessory muscles Muscle retraction – intercostal and suprasternal muscles Nasal flaring	Pneumonia Airway inflammation/ obstruction Emphysema Trauma
Colour	Skin colour – check the skin, nail beds, lips, tongue, ears and nose		Cyanosis – central or peripheral	Central – hypoxaemia Peripheral – perfusion abnormality
Chest	Shape		Barrel chest	Emphysema
			Pigeon chest	Rickets
	Movement	Symmetrical	Asymmetrical	Pneumothorax – air trapped in the pleura Extreme atelectasis

Box 12.2 Nursing assessment of dyspnoea

- Is the breathlessness episodic or persistent?
- Is it associated with seasonal change, exposure to environmental irritants, anxiety, emotion?
- Is it associated with any other symptoms: cough/wheeze/stridor?
- Does it occur at rest or on exertion? Is there nocturnal dyspnoea? Or orthopnoea?
- What is the exercise tolerance? For example, how does it affect daily activities such as washing, dressing or walking?
- Is it associated with chronic fatigue?
- How does the dyspnoea affect social activities with family and friends?
- Does the dyspnoea make the patient feel anxious or depressed?
- What is the patient's perception of the severity of their dyspnoea?

Table 12.3 Assessment of productive cough

Characteristic	Monitor	Observe	Indication/action
Effective or ineffective	Breath sounds Fatigue	Improvement, lack of improvement or deterioration in condition Signs of decreased effort without clinical improvement	Increase respiratory support as necessary to avoid respiratory failure
Productive or dry	Amount	Teaspoon/tablespoon/cup	Record amount
	Colour	Clear	Non-infective
		Yellow Green Brown	Infection Send sample for culture and sensitivity
		White – frothy	Pulmonary oedema – monitor fluid intake and output, restrict intake, give diuretics Pulmonary TB – send a sample for isolation of acid-fast bacilli Lung cancer – send a sample for cytology
		White or pink-tinged frothy sputum	Pulmonary oedema, lung cancer
	Consistency	Watery	Easy to expectorate
		Thick and tenacious	Difficult to expectorate – give warmed humidified inhalations, keep the patient well hydrated
	Smell	None	
		Purulent	Infection

Table 12.4 Breath sounds

Sound	Characteristic	Signs of
Wheezing	Whistling sound, generally heard on expiration	Asthma and airway obstruction
Stridor	Snoring sound heard on inspiration	Typical of obstruction, sputum plug or foreign body, anaphylactic reaction
Crackles	A crackling or popping sound	Collapsed alveoli popping open on inspiration
Rhonchi	Snoring or rattling sounds	Fluid partly blocking the bronchi; generally heard on expiration
Pleural friction	A grating or rubbing sound heard on inspiration and expiration	Indicative of pleural inflammation

Chest pain

Chest pain with a respiratory origin may be related to painful coughing, pleural inflammation, pulmonary embolism or lung cancer. It may be persistent, dull and aching, which is associated with lung cancer, or sharp and stabbing, as with pleural inflammation and pulmonary embolism. Pleuritic pain is typically felt on inspiration and often results in the client taking only shallow breaths, which will lead to a worsening of pleural inflammation and any associated respiratory tract infection. The pain may be musculoskeletal in origin, sharp or dull, and may be the result of traumatic injury.

Abnormal breath sounds

Breath sounds are an important part of respiratory assessment and are usually assessed by the respiratory team (Table 12.4).

Clubbing of the fingers, tremor and pitting oedema

It is essential to assess the patient's general health and look for non-respiratory signs of respiratory-related illness:

- **Clubbing of the fingers** is found where there is persistent hypoxia, as in chronic respiratory disease and lung cancer.
- **Tremor** is associated with salbutamol use, which also causes tachycardia and cardiac arrhythmias. Flapping of the wrists when the arms are held outstretched is indicative of carbon dioxide retention. Warm, red skin and hands with a bounding pulse and headache are also indicative of hypercapnia.
- **Pitting oedema** in dependent areas, such as the ankles, sacrum and lower arms, is associated with heart failure.

Smoking history

It is essential to check whether the patient smokes and assess their smoking history, including their exposure to passive smoking. The number of pack–years should be calculated, one pack year corresponding to 20 cigarettes smoked per day for 1 year. The total number of pack–years is therefore calculated as follows:

$$\frac{(\text{Number of cigarettes smoked per day}) \times (\text{Number of years smoking})}{20}$$

Previous attempts at smoking cessation should be explored, and the level of success and facilitators and barriers should be identified.

Medications

Determine whether the patient is receiving any medications or treatments, including oxygen and non-invasive ventilation (NIV). Note the drug, dose, frequency, effectiveness and side effects if any. Patient education is imperative to ensure that patients are competent to manage their medications, adjusting the dosage and medications as necessary so they can best manage their condition. The use of symptom diaries or measures of function should be encouraged to gain an accurate picture of the impact of the disease. Oxygen use should be assessed in relation to the amount and the duration of use. Assessing patients' technique when using inhalers or nebuliser preparations is essential to maximise the benefit of the treatment.

Respiratory function testing

Peak expiratory flow

Peak expiratory flow (PEF) measures maximum expiratory flow following a forced expiration (Figure 12.8); it can provide a crude record of respiratory function over time if a diary of the results is kept. Morning and evening daily monitoring of PEF rate for 2–4 weeks can identify variability in airflow limitation for diagnosis and monitoring.

Pulse oximetry

Pulse oximetry (Figure 12.9) provides an estimated measure of oxygen saturation that is accurate within 5% for the range above 70% (Robinson & Scullion 2009); below 70% saturation, it is not reliable. Poor peripheral circulation or coldness will also reduce reliability.

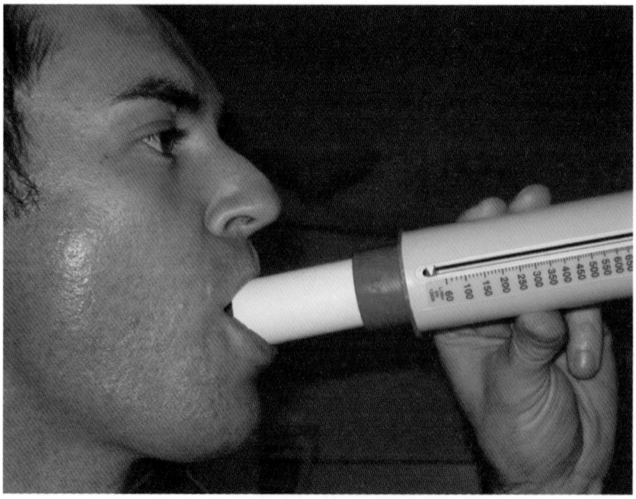

Figure 12.8 Measurement of peak flow. Reproduced from Dougherty, L. & Lister, S. (2011) *The Royal Marsden Hospital Manual of Clinical Nursing Procedures*, with kind permission from Wiley Blackwell.

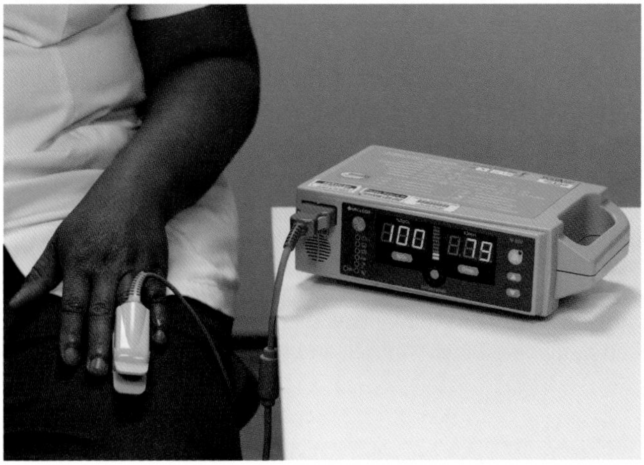

Figure 12.9 Pulse oximetry. Reproduced from Dougherty, L. & Lister, S. (2011) *The Royal Marsden Hospital Manual of Clinical Nursing Procedures*, with kind permission from Wiley Blackwell.

Spirometry

Spirometry is used to diagnose patients as well as to monitor disease progression and the response to medication. Measures include forced expiratory volume in 1 second (FEV_1), forced vital capacity (FVC), lung capacity and FEV_1/FVC ratio, which is a measure of the amount of air in the full lungs that has been expired after 1 second.

Reversibility testing

Reversibility testing with bronchodilators or corticosteroids can be used to establish the reversibility of airflow obstruction that is typically seen in asthma (Robinson & Scullion 2009).

Sputum

If there is an indication of respiratory tract infection, sputum is sent for culture and sensitivity (C & S) so that appropriate antibiotics can be prescribed.

Radiological investigations

Radiological investigations are used for diagnosis and monitoring. They include chest X-ray, computed tomography (CT) and magnetic resonance imaging.

Bronchoscopy

Bronchoscopy is used to directly visualise the lungs. A fibreoptic camera is passed into the patient's trachea and lungs, and the lungs can then be assessed for signs of lung disease. Samples can be taken for histological and cytological examination.

ABG readings

Arterial blood is taken to measure PaO_2, $PaCO_2$ and pH (see Table 12.1 earlier in the chapter). ABG values demonstrate the level of functioning of the lungs and are used to diagnose, assess and monitor critically ill patients. Abnormal ABGs can indicate respiratory acidosis, respiratory alkalosis, metabolic acidosis and metabolic alkalosis.

Skin prick testing

Skin prick testing is used to test for specific allergies in asthma or rhinitis. Various potential allergens are tested, for example house dust mite, animal dander and grass pollen.

Body mass index

Patients with advanced lung disease may be underweight as a result of the increased energy expenditure associated with dyspnoea, and reduced tolerance to eating from a full stomach pressing on the diaphragm. A low body mass index (BMI) is associated with an increased risk of death in patients with advanced respiratory disease, while patients with a high BMI generally have decreased exercise tolerance and increased dyspnoea. Dietary advice and referral to a dietitian are advised for those with an abnormal BMI.

Respiratory interventions

Patients with decreased mobility, decreased neurological or immunological functioning, underlying respiratory illness or chronic conditions are at increased risk of developing respiratory tract infections. Respiratory interventions that enhance lung function and decrease lung stasis and the risk of respiratory tract infection include positioning, oxygen administration and breathing exercises.

Positioning

Positioning can help patients to maximise their lung function. The high side-lying position facilitates maximum lung expansion while the patient in bed (Figure 12.10a). The tripod position (Figure 12.10b) increases the potential for thoracic expansion with minimal effort; in this, the patient leans forward with their arms on a table. Chest clearance can be enhanced with the use of postural drainage. Relaxed sitting (Figure 12.10c), forward-lean standing (Figure 12.10d) and relaxed standing against a wall (Figure 12.10e) also provide support for the body by minimising the use of postural muscles and reducing oxygen requirements. Alternating positions in critically ill and immobile patients can help to prevent and treat atelectasis and pneumonia.

Oxygen administration and nebuliser use

Oxygen can be administered via a nasal cannula (Figure 12.11), oxygen mask (Figure 12.12) or mask with Venturi valve (Figure 12.13) to enhance the amount of oxygen delivered to the tissues. Oxygen can be humidified to offset its drying effects and loosen secretions; this is particularly useful for patients with tenacious sputum. Showers and baths or steam inhalation in the home setting also help to liquefy secretions, aiding expectoration. Nebulisers can be used to moisten the air and deliver medications to the respiratory tract.

Breathing exercises

Breathing exercises help patients to manage their breathlessness and maximise the amount of oxygen delivered to the tissues. Pursed lip breathing, in which the lips are pursed on exhalation to slow breathing, prevents airway collapse in emphysema. Practising huffing and coughing clears lung secretions. Incentive spirometry can be used to increase the inspiratory volume and to induce coughing.

Mobilisation and exercise

Mobilisation, especially early mobilisation following surgery, is essential in maximising chest clearance. A passive range of movement exercises will stimulate deep breathing and be effective in reducing atelectasis and respiratory tract infections in immobile patients.

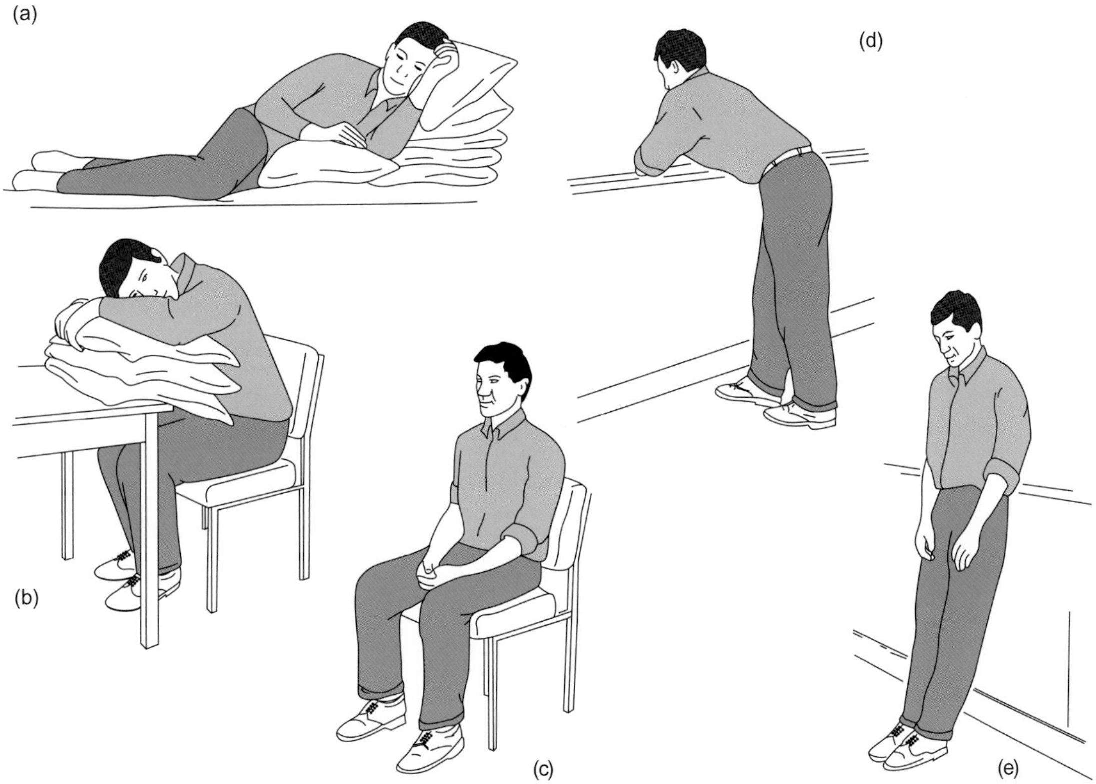

Figure 12.10 Optimal positions to reduce breathing effort (see the text for a description). Reproduced from Dougherty, L. & Lister, S. (2011) *The Royal Marsden Hospital Manual of Clinical Nursing Procedures*, with kind permission from Wiley Blackwell.

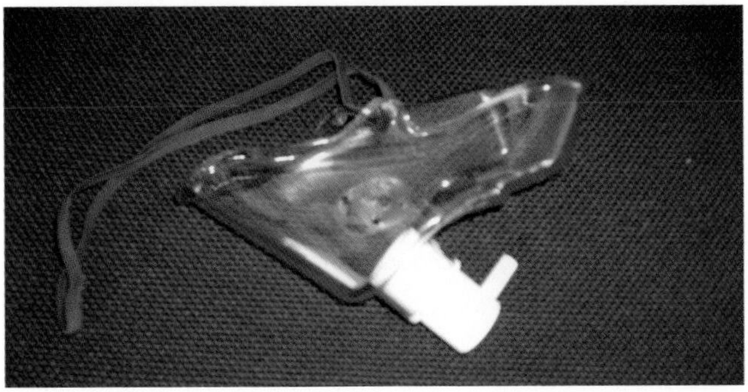

Figure 12.11 Nasal cannula. Reproduced from Dougherty, L. & Lister, S. (2011) *The Royal Marsden Hospital Manual of Clinical Nursing Procedures*, with kind permission from Wiley Blackwell.

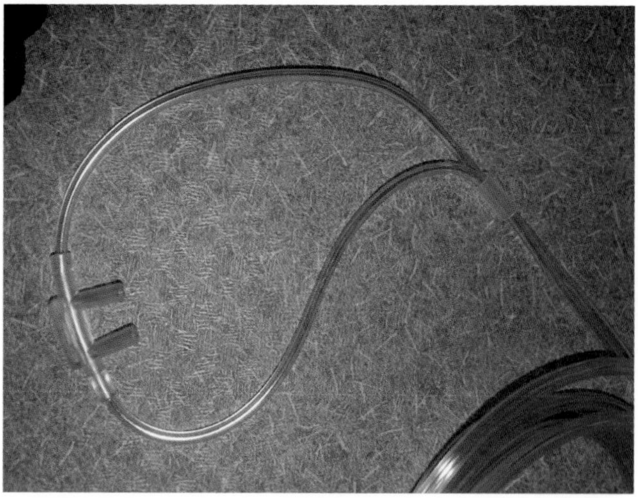

Figure 12.12 Oxygen mask. Reproduced from Dougherty, L. & Lister, S. (2011) *The Royal Marsden Hospital Manual of Clinical Nursing Procedures*, with kind permission from Wiley Blackwell.

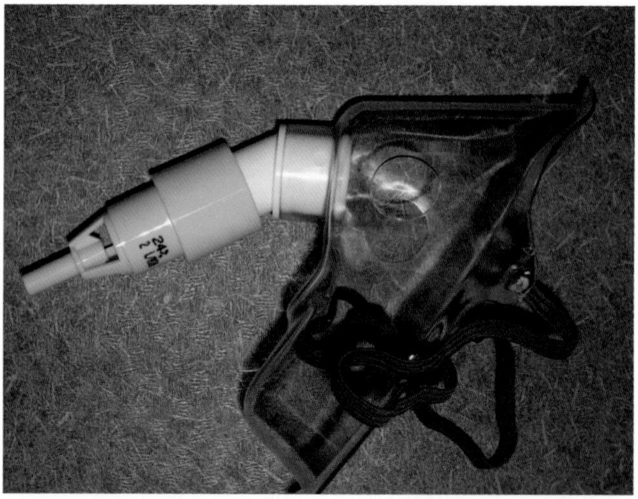

Figure 12.13 Mask with Venturi valve. Reproduced from Dougherty, L. & Lister, S. (2011) *The Royal Marsden Hospital Manual of Clinical Nursing Procedures*, with kind permission from Wiley Blackwell.

Hydration and dietary advice

Ensuring that the patient is well hydrated makes it easier for them to expectorate respiratory secretions. Oral fluid intake should be encouraged as tolerated but with caution if any cardiac disease is present. Dyspnoea impacts on a patient's eating tolerance, and advice should be given to those with a low BMI to eat frequent small, high-calorie meals.

Smoking cessation

Smoking cessation is arguably the single greatest intervention that any patient with respiratory illness can do to enhance their health and reduce the burden of illness. Even in advanced chronic respiratory illness, smoking cessation can arrest the decline in lung function.

Brief interventions to promote cessation have been shown to increase smoking cessation (Milner 2004; National Institute for Clinical Excellence 2006) and should be used on assessment and documented; they need to be sensitive to the person's situation, needs and preferences.

Smoking status, advice offered and client preferences should be recorded annually. Provide details of local smoking cessation groups and national helplines. Changing routine or quitting with a friend can also help increase the likelihood of the individual successfully quitting (Scullion 2007). Information should also be provided to patients on both pharmacological and non-pharmacological smoking cessation aids. Nicotine replacement therapy, for example, can be used to help reduce nicotine cravings when the patient initially stops smoking.

Pulmonary rehabilitation

Pulmonary rehabilitation refers to a programme of education and exercise specifically designed for the patient by the multidisciplinary team to increase self-management and self-efficacy, increase exercise tolerance, decrease symptom burden, decrease anxiety and depression, enhance quality of life through enhanced physical, mental, social and emotional well-being, and maximise work potential (Williams 2009). The programme will involve a tailored exercise regime, an assessment of BMI and dietary advice, smoking cessation advice, education about the patient's illness, self-management, coping strategies, energy conservation, establishing priorities, pacing, anxiety management, pharmacological review and psychological and behavioural interventions.

Management of specific conditions

Pneumonia

Pathophysiology

Pneumonia is an infection of the lungs involving an acute inflammatory response that impairs the work of the alveoli and interferes with ventilation.

Classification

Pneumonia can be classified as:

- community-acquired pneumonia;
- hospital-acquired pneumonia;
- aspiration pneumonia;
- pneumonia in immunocompromised patients.

Clinical manifestations

The clinical manifestations of pneumonia are:

- fever;
- pleuritic chest pain;
- tachypnoea (25–45 breaths per minute) and possibly orthopnea;
- tachycardia;
- a productive cough with purulent, blood-stained sputum;
- general symptoms including anorexia, headaches and muscle pains;
- on auscultation, there may be reduced breath sounds, crackles or dullness.

Diagnosis

The following investigations are used in diagnosis (Woodhead 2010):

- chest X-ray;
- blood analysis, typically showing a raised white cell count;
- blood pressure monitoring;
- blood urea measurement;
- pulse oximetry;
- ABGs;
- blood culture;
- sputum samples for C & S.

Assessment and management

Assessment of severity is important to determine the management of the patient with pneumonia, and the CURB65 score can be used for this. This scores 1 point for each of:

- C (confusion);
- U (blood urea >7 mmol/L);
- R (respiratory rate >30/min);
- B (blood pressure: systolic <90 mmHg, diastolic <60 mmHg);
- 65 (>65 years of age).

Medical management includes the prompt and appropriate administration of intravenous antibiotic therapy, oxygen and intravenous fluids to correct the fluid balance. If an oxygen saturation of more than 92% is not achieved using oxygen, NIV may be considered.

Nursing assessment and management

Respiratory assessment should include a particular focus on observing the patient's temperature, respiration, blood pressure, mentation and hydration. Signs of confusion are important markers of disease severity and response to treatment.

The patient may require pain relief and management of dyspnoea. A high semi-Fowler's position can relieve dyspnoea and the patient's position should be alternated to enhance oxygenation and sputum clearance. Oxygen should be humidified and the patient well hydrated to facilitate sputum clearance. Pulse oximetry should be monitored closely and any abnormalities treated promptly. Breathing and coughing exercises and mobilisation as tolerated can be used to maximise expectoration. Supportive care is necessary, so manage pyrexia, assist with hygiene needs, alternate rest with activity and encourage a high-protein, high-calorie diet as far as the patient can tolerate it.

Tuberculosis

TB is an infectious disease that, in humans, is caused by *Mycobacterium tuberculosis*. Mycobacteria are transmitted from person to person by droplet infection through coughing or sneezing. The response to infection can result in latent or active TB (Sotgiu & Migliori 2010). Prevention requires the rapid identification of new cases, effective treatment and contact tracing.

Aetiology

TB can affect any organ but the focus here is on pulmonary TB. Extrapulmonary or disseminated TB occurs when infection is through the blood or lymphatic system.

Clinical manifestations

These can include:

- a persistent cough, possibly with haemoptysis, that may initially be dry but can become productive with blood-streaked sputum;
- weight loss;
- low-grade fever with night sweats;
- loss of appetite;
- dyspnoea;
- on blood sample analysis, usually anaemia and a raised erythrocyte sedimentation rate and lymphocyte count.

Diagnosis

Investigations can include:

- sputum smear microscopy (mycobacterial culture being the gold standard test, although it can take several weeks for results to be obtained);
- chest X-ray (Sotgiu & Migliori 2010);
- tuberculin skin testing, commonly referred to as the Mantoux test, which is used for screening purposes and can detect those who have been infected or have received vaccination (BCG) but do not have active disease.

Assessment and management

- Test for sensitivity of the bacillus to the medication regimen.
- Monitor the sputum results.
- Promptly identify and manage any side effects from medication and medication adherence by talking to the patient and monitoring medication containers to ensure that the expected quantities have been used.

A standard course of treatment typically involves a 6-month regimen of a combination of anti-TB medications, such as isoniazid and rifampicin with pyrazinamide and ethambutol for 2 months, followed by isoniazid and rifampicin for a further 4 months. This regimen is extended to 9 months in certain circumstances, including persistent positive sputum cultures and resistance of the organism to pyrazinamide.

Multi-drug-resistant (MDR) TB is an increasing problem, with risk factors including a history of TB treatment prior to the current diagnosis, contact with known MDR TB, HIV infection, and birth in a country where the World Health Organization has reported a high incidence of MDR TB. Treatment is complex and needs to be directed by an specialist respiratory infectious diseases physician.

Directly observed therapy

Directly observed therapy is a recognised approach to enhancing adherence. It involves a health worker meeting with and observing the patient taking the medication. This demands daily or weekly visits as required by the treatment regimen. Although it is resource-intensive, directly observed therapy has been shown to be a key mechanism for the control of TB (Maguire *et al*. 2011).

Nursing management

Most TB management is organised through national TB centres, where public health teams and specialist respiratory TB nurses collaborate on TB control. The nurse plays an essential role in supporting the patient through individual assessment, relationship-building, education and monitoring. TB is associated with stigma, and the nurse's sensitivity to the patient's distress is essential. Ongoing treatment after the symptoms have disappeared and monitoring for adverse reactions to anti-TB medications are priorities.

Nursing care for patients with infectious TB requires collaboration with infection control specialists and adherence to procedures aimed at eliminating the risk of TB transmission. It must be remembered that the risk of healthcare-associated transmission is increased during aerosol-producing procedures, including coughing, suctioning, bronchoscopy, endotracheal intubation, open abscess irrigation and autopsy.

Breathing and coughing exercises, with close attention to infection control and hygiene needs, can be used to facilitate expectoration. Supportive care with the management of pyrexia and assistance to manage night sweats may be necessary. Ensure the patient is well hydrated, and alternate rest with activity. A high-protein, high-calorie diet and oxygen as necessary can be used to manage loss of appetite, weight loss and any consequent fatigue.

Visit www.wileyfundamentalseries.com/medicalnursing and read Reflective Question 12.1 to think more about this topic.

Asthma

Definition

Asthma is a chronic inflammatory disease of the airways, associated with airway hyperresponsiveness causing widespread, but variable, airflow obstruction within the lung that is often reversible, either spontaneously or with treatment (Global Initiative for Asthma Management [GINA] 2010).

Triggers and risk factors

The exact cause(s) of asthma are not fully known. Risk factors include:

- a familial predisposition;
- atopy (an inherited trait in which the immune system is highly responsive to allergens);
- exposure to allergens and irritants;
- smoking;
- frequent respiratory tract infections, such as with respiratory syncytial virus.

Common triggers for symptoms and exacerbations of asthma include exercise, cold air, strong odours, perfume, rhinosinusitis and stress.

Pathophysiology

Airway inflammation, with associated airway hyperresponsiveness, is the underlying feature of asthma irrespective of whether symptoms are triggered by exposure to allergy, irritants or a combination of both. Airway hyperresponsiveness causes an 'overresponse' of the airways to a wide range of stimuli such as allergens and irritants, resulting in a narrowing of the airways and variable airflow limitation with intermittent symptoms.

Persistent inflammation results in increased smooth muscle, a proliferation of blood vessels in the airway walls and an increased number of mucus-producing goblet cells.

Clinical manifestations

These include:

- breathlessness with wheezing and/or cough;
- chest tightness;

- symptoms that are usually worse at night and in the early morning;
- cyanosis and abnormal ABGs;
- respiratory effort marked by nasal flaring and the use of accessory muscles;
- wheezing that may be absent on auscultation, indicating that the airways are too constricted for air to flow;
- in very severe attacks, respiratory failure; PaO_2 (on air) will be <60 mmHg and $PaCO_2$ >45 mmHg.

Diagnosis

Diagnosis involves:

- a medical history;
- a physical examination;
- respiratory function tests.

Respiratory function tests

Spirometry is recommended to diagnose and assess the severity of asthma by measuring airflow limitation and reversibility. With bronchodilators, a reversibility of airflow limitation of >12% and of FEV_1 >200 mL confirms a diagnosis of asthma.

Daily monitoring of PEF every morning and evening for 2–4 weeks can identify any variability in airflow limitation for diagnosis and monitoring. A diurnal variability of over 20% is diagnostic of asthma, the magnitude of the variability reflecting the severity.

Assessment and management

The aim of management is to relieve the immediate symptoms and reduce and control inflammation, to prevent restructuring of the airways. Initial treatment should be adjusted according to the level of control being achieved. Treatment is then stepped up and stepped down to achieve and maintain control with minimum medication, thereby minimising the risk of adverse effects.

Pharmacological management

Asthma medication is categorised into two groups: controllers and relievers.

Controllers are usually anti-inflammatory medications taken daily on a long-term basis to maintain clinical control. Controllers include inhaled glucocorticosteroids taken alone or in combination with long acting beta-2-agonists. Secondary agents, including anti-leukotrienes, can be used in addition if necessary. Glucocorticosteroids work by reducing oedema and airway spasm. Anti-leukotrienes work by blocking the action of leukotrienes, which attract inflammatory-promoting eosinophils to the airway mucosa.

Relievers or rapidly acting beta-2-agonists are bronchodilator medications that stimulate beta-adrenergic receptors to dilate the airways. Beta-2-agonists are taken on an as-needed basis to reverse the bronchoconstriction and relieve the symptoms. Ideally, relievers should not be required if the asthma is well controlled, and an increased use of reliever medication is a sign of deteriorating control and increased inflammation.

Asthma treatment can be administered in inhaled, oral or injectable forms. A range of different inhaler devices are available that allow greater choice in meeting patients' preferences and maximising their adherence to treatment. However, all inhalers require coordination, training and skill for effective use. Poor inhaler technique results in an inadequate delivery of medication to the airways and an increased deposition of medication in the mouth, resulting in poor symptom control. Deposition of glucocorticoids in the mouth can also lead to oral candidiasis.

Management of exacerbations

Guidelines for the management of exacerbations of asthma provide a step-wise management programme based on the symptoms and the response to beta-2-agonists, involving a combination of controllers and relievers to relieve the symptoms and reduce inflammation (see http://www.ginasthma.org for up-to-date international management guidelines).

Nursing assessment and management

Assessment of the patient's clinical condition, level of control and risk of exacerbation are essential aspects of the nurse's role, as are educating and supporting patients to manage their treatment.

Effective management is reliant on developing a partnership between the patient and the healthcare professional; knowledge, skills and confidence in self-care are essential to this partnership (GINA, 2010). Guided self-management reduces asthma morbidity (GINA, 2010) and features:

- education
- joint goal-setting
- regular review
- a written action plan
- self-monitoring.

Asthma education includes being sensitive to the particular information needs and difficulties of individual patients. Attending to their fears, exploring their expectations and sharing information underpin a partnership approach to guided self-management.

Specific information should be provided on the condition and the reliever and controller medication. By demonstrating and checking, the nurse must ensure that all patients use their inhalers correctly as poor inhaler technique is associated with deteriorating asthma. It is important to check inhaler and PEF technique regularly in the ward, clinic and emergency department. Information on inhaler devices and techniques is also provided on the GINA website (http://www.ginasthma.org). Verbal information should be supported by written information and contact details for the local asthma support group.

Morbidity can be reduced by a guided self-management with a personalised written asthma action plan to adjust the treatment in response to changes in asthma control (GINA, 2010).

Visit www.wileyfundamentalseries.com/medicalnursing and read Reflective Question 12.2 to think more about this topic.

Chronic obstructive pulmonary disease

Definition

Chronic obstructive pulmonary disease (COPD) is currently the fourth leading cause of mortality in the world and includes chronic bronchitis and emphysema. COPD is characterised by airflow obstruction that is not fully reversible and is usually progressive. The airflow limitation is associated with inflammatory responses of the lung to noxious particles or gases, especially cigarette smoke (Global Initiative for Chronic Obstructive Disease [GOLD] 2010). Other risk factors include exposure to significant air pollutants.

COPD is a treatable and preventable disease that is also associated with extrapulmonary effects that can, in some patients, contribute to the severity of their condition. The extrapulmonary effects of COPD include weight loss, skeletal muscle dysfunction and nutritional abnormalities. In addition, COPD is also associated with an increased risk of myocardial infarction and angina, osteoporosis, anxiety and depression, respiratory infections, lung cancer, diabetes and anaemia (GOLD, 2010).

Classification of COPD

COPD is classified by GOLD (2010) into four stages reflecting the degree of severity – mild, moderate, severe and very severe – with the FEV_1 ranging from 80% or more to less than 30%. Although mild COPD generally remains undiagnosed, severe and very severe COPD have a major impact on quality of life, with fatigue and frequent exacerbations commonplace. Very severe COPD may also involve respiratory and cardiac failure with life-threatening exacerbations (GOLD, 2010).

Risk factors

The following are risk factors for COPD:

- noxious gases including tobacco smoke;
- the total number of pack–years of smoking, the age at which smoking started and current smoking are risk factors for mortality in COPD. Not all smokers develop clinically significant COPD, indicating the importance of other factors at play;
- alpha-1-antitrypsin deficiency.

COPD rarely gives rise to troublesome symptoms before the age of 40 years. One exception to this rule is when it is linked with an inherited deficiency of alpha-1-antitrypsin.

Pathophysiology

Pathological changes include chronic inflammation, an increased number of inflammatory cells and structural changes as a result of injury and repair. These changes are arrested but not reversed following smoking cessation.

Inflammation, fibrosis (structural changes) and exudate in COPD result in and correlate with a reduced FEV_1 and FEV_1/FVC ratio, while destruction of the lung tissue results in decreased gas transfer. As a consequence of destruction at the alveolar level and loss of airway recoil, air trapping occurs, resulting in hyperinflation. Abnormal gas exchange results in hypoxaemia and hypercapnia.

Clinical manifestations

These include:

- increasing breathlessness;
- a breathing pattern that involves a long expiration phase using pursed lips;
- a prolonged forced expiratory phase may extend to longer than 5 seconds in advanced disease;
- an increased use of the accessory muscles during respiration;
- the patient visibly leaning forward;
- cough with production of sputum;
- a wheeze;
- weight loss;
- fatigue;
- hyperinflation of the lungs and a 'barrel-shaped' chest;
- Hoover's sign – flattening of the diaphragm and pulling in of the lower ribs on inspiration;
- jugular vein distension, liver enlargement and peripheral oedema indicating right-sided heart failure associated with pulmonary hypertension.

Diagnosis

Diagnosis involves:

- a medical history;
- the patient's occupation;
- a physical examination;
- the symptoms;
- spirometry – COPD is indicated if the FEV_1/FVC ratio is <0.7 after administration of a bronchodilator;
- breathlessness, wheeze, persistent cough and sputum production.

Assessment and management

The overall aim of COPD management is to relieve symptoms, assess severity, improve exercise capacity and health status, prevent disease progression, and prevent and treat complications and exacerbations

(GOLD 2010; National Clinical Guideline Centre 2010). Bronchodilator medications form the basis of symptom relief and improvement of exercise tolerance. These include beta-2-agonists, anticholinergic agents and methylxanthines, which may be used in combination. Inhalational treatment is preferred both for its effectiveness and to minimise side effects. Long-acting inhaled anticholinergics reduce the rate of exacerbations and improve the effectiveness of pulmonary rehabilitation. Regular assessment of inhaler technique is essential.

Acute exacerbations

An acute exacerbation of COPD is identified by an increase in respiratory symptoms beyond normal everyday variations that possibly requires hospitalisation (GOLD 2010; National Clinical Guideline Centre 2010). Acute exacerbations are also associated with an increased risk of readmission to hospital (10–14%) and mortality, with a mean survival time after the first admission to hospital of just under 6 years (GOLD, 2010; Miravitlles 2010; National Clinical Guideline Centre 2010). Up to 75% of exacerbations are infective (bacterial or viral); other causes include air pollution, increased comorbidity and poor medication adherence (Miravitlles 2010).

Presentation includes increased breathlessness with increased purulence and volume of the sputum. Cough, wheeze, exercise intolerance and fatigue are also common features. In addition, patients may also experience chest tightness, fluid retention and confusion.

Management of exacerbations

Antibiotic therapy is usually prescribed. A course of oral corticosteroids is prescribed to reduce inflammation. However, this has to be balanced against the risk of complications from their regular use. Oxygen therapy is indicated for the management of hypoxaemia; an oxygen saturation of over 90% is acceptable. ABG analysis is essential to detect carbon dioxide retention. Rapid assessment units, early discharge and hospital at home programmes are increasingly being developed to support the treatment of patients with acute exacerbations at home.

Nursing assessment and management care plan for COPD

A care plan for the nursing assessment and management of COPD is shown in Table 12.5.

Patients with advanced disease experience poor symptom control, isolation, guilt, stigma, anxiety and depression (Andenaes *et al.* 2004; Bailey 2004; Fraser *et al.* 2006; Gudmundsson *et al.* 2006; Jones 2009). There are also clear links between a deteriorating health status in COPD and a need for admission to hospital (Groenewegen *et al.* 2003; Oostenbrink & Rutten-van Mölkena 2004). Thus, the nursing diagnosis and management need to be sensitive to the immediate care needs of the patient and also mindful of changes in the patient's overall health status over time.

Palliative care

Palliative care is an approach to care that, through the prevention and relief of suffering, seeks to improve the quality of life of patients and their families facing problems associated with life-threatening illness. Palliative care is indicated for the management of severe and very severe COPD. Elkington *et al.* (2005) found that approximately 40% of carers of individuals who had recently died from COPD had been unaware that the patient was likely to die.

There are well-recognised challenges in end of life communication in COPD (Russell & Russell 2007). Open communication between healthcare professionals, the patient and the carers allows an exploration of the patient's prognosis and current and anticipated fears and concerns. Conversations of this nature develop over time and should be encouraged when the patient is stable and able to participate fully in exploring possible treatment interventions, such as mechanical ventilation.

In addition to communication needs, the patient may also require nursing care to address breathlessness, relaxation and breathing exercises, sputum clearance, cough, smoking cessation, oxygen and medication management, anxiety and depression, pain, nutritional support and social, psychological and emotional support. The use of opiates, benzodiazepines, tricyclic antidepressants, major tranquillisers and oxygen may be indicated when a patient in end-stage COPD has not responded to other medical treatment (National Clinical Guideline Centre 2010).

Table 12.5 Nursing assessment and management care plan for COPD

Assessment and management	Action	Outcome
Dyspnoea	Monitoring of respiratory rate and pattern, oximetry, mental state and orientation	Prompt recognition of and response to deteriorating respiratory function, anxiety and distress
	Positioning the patient in an upright position	An upright position enables breathing
	Spirometry	Establishes respiratory function status
	Administering medication	Inhaled or nebulised bronchodilators to relax bronchial smooth muscle
	Monitoring inhaler and nebuliser technique	Ensure optimum deposition of medication and minimise unwanted side effects such as tremor and tachycardia
Oxygenation saturation	Oximetry	Prompt recognition of and response to desaturation
	Monitoring ABGs	Prompt recognition and treatment of hypoxemia and carbon dioxide retention
	Administering oxygen therapy as prescribed when saturation is <90%	Avoidance of suppression of respiratory drive
Cough and mucous clearance	Encouraging an effective coughing technique	Effective clearance while conserving energy
	Encouraging fluid intake	Adequate hydration to help thin secretions
	Oral care	Removal of mucus deposits in the mouth
Anxiety	Remaining with the patient who is experiencing increased dyspnoea	Minimising anxiety and its effects on an increasing sense of breathlessness
		Reduction in risk of panic attacks associated with severe dyspnoea
	Enhancing the environmental impact on dyspnoea-related anxiety: provide care in a calm and reassuring manner; reduce the impact of noise; position the patient near a window or door if possible	Minimise the sense of suffocation and feeling of being trapped in an enclosed area
	Encouraging deep breathing and relaxation exercises	Enhance self-care

(*Continued*)

Table 12.5 (*Continued*)

Assessment and management	Action	Outcome
Activity and exercise tolerance, fatigue	Monitoring dyspnoea and oxygenation	Prompt recognition of and response to activity-related desaturation
		Conservation of energy
	Planning exercise activity, increasing exercise tolerance and returning to the (pre-exacerbation) baseline activities of daily living	Synchronisation of exercise with administration of medication for maximum benefit
	Seeking physiotherapy support	Redress and improve exercise tolerance and management of dyspnoea
	Assisting patients with a gradual return towards (pre-exacerbation) baseline activities of daily living	Minimise loss of overall health status and independence
	Supporting and teaching the patient about energy conservation through pacing activities, alternating high- and low-energy activities; pursed-lip breathing	Minimise loss of overall health status and independence while also enhancing self-care in the longer term
	Support patient to identify priorities	Energy is focused on priorities
Nutritional status	Monitoring the patient's weight	Prompt recognition of and response to changes in both fluid retention and nutritional status
	Seeking the nutritionist's support	Dietary support in terms of high-protein and low-carbohydrate meals
	Improving intake (Odencrants *et al.* 2005, 2007) and meal experience through ordering small frequent meals during the patient's hospital stay and teaching the patient about planning small meals	Improvement in dietary intake in both the short and long term; improvement in nutritional status and reduction in risk of mortality
Emotional, social and psychological well-being	Opening a conversation with the patient and carer about illness experiences	Prompt recognition of and response to signs of depression; address fears and concerns about the future
	Providing information on community support groups	Help to minimise the risk of increased social isolation
	Seeking an occupational therapist, social worker and/or psychologist for information and support	Optimisation of the capacity to self-care and remain independent; ensuring access to social benefits and supports

Table 12.5 (*Continued*)

Assessment and management	Action	Outcome
Palliative care needs	Communication – prognosis and fears	Open communication between the patient, family and carers
	Providing a supportive environment	The patient and family feel supported
	Establishing priorities	The patient and family focus on the patient's identified priorities
	Establishing a plan for advanced care, use of opiates and ventilation	Patients' and families' wishes in relation to management are adhered to where possible

Bronchiectasis

Pathophysiology

Bronchiectasis is an obstructive lung condition in which there is destruction and widening of the large airways and abnormal bronchial wall thickening as a result of a recurring cycle of infection and inflammation (Ten Hacken 2010). Bronchiectasis is usually localised to one lung segment or lobe but may spread over time to other parts of the same lung as a result of unresolved infections. Exacerbations are associated with infections.

A number of conditions lead to bronchiectasis, including structural lung conditions, CF and other conditions associated with abnormal mucocillary clearance; retained inhaled foreign objects, tumours and obstructive lung conditions including COPD; an abnormal immune response; infections including tuberculosis, pneumonia, measles and whooping cough; and inflammatory bowel disease (Bilton & Jones 2011).

Clinical manifestations

Signs and symptoms include:

- a productive cough;
- breathlessness with chest pain;
- increased sputum production, possibly with haemoptysis;
- fatigue;
- clubbing of the fingers in severe cases.

Diagnosis

This will involve:

- high-resolution CT;
- spirometry and demonstration of a reduced FEV_1 and reduced FEV_1/FVC ratio.

Assessment and management

Management of the underlying cause is important for both the short-term and long-term outcome. A prompt treatment and resolution of infective exacerbations, the prevention of further infections, possibly with the prolonged use of antibiotics, and bronchial clearance underpin treatment plans (Drain & Elborn 2011). Nursing assessment and care is similar to that for COPD.

Cystic fibrosis

Pathophysiology

CF is a life-threatening inherited multisystem disease that results from a genetic mutation; it is common in white individuals, affecting 1 in 2500 births in the UK. The abnormal gene is subject to autosomal recessive inheritance, meaning that both parents must be carriers for the condition to be inherited by their child.

Diagnosis and clinical manifestations

Examination will identify:

- a positive sweat test;
- typically, a patient who is small in stature and underweight, and has finger clubbing;
- failure to thrive in infants;
- steatorrhoea;
- respiratory symptoms;
- infertility in males.

Assessment and management

As a consequence of the multisystem involvement, patients require management of gastrointestinal, pancreatic and hepatic complications in addition to respiratory problems. Poor secretion clearance from the airways results in recurrent infections, damage to the bronchi, the development of bronchiectasis and respiratory failure. The respiratory tract is colonised with bacteria that must frequently be treated combinations of antibiotics; resistance is a significant challenge.

With bronchiectasis and as a result of exacerbations, there is progressive scarring of the lungs and colonisation with pathogens. Antibiotic resistance develops, and management of exacerbations requires the involvement of a microbiologist to explore treatment options.

A specialist multidisciplinary CF team should provide care, but where this is not possible, a shared care approach involving specialist team support is necessary. Historically, CF was a disease of childhood. Over the past decade, however, early diagnosis and significant advances in treatment have resulted in more patients surviving early adulthood. As a consequence, new challenges have emerged in terms of care transition from paediatric to adult care and the emerging complications of CF, including diabetes, in adult life.

Respiratory-specific care

A high–energy, high-protein diet is a cornerstone of CF management. As respiratory symptoms increase with loss of lung function, intensive nutritional support is needed. Physiotherapy support for help with airway clearance, maintenance of exercise capacity and management of dyspnoea is a key component of care in CF (Robinson & Scullion 2009).

When respiratory failure and end-stage lung disease develop, patients are assessed for lung transplant, but many do not meet the criteria. Some 50% of patients die while waiting for a transplant. Patients approaching end-stage disease experience loss of lung function and oxygen dependency, and may require NIV. End of life care may be especially challenging as patients may be focused on lung transplantation and unable to consider death and dying.

In 2001, the Cystic Fibrosis Trust (UK) published a national consensus on standards for the nursing management of CF (UK Cystic Fibrosis Nurse Specialist Group 2001). Although this is now dated, the standards highlight the nursing role in advocacy, support and education, assessment, the transition from paediatric to adult care, and audit of CF care.

Table 12.6 Respiratory failure and ABG values

ABG parameter	Normal values	Values in type I respiratory failure	Values in type II respiratory failure
pH	7.35–7.45	7.35–7.45	<7.35–7.45
PaO_2	12–14 kPa	<8 kPa	<8 kPa
$PaCO_2$	4.6–6.0 kPa	4.6–6.0 kPa	>6 kPa
SaO_2	>95%	<92%	<92%

SaO_2, arterial oxygen saturation.

Respiratory failure

Definition

Respiratory failure is defined as a PaO_2 <8 kPa (<60 mmHg) or a $PaCO_2$ >7 kPa (>55 mmHg).

Pathophysiology

When the lungs fail to maintain sufficient arterial oxygenation or carbon dioxide elimination, respiratory failure can occur. Carbon dioxide retention as a result of insufficient ventilation results in hypercapnia or respiratory acidaemia; the $PaCO_2$ will be raised above the normal limits of 35–45 mmHg. Low amounts of carbon dioxide as a result of hyperventilation result in hypocapnia or respiratory alkalaemia.

Respiratory failure may be type I or type II (Table 12.6). In type I respiratory failure, hypoxaemia is present but there is no associated hypercapnia. This occurs in acute asthma attacks, pneumonia or chest trauma. In type II failure, both hypoxaemia and hypercapnia are present. This occurs during acute exacerbations of COPD and conditions associated with severe neuromuscular weakness. Oxygenation failure is most commonly the result of a V/Q mismatch. Ventilatory failure (e.g. hypoventilation) may be a result of medications such as opiates, chest trauma, muscular dystrophy and Guillain–Barré syndrome.

Assessment and management

Type I respiratory failure is managed by oxygen therapy and treatment of the underlying condition. The concentration of oxygen prescribed varies from patient to patient but may be as high as 60–100%. However, oxygen therapy should be reduced as the patient shows clinical improvement.

Type II respiratory failure may develop over a period of time. These patients may have developed compensatory mechanisms for hypercapnia. Hypercapnia may play a more limited role in triggering inspiration, but instead a fall in oxygen concentration will trigger inspiration. For such patients, oxygen therapy may be counterproductive by:

- reducing the rate and depth of respiration;
- further raising carbon dioxide levels and the problem of hypercapnia.

Thus, in type II respiratory failure, oxygen must be used with caution and is usually commenced at low levels of 24–28%. Monitoring of ABG analysis is important in type II respiratory failure and guides the titration of oxygen therapy.

Medication management also includes inhaled and possibly intravenous bronchodilators, beta-2-agonists and anticholinergic agents, and intravenous and inhaled corticosteroids. Diuretics may be required, and opiates and anxiolytics may be necessary for breathlessness and anxiety.

Oxygen therapy and ventilation

Oxygen is a drug that is prescribed to correct hypoxaemia. In hypercapnic respiratory failure, when there is a risk of impairing ventilator compensation, the target for arterial oxygen saturation (SaO_2) is 88–92% (Simonds 2010). Venturi masks are a more accurate means of delivering oxygen than nasal prongs, but this must be balanced against patient comfort.

Long-term oxygen

Long-term oxygen therapy (LTOT) for more than 15 hours per day for patients who have chronic respiratory failure increases survival and improves exercise capacity and well-being (GOLD 2010). Oxygen must be used with care because, for some patients, their respiratory drive depends on their degree of hypoxia rather than the usual dependence on hypercapnia. Uncontrolled oxygen therapy can therefore lead to a suppression of respiratory drive, carbon dioxide narcosis and respiratory arrest. Ideally, oxygen is delivered via a facemask at an inspiratory flow rate of between 24% and 35%. The face mask enables more accurate titration, which is important for patients who are prone to carbon dioxide retention (GOLD 2010; Simonds 2010).

LTOT is indicated for those patients with an FEV_1 <1.5 L, or <40% of predicted normal values. LTOT should be prescribed for a minimum of 15 hours per day, although survival improves when LTOT is used for more than 20 hours per day (National Clinical Guideline Centre 2010). LTOT should not prevent patients leaving home, and the nurse will play an important role in encouraging patients on LTOT to maintain their normal activities. However, there appears to be no benefit in the use of LTOT for patients whose PaO_2 is above 8 kPa.

Non-invasive ventilation

Positive-pressure NIV is prescribed for persistent hypercapnic ventilatory failure in the acute stages of exacerbations and when other treatment has not been effective (National Clinical Guideline Centre 2010). Although it does not improve overall lung function, NIV can reduce carbon dioxide retention and shortness of breath in some patients (GOLD 2010). It has been shown to reduce mortality in acute hypercapnic exacerbations of COPD and reduce the need for invasive ventilation and referral to intensive care (Simonds 2010). NIV is increasingly used in the ward setting, and competency in NIV support requires training. When patients are commenced on NIV, their care plans must include what actions are to be taken in the event of deterioration and agreed therapy ceilings (National Clinical Guideline Centre 2010).

Nursing assessment and management

Nursing care needs include observations with a particular emphasis on respiration and the signs of hypoxaemia and hypercapnia, mentation, the ability to tolerate an increased work of breathing, ABGs and oxygen saturation levels. The management of dyspnoea, airway clearance and impaired gas exchange is essential. Administration of bronchodilators, corticosteroids, diuretics and possibly opiates and anxiolytics should be as prescribed.

Lung cancer

Definition

Lung cancer refers to malignancies that originate in the airways or pulmonary parenchyma.

Epidemiology

Lung cancer is the third most common form of cancer across Europe and is the most lethal (Wilking & Jönsson 2008). In the UK alone, there are 39,000 new cases and more than 35,000 deaths from lung cancer each year (National Institute for Health and Clinical Excellence 2011). Lung cancer is associated with late diagnosis and poor prognosis. For those patients who are diagnosed early and before symptoms occur, the 5-year survival is greater.

Table 12.7 Classification of malignant lung tumours

Pre-invasive lesions	These are typically precursors to squamous cell carcinoma
Small cell lung cancer (SCLC)	Carcinoma with small cells is most commonly associated with smoking. It accounts for 20–25% of all lung cancers and has usually spread by the time it is diagnosed. If not treated, SCLC spreads rapidly often to the bone, liver, head and adrenal glands
Non-small cell lung cancer (NSCLC)	NSCLC accounts for over 75% of all lung cancers and includes four categories: • Squamous cell lung cancer (most common), which often occurs centrally in segmental or main bronchi • Adenocarcinoma (which is increasing in incidence) • Large cell carcinoma • Bronchial alveolar cell (the least common)

Risk factors

Smoking accounts for 80–90% of all lung cancers (Vansteenkiste & Derijcke 2010). Other factors also play an important role in risk of lung cancer, including underlying acquired lung disease such as COPD or pulmonary fibrosis, and environmental exposure to agents such as asbestos and radiation. An increased understanding of the biology of lung cancer in tandem with recent developments in both diagnostic techniques and treatments raises hopes for improved prognosis, if not cure.

Classification

Malignant lung tumours are classified into three major groups, as shown in Table 12.7.

Clinical manifestations

Symptoms of lung cancer include cough, haemoptysis, chest pain and/or shortness of breath. Breathlessness may be a consequence of airflow obstruction or pleural effusion. More general symptoms include weight loss and fatigue. Symptoms of metastatic lung cancer depend on the site(s) of metastasis. Haemoptysis in lung cancer is associated with vascular invasion by the tumour. Breathlessness may be accompanied by stridor as a result of the tumour pressing on the trachea or main bronchi. Chest pain may typically be central and persistent.

Diagnosis

The National Institute for Health and Clinical Excellence (now the National Institute for Health and Care Excellence) has set out guidelines for the diagnosis and management of lung cancer (http://www.ice.org.uk) that include the staging of the disease. 'Staging' is a term used to the tumour's overall size and spread to surrounding areas, and is described in terms of tumour (T), node (N) and metastasis (M).

A chest X-ray or CT scan is indicated for patients with suspicious symptoms such as haemoptysis, persistent central chest pain, hoarseness or stridor. Diagnostic procedures include bronchoscopy, sputum analysis, cytology, positron emission tomography, CT-guided biopsy, mediastinoscopy and, more recently, autofluorescence bronchoscopy.

Assessment and management

Patients with small cell lung cancer are treated with chemotherapy in combination with thoracic radiotherapy. Patients with non-small cell lung cancer may be assessed for surgical resection followed by chemotherapy. Management is determined by the performance status of the patient. Performance status is a measure to determine the overall health of the patient and is linked with prognosis and treatment choices. Palliative radiotherapy may also be offered for symptom relief.

Communication

Given the poor prognosis and often late diagnosis, the initial breaking of bad news and exploration of treatment options is particularly challenging for healthcare professionals, patients and their loved ones. Treatment options may include radical surgery and chemotherapy but offer limited hope for 1–5-year survival. Added to this, some patients also have advanced COPD and may be experiencing considerable fatigue. For these reasons, guidelines on communication in lung cancer promote the use of decision aids, the ready availability of a lung cancer nurse specialist, and the documentation of any discussion on treatment options.

Nursing management

Nursing management needs to include a focus on the patient's understanding of the diagnosis and treatment options, and to respond to support needs for coping with what is often devastating news and complex information. Once a diagnosis of lung cancer has been confirmed, the patient faces uncertainty, and possibly extensive and radical medical treatment, with all its intended and unintended consequences.

Nursing assessment is therefore of significant importance in developing a plan of care that can anticipate needs and offer support. Symptoms of dyspnoea, recurrent infection, fatigue, pain and weight loss should be explored with the patient. Family history, smoking and occupational history should be recorded. Assessment and care should determine the available support at home and in the community for dealing with the condition and its effects in the short, medium and longer term, including the effects of treatment regimens.

Palliative care

Palliative care should be incorporated into the care needs assessment once the diagnosis has been confirmed. This enables the management and support of complex symptoms even if the patient is responding to treatment and has a promising prognosis. Early involvement of the palliative care team facilitates communication and the exploration of treatment options with the patient and family while also enabling a discussion about advanced care planning and discussion about the patient's fears.

Conclusion

This chapter provides an overview of the anatomy and physiology related to various respiratory infections and more chronic conditions such as COPD, respiratory failure, and cystic fibrosis that require frequent admissions to hospital. The treatment and nursing care addresses physical and psychological issues that can have a negative impact on a patient's quality of life.

Now visit the companion website and test yourself on this chapter:
www.wileyfundamentalseries.com/medicalnursing

References

Andenaes, R., Kalfoss, M.H. & Wahl, A. (2004) Psychological distress and quality of life in hospitalized patients with chronic obstructive pulmonary disease. *Journal of Advanced Nursing*, **46**(5):523–30.

Bailey, P.H. (2004) The dyspnea-anxiety-dyspnea cycle – COPD patients' stories of breathlessness: 'It's scary/when you can't breathe'. *Qualitative Health Research*, **14**(6):760–78.

Bilton, D. & Jones, A.L. (2011) Bronchiectasis: epidemiology and causes. *Bronchiectasis: European Respiratory Society Monograph*, **52**:1–10.

Conway, A. (2007) Respiratory assessment. In: Scullion J. (ed.), *Fundamental Aspects of Nursing Adults with Respiratory Disorders* (pp. 156–66). London: Quay Books.

Drain, M. & Elborn, J.S. (2011) Assessment and investigation of adults with bronchiectasis. *Bronchiectasis: European Respiratory Society Monograph*, **52**:32–43.

Dougherty, L. & Lister S. (2011) *The Royal Marsden Hospital Manual of Clinical Nursing Procedures*, 8th edn. Oxford: Wiley Blackwell.

Elkington, H., White, P., Addington-Hall, J., Higgs, R. & Edmonds, P. (2005) The healthcare needs of chronic obstructive pulmonary disease patients in the last year of life. *Palliative Medicine*, **19**:485–91.

Fraser, D.D., Kee, C.C. & Minick P. (2006) Living with chronic obstructive pulmonary disease: insiders' perspectives. *Journal of Advanced Nursing*, **55**(5):550–8.

Global Initiative for Asthma Management (2010) *Global Strategy for Asthma Management and Prevention 2010 (update)*. Retrieved 6th June 2013 from http://www.ginasthma.org.

Global Initiative for Chronic Obstructive Disease (2010) *Global Strategy for the Diagnosis, Management, and Prevention of Chronic Obstructive Pulmonary Disease (Updated 2010)*. NHLB/WHO. Retrieved 6th June 2013 from http://www.goldcopd.com/GuidelinesResources.asp.

Groenewegen, K.H., Schols, A.M.W.J. & Wouters, E.F.M. (2003) Mortality and mortality-related factors after hospitalization for acute exacerbation of COPD. *Chest*, **124**:459–67.

Gudmundsson, G., Gislason, T., Janson, C. *et al.* (2006) Depression, anxiety and health status after hospitalisation for COPD: a multicentre study in the Nordic countries. *Respiratory Medicine*, **100**:87–93.

Jones, P.W. (2009) Health status and the spiral of decline. COPD: *Journal of Chronic Obstructive Pulmonary Disease*, **6**(1):59–63.

Scullion, J. (2007) *Fundamental Aspects of Nursing Adults with Respiratory Disorders*. London: Quay Books.

Maguire, H., Brailsford, S., Carless, J. *et al.* (2011) Large outbreak of isoniazid-monoresistant tuberculosis in London, 1995 to 2006: case–control study and recommendations. *Euro Surveillance*, **16**(13):pii=19830. Available online at http://www.eurosurveillance.org/ViewArticle.aspx?ArticleId=19830.

Milner, D. (2004) The physiological effects of smoking on the respiratory system. *Nursing Times*, **100**(24): 56–9.

Miravitlles, M. (2010) Infective exacerbations of COPD. In: Palange, P. & Simonds A. (eds), *ERS Handbook Respiratory Medicine* (pp. 172–5). Sheffield: European Respiratory Society.

National Clinical Guideline Centre (2010) *Chronic Obstructive Pulmonary Disease: Management of Chronic Obstructive Pulmonary Disease in Adults in Primary and Secondary Care*. London: National Clinical Guideline Centre. Retrieved 10th June 2013 from http://guidance.nice.org.uk/CG101/Guidance/pdf/English.

National Institute for Clinical Excellence (2006) *Brief Interventions and Referral for Smoking Cessation in Primary Care and Other Settings*. London: NICE.

National Institute for Health and Clinical Excellence (2011) *The Diagnosis and Treatment of Lung Cancer (Update)*. Clinical Guideline No. 121. London: NICE.

Odencrants, S., Ehnfors, M. & Grobe, S.J. (2005) Living with chronic obstructive pulmonary disease. I. Struggling with meal-related situations: experiences among persons with COPD. *Scandinavian Journal of Caring Sciences*, **19**(3):230–9.

Odencrants, S., Ehnfors, M. & Grobe, S.J. (2007) Living with chronic obstructive pulmonary disease (COPD). II. RNs' experience of nursing care for patients with COPD and impaired nutritional status. *Scandinavian Journal of Caring Science*, **21**(1):56–63.

Oostenbrink, J.B. & Rutten-van Mölkena, M.P.M.H. (2004) Resource use and risk factors in high-cost exacerbations of COPD. *Respiratory Medicine*, **98**:883–91.

Robinson, T. & Scullion, J.E. (2009) *Oxford Handbook of Respiratory Nursing*. Oxford: Oxford University Press

Russell, S.J.F. & Russell, R.E.K. (2007) Challenges in end-of-life communication in COPD. *Breathe*, **4**(2):133–9.

Simonds, A. (2010) Oxygen therapy and ventilatory support. In: Palange, P. & Simonds, A. (eds), *ERS handbook Respiratory Medicine* (pp. 151–3). Sheffield: European Respiratory Society.

Sotgiu, G. & Migliori, G.B. (2010) Pulmonary tuberculosis. In: Palange, P. & Simonds, A. (eds), *ERS Handbook Respiratory Medicine* (pp. 202–8). Sheffield: European Respiratory Society.

Ten Hacken, N.H. (2010) Bronchiectasis. In: Palange, P. & Simonds, A. (eds), *ERS Handbook Respiratory Medicine* (pp. 252–5). Sheffield: European Respiratory Society.

Tortora, G.J. & Derrickson, B. (2011) *Principles of Anatomy and Physiology Maintenance and Continuity of the Human body*, Vol. 2. Danvers, MA: John Wiley & Sons.

UK Cystic Fibrosis Nurse Specialist Group (2001) *National Consensus Standards for the Nursing Management of Cystic Fibrosis*. Bromley: Cystic Fibrosis Trust.

Vansteenkiste, J. & Derijcke, S. (2010) Lung cancer. In: Palange, P. & Simonds, A. (eds), *ERS Handbook Respiratory Medicine* (pp. 372–6), Sheffield: European Respiratory Society.

Wilking N. & Jönsson, B. (2008) *Karolinska Institutet/i3 Innovus Benchmarking Report of Lung Cancer Care in Selected European Countries*. Stockholm: Karolinska Institute.

Williams, J.E.A. (2009) The challenge of increasing uptake of pulmonary rehabilitation: what can we do to maximise the chances of success? *Chronic Respiratory Disease*, **8**(2):87–8.

Woodhead, M. (2010) Pneumonia. In: Palange, P. & Simmonds, A.H. (eds), *ERS Handbook Respiratory Medicine* (pp. 176–9). Sheffield: European Respiratory Society.

Woodrow, P. (2004) Arterial blood gas analysis. *Nursing Standard*, **18**(21):45–52, 54–5.

13

Nursing care of conditions related to the circulatory system

Kate Olson and Tracey Bowden

School of Health Sciences, City University London, London, UK

Contents

Introduction	211
Anatomy and physiology	211
Assessment	218
Diagnostic investigations	220
Coronary artery disease	222
Arrhythmias	227
Cardiac surgery	229
Valvular heart disease	230
Heart failure	232
Vascular disorders	234
Conclusion	237
References	238

Learning outcomes

Having read this chapter, you will be able to:

- Describe the basic anatomy and physiology of the heart and circulatory system
- Understand how to complete an assessment of a patient with cardiovascular disease
- List common diagnostic investigations
- Understand the acute nursing care of a patient with acute coronary syndrome
- Understand the treatment options for a patient with coronary heart disease
- Describe other cardiac conditions such as valvular disease, rhythm problems and heart failure
- Understand the management of a patient with a vascular disorder

Fundamentals of Medical-Surgical Nursing: A Systems Approach, First Edition. Edited by Anne-Marie Brady, Catherine McCabe, and Margaret McCann.

Introduction

Diseases of the heart and circulatory system are one of the major causes of death in the UK and Ireland. There were over 180,000 deaths from cardiovascular disease (CVD) in the UK in 2009, which accounts for 1 in 3 deaths; 45,000 of these were in the under-75-years age group (Scarborough *et al.* 2010). CVD is the most common cause of death in Ireland, with over 10,000 people dying of CVD each year (Irish Heart Foundation 2011). The largest number of deaths in all cases comes from coronary heart disease. This chapter looks at the anatomy and physiology, assessment, diagnosis, clinical management and nursing care of individuals with CVD.

Anatomy and physiology

The cardiovascular system consists of two main components: the heart and the blood vessels. The heart is a muscular pump that provides the pressure necessary to propel blood throughout the body. The blood vessels are a closed system of tubes that carries blood away from the heart, transports it to the tissues of the body and then returns it to the heart.

The heart

The heart is a hollow, four-chambered organ that rests on the diaphragm near the midline of the thorax, between the lungs. It is surrounded by a protective membrane called the pericardium. The walls of the heart are composed of a thick layer of cardiac muscle known as the myocardium. The myocardium is covered externally by the epicardium and internally by the endocardium. The heart is divided into four chambers: two upper atria and two lower ventricles (Figure 13.1). The two atria and two ventricles are separated by the septum (Tortora & Derrickson 2009).

The heart contains four valves (Figure 13.1) that open and close in response to pressure changes during contraction and relaxation. The atrioventricular valves are located between the atria

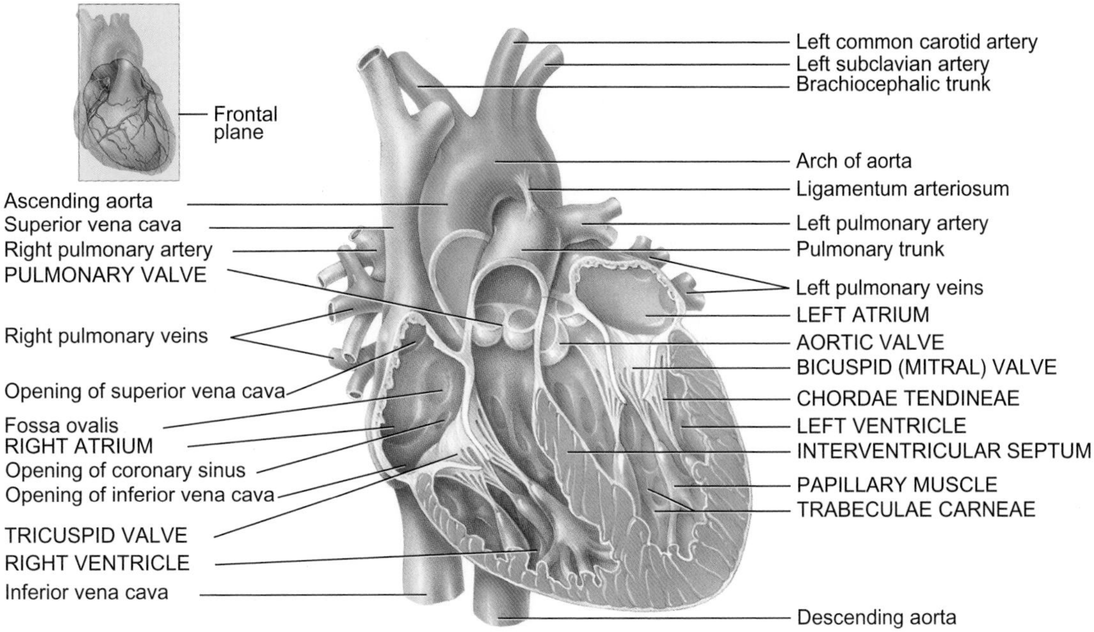

Figure 13.1 The heart: internal structures. Reproduced from Tortora, G.J., Derrickson, B. (2011) *Principles of Anatomy and Physiology*, with kind permission of Wiley Blackwell.

and ventricles on both sides of the heart. The tricuspid valve is located on the right-hand side, and the bicuspid, often called the mitral valve, is located on the left. The other two valves are located where the aorta (aortic valve) and pulmonary artery (pulmonary valve) join the heart, and are referred to as the semilunar valves. The purpose of heart valves is to ensure that the blood flows through the heart in one direction by opening to let blood flow through, and then closing to prevent it flowing backwards.

The heart requires a constant supply of blood to maintain its cellular activity. This is delivered via the coronary arteries. Two coronary arteries arise from the aorta immediately above the aortic valve, each of which has several branches (Figure 13.2).

The heart contains a small proportion of specialised muscle fibres that are self-excitable, meaning that they are able to spontaneously generate an electrical impulse. These cells form the conduction system (Figure 13.3). In normal circumstances, the impulse is generated in the sinoatrial node (the pacemaker). The impulse travels down the rest of the conduction system and then to different regions of the heart, producing a coordinated contraction of the four chambers of the heart (Tortora & Derrickson 2009). The sequence of electrical events can be captured and recorded on an electrocardiogram (ECG).

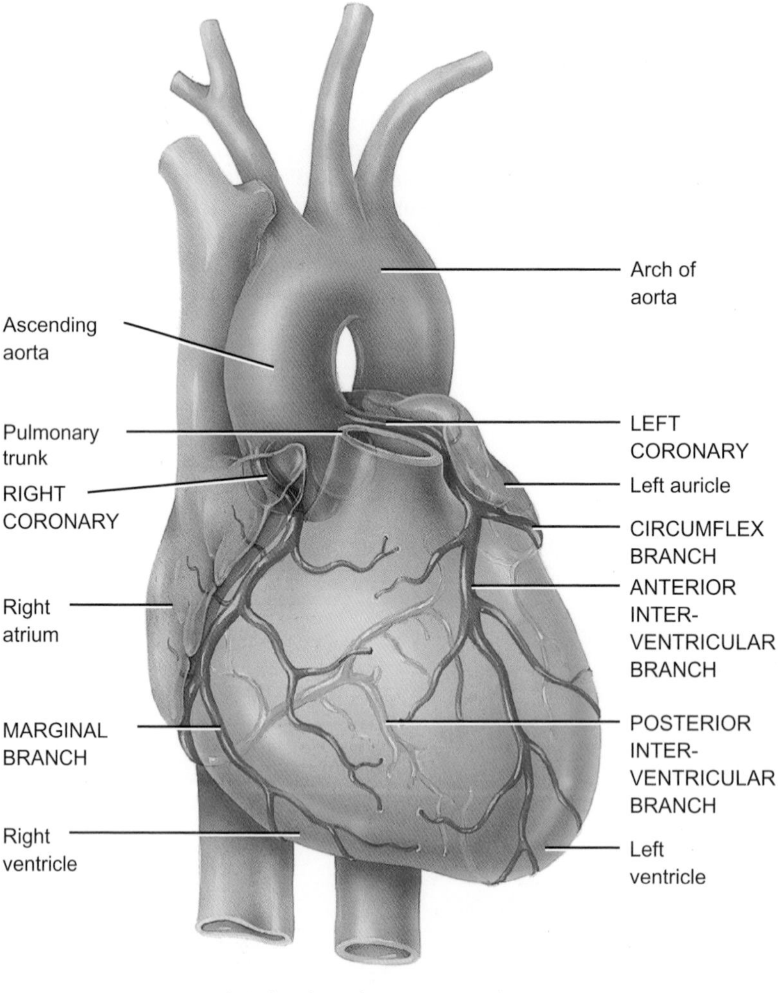

Figure 13.2 The heart: coronary circulation. Reproduced from Tortora, G.J., Derrickson, B. (2011) *Principles of Anatomy and Physiology*, with kind permission of Wiley Blackwell.

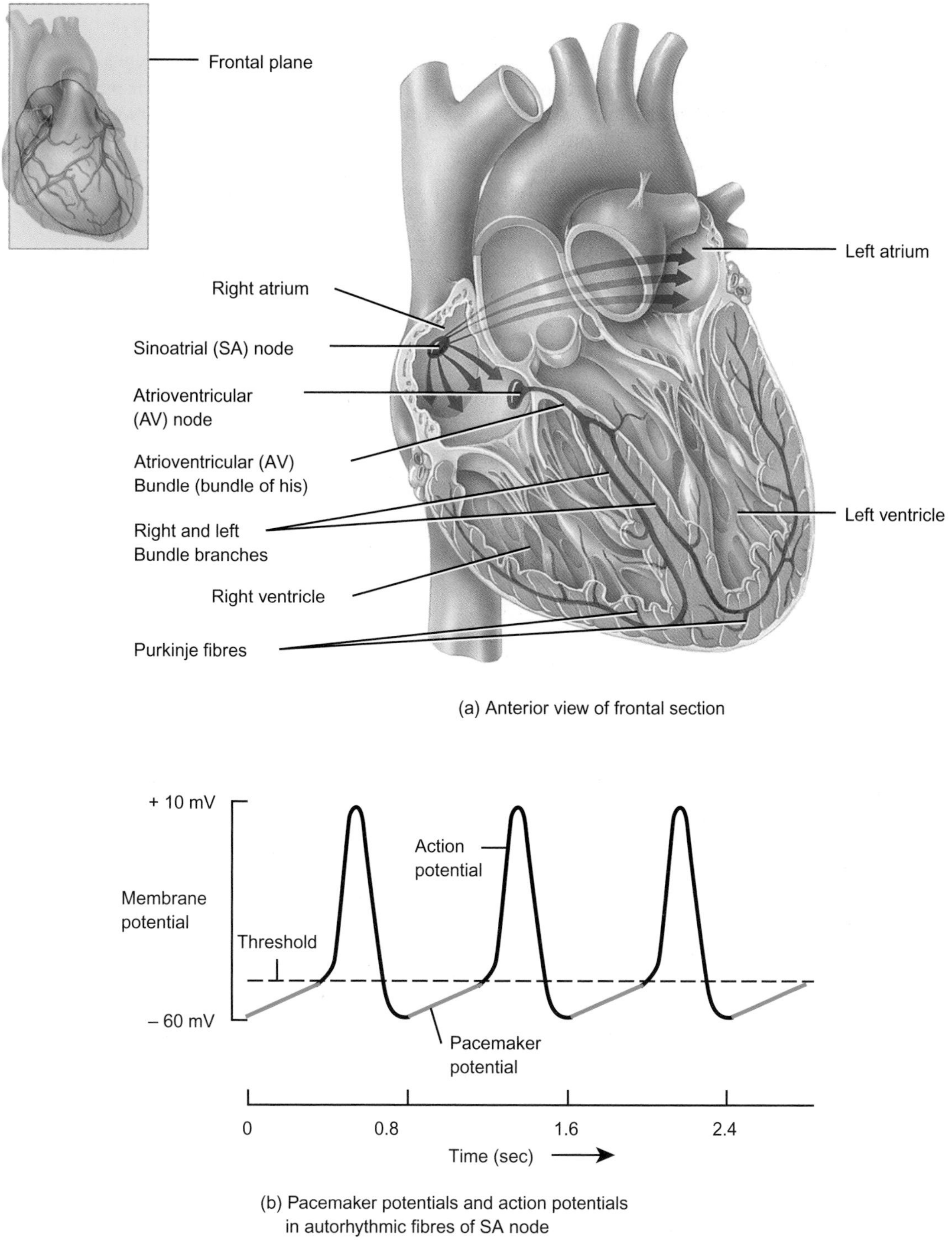

Figure 13.3 The heart: conduction system. Reproduced from Tortora, G.J., Derrickson, B. (2011) *Principles of Anatomy and Physiology*, with kind permission of Wiley Blackwell.

Blood flow through the heart

Deoxygenated blood enters the right atrium of the heart via the inferior and superior venae cavae and coronary sinus (Figure 13.4). Blood then flows to the right ventricle through the tricuspid valve. The ventricle is stimulated to contract, pumping blood to the lungs through the pulmonary valve and pulmonary arteries, at which point gaseous exchange occurs. Carbon dioxide is exchanged for oxygen. Oxygen-rich red blood cells are then transported back to the heart (left atrium) to be distributed to the rest of the body. Blood flows through the mitral valve into the left ventricle. Oxygenated blood is then pumped into the aorta via the aortic valve to be transported around the body. Deoxygenated body returns to the right atrium and the process is repeated.

Regulation of the heart

The sinoatrial node is responsible for initiating the impulse and the heart rate. The heart rate may, however, be influenced by the autonomic nervous system. The sympathetic nerve supply is responsible for increasing the heart rate, whereas the parasympathetic (vagus) nerve decreases the heart rate. The nerve supply originates in the cardiorespiratory centre, which is located in the medulla oblongata. Other factors that affect the heart rate include hormones, stress, drugs, body temperature, electrolyte imbalance and circulating blood volume.

Blood vessels

There are several types of blood vessel within the body (Figure 13.5):

- Arteries and arterioles carry oxygenated blood away from the heart, with the exception of the pulmonary artery, which carries deoxygenated blood.
- Veins and venules carry deoxygenated blood towards the heart, with the exception of the pulmonary vein, which carries oxygenated blood.
- Capillaries are tiny, thin-walled vessels that allow an exchange of substances between the blood and body tissues.

With the exception of the capillaries, blood vessels are composed of three layers of the vessel wall (Figure 13.6) surrounding a central lumen through which blood flows (Tortora & Derrickson 2009). The layers are:

- the tunica intima – the epithelial lining;
- the tunica media – the middle layer of smooth muscle and elastic connective tissues;
- the tunica externa – a connective tissue outer covering with a plentiful nerve supply.

Blood pressure

As blood is pumped out of the left ventricle into the aorta, the circulating blood exerts pressure on the walls of the blood vessels; this is referred to as the blood pressure (Nicol *et al.* 2008). Blood pressure varies in different vessels, and in clinical practice the systemic arterial pressure is measured. Blood pressure varies throughout the day. It is often lower during sleep and higher during periods of activity. Several factors affect blood pressure, including cardiac output, circulating blood volume, peripheral resistance, stress, hormones and drugs.

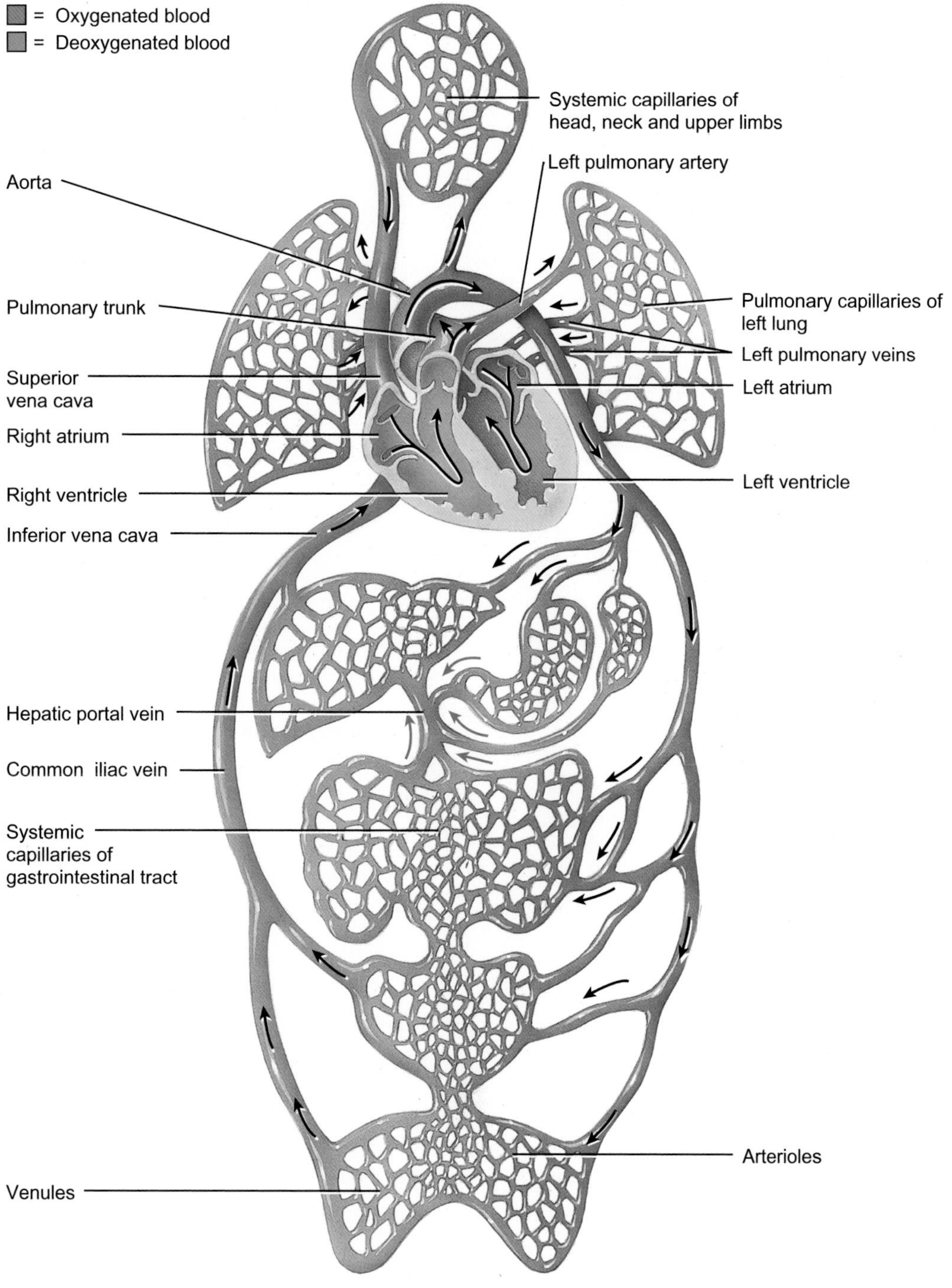

Figure 13.4 Blood flow through the heart. Reproduced from Tortora, G.J., Derrickson, B. (2011) *Principles of Anatomy and Physiology*, with kind permission of Wiley Blackwell.

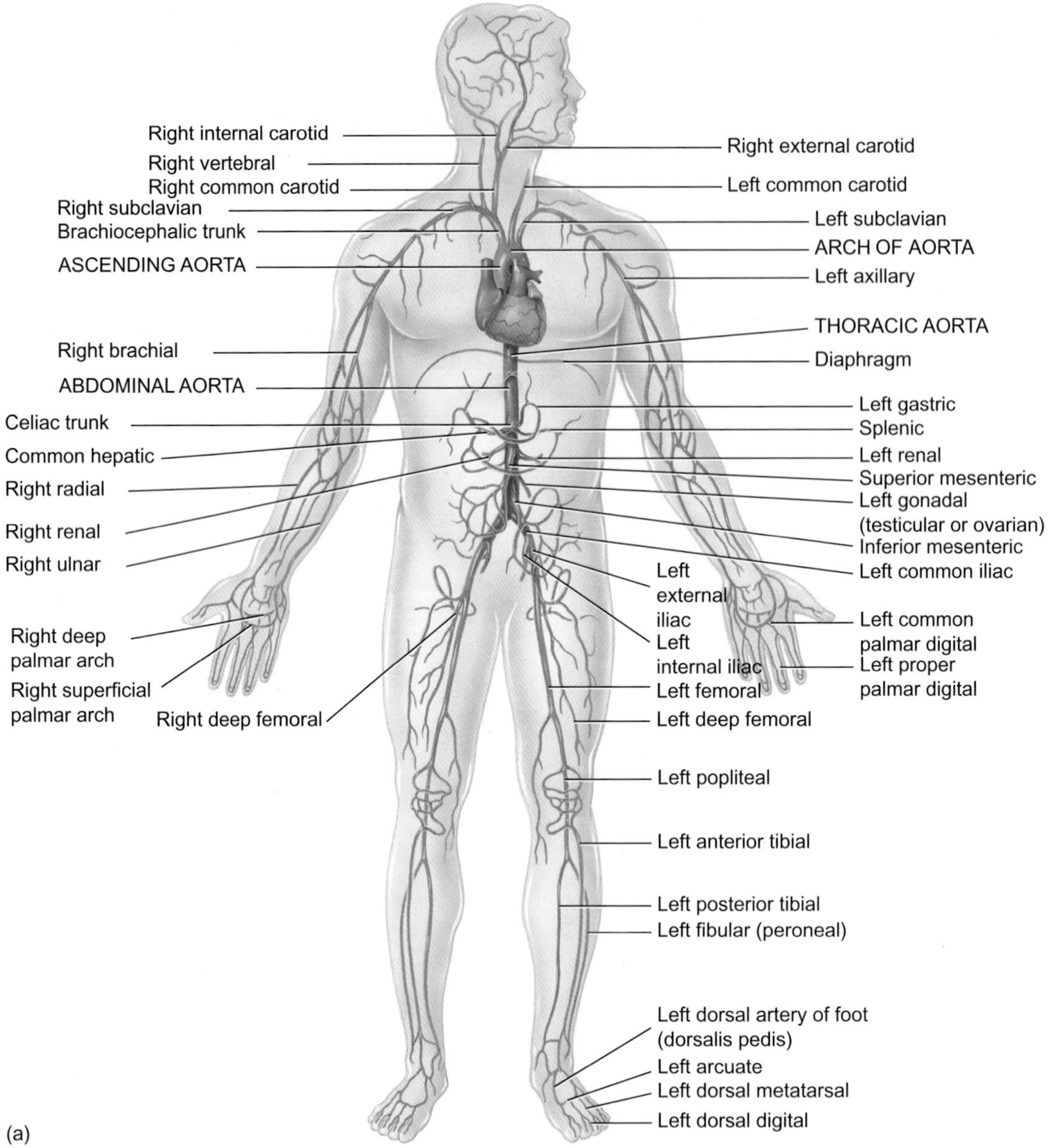

Figure 13.5 The main arterial and venous systems of the body. (a) Overall anterior view of the principal branches of the aorta. (b) Overall anterior view of the principal veins. Reproduced from Tortora, G.J., Derrickson, B. (2011) *Principles of Anatomy and Physiology*, with kind permission of Wiley Blackwell.

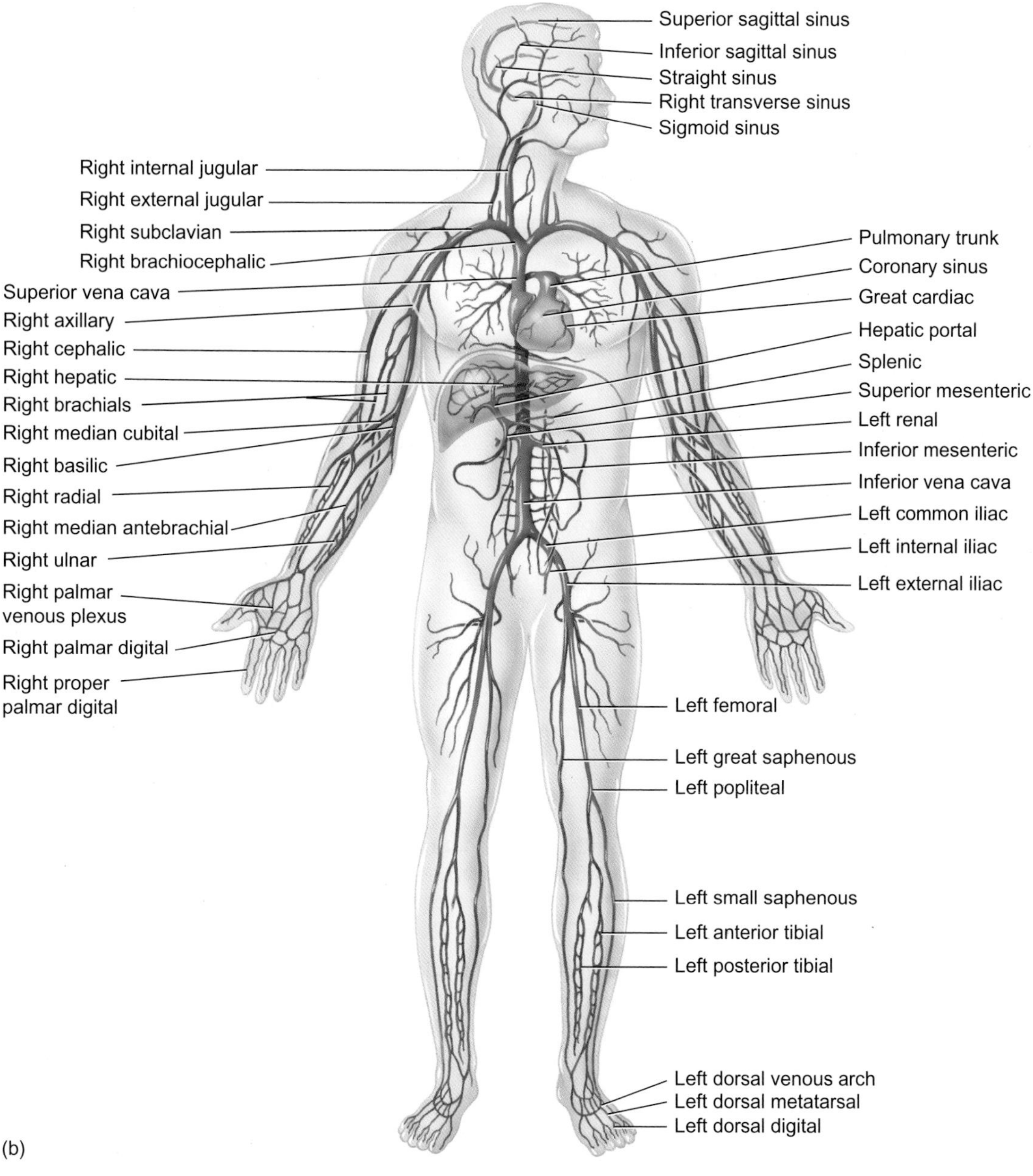
Superior sagittal sinus
Inferior sagittal sinus
Straight sinus
Right transverse sinus
Sigmoid sinus
Right internal jugular
Right external jugular
Right subclavian
Right brachiocephalic
Superior vena cava
Right axillary
Right cephalic
Right hepatic
Right brachials
Right median cubital
Right basilic
Right radial
Right median antebrachial
Right ulnar
Right palmar venous plexus
Right palmar digital
Right proper palmar digital
Pulmonary trunk
Coronary sinus
Great cardiac
Hepatic portal
Splenic
Superior mesenteric
Left renal
Inferior mesenteric
Inferior vena cava
Left common iliac
Left internal iliac
Left external iliac
Left femoral
Left great saphenous
Left popliteal
Left small saphenous
Left anterior tibial
Left posterior tibial
Left dorsal venous arch
Left dorsal metatarsal
Left dorsal digital
(b)

Figure 13.5 (*Continued*)

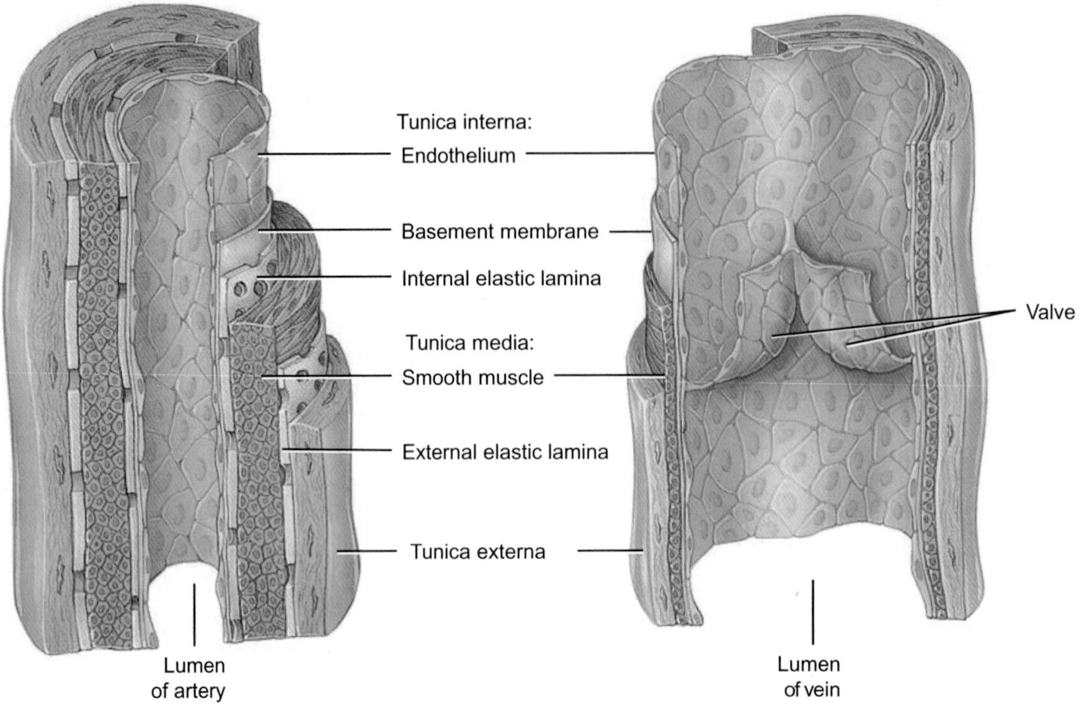

Figure 13.6 Structure of a blood vessel. Reproduced from Nair, M. & Peate, I. (2009) *Fundamentals of Applied Pathophysiology*, with kind permission from Wiley Blackwell.

Assessment

Although student nurses and junior staff can carry out many of the elements discussed below, parts of the assessment such as chest auscultation will be carried out either by doctors or by specialist nurses. Effective and accurate assessment should be systematic and requires good communication skills. The assessment will include:

- the patient's current and previous medical and surgical history, including medications;
- assessment of the presenting complaint, including symptoms, aggravating and relieving factors, and duration, for example:
  - dizziness and/or syncope;
  - chest pain (location, type and intensity);
  - palpitations;
  - fatigue;
  - heartburn;
  - shortness of breath;
  - nausea and vomiting;
- social history – social isolation can be an important factor in determining mortality and morbidity following a cardiovascular event, and is also useful to know in terms of discharge planning;
- family history – any incidence of CVD, diabetes or hyperlipidaemia in close family members should be noted.

Cardiovascular risk factors

Physical assessment

This starts with recording of the vital signs, including temperature, pulse, blood pressure, respiration and peripheral oxygen saturation. The nurse should pay careful attention to the patient's general

Box 13.1 The ABCDE approach to assessment

- **Airway** – look for signs of total or partial obstruction, e.g. snoring or gurgling; can the patient talk?
- **Breathing** – rate, depth and rhythm of breathing, peripheral oxygen saturation, breath sounds, evidence of cyanosis, use of accessory muscles
- **Circulation** – rate, rhythm and volume of pulse, blood pressure, capillary refill time, urine output, signs of bleeding, ECG
- **Disability** – assessment of neurological function
- **Exposure** – other factors not already considered, e.g. temperature, presence of a rash

appearance, for example pallor, positioning and increased work of breathing. Other areas of assessment (Johnson & Rawlings-Anderson 2007) include:

- urine output and urinalysis;
- height, weight and body mass index;
- waist circumference;
- allergies;
- pain assessment (see the section on angina for assessment tools);
- blood glucose monitoring (if appropriate).

The assessment needs to be carefully documented, and reassessment should take place as the patient's condition dictates.

If the patient is acutely unwell, the ABCDE approach may be used (Resuscitation Council 2010; Box 13.1).

Assessment of cardiovascular risk factors

Risk factors can be divided into non-modifiable, modifiable, behavioural and psychosocial (Table 13.1; Kucia & Birchmore 2010; Webster & Thompson 2011).

The probability of an individual developing the disease can be estimated using a cardiovascular risk assessment tool such as the European Systemic Coronary Risk Estimation (SCORE). SCORE charts are available at http://www.escardio.org/communities/EACPR/toolbox/health-professionals/Pages/SCORE-Risk-Charts.aspx.

During a risk assessment, the nurse should ensure that the patient understands not only the nature of the risk, but also the likelihood that behavioural change may occur. Health promotion interventions can then be tailored to this.

Table 13.1 Risk factors for CVD

Non-modifiable	Modifiable	Behavioural	Psychosocial
Family history of premature CVD (<75 years) South Asian origin Age Male Premature menopause	Increased serum cholesterol (in particular low high-density lipoprotein levels, and high low-density lipoprotein) Insulin resistance Obesity (in particular waist circumference) Renal disease Hypertension	Smoking Physical inactivity Increased alcohol intake	Depression Stress and anxiety Social isolation

Diagnostic investigations

Blood tests

Biochemical markers are particularly important to help diagnose acute coronary syndromes (ACSs). Myocardial necrosis (death of heart muscle) results in and can be recognised by the appearance in the blood of different proteins released into the circulation from the damaged myocytes, including cardiac troponin T, cardiac troponin I, creatine kinase and lactate dehydrogenase. Cardiac troponins are now considered to be the gold standard biochemical marker for myocardial necrosis, and measurement of troponin levels has largely superseded the measurement of creatine kinase and lactate dehydrogenase. Troponin is detectable in the bloodstream within 4 hours of ischaemic injury, peaks at around 24 hours and remains elevated for up to 14 days (Bowden & McLeod 2010). Other routine blood tests include urea and electrolytes, clotting, glucose and lipids.

Electrocardiography

The ECG is a graphic representation of the electric current generated by the wave of depolarisation that progresses through the atria and ventricles (the P wave and QRS complex), followed by the wave of repolarisation (the T wave) (Huszar 2007). The electrical current is detected by electrodes placed on the patient's body and amplified through the electrocardiography machine (see Figure 13.7 for details of electrode placement and how to record a 12-lead ECG). The image is displayed on a cardiac monitor or recorded on ECG paper.

Cardiac monitoring provides continuous information relating to the heart rate and rhythm, whereas the 12-lead ECG provides a 'snapshot' of multiple surfaces of the heart. The 12-lead ECG is an essential tool in the diagnosis of ACS. It also has a role to play in the detection of chamber enlargement and certain electrolyte imbalances.

Ambulatory monitoring

Ambulatory ECG devices such as Holter monitors and patient-activated devices allow patients to be monitored while they carry out their normal activities. They are often used to determine the cause of intermittent symptoms thought to be due to a cardiac arrhythmia. The data retrieved are interpreted retrospectively and cannot be viewed in real time. Alternatively, intermittent monitoring may be preferred, for example if the patient's symptoms are infrequent. Patients are required to activate the recorder when they experience symptoms. Patients should ideally be asked to keep a record of their activities and any symptoms to determine whether there is any correlation with an arrhythmia.

Exercise tolerance test

The exercise tolerance test is a non-invasive investigation used to assess a patient's response to exercise. The test involves the patient exercising on a treadmill with a progressive increase in speed and elevation (incline). The heart rate and rhythm are monitored continuously throughout, and a 12-lead ECG and blood pressure reading are obtained at the end of each stage of the test. Significant stenosis of a coronary artery results in ischaemia, which provokes angina and subsequent changes in the ECG, heart rate and blood pressure. The exercise tolerance test is currently being phased out in favour of computed tomography (CT) calcium scoring (Oriolo & Albarran 2010).

CT calcium scoring

CT calcium scoring is a non-invasive test using CT scanning to detect and measure the number of calcified plaques within the coronary arteries (National Institute for Health and Clinical Excellence

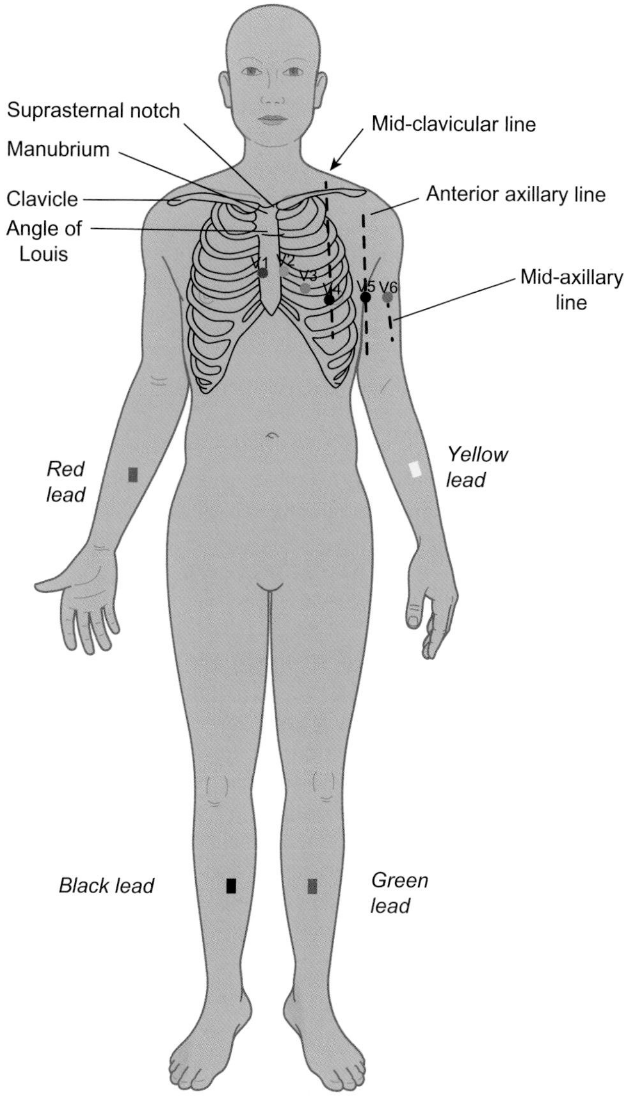

Figure 13.7 Electrocardiographic anatomy of the thorax and 12-lead ECG electrode placement.

[NICE] 2010c). The plaques are formed by the build-up of substances such as fat in the inner layer of the coronary arteries. Calcification of this substance is known as atherosclerosis. The amount of calcium evident on the cardiac CT scan is converted to a calcium score, which correlates with the severity of the blockage. Since publication of the NICE guidelines on the assessment and diagnosis of recent-onset chest pain (NICE 2010a), calcium scoring has been playing an increasingly important role in the diagnosis, management and risk stratification of patients with coronary artery disease (CAD).

Echocardiography

Echocardiography uses ultrasound technology to provide information on the anatomy and physiology of the heart and great veins. It assesses structural and functional abnormalities such as left ventricular failure and valve disease.

Coronary angiography

Coronary angiography is an invasive test used to diagnose the presence or absence of CAD. The procedure involves the insertion of a specially shaped catheter into the coronary arterial system. This is performed under fluoroscopic X-ray guidance. The catheter is advanced through the arterial system until it reaches the ostium, or opening, of the coronary arteries. Contrast is then injected into each coronary artery, allowing visualisation of the lumen and any narrowings or blockages that exist. Arterial access may be achieved via the femoral, brachial or radial artery.

Nurses have an important role in caring for patients undergoing angiography, particularly in relation to physical and psychological preparation. Post-procedural care is equally important to ensure that complications related to arterial access and systemic or disease-related events are detected as early as possible.

Other tests

Other diagnostic tests include myocardial perfusion imaging (scintigraphy), cardiac magnetic resonance imaging (MRI), transoesophageal echocardiography and electrophysiology studies.

Coronary artery disease

CAD, also known as coronary heart disease, is characterised by the development of atherosclerotic plaques within the coronary arteries. Atherosclerosis is a thickening or hardening of the arteries. It is a slow and progressive disease resulting in a reduction of blood flow to the myocardium and the development of angina (Figure 13.8). In addition, atherosclerotic plaques result in endothelial injury and dysfunction, which affects the normal vasomotor response to changes in myocardial oxygen demand (Aouizerat *et al.* 2010). The development of CAD varies depending on the individual's risk factors (see Table 13.1) and the coronary arteries affected. Manifestations of CAD include stable angina and ACS. ACS is a life-threatening manifestation of atherosclerosis induced by a ruptured atherosclerotic plaque, which causes a sudden complete or critical reduction in blood flow (Bassand *et al.* 2007).

Stable angina

Angina is the most common manifestation of CAD. It is a symptom describing the pain or discomfort resulting from a transient, reversible reduction in blood supply to the myocardium. It is often associated with exertion and relieved by rest. Angina is regarded as stable if it has been recurring over several weeks without any major deterioration.

Angina develops when the atherosclerotic plaque within the affected coronary artery causes an obstruction of at least 70%. When the myocardium requires an increased oxygen supply, for example during exercise, the vessel is unable to meet this demand because the plaque is severely limiting the coronary blood flow. In addition, the plaque damages the endothelium, resulting in an inability of the vessel to control the blood flow by local vasoconstriction or vasodilatation.

The diagnosis of angina may be based on clinical assessment alone, as outlined above, but further diagnostic investigations are often required. Angina is diagnosed when the pain is described as constricting in the front of the chest, neck, shoulders, jaw or arms, is precipitated by physical exertion and is relieved by rest or glyceryl trinitrate (GTN) within 5 minutes (NICE 2010b).

The PQRST chest pain assessment tool is useful for ensuring that adequate information is obtained relating to the characteristics of the chest pain (Box 13.2).

NICE (2010b) recommends that the perceived likelihood of CAD in a particular individual should be estimated to determine the most appropriate investigations. Factors such as age, gender, risk factors and previous coronary events (e.g. myocardial infarction) should be considered when estimating the likelihood of CAD.

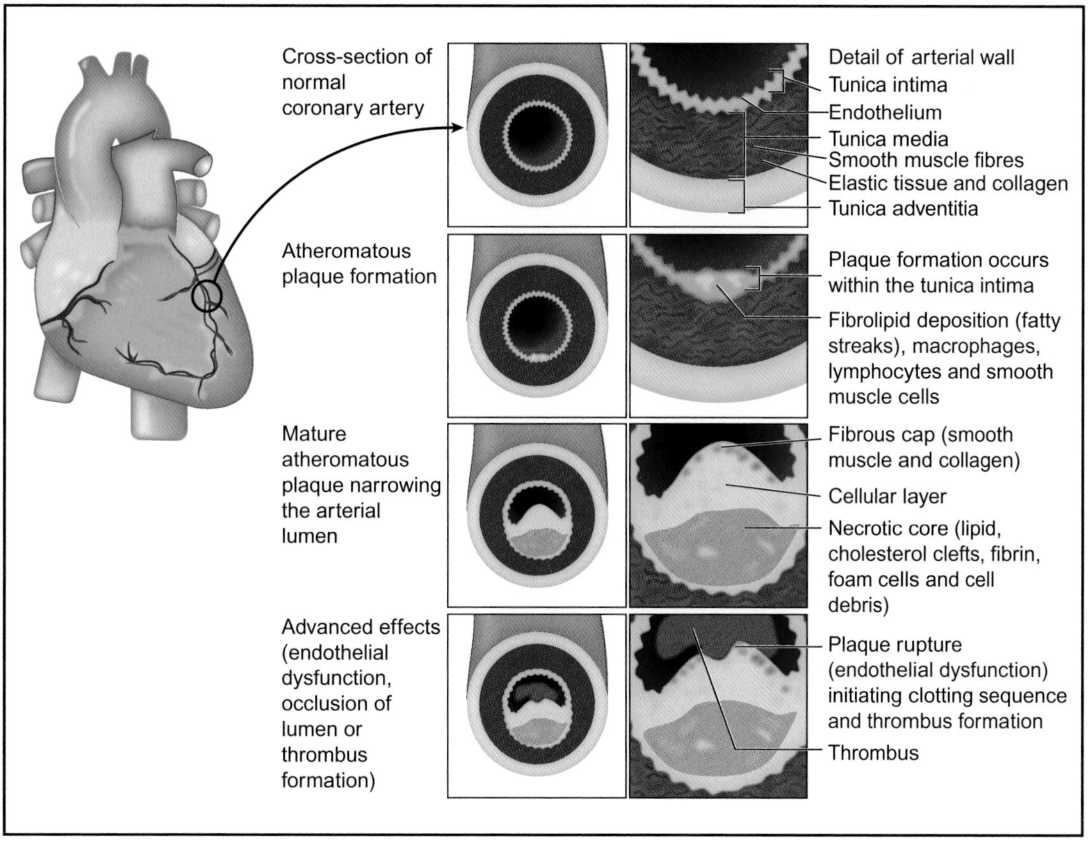

Figure 13.8 The development of atherosclerosis. Reproduced with permission of Peter Lamb, HFS Imaging.

Box 13.2 The PQRST chest pain assessment tool (Kelly 2004)

P *Precipitating and palliative factors*
What brought on the chest pain? What were you doing when the chest pain started? What measures have helped to relieve the pain (position, medication, relaxation)?

Q *Quality*
Can you describe your pain in your own words? What does it feel like?

R *Region and radiation*
Can you show me where the pain is? Do you have pain anywhere else?

S *Severity*
On a scale of 0 (no pain) to 10 (worst pain ever experienced), how would you rate your pain?

T *Timing*
How long did it last?

Clinical and nursing management

The main treatment options include:

- medical management and modification of risks;
- revascularisation by percutaneous coronary intervention (PCI) or coronary artery bypass grafting (CABG).

Patients with stable angina do not usually require hospitalisation. Instead, they may be referred by their GP to a chest pain clinic, where they are often assessed by specialist nurses. Clinical and nursing management is aimed at improving patients' prognosis and minimising their symptoms. This is achieved by a secondary prevention of cardiac events: medication is prescribed to reduce the risk of death or ACS and often includes a nitrate, antiplatelet agent (aspirin or clopidogrel), statin, beta-blocker and calcium-channel blocker.

Percutaneous coronary intervention

PCI is a term that collectively describes a group of procedures that aim to restore or improve the blood flow to the myocardium following a period of ischaemia or injury. PCI includes percutaneous transluminal coronary angioplasty (PTCA) and intracoronary stenting. It is often performed electively in patients who continue to have symptoms of angina despite medication. PCI may also be performed urgently as a treatment option for patients presenting with ST elevation myocardial infarction (STEMI).

PTCA involves widening a coronary artery from within using a balloon catheter in an attempt to increase the blood supply to the myocardium. The catheter is inserted into the artery (femoral, radial or less commonly brachial) and guided through the arterial system under X-ray guidance. Contrast medium is injected into the coronary artery to determine the size and location of the atherosclerotic plaque(s). The balloon is then advanced and inflated to compress the plaque against the arterial wall, resulting in widening of the coronary artery.

Stents are thin mesh wire structures that act as 'scaffolding' to keep the artery open. NICE guidelines (2004) suggest that stents should be used routinely if PCI is clinically appropriate. One of the major problems with stent insertion is re-stenosis of the artery. Drug-eluting stents have been developed to counteract this. In addition to the pre-procedural care discussed for coronary angiography, patients usually require the administration of a thienopyridine antiplatelet drug. Following the procedure, frequent observations are taken to ensure that complications related to arterial access and systemic or disease-related events are detected as early as possible. Complications are listed in Box 13.3.

Acute coronary syndromes

The definition of, and distinction between, these syndromes is based on clinical presentation (Box 13.4), serial ECGs and biochemical markers of necrosis. If ACS is suspected after the initial assessment of signs and symptoms (Box 13.5), an ECG is conducted. Following the ECG, patients will be categorised as having an ST elevation ACS or a non-ST elevation ACS. This is an important distinction to make as treatment options are initially based on the patient's symptoms and ECG changes (Marshall 2011).

Box 13.3 PCI: complications

Recurrent chest pain
Non-STEMI/STEMI
Arrhythmias and conduction disturbances
Vagal reaction
Occlusive thrombus at the puncture site
Abrupt closure of the artery
In-stent re-stenosis
Cerebrovascular complications
Bleeding at the puncture site
Coronary artery dissection

NSTEMI, non-ST elevation myocardial infarction.

Box 13.4 Differentiation of ACS at a glance

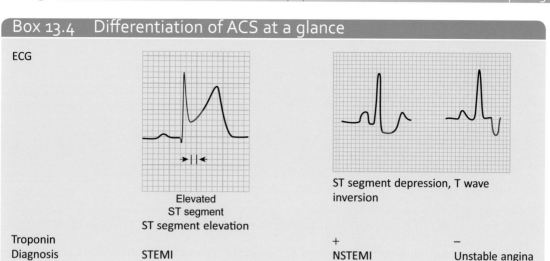

ECG	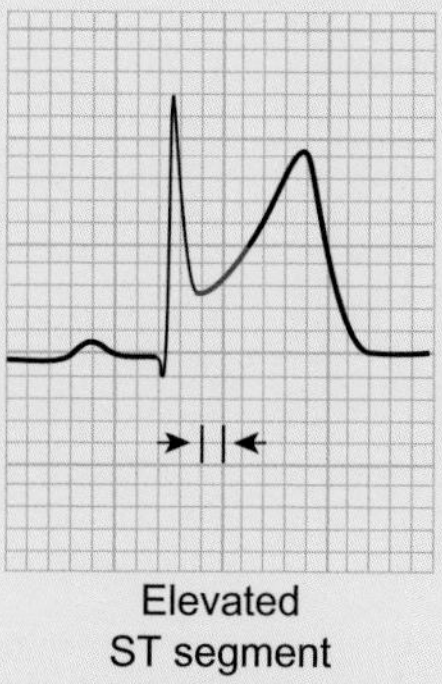 ST segment elevation	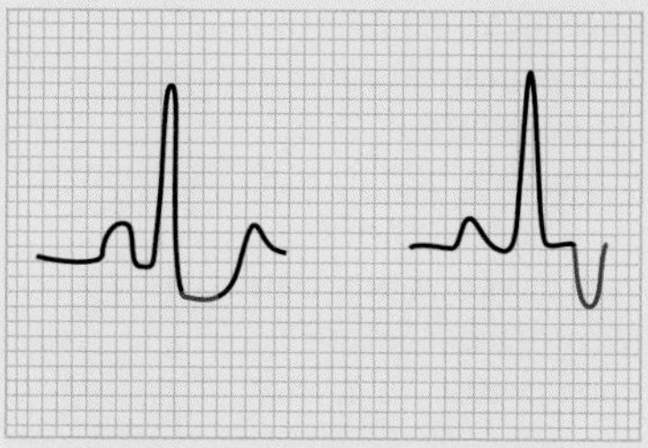 ST segment depression, T wave inversion	
Troponin		+	–
Diagnosis	STEMI	NSTEMI	Unstable angina

Box 13.5 Signs and symptoms of ACS

Signs

Pallor

Cool and clammy peripheries

Blood pressure may be lower than normal (reduced cardiac output) or higher than normal (pain and anxiety)

Heart rate may be normal or outside normal parameters depending on several factors such as pain, ischaemia of the conduction system and arrhythmias

Symptoms

Chest pain (see below)

Shortness of breath

Nausea

Sweating

Dizziness

Fear and anxiety

Chest pain is the most common symptom of ACS. It is often described as a tightness ('vice-like'), pressure, heaviness or crushing, and is often mistaken for indigestion. It is usually located in the central chest but often radiates to the arms, jaw, back and/or shoulder

Non-ST elevation myocardial infarction

This type of infarction results in the formation of a thrombus that does not result in a sustained complete occlusion of the coronary artery. These patients usually present with prolonged chest pain. Biochemical markers (via a blood test) will be elevated outside the normal parameters, and a diagnosis of non-ST elevation myocardial infarction (NSTEMI) will be made. If the ischaemia does not result in myocardial cell necrosis, biochemical markers will not be elevated outside the normal parameters, and a diagnosis of unstable angina is made.

STEMI

This results in the formation of a fixed and persistent clot that causes a complete sustained occlusion of the affected coronary artery and subsequent cellular necrosis and damage to the cardiac muscle. These patients usually present with prolonged (more than 20 minutes) chest pain and persistent ST segment elevation. Urgent revascularisation is required.

Box 13.6 Complications of ACS (Verrier & Deelstra 2010)

- Cardiac arrest
- Arrhythmias
- Heart failure
- Hypoxia
- Cardiogenic shock
- Ventricular septal defect
- Myocardial rupture
- Pericarditis

Immediate clinical and nursing management of patients with ACS

All patients with confirmed or suspected ACS should be managed in a coronary care unit. Although there are some distinct differences in the treatment of ST elevation ACS and non-ST elevation ACS, all patients require the following;

- Continuous cardiac monitoring to observe for any arrhythmias. Vital signs should also be monitored closely to detect any changes in the patient's condition and life-threatening complications (Box 13.6).
- Bed rest to reduce myocardial oxygen demand.
- Oxygen therapy. Current recommendations dictate that oxygen should not be given routinely, and that the oxygen saturation (SpO_2) levels should be monitored and used to guide oxygen therapy. Optimum SpO_2 levels are >94% in patients without chronic obstructive pulmonary disease (COPD) and between 88% and 92% in those with COPD (Bowden & McLeod 2010).
- Venous access and blood samples.
- 12-lead ECG monitoring when the patient is experiencing symptoms and following every episode of chest pain when the symptoms have subsided.
- Pain relief. Pain is associated with sympathetic activation, which causes vasoconstriction and increases the workload of the heart. The administration of morphine or diamorphine relieves pain as well as anxiety and may lead to a lowered threshold for cardiac arrhythmias (Kelly 2004). An antiemetic should also be given.
- Sublingual GTN if the systolic blood pressure is greater than 90 mmHg.
- Antiplatelet agents (which prevent platelets from adhering to each other and to the atherosclerotic plaques, thereby preventing the formation or extension of thrombus; Johnson & Rawlings-Anderson 2007). A thienopyridine antiplatelet drug is often simultaneously prescribed to help prevent further cardiovascular events.
- Early risk stratification to assess the extent to which patients are at risk of an adverse event such as myocardial infarction, stroke or death. Several validated risk scores are available for use in clinical practice, but NICE (2010b) recommends the Global Registry of Acute Coronary Events (GRACE) risk score.
- Secondary prevention of subsequent cardiac events.
- Relief of anxiety and support for the patient.

Clinical and nursing management specific to STEMI

The aim of treatment is to restore the blood flow to the myocardium in attempt to salvage any viable cardiac muscle. Reperfusion can be attempted:

- pharmacologically, by the administration of an intravenous thrombolytic drug, such as tenecteplase, which is administered in attempt to dissolve the clot;
- mechanically, by primary PCI.

Clinical and nursing management specific to NSTEMI

The management of patients with NSTEMI is guided by the individual patient's risk of future adverse coronary events and may include (NICE 2010d; Marshall 2011):

- fondaparinux if the patient does not have a high risk of bleeding;
- intravenous heparin infusion;
- a glycoprotein IIb/IIIa inhibitor.

Revascularisation options should be considered and tailored to the individual patient, and should include conservative management, PCI or CABG.

Arrhythmias

An arrhythmia is any cardiac rhythm that is not normal sinus rhythm at a normal rate (Jacobson 2010). There is a deviation from the normal pattern of electrical activity in which the heart beats too slowly (bradycardia), too fast (tachycardia) or irregularly. Symptoms experienced with an arrhythmia include:

- palpitations
- dizziness
- a feeling of faintness
- shortness of breath
- chest pain
- anxiety
- reduced exercise tolerance.

Cardiac monitoring should be established as early as possible. A 12-lead ECG should also be obtained as this will provide documented evidence of the arrhythmia and will enable a more detailed interpretation by an appropriate experienced practitioner. Adverse features include:

- hypotension (systolic blood pressure <90 mmHg);
- syncope;
- signs of heart failure;
- chest pain or signs of ischaemia on the ECG;
- an extreme heart rate: >150 beats per minute or <40 beats per minute.

Tachyarrhythmias

A tachyarrhythmia is an arrhythmia with a heart rate of more than 100 beats per minute. It does not include sinus tachycardia, which is a normal pattern of electrical activity with an abnormally high heart rate, often due to an alternative physiological or pathological state, for example exercise, anxiety or fever. Tachyarrhythmias are often categorised by (and treated according to) the width of the QRS complex: narrow or broad.

Narrow complex tachycardias usually originate above the ventricle and include the following:

- **Atrial fibrillation.** This is the most common arrhythmia encountered in clinical practice. It is recognised by an absence of atrial activity and an irregular rhythm. The heart rate may be slow, normal or fast.
- **Atrial flutter.** This rhythm is characterised by its unique atrial activity; it is often described as a 'sawtooth' pattern. The ventricular activity is often normal. The heart rate is dependent on the degree of block at the atrioventricular node; this is described by a ratio, for example 4:1, meaning the atria are activated four times for each ventricular activation.

Broad complex tachycardias are any rhythm with a fast heart rate and a broad complex. Always treat the patient and not the monitor or the rhythm. The most common broad complex tachycardia is ventricular tachycardia. The patient may be asymptomatic, symptomatic and haemodynamically compromised, or pulseless. Treatment is determined by the patient's condition.

Clinical and nursing management

Treatment is aimed at either controlling the heart rate (rate control) or restoring sinus rhythm (cardioversion). Generally speaking, if the patient is stable during the arrhythmia, the use of pharmacological agents is preferred over electrical intervention. Amiodarone is a common antiarrhythmic medication for both narrow and broad complex tachycardias, but others are used.

If the patient is unstable or displaying adverse signs, DC cardioversion is the treatment of choice. This is the process of delivering an electric current, in a controlled manner, externally to the heart via a defibrillator. Anaesthesia or sedation is usually administered to the patient. Alternative electrical therapies for arrhythmias include ablation and implantable cardioverter defibrillator implantation.

Bradyarrhythmias

A bradyarrhythmia is an arrhythmia with a heart rate of less than 60 beats per minute. It does not include sinus bradycardia, which is a normal pattern of electrical activity with an abnormally slow heart rate, as in seen in athletes, during sleep or as an effect of medication such as beta-blockers. Bradyarrhythmias usually develop because the conduction from the atria to the ventricles is either slowed or blocked, resulting in atrioventricular block. There are three degrees of heart block: first, second and third degree.

Clinical and nursing management

Treatment options for bradyarrhythmias include the following:

- With pharmacological management, intravenous atropine is administered as a first-line treatment to patients who are displaying adverse features.
- Cardiac pacing is the delivery of a small electrical current to the heart to stimulate myocardial contraction. Pacing may be required temporarily or permanently. The most common form of temporary pacing is transvenous pacing. This is when pacing wires are inserted into the veins via an introducer sheath and passed through the venous system to the heart. Common insertion sites include the internal jugular, subclavian and femoral veins (Gibson 2008). Alternative temporary pacing is achieved externally as an emergency or following cardiac surgery (epicardial pacing wires). A permanent pacemaker is a small implantable device used to maintain a sufficient heart rate when natural mechanisms fail (Jackson 2010).

Cardiac arrest rhythms

The cessation of effective pumping of the heart will result in cardiac arrest. Once cardiac arrest has been established, cardiopulmonary resuscitation should be commenced immediately. A cardiac monitor should be attached at the earliest opportunity to determine the cardiac rhythm as this will determine the appropriate treatment. Rhythms encountered during a cardiac arrest include the following (Resuscitation Council 2010):

- **Shockable rhythms.** The definitive treatment for the following rhythms is defibrillation by an appropriately trained practitioner:
  - *Ventricular fibrillation*. This is the only rhythm that does not require systematic interpretation. It is characterised by its chaotic appearance without any distinguishable complexes.
  - *Ventricular tachycardia*. This rhythm appears as a regular, fast rhythm with broad QRS complexes. The patient in ventricular tachycardia may or may not have a pulse.
- **Non-shockable rhythms.** Defibrillation is not effective in the treatment of the following rhythms:
  - *Asystole*. No electrical activity is present, and there is an absence of identifiable waveforms. This has been referred to as a 'flat line' but there is usually a degree of baseline wander. A completely flat line usually indicates that the monitor has become disconnected.
  - *Pulseless electrical activity*. This term is used when there is a clinical absence of cardiac output despite electrical activity being seen on the monitor.

Box 13.7 Potential complications of cardiac surgery (Johnson & Rawlings-Anderson 2007)

- Cardiovascular – bleeding, arrhythmias, conduction problems, hypertension, hypotension, left ventricular failure, anaemia
- Respiratory – pulmonary oedema, pleural effusion, atelectasis, basal collapse
- Renal – decreased urinary output
- Neurological – stroke, memory loss, confusion
- Gastrointestinal – nausea and vomiting, loss of appetite
- Other – pain, wound infection

Cardiac surgery

For patients who have triple vessel disease and/or left main stem stenosis not suitable for PCI and stent insertion, CABG may be performed instead. Grafts are used to bypass the patient's diseased coronary arteries and therefore improve the blood supply to the myocardium, alleviate the symptoms of angina and improve quality of life (Webster & Thompson 2011). A patient may have a number of bypass grafts (usually between three and six) depending on their disease process. One end of the graft is attached to the aorta, and the other end is attached beyond the diseased area. Veins such as the long saphenous vein from the leg may be used as grafts, as may arteries such as the radial artery or internal mammary artery.

During surgery, the patient's heart is stopped, the body temperature is lowered, and the work of the heart and lungs is carried out by a cardiopulmonary bypass machine. The combination of the effects of the cardiopulmonary bypass and the sternotomy approach can lead to complications (Box 13.7). Although this method is still widely used, more minimally invasive techniques and beating heart surgery have become more common.

Clinical and nursing management

Preoperatively

Many patients will attend a pre-admission clinic where they are psychologically and physically prepared for surgery. As well as the nurse and surgeon, they may also be assessed by an anaesthetist and physiotherapist. Tests include:

- an ECG;
- a chest X-ray;
- echocardiography (for those having valve surgery);
- blood tests;
- the calculation of a risk stratification score, for example the EuroSCORE or Parsonnet score (Riley 2007);
- screening for multiresistant *Staphylococcus aureus*;
- baseline observations;
- height and weight.

Other comorbidities that may affect the outcome of surgery are also assessed. A discussion of what the surgery entails and the recovery afterwards will also be included. In some cases, patients may be shown the intensive care or high-dependency area to prepare them and their families for this. Issues affecting discharge should also be assessed. Some medications, such as digoxin, diuretics, beta-blockers, warfarin and aspirin, have to be stopped prior to surgery, and patients should be advised of this.

Patients are then usually admitted the day before surgery. Hair removal (if necessary) is carried out using a depilatory cream, and the patient will also have a shower using surgical soap. They will be nil by mouth in line with the usual hospital policy.

Postoperatively

Postoperative objectives include cardiovascular monitoring and support, pain relief, detection and management of complications, fluid management, respiratory support, wound care, assistance with activities of living, psychological support and preparation for discharge.

Some patients will remain intubated following surgery and may stay on a ventilator in intensive care for a few hours. In order to perform the surgery, the patient is put into a hypothermic state to protect the myocardial cells. The patient is then slowly warmed using warming blankets. There will usually be two or three chest drains, a catheter, one or more central lines and an arterial line *in situ*. Central venous pressure, heart rhythm, peripheral oxygen saturation and arterial blood pressure are continuously monitored. Urine output and blood loss in the drains will be checked carefully. Intravenous antibiotics are also given (Johnson & Rawlings-Anderson 2007).

Once patients are awake and off the ventilator, they are usually transferred to a high-dependency unit where their cardiovascular status is still carefully monitored. Fluids will be titrated to urine output and blood pressure. Approximately one-third of patients may develop atrial fibrillation, so close monitoring to detect this is important. Pain may initially be controlled by an intravenous infusion of morphine, but this will be replaced by patient-controlled analgesia once the patient is awake.

In the following days, drains will be removed, infusions including patient-controlled analgesia will be discontinued, and the catheter will also be removed. Oxygen is discontinued and the patient is encouraged to mobilise. Physiotherapists will also assess to check for signs of chest infection and encourage to the patient to breath deeply and cough. The patient will usually be discharged 5–7 days after surgery. In some cases, they may be invited to attend a cardiac rehabilitation programme 6 weeks after discharge.

Valvular heart disease

Any of the four heart valves can develop a problem, although this is more common on the left side of the heart – the mitral and aortic valves. Valves may become too tight (stenosis) or may leak (regurgitation). The most common valve problem is aortic stenosis ,which affects 2–7% of the population over the age of 65 (Davies & Lucas 2009).

Aortic stenosis

The aortic valve has three semilunar cusps. Aortic stenosis may be a result of narrowing below the cusps in the left ventricular outflow tract (subvalvular) or could be a constriction of the aorta (supravalvular).

Although there may be acute cases of aortic stenosis, in most cases the cusps stiffen over time and movement becomes limited. This then leads to concentric hypertrophy of the left ventricle, which increases the myocardial oxygen demand. The oxygen supply may be limited by compression of the coronary epicardial vessels, which can lead to angina. Other symptoms are syncope on exertion as the cardiac output is decreased due to the stenosis, shortness of breath on exertion, tiredness, weakness and occasionally palpitations due to rhythm abnormalities such as atrial fibrillation (Barrett 2006). As aortic stenosis may take many years to develop, it is mainly seen in older adults; once the condition is symptomatic, prognosis is poor without treatment. Patients with aortic stenosis may also develop aortic regurgitation.

Aortic regurgitation

Aortic regurgitation results in a leakage of blood from the aorta to the left ventricle during diastole. This will eventually cause the left ventricle to dilate and can eventually lead to left ventricular failure.

When recording the blood pressure, an increase in pulse pressure (a large difference between the systolic and diastolic blood pressure; Barrett 2006) may be found.

Mitral valve prolapse

Mitral valve prolapse can occur as a result of Marfan's syndrome, pregnancy or a hereditary condition. It does not usually require treatment unless symptomatic mitral regurgitation develops.

Mitral valve regurgitation

In mitral valve regurgitation, blood leaks back into the left atrium during systole. This leads to an increase in left ventricular volume, a decreased afterload and eventually left ventricular dilatation and left ventricular remodelling. Mitral valve regurgitation can be due to abnormalities of the valve leaflets, annulus, chordae tendinae or ventricle. Symptoms include shortness of breath, atrial fibrillation (in around a third of patients), night cough, fatigue and signs of right heart failure such as peripheral oedema.

Mitral stenosis

Due to the drop in rate of rheumatic fever, the rate of mitral valve stenosis has also decreased. As the orifice narrows, the pressure in the left atrium will increase. The walls will stretch, which can then lead to pulmonary oedema and eventually signs of right ventricular failure.

Symptoms will develop slowly but include shortness of breath, cough, frothy sputum (if pulmonary oedema is present), atrial arrhythmias and tiredness.

Investigations

Investigations include:

- an ECG
- an echocardiogram
- a chest X-ray
- a coronary angiogram
- heart sounds.

Clinical and nursing management

While patients are asymptomatic, their condition is monitored on a regular basis. Once symptoms develop, the patient will be considered for surgery (see below) as in some cases the prognosis is poor.

Management will therefore be tailored to the symptoms that the patient is experiencing; for example, those with aortic stenosis should be advised to avoid excessive activity as this may cause syncope or possible collapse. Arrhythmias are treated with an appropriate antiarrhythmic, and an anticoagulant such as warfarin is given if there is a risk of thrombotic events.

Where valvular conditions lead to heart failure, the patient will be managed in the same way with diuretics and other appropriate pharmacological therapy.

Surgery

Valves may be repaired or replaced. Valvular surgery was traditionally performed via a sternotomy with the patient on cardiopulmonary bypass. In the last few years, however, new minimally invasive techniques have been developed, such as thoracoscopically assisted mitral valve surgery and transcatheter

Box 13.8 Causes of heart failure (Johnson & Rawlings-Anderson 2007)

Right ventricular failure

- Right ventricular myocardial infarction
- Pulmonary disorders
- Valvular disease
- COPD
- Congenital defect

Left ventricular failure

- ACS
- Ischaemia
- Valve disease
- Hypertension
- Cardiomyopathy
- Arrhythmias

aortic valve implantation (Gibbins *et al.* 2009). These techniques are particularly good for those who are high risk with traditional surgery.

Types of valve replacement include mechanical valves, homografts (human) and bioprosthetic valves (tissue valves) (European Cardiovascular Society 2012).

Heart failure

Heart failure is a generic term for the heart's inability to pump blood to meet the body's requirements (Johnson & Rawlings-Anderson 2007). The type of heart failure will determine the symptoms exhibited and the subsequent management. However, heart failure is usually characterised by shortness of breath (dyspnoea), fluid retention, effort intolerance, fatigue and eventually death. Causes of heart failure are outlined in Box 13.8.

Left ventricular failure

If the left ventricle is not functioning properly, some blood will remain in it at the end of systole. This will initially lead to an increase in left ventricular size and pressure. However, as time goes on, there will be a backflow of blood into the left atrium, which will cause an increase in pulmonary pressure and result in fluid entering the alveolar sacs, leading in turn to pulmonary oedema. Left ventricular failure is classified by the NICE (2010e) as either heart failure with left ventricular systolic dysfunction or heart failure with a preserved ejection fraction.

Right ventricular failure

This is less common than left ventricular failure. It can occur on its own or as a consequence of left ventricular failure. Right ventricular failure leads to peripheral oedema and abdominal ascites.

Signs and symptoms

The patient may exhibit any of the following signs and symptoms depending on the origins of the heart failure and whether it is acute or chronic:

- Shortness of breath on exertion
- Frothy white sputum
- Paroxysmal nocturnal dyspnoea
- Swollen ankles
- Abdominal discomfort and ascites
- Fatigue
- Cough
- Tachycardia
- Jugular vein distension.

Diagnosis and investigations

The diagnosis of heart failure is usually based on the patient's history and symptoms, and is then confirmed by an echocardiogram. The patient will also have an ECG, chest X-ray and blood tests. In addition, an assessment needs to be made of the patient's cardiac output, heart rhythm, cognitive function, nutritional status and functional capacity.

Clinical and nursing management

Acute heart failure

Acute heart failure is usually rapid in onset and can be the result of an acute myocardial infarction, occurring in 25–50% of patients following ACS (Webster & Thompson 2011); alternatively, it may be an exacerbation of chronic heart failure. This can then deteriorate into cardiogenic shock if it is not treated quickly and appropriately. Therefore patients should be nursed in either coronary care or other suitable critical care settings.

The patient may become hypotensive and could develop rhythm abnormalities. This is likely to be tachycardia as the heart struggles to maintain cardiac output. Therefore patients need cardiovascular monitoring including cardiac monitoring, blood pressure, respiratory rate, SpO_2 and in some cases central venous pressure monitoring.

Patients should be nursed upright, supported by pillows in either a bed or a chair. Supplemental oxygen is given to maintain the SpO_2 above 95%. Regular blood gas readings will also be taken. If the SpO_2 cannot be maintained with oxygen therapy, the patient may require non-invasive ventilation either via continuous positive airway pressure or bilevel positive airway pressure (Quinn 2010). Regular oral hygiene needs to be given to combat the effects of humidified oxygen. The oxygen demand on the myocardium needs to be minimised as much as possible, so patients will need assistance with activities of living. The patient and family may be very distressed and anxious; therefore reassurance and psychological care are very important.

The aim of pharmacological care is to reduce both preload and afterload using a combination of intravenous vasodilators and diuretics. Other therapies that may be indicated include cardiac resynchronisation therapy (pacing of both ventricles), inotropes or even the insertion of an intra-aortic balloon pump or left ventricular assist device. These last two therapies should, however, only be considered as either a bridge to cardiac transplantation or if recovery is likely (Quinn 2010).

Chronic heart failure

There are a number of pharmacological therapies that can be used to help alleviate symptoms and improve prognosis in those with chronic heart failure. Current pharmacological guidelines are shown in Box 13.9.

The current guidance means that patients could be on at least six different medications a day, which may cause problems with both medication interactions and patient compliance. Nurses have a very important role in helping patients to understand what each of the medications is for and the

Box 13.9 Medication for heart failure (NICE 2010e)

- Angiotensin-converting enzyme inhibitors
- Beta-blockers
- Diuretics
- Angiotensin receptor blockers
- Aldosterone antagonists
- Digoxin

importance of taking them as prescribed (see http://www.healthtalkonline.org/heart_disease/Heart_Failure for patients' stories about coping with medication).

Vascular disorders

Aortic aneurysm

An aneurysm is defined as a permanent dilation of the aorta with a diameter that is more than 50% bigger than expected (Webster & Thompson 2011). Aneurysms can occur in one area or along a length of the aorta and may be completely circumferential (known as fusiform) or a pouch out from a weakened area (known as saccular). The most common site is the abdomen. The Stanford classification is often used for thoracic aneurysms (Johnson & Rawlings-Anderson 2007):

- Type A – in the proximal ascending aorta, with or without extension into the descending aorta (seen in two-thirds of patients).
- Type B – distal – descending aorta without involvement of ascending aorta.

Causes of aneurysm include:

- hypertension
- male sex
- Marfan's syndrome
- increasing age
- coarctation of the aorta
- trauma
- intra-aortic balloon pump
- pregnancy
- atherosclerosis
- infection, for example syphilis.

An aneurysm may not initially cause any symptoms or may mimic other problems. An abdominal aortic aneurysm may cause a pulsatile bulge in the abdomen when the patient is lying flat. A screening programme is being rolled out in the UK for men over the age of 65 as this is the group who are most susceptible. Ruptured abdominal aortic aneurysm causes 6000 deaths a year (Scott 2011). Other signs and symptoms may include back pain, pain from the compression of other organs and ischaemia of the end organs.

The signs and symptoms of a thoracic aneurysm will depend on the location. Pressure on other structures such as the oesophagus may lead to problems. If the aneurysm ruptures, patients are likely to feel an intense tearing pain. They may also experience neurological or renal problems if the blood supply to these areas is affected. Signs of a low cardiac output will be found, and peripheral pulses may be lost. Blood pressure recordings may be different for the two arms.

Investigations

Investigations will include ultrasound, MRI and CT scans.

Clinical and nursing management

The size, type and location of the aneurysm will determine the treatment given. Abdominal aortic aneurysms may be repaired by either major abdominal surgery with a graft inserted or a procedure called an endovascular aneurysm repair, in which catheters are inserted into both groins and stents are placed at the site of the aneurysm. Although this second procedure is less invasive and recovery is much quicker, not all patients will be suitable for it (Scott 2011).

A fusiform aneurysm will usually require excision and replacement with a tubular graft. If the ascending aorta is affected, an aortic valve replacement may be required. A saccular aneurysm may be tied at the neck of the sac (Webster & Thompson 2011).

If a rupture is suspected, the patient will need to be cared for in a critical care area with close monitoring. Intravenous opiates may be given to control pain, and intravenous vasodilators or beta-blockers may be required if the patient is severely hypertensive. The patient and family may be extremely anxious so good psychological care is very important. Urgent surgery is usually required, and the post-operative care is similar to that of cardiac surgery.

Peripheral vascular disease

Arterial and venous disease can occur alone or together. Many of the risk factors for heart disease will be the same for vascular disease.

Arterial disease

Atherosclerosis can occur within the peripheral arteries and plaques may form. As this happens over a period of time, a collateral circulation may develop, providing a blood supply to the extremities. Symptoms may therefore be slow to develop.

In atherosclerosis obliterans, there is chronic occlusive atherosclerosis of an artery supplying an extremity. Thrombosis of the deep veins can then occur secondary to arterial thrombosis as the blood becomes hypercoagulable. Ischaemic neuropathy and even gangrene can eventually occur. Inflammation can occur in the area between necrotic and viable tissue. Diabetic patients are more prone to an infected ulcer in association with gangrene (Webster & Thompson 2011).

Signs and symptoms

The patient may experience intermittent claudication, in which pain in the limb is experienced during exercise. This may start as fairly mild but can be very severe, and will initially be relieved by rest. However, as the disease progresses, pain may be experienced at rest. The distance a patient can walk on the flat before pain occurs is a good indicator of the progress of the disease.

Investigations

Peripheral circulation is assessed by looking at the pulses, colour, warmth and sensation. The tibial, popliteal and femoral pulses are assessed, but as the dorsalis pedis pulse may not be present in all people, it is not a reliable indicator. The presence or absence of the pulse and its strength should be compared between the two legs. As occlusion progresses, the toes may become quite bluish and mottled in appearance. If the legs are elevated, the feet will become extremely pale, with colour only resuming once they have been lowered again.

Other investigations include X-ray scanning, Doppler ultrasonography (including an ankle–brachial pressure index), helical computed tomography and arteriograms. Exercise testing will provide an indication of how far the patient can walk without pain.

Clinical and nursing management

The patient should be advised to avoid extremes of temperature and also tight clothes. Lack of sensation means that they can be at risk of burns so their lower limbs should be kept away from sources of direct heat such as hot water bottles and they should avoid sitting close to a fire or soaking their feet in hot water. Ill-fitting shoes also need to be avoided. Exercise should be encouraged where possible.

Treatment includes aspirin or antiplatelet agents, percutaneous transluminal balloon angioplasty or even a femoral popliteal bypass. An embolectomy may be performed for a localised embolus. In extreme cases, an amputation may be performed if gangrene is present.

Venous disease

Incompetence of the valves or an obstruction can lead to venous disease.

Venous thromboembolism

A thrombus is more likely to form when there is a decrease in blood flow, for example with an obstruction, stasis or damage to the endothelial wall. Factors predisposing to venous thromboembolism (VTE) are shown in Box 13.10. VTE is more likely to occur in the deep veins of the legs (deep vein thrombosis), but if it dislodges it can travel to the lungs and cause a pulmonary embolus, which can be fatal.

Symptoms

The patient will usually have a hot, tender and swollen calf (although more than 25% of patients with deep vein thrombosis have no symptoms).

Diagnosis

Diagnosis is made by considering:

- Homan's sign – pain in the calf when dorsiflexing the foot of a patient who is lying flat with their legs straight indicates a positive result;
- the level of D-dimer – a by-product of fibrin production measured by a blood test; this can be done during compression ultrasonography;
- a history of any of the predisposing factors, which will also be useful in reaching a diagnosis.

Box 13.10 Factors predisposing to VTE (Scottish Intercollegiate Guidelines Network 2010)

- Thrombophilia
- Obesity
- Trauma
- Pregnancy
- Contraceptive agents
- Dehydration
- Cancer
- Long-haul travel
- Varicose veins
- Hormone replacement therapy
- Immobility
- Central venous catheters

Clinical and nursing management

Both the Scottish Intercollegiate Guidelines Network (2010) and NICE (2010f) guidance recommends that all patients admitted to hospital should be assessed using a checklist for their risk of developing VTE. The risks and benefits of prophylaxis such as antiembolic stockings, leg exercises and subcutaneous heparin should also be discussed. For those with an established VTE, pain relief and anticoagulants (heparin followed by warfarin) are the recommended treatment.

Health promotion is a key part of the nurse's role, and patients should be encouraged to avoid dehydration, external pressure and immobility. Awareness of risk factors such as smoking and the contraceptive pill also needs to be raised.

Varicose veins

Varicose veins occur when valves in the veins become incompetent and tortuous. They are usually found in those who stand for long periods. Other causes include pregnancy, obesity and genetic predisposition. Thrombophlebitis may also lead to an increase in venous pressure as well as a destruction of valve tissue.

Valves become incompetent and veins dilate. Eventually, patients may complain of aching legs. Although there are not usually serious complications of varicose veins, discomfort or cosmetic reasons cause people to seek treatment. Varicose veins can also lead to venous ulcers.

Investigations

Ultrasonography may be carried out to assess the veins.

Clinical and nursing management

A number of treatment options are available depending upon the size and location of the varicose veins and the symptoms a patient may be experiencing. Support stockings may initially be recommended.

Traditionally, surgical removal of the veins by ligation and stripping was the main treatment. This involved a general anaesthetic and patients would have several small cuts in their leg. There are now less invasive procedures such as radiofrequency ablation, laser therapy or the injection of a sclerotherapy agent. These can all usually be carried out under local anaesthetic, but they may not be suitable for all patients and the long-term effectiveness of some of these treatments is not yet known.

Whatever treatment is used, patients are usually only in hospital for 1 day and are normally required to wear compression stockings for a period of time afterwards. Patients may have some tenderness and swelling after the procedure. They can usually drive a week afterwards and return to work after 1–3 weeks.

Conclusion

CVD is one of the major causes of death in the UK and Ireland, therefore it is important that nursing students gain an understanding of the assessment and treatment of conditions related to the heart such as valvular disease, rhythm problems, vascular disorders and coronary heart disease. High-quality nursing care before, during and after cardiac/vascular investigations and treatment is essential in ensuring a safe recovery.

Visit www.wileyfundamentalseries.com/medicalnursing and read Reflective Questions 13.1 and 13.2 to think more about this topic.

Now visit the companion website and test yourself on this chapter:
www.wileyfundamentalseries.com/medicalnursing

References

Aouizerat, B.E., Gardner, P.E. & Altman, G. (2010) Atherosclerosis, inflammation, and acute coronary syndrome In: Woods, S.L., Forelicher, E.S.S., Motzer, S.U. & Bridges, E.J. (eds), *Cardiac Nursing*, 6th edn. London: Lippincott Williams & Wilkins.

Barrett, D. (2006) Valve disease, cardiomyopathy and inflammatory disorders. In: Barrett, D., Gretton, M. & Quinn, T. (eds), *Cardiac Care: An Introduction for Healthcare Professionals*. Chichester: John Wiley & Sons.

Bassand, J.P., Hamm, C.W., Ardissino, D. *et al* (2007) Guidelines for the diagnosis and treatment of non ST segment elevation acute coronary syndromes. *European Heart Journal*, **28**(13):1598–660.

Bowden, T. & McLeod, A. (2010) The patient in haemodynamic compromise leading to renal dysfunction. In: McGloin, S. & McLeod, A. (eds), *Advanced Practice in Critical Care: A Case Study Approach* (pp. 26–70). Oxford: Wiley Blackwell.

Davies, K. & Lucas, R. (2009) Transcatheter aortic valve implantation: a review of clinical outcomes. *British Journal of Cardiac Nursing*, **4**(12): 583–7.

European Cardiovascular Society (2012) Guidelines on the management of valvular heart disease. *European Heart Journal*, **33**:2451–96.

Gibbins, A., Gannaway, A., Parker, J., Hyde, K., Brown, J. & Young, S. (2009) Transcatheter aortic valve implantation: developing nursing practice. *British Journal of Cardiac Nursing*, **4**(12):576–81.

Gibson T. (2008) A practical guide to external cardiac pacing. *Nursing Standard*, **22**(20):45–8.

Huszar R.J. (2007) *Basic Dysrhythmias: Interpretation and Management*, 3rd edn. St Louis: Mosby.

Irish Heart Foundation (2011) *Facts on Heart Disease and Stroke*. Retrieved 18th July 2011 from http://www.irishheart.ie/iopen24/facts-heart-disease-stroke-t-7_18.html.

Jackson, A. (2010) An overview of permanent cardiac pacing. *Nursing Standard*, **25**(12):47–57.

Jacobson, C. (2010) Arrhythmias and conduction disturbances In: Woods, S.L., Forelicher, E.S.S., Motzer, S.U. & Bridges, E.J. (eds), *Cardiac Nursing*, 6th edn (pp. 333–87). London: Lippincott Williams & Wilkins.

Johnson, K. & Rawlings-Anderson, K. (2007) *Oxford Handbook of Cardiac Nursing*. Oxford: Oxford University Press.

Kelly, J. (2004) Evidence-based care of a patient with a myocardial infarction. *British Journal of Nursing*, **13**(1):12–18.

Kucia, A.M. & Birchmore, E. (2010) Risk factors for cardiovascular disease. In: Kucia, A.M. & Quinn, T. (eds), *Acute Cardiac Care: A Practical Guide for Nurses* (pp. 26–49). Oxford: Wiley Blackwell.

Marshall, K. (2011) Acute coronary syndrome: diagnosis, risk assessment and management. *Nursing Standard*, **25**(3):47–57.

National Institute for Health and Clinical Excellence (2004) *Guidance on the Use of Coronary Artery Stents*. Technology Appraisal Guidance No. 71. Retrieved 18th July 2011 from http://guidance.nice.org.uk/TA71/Guidance/pdf/English.

National Institute for Health and Clinical Excellence (2010a) *Prevention of Cardiovascular Disease – A National Framework for Action*. NICE Public Health Guidance No. 25. Retrieved 12th June 2011 from http://www.nice.org.uk/nicemedia/live/13024/49273/49273.pdf.

National Institute for Health and Clinical Excellence (2010b) *Chest Pain of Recent Onset: Assessment and Diagnosis of Recent Onset Chest Pain or Discomfort of Suspect Cardiac Origin*. NICE Clinical Guideline No. 95. Retrieved 18th July 2011 from http://guidance.nice.org.uk/CG95/QuickRefGuide/pdf/English.

National Institute for Health and Clinical Excellence (2010c) *Chest Pain of Recent Onset. CT Calcium Scoring Factsheet Implement NICE Guidance*. Retrieved 18th July 2011 from http://www.nice.org.uk/nicemedia/live/12947/47987/47987.pdf.

National Institute for Health and Clinical Excellence (2010d) *Unstable Angina and NSTEMI: The Early Management of Unstable Angina and Non-ST-Segment-Elevation Myocardial Infarction*. NICE Clinical Guideline No. 94). Retrieved 18th July 2011 from http://guidance.nice.org.uk/CG94/QuickRefGuide/pdf/English.

National Institute for Health and Clinical Excellence (2010e) *Chronic Heart Failure: Management of Chronic Heart Failure in Adults in Primary and Secondary Care*. NICE Clinical Guideline No 108. Retrieved 20th June 2011 from http://www.nice.org.uk/nicemedia/live/13099/50514/50514.pdf.

National Institute for Health and Clinical Excellence (2010f) *Venous Thromboembolism: Reducing the Risk of Venous Thromboembolism (Deep Vein Thrombosis and Pulmonary Embolism) in Patients Admitted to Hospital*. NICE Clinical Guidance No. 92. Retrieved 3rd July 2011 from http://www.nice.org.uk/CG92.

Nicol, M. Bavin, C. Cronin, P. & Rawlings-Anderson, K. (2008) *Essential Nursing Skills*, 3rd edn. London: Mosby Elsevier.

Oriolo, V. & Albarran, J.W. (2010) Assessment of acute chest pain. *British Journal of Cardiac Nursing*, **5**(12):587–93.

Quinn, T. (2010) Acute heart failure. In: Kucia, A.M. & Quinn, T. (eds), *Acute Cardiac Care: A Practical Guide for Nurses* (pp. 257–68). Oxford: Wiley Blackwell.

Resuscitation Council (UK) (2010) *Resuscitation Guidelines*. London: Resuscitation Council.

Riley, J. (2007) Breathing and circulation. In: Brooker, C. & Waugh, A. (ed.), *Foundations of Nursing Practice*. Edinburgh: Elsevier.

Scarborough, P., Bhatnagar, P., Wickramasinghe, K., Smoina, K., Mitchell, C. & Rayner, M. (2010) *Coronary Heart Disease Statistics 2010 Edition*. Retrieved 18th July 2011 from http://www.bhf.org.uk/heart-health/statistics.aspx.

Scott, J. (2011) Focus on abdominal aortic aneurysm. *Heart Matters*, June/July:26–7.

Scottish Intercollegiate Guidelines Network (2010) *Prevention and Management of Venous Thromboembolism*. SIGN 122. Retrieved 1st July 2011 from http://www.sign.ac.uk/guidelines/fulltext/122.

Tortora, G.J. & Derrickson, B.H. (2009) *Principles of Anatomy and Physiology*, 12th edn. Danvers, MA: John Wiley & Sons.

Verrier, J.M.B. & Deelstra, M.H. (2010) Acute coronary syndromes syndrome. In: Woods, S.L., Forelicher, E.S.S., Motzer, S.U. & Bridges, E.J. (eds), *Cardiac Nursing*, 6th edn (pp. 511–36). London: Lippincott Williams & Wilkins.

Webster, R.A. & Thompson, D.R. (2011) Nursing patients with cardiovascular disorders. In: Brooker, C. & Nicol, M. (eds), *Alexander's Nursing Practice*, 4th edn (pp. 9–50). London: Churchill Livingstone.

14

Nursing care of conditions related to the digestive system

Joanne Cleary-Holdforth and Therese Leufer

School of Nursing, Dublin City University, Dublin, Ireland

Contents

Introduction	241
Nursing assessment	241
Nursing care	242
Diagnostic investigations	246
Conditions of the digestive system	249
The biliary system	254
Irritable bowel disease	257
Appendicitis	259
Bariatric surgery	260
Conclusion	260
References	261

Learning outcomes

Having read this chapter, you will be able to:

- Describe the anatomical structures of the digestive system
- Define and describe common conditions affecting the digestive system
- Recognise the common presenting symptoms of conditions affecting the digestive system
- Identify the investigations that may be necessary to aid diagnosis
- Undertake a nursing assessment and plan, implement and evaluate the care required by individuals with conditions affecting the digestive system

Fundamentals of Medical-Surgical Nursing: A Systems Approach, First Edition. Edited by Anne-Marie Brady, Catherine McCabe, and Margaret McCann.

Introduction

This chapter provides an overview of disorders affecting the digestive system. The specific nursing care of individuals with disorders of the digestive system is presented, alongside the related anatomy and physiology where appropriate. Nursing priorities when assessing individuals with disorders of the digestive system are then addressed, followed by a consideration of the nursing care required from both a conservative and a surgical approach as indicated. The aetiology, pathophysiology, investigations, diagnosis and clinical treatment of these conditions are outlined.

The digestive system extends from the mouth through the pharynx, oesophagus, stomach, duodenum and small and large intestines, terminating in the anal canal and rectum. The accessory organs of the digestive system include the teeth, salivary glands, liver, pancreas and gallbladder (Figure 14.1). The primary functions of the digestive system (including both the main and the accessory organs) include the ingestion, mastication and digestion (mechanical and chemical) of the food, the absorption of nutrients and the elimination of waste products of digestion.

Nursing assessment

Detailed assessment is essential in determining an appropriate plan of nursing care for all individuals with conditions affecting the digestive system. Assessment should include, but is not limited to, the following key areas:

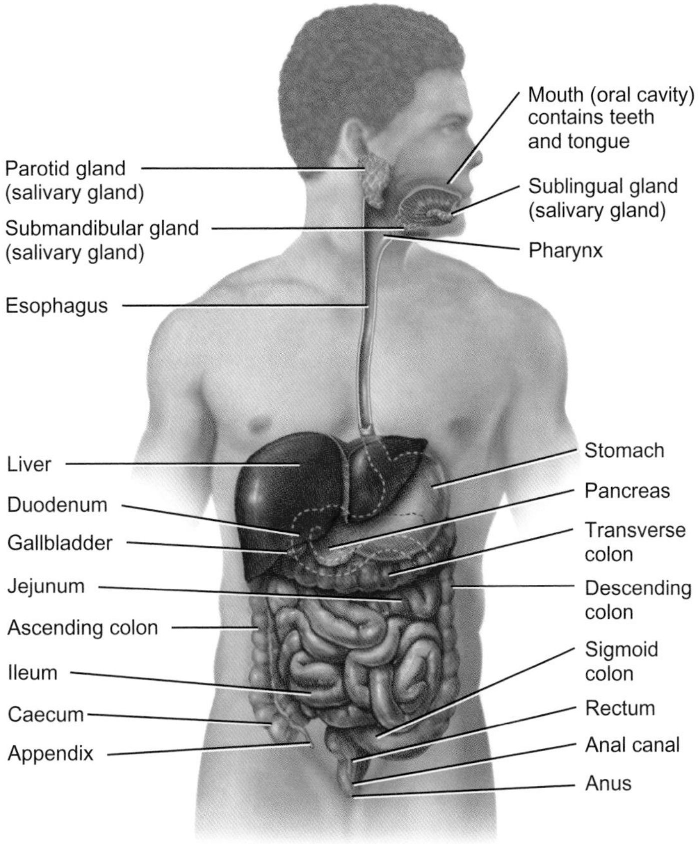

Figure 14.1 Organs of the digestive system. Reproduced from Tortora, G.J., Derrickson, B. (2011) *Principles of Anatomy and Physiology*, with kind permission of Wiley Blackwell.

- a general observations of the patient, including the vital signs;
- the patient's medical, surgical and social history;
- identification of the presenting signs and symptoms.

Chapter 1 addressed nursing assessment in detail. However, specific observations and clinical features of conditions related to the digestive system are addressed in this chapter:

- **General appearance:**
  - Skin – dehydration, pallor, jaundice, bruising, itching
  - Eyes – sunken eyes, yellow sclera, pale conjunctivae
  - Mouth – halitosis; lips – dry, chapped, pale, presence of sores; tongue – dry and coated, ulcerations; condition of the gums and teeth
  - Weight – current weight in addition to any recent unexplained changes in weight
- **Vital signs** – blood pressure, temperature, pulse, respiration
- **Diet** – any changes in dietary habits or appetite, altered bowel pattern, food intolerances
- **Medical/surgical history** – any pre-existing conditions or previous surgery
- **Medication history** – usual medications, any recently commenced medications, drug allergies
- **Social/personal history** – any recent travel to tropical regions, use of recreational drugs including alcohol and smoking, significant life events, occupation
- **Symptoms** – the presence or absence of any of the following specific symptoms:
  - Nausea and vomiting – note the onset, duration and triggers of vomiting in addition to the characteristics of any vomitus
  - Dyspepsia (indigestion)
  - Dysphagia (difficulty swallowing)
  - Abdominal pain – note the site, onset, nature and severity, the course and any precipitating and relieving features
  - Haematemesis (the presence of blood in the vomitus).
  - Diarrhoea – note the onset, duration and frequency, the characteristics of the stools and any exacerbating or relieving features
  - Constipation – note the onset and duration, the characteristics of the stool, whether the condition is chronic or irregular in nature, and whether there is any associated pain or discomfort
  - Melaena (a black tarry stool resulting from bleeding in upper gastrointestinal tract)
  - Palpable lump(s) – note the site, onset and characteristics.

It is imperative to ascertain from the patient the characteristics of specific symptoms, including their onset, nature, severity and duration, in order to make a comprehensive nursing assessment and provide an accurate and prompt medical diagnosis.

Nursing care

A systematic approach to the planning and implementation of nursing care will ensure that the individual's needs are comprehensively addressed. The pertinent nursing care is outlined here.

Communication

It is crucial to have clear communication with patients at all times in order to establish trust and a good nurse–patient relationship. This should ensure that patients' needs are identified and met as quickly and effectively as possible, so that patient outcomes are maximised.

Observations

In addition to the signs and symptoms outlined above, the patient should also be monitored closely for any deterioration in condition. The vital signs (blood pressure, temperature, pulse and respiration) should be monitored regularly, the frequency of readings being determined by the patient's condition and by medical advice. Any deviation from baseline observations should be documented and reported immediately.

Nutrition and hydration

It is imperative to ensure that any patient with a digestive disorder is adequately hydrated at all times. If, as is frequently the case with this patient group, oral intake is not permitted due to the presenting symptoms, intravenous access must be established and hydration facilitated by an intravenous infusion. A strict fluid balance record must be maintained. In addition, meticulous attention to oral hygiene is a priority when oral intake is prohibited.

Where oral intake is possible, a balanced nutritional intake should be encouraged. It is helpful to enlist the assistance of the hospital dietitian, who can provide appropriate dietary advice and guidance. Symptoms such as dyspepsia, dysphagia, nausea and loss of appetite can interfere with the patient's nutritional intake, and such symptoms should be reported, investigated and managed appropriately. The management of these symptoms may be conservative in nature, for example the prescription of antacids such as calcium carbonate, histamine (H2) receptor antagonists such as ranitidine, or proton pump inhibitors such as omeprazole in the case of dyspepsia (Barber & Robertson 2009), but further interventions may also be required. It is essential to provide adequate patient education on the effects, side effects and potential interactions of any medications.

Elimination

Common presenting features of digestive disorders include nausea, vomiting, diarrhoea and constipation. As already mentioned, it is important to observe the nature, course and characteristics of these symptoms in order to get a clear insight into the patient's condition and to determine the best course of treatment. An accurate record of the patient's output (vomitus, diarrhoea and urinary output) is essential to help determine hydration needs and prevent dehydration. A patient who is experiencing frequent diarrhoea should, where possible, be located in close proximity to the bathroom in order to maintain their privacy and dignity during both elimination and hygiene needs. Stool samples should be obtained for investigations including faecal occult blood and culture and sensitivity of any organisms present.

Pain relief

Patients with a digestive disorder are likely to experience varying degrees of pain. An accurate pain assessment using a recognised pain assessment tool is integral to adequate pain management and should include an observation of both verbal and non-verbal cues. It is important for the nurse to act promptly on any complaints of pain the patient may have. In certain emergency situations, it may be necessary to establish a definitive diagnosis before pain relief can be administered. In these cases, it is important to communicate this clearly to patients and to offer them reassurance that the situation will be resolved as quickly as possible. All efforts should also be made to maximise the patient's comfort. Clear reporting and documenting of the patient's pain, prescription medication(s) and administration and evaluation of pain relief is paramount in diagnosis and management. Any drug allergies must be ascertained prior to administering any medication.

Preparation for investigations

A variety of investigations may be necessary to make a diagnosis. Specific examples include plain X-rays, ultrasound scanning, gastroscopy, barium swallow, colonoscopy and laparoscopy (see Figures 14.3 and 14.4 later in the chapter). Some of these require no particular preparation. However, investigations such as colonoscopy and laparoscopy require very specific preparation, which may include bowel clearance and/or fasting in advance. Local policy regarding the preparation for such investigations must be adhered to.

Mobilisation

The patient's mobility may be limited, so in order to prevent complications of prolonged bed rest such as chest infection, constipation, pressure ulcer development and deep vein thrombosis, for example, it is important to encourage active mobilisation if the patient's condition permits. Otherwise, active limb exercises, repositioning and deep breathing exercises should be encouraged.

Psychosocial support

Admission to hospital can be traumatic and frightening for the patient and indeed for their family members, and this anxiety may be compounded by a fear of any impending diagnosis and treatment. A friendly approach and clear, regular communication may help to reassure the patient and their family. Keeping the patient (and where appropriate the next of kin) informed on their progress with prompt updates regarding any test results and the plan of care can help to alleviate unnecessary worry. It is also imperative to ask for the patient's social history including their next of kin and any social support network as such information is a vital part of optimal discharge planning.

Patients undergoing surgery

Surgery on the digestive system can range from laparoscopic ('keyhole') surgery to open abdominal surgery (Figure 14.2). It can be for the purpose of:

- investigation (e.g. laparoscopy);
- excision (e.g. appendix, gallbladder or intestine);
- repair (e.g. hernia);
- transplantation (liver or pancreas).

Surgery may be elective (planned) in nature or it may be carried out as an emergency. In some cases, it may have life-changing consequences, such as the formation of a stoma, as in the case of an ileostomy.

Perioperative management

The general principles of perioperative management can be found in Chapter 8, but perioperative management specific to patients with a digestive disorder will be outlined here.

The patient will need to fast in preparation for gastrointestinal surgery. In theory, this means that the patient may have light food up to 6 hours and water and clear fluids up to 3 hours preoperatively (Westby *et al.* 2005). However, depending on the digestive disorder and the nature and site of the surgery, the patient may have to fast for longer. The patient's hydration and nutritional status must be monitored closely and appropriate measures taken to prevent dehydration and malnutrition. This may include administering intravenous fluids or even total parental nutrition.

In addition to preoperative fasting, the patient who is undergoing intestinal surgery will require bowel clearance. This may involve a low-residue diet or clear fluid intake and the oral ingestion of a purgative preparation such as sodium picosulphate over the 24–48 hours prior to surgery to cleanse the bowel of faecal matter (Norton *et al.* 2008). Local guidelines could be consulted for details of the policy and procedure involved. The patient should be supported during this preparation as it can be unpleasant and uncomfortable, and care should be taken to ensure that the patient's dignity is maintained. Reassurance that this preparation will contribute to safe and successful surgery may encourage the patient to adhere to it.

Along with the usual risks associated with surgery, such as infection and haemorrhage, gastrointestinal surgery carries the additional risk of peritonitis, as well as negative outcomes such as stoma formation or a poor prognosis in the case of a malignancy. It is vital to provide patients with clear, comprehensive explanations of the condition, its treatment and its prognosis and to ensure that they fully understand what they will be asked to consent to. The stoma care specialist will need to be consulted over the location of the stoma and the patient's physical and psychological preparation. Setting

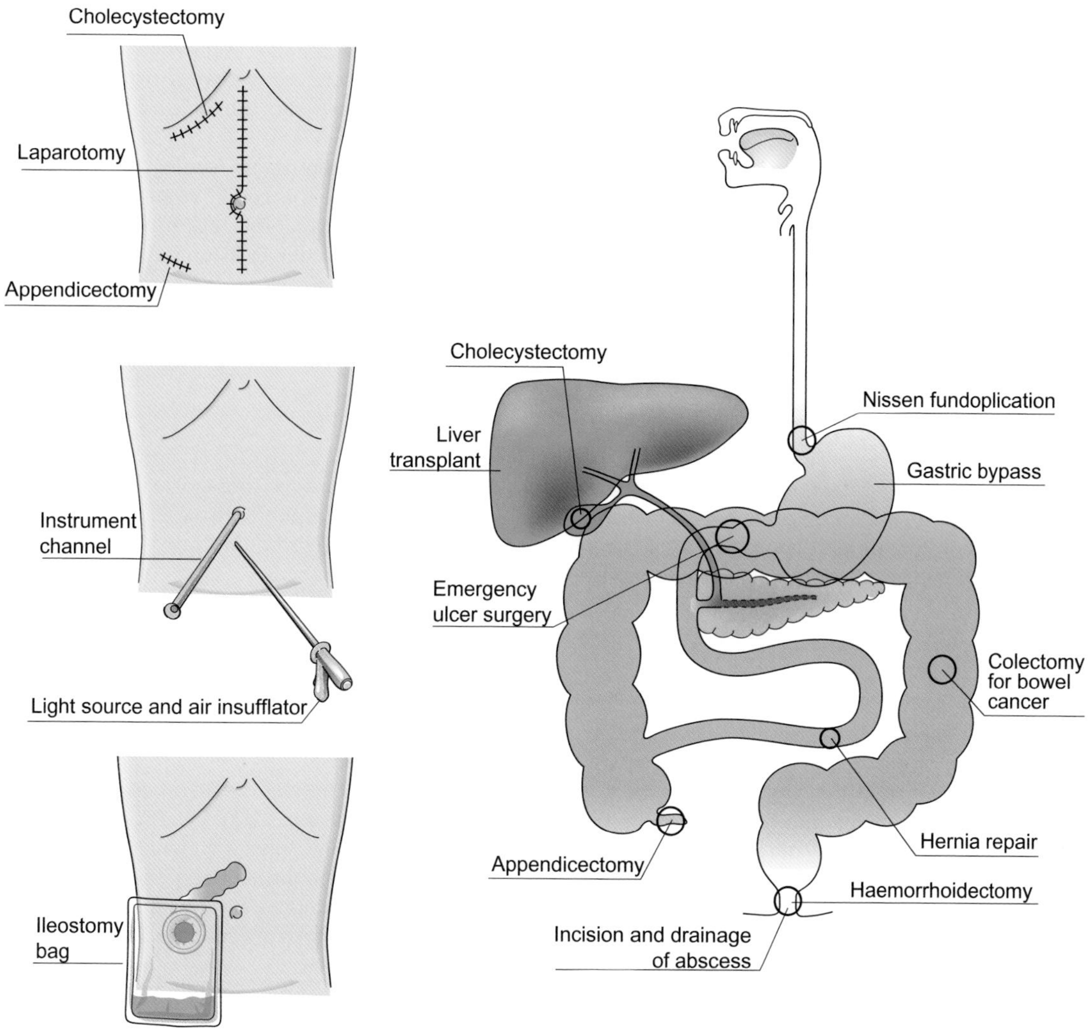

Figure 14.2 Gastrointestinal surgery. Reproduced from Keshav, S. (2004) *Gastrointestinal System at a Glance*, with kind permission of Wiley Blackwell.

up a meeting with a person who already has a stoma may also be helpful. Spend time with the patient listening to their concerns and answering their questions where possible.

Postoperative management

The patient may return from theatre with an intravenous infusion line, nasogastric tube, urinary catheter, wound drain and/or stoma in place. The purpose of these should be explained clearly to the patient, along with an indication of how long they may be in place and any specific care that will be required. Monitoring and documentation of vital signs and fluid balance are of the utmost priority after gastrointestinal surgery so that complications such as shock, infection, haemorrhage, dehydration and peritonitis can be detected early. The patient may experience nausea and vomiting postoperatively and will require an antiemetic; the effect of this should also be monitored.

Pain management is crucial in the postoperative period. Assess the patient's pain level using a pain assessment tool and note any physiological signs of pain or body cues indicating pain. It is imperative that the patient's reports of pain are responded to promptly. Administer analgesia as prescribed. Observe and document the patient's response and any side effects. Make sure that patients on patient-controlled analgesia know how to use it safely and effectively. Make sure that patient is in a comfortable position, that the wound is not under strain and that any drain or catheter tubing is not compressed or kinked.

Gastrointestinal surgery often results in a temporary cessation of peristalsis leading to a condition called paralytic ileus. The patient may not eat or drink anything while this condition persists as doing so may result in profuse vomiting and unnecessary discomfort or pain. The return of peristalsis is monitored by the doctor by auscultating the abdomen using a stethoscope to listen for bowel sounds. Once the bowel sounds have returned and the patient is no longer vomiting, they are usually commenced on sips of clear fluids followed by a light diet as tolerated, depending on the type of surgery and the surgeon's postoperative instructions.

Diagnostic investigations

A wide variety of tests can contribute to the diagnosis of digestive disorders. These include radiological, ultrasound, endoscopic and serum investigations (Figure 14.3). The results of these investigations, in addition to a physical examination of the patient, a description of the symptoms and a consideration of the patient's history, will, in most cases, lead to a definitive diagnosis.

Radiological investigations

A plain film of the abdomen, also referred to as an abdominal X-ray, and contrast studies are common investigations. The plain film allows the identification of gas and fluid levels that may indicate bowel disease or obstruction. No specific preparation or aftercare is required.

Imaging studies of the gastrointestinal tract commonly use the contrast medium barium sulphate and include the barium swallow, barium meal, barium follow-through and barium enema. The barium is administered orally or rectally, depending on the part of the gastrointestinal tract being investigated. Barium is radio-opaque and therefore visible on an X-ray. This enables abnormalities of the oesophagus, stomach and intestinal tract to be visualised. Air can also be used as a contract medium for gastrointestinal investigations, but this is less common. However, these procedures are contraindicated in cases of suspected obstruction or perforation of any part of the digestive tract.

The preparation for these investigations varies. In the case of a barium swallow, meal or follow-through, the patient will need to fast for 4–6 hours in advance. In the case of the barium enema, however, the patient will require a low-residue diet and high fluid intake for 48 hours prior to the test, in addition to bowel clearance (Norton *et al.* 2008). In all cases, the barium should pass from the patient's system unaided, but occasionally a mild laxative may be required to assist its evacuation. Patients should also be encouraged to increase their oral fluid intake, where appropriate, to prevent constipation.

Abdominal ultrasound

This non-invasive investigation involves imaging the abdominal cavity using sound wave technology to produce two-dimensional images. It allows the abdominal organs and structures to be examined for inflammation and abnormalities, and is particularly useful for the detection of gallstones (Smith & Watson 2005). It aids the diagnosis of a number of conditions including cholecystitis, irritable bowel disease (IBD), abdominal masses and hepatomegaly.

Endoscopy

Endoscopic investigations allow direct visualisation of the mucosal lining and organs of the gastrointestinal tract using rigid or flexible scopes equipped with a light source and camera (Figure 14.4). Such investigations include:

Test	Structure
Barium swallow	Pharynx, oesophagus
Barium meal	Stomach, duodenum
Barium meal and follow-through	Duodenum, jejunum, ileum
Barium enema	Large intestine, terminal ileum
ERCP	Gallbladder, bile ducts, pancreas

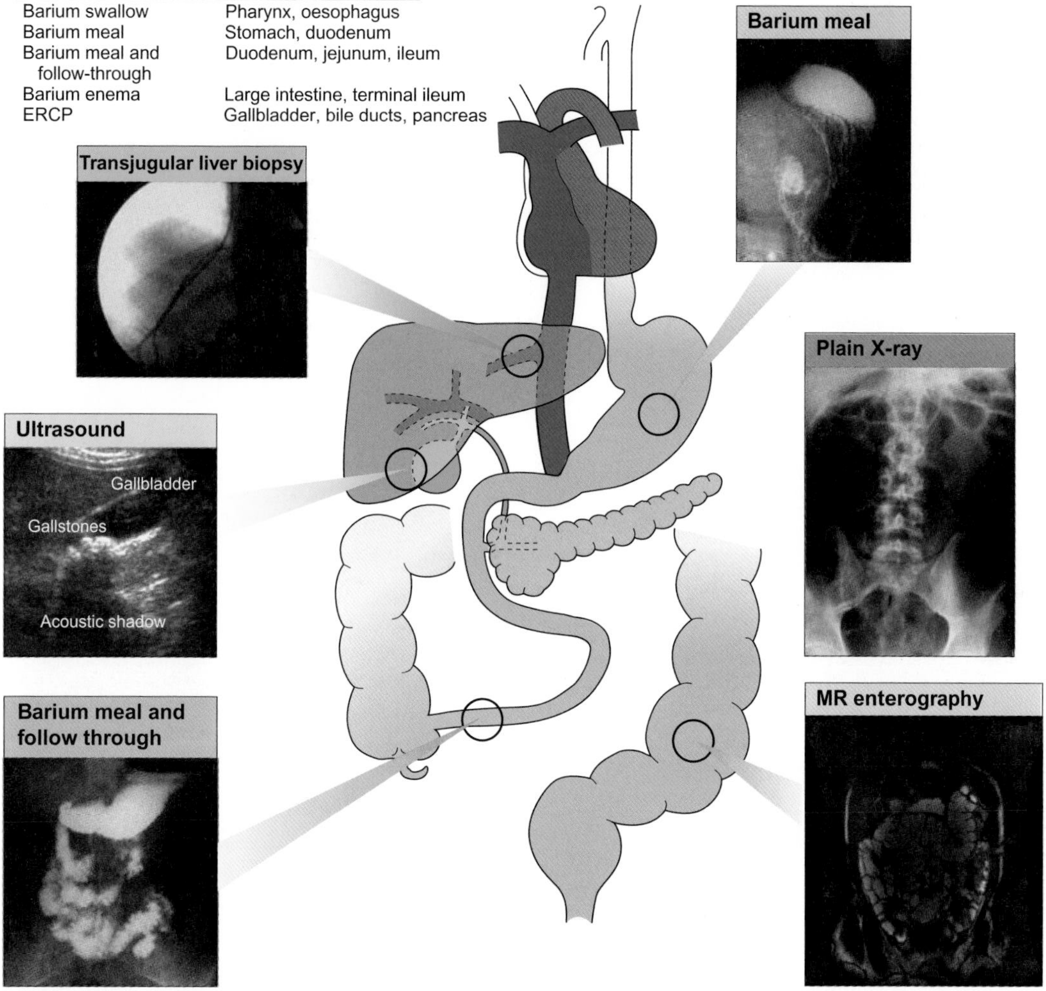

Nuclear medicine scans	
Scan name	**Principle and uses**
Gastric emptying scan	The rate of passage of a labelled meal measures gastric motility
Meckel's scan	Labelled pertechnetate taken up by parietal cells localises ectopic gastric tissue
Red cell scan	Labelled red cells reinjected into the patient localise rapidly bleeding lesions
White cell scan	Labelled white cells reinjected into the patient accumulate at sites of inflammation
Octreotide scan	Labelled octreotide binds to somatostatin receptors, localising neuroendocrine tumours that strongly express these receptors
SeHCAT scan	Measures retention of exogenous labelled bile acid (homocholic acid taurine) to diagnose bile acid malabsorption

Figure 14.3 Radiology and imaging. CCD, charge-coupled device; ERCP, endoscopic retrograde cholangiopancreatography. Reproduced from Keshav, S. (2004) *Gastrointestinal System at a Glance*, with kind permission of Wiley Blackwell.

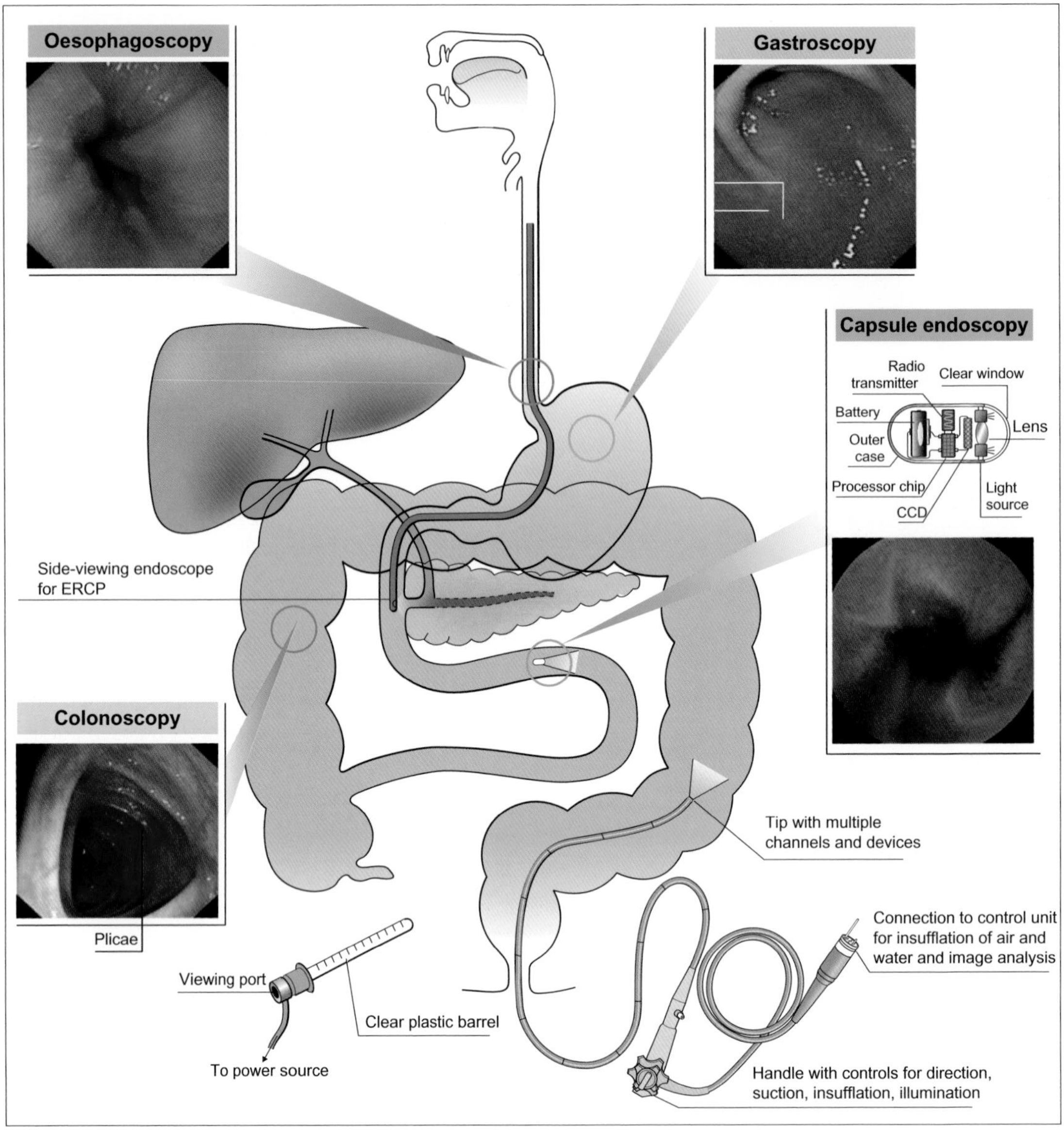

Figure 14.4 Endoscopy. MR, magnetic resonance. Reproduced from Keshav, S. (2004) *Gastrointestinal System at a Glance*, with kind permission of Wiley Blackwell.

- oesophago-gastroduodenoscopy (visualising the oesophagus, stomach and duodenum);
- endoscopic retrograde cholangiopancreatography (ERCP; for the gallbladder and biliary and pancreatic ducts);
- proctoscopy (the rectum);
- sigmoidoscopy (the distal colon);
- colonoscopy (the entire large bowel).

In addition to directly visualising and capturing images of the gastrointestinal tract and organs, endoscopies also allow biopsies and fluid samples to be obtained to help in the diagnosis. Endoscopy can also be used to remove polyps (abnormal tissue growth in the intestinal mucosa) and to treat certain conditions such as bleeding ulcers, oesophageal varices, bleeding intestinal lesions and some gastro-oesophageal obstructions caused by tumours, strictures or foreign bodies (Norton *et al.* 2008).

Patients are usually sedated for endoscopic investigations, and these can, if necessary, be performed under anaesthetic. Preparation of the patient varies depending on the endoscopic investigation being undertaken. Informed consent must be obtained from the patient before undergoing any endoscopic procedure. As sedation is usually required, an intravenous cannula should be inserted in advance. In the case of a colonoscopy, the patient will be required to have a low-residue diet for 2 days prior to the procedure and bowel clearance on the day before, and to fast for 2 hours before the colonoscopy (Norton *et al.* 2008). It is important to consult local policy for any additional preparation that may be warranted. The patient's condition and vital signs should be monitored closely during and after all endoscopic investigations to detect signs of haemorrhage, perforation or aspiration.

Computed tomography scanning

This technology produces cross-sectional images of the organs of the gastrointestinal tract. It is usually performed if the ultrasound scan has been unsuccessful or inconclusive. A contrast medium may be used to enhance the images of the abdominal organs, but this can impair renal function and cause anaphylaxis. Where these risks may prove too high, alternative means of investigation and diagnosis should be considered.

Laparoscopy

This investigation is very useful in the diagnosis of digestive disorders. It is performed under anaesthetic, involving a small incision ('keyhole') through the abdominal wall to allow the injection (insufflation) of carbon dioxide into the peritoneal cavity; this moves the organs and structures away from each other so that they can be visualised more easily (Smeltzer *et al.* 2008). This technique helps in obtaining tissue and fluid samples from the abdominal structures and organs, as well as in detecting inflammation, masses, gallbladder and liver disease and other abnormalities. In certain circumstances, it may be necessary to proceed to therapeutic measures such as laparoscopic excision, for example of the gallbladder, or indeed to open abdominal surgery if needed. This possibility must be clearly stated and explained to the patient preoperatively when informed consent is being sought.

Stool analysis

Stool samples can be examined for their volume, consistency, odour and colour. Laboratory tests include checking for the presence of blood, bacteria, viruses, parasites, cysts, ova, toxins, pus cells and white cells, all of which can produce symptoms of diarrhoea and intestinal inflammation.

Blood tests

A variety of blood tests may be ordered depending on the patient's presenting clinical features:

- full blood count;
- urea and electrolytes (U & E);
- clotting factors;
- liver function tests.

Conditions of the digestive system

Constipation

Constipation can be defined as the incomplete or infrequent passage of hard stools, a reduced volume of stools or difficulty passing stools, and is often associated with straining and/or pain on defaecation (Norton *et al.* 2008). The normal pattern of defaecation varies from person to person and ranges from three times a day to once every 3 days. It is important to establish with the patient what their normal bowel pattern is and to document this in the nursing assessment.

The causes of constipation can be differentiated into two broad categories: mechanical and functional. Mechanical causes of constipation include obstruction due to IBDs, postponing defaecation, lesions, and scar tissue after previous surgery. Examples of functional causes of constipation include reduced gut motility due to immobility and paralytic ileus after surgery, a poor intake of dietary fibre, poor fluid intake, certain drugs such as iron preparations and codeine phosphate, which have a constipating effect, and abuse of laxatives. Other symptoms associated with constipation include abdominal distension and discomfort, reduced appetite, headache and indigestion (Smeltzer *et al.* 2008).

Constipation is diagnosed by collating the patient's history and symptoms, coupled with a physical examination and investigations such as an abdominal X-ray. Particular attention is paid to the patient's normal bowel pattern and whether the constipation is a deviation from that pattern. Any recent changes to the patient's lifestyle or dietary intake that may have led to constipation are also of particular interest. Treatment of constipation involves administering oral laxatives in the first instance, along with advice on a nutritious diet high in fibre and fluid intake if appropriate, regular exercise and lifestyle modifications to prevent a recurrence. Prolonged constipation can lead to a variety of complications including haemorrhoids, impaction, hypertension and bowel perforation in extreme cases (Smeltzer *et al.* 2008).

Diarrhoea

Diarrhoea, on the other hand, can be described as an increase in the number of bowel motions per day compared with what is normal for the individual (Young Johnson 2008). This increased frequency is usually accompanied by increased volume, increased urgency and increased liquidity of the stool. Some individuals may also experience pain that may be abdominal and/or rectal in nature.

Diarrhoea can be acute or chronic depending on the cause and/or condition. For example, diarrhoea caused by infective agents (as in the case of food poisoning) is acute and usually self-limiting, whereas diarrhoea secondary to an underlying condition such as ulcerative colitis may be more chronic in nature. Complications of diarrhoea can include fluid and electrolyte imbalance, which can in extreme cases lead to cardiac arrhythmias and other cardiac complications. If diarrhoea is extreme or prolonged, intravenous fluid replacement may be required.

Priorities of nursing management focus on maintaining the patient's dignity, facilitating good personal hygiene, ensuring and encouraging adequate fluid replacement and offering reassurance and support as necessary. Where possible, it is prudent to identify the underlying cause of the diarrhoea by sending a stool sample to the laboratory for analysis, among other diagnostic tests. Treatments for diarrhoea may include fluid replacement and electrolyte replacement, antidiarrhoeal agents such as loperamide or codeine preparations to reduce intestinal motility, and antimicrobial agents if an infective organism has been identified (Young Johnson 2008).

Nausea and vomiting

Nausea is the feeling or sensation of sickness and the desire to vomit, which may or may not result. Vomiting is forceful expulsion of the gastric contents, which is usually preceded by nausea. It is important to note that vomiting can be a significant presenting feature of a number of conditions and can provide a useful indication of potential underlying conditions or the end diagnosis. Other symptoms that often accompany nausea and vomiting include sweating, increased salivation and tachycardia.

The causes of nausea and vomiting are numerous and may include ingested infective organisms or irritants, reduced gastric emptying and intestinal motility, peritoneal irritation, hepatobiliary or pancreatic disorders, bowel obstruction, reduced intestinal motility secondary to anaesthesia, disorders of the vestibulocochlear (VIIIth cranial) nerve, neurological conditions involving raised intracranial pressure or infections of the central nervous system, and cancer treatments such as chemotherapy or radiotherapy (Smeltzer *et al.* 2008). If nausea and/or vomiting are prolonged or severe, a number of potential outcomes can result, such as dehydration, electrolyte imbalance, weight loss, acid erosion of the teeth and oesophageal tears leading to haematemesis (vomiting blood), although these are usually superficial and heal quickly.

Priorities of nursing care are directed towards identifying the underlying cause so that specific treatment can be initiated, in addition to correcting fluid and electrolyte imbalance and reassuring and supporting the patient. Antiemetic medications such as ondansetron or metoclopramide may be prescribed in an attempt to alleviate nausea and vomiting.

Cancers of the digestive system

Cancer can affect any part of the digestive system, with varying disease manifestations, progression and consequences. Most of the recent statistics reported by the National Cancer Registry of Ireland (2009) and Cancer Research UK (2008) indicate that colorectal cancer is one of the most common invasive cancers and was the second most common cause of all cancer deaths (12%) in the Republic of Ireland in the period 1994–2007. Early detection is key to optimising the management and outcome for the patient.

Diagnosis

The number and nature of investigations undertaken to reach a diagnosis will be determined by the patient's presenting features and the location of the presenting complaint. Investigations additional to those already outlined include magnetic resonance imaging (MRI) and positron emission tomography scans, both of which offer a more detailed visualisation of the relevant tissues and structures.

The signs and symptoms of cancers of the digestive tract will vary depending on the part or area affected. Commonly presenting signs and symptoms include weight loss, loss of appetite, an altered eating pattern, tiredness, nausea and vomiting, and anaemia. More specific signs and symptoms related to the specific part or area affected may include dysphagia, dyspnoea, dyspepsia, a feeling of fullness, haematemesis, abdominal pain and/or distension, an altered bowel pattern, altered stools including malaena, rectal bleeding, tenesmus (the feeling of a need to pass stool even when the rectum is empty) and a palpable mass in the affected region.

In addition to reaching a diagnosis of cancer, it is also normal practice to ascertain the extent of the cancer. This is termed staging. Stages of cancer progression generally range from stage 1, in which the tumour is confined to its primary site, through to stage 5, which involves extensive spread of the cancer to tissues and organs in other parts of the body. The earlier the stage of the cancer at the time of diagnosis, the better the prognosis for the patient.

Treatment

Treatment of cancer will be determined by a number of factors including the site, type and stage of the cancer, the impact it has had on the patient, the anticipated efficacy of interventions, their effects on the patient and any comorbidity. Standard cancer treatments that are usually employed include surgery, where appropriate, chemotherapy, radiotherapy, photodynamic therapy or indeed any combination of these. A holistic and multidisciplinary approach to patient care is essential when caring for a patient with a diagnosis of cancer of the digestive system who is undergoing treatment. The plan of nursing care depends on the individual patient's specific diagnosis, the particular treatment regimen prescribed and the patient's response to that treatment. Priorities of nursing care focus on:

- psychological care;
- reassurance and promotion of the patient's dignity;
- observing and documenting the vital signs and the patient's condition;
- preventing infections;
- maintaining a high level of personal hygiene;
- managing symptoms such as pain, nausea, vomiting, diarrhoea, poor appetite and dehydration;
- maintaining skin integrity;
- encouraging sleep and rest.

It is essential to involve members of the multidisciplinary team such as the dietitian, stoma care specialist, chaplain, social worker, counsellor and, where necessary, palliative care team. It is also

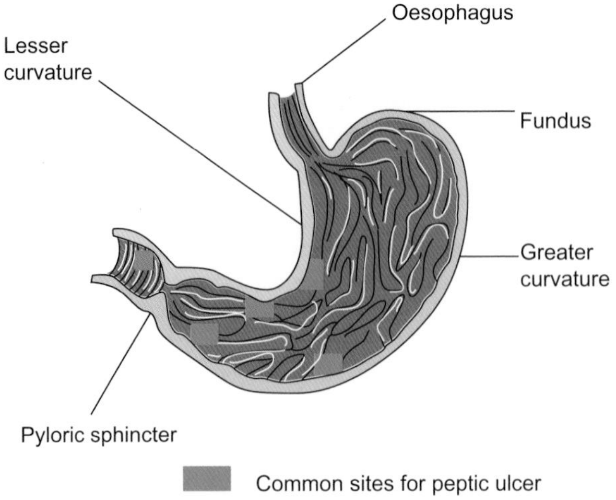

Figure 14.5 Common sites for peptic ulcer development. Reproduced from Nair, M. & Peate, I. (2013) *Fundamentals of Applied Pathophysiology*, with kind permission from Wiley Blackwell.

essential to support and care for the patient before, during and after any prescribed treatments and, in so doing, respect their wishes at all times.

Peptic ulcer disease

Peptic ulcer disease can affect the oesophagus, stomach and duodenum. The lining of affected area is damaged, usually by increased acid secretion, leading to inflammation and ulceration (Figure 14.5). Peptic ulcer disease can range from mild, causing few symptoms, to severe and even life-threatening, as in the case of perforation of the gastrointestinal wall. Duodenal ulcers occur more commonly than gastric ulcers, with gastric ulcers occurring most commonly on the lesser curvature of the stomach (Nair, 2009a). Peptic ulcer disease can affect individuals of any age but occurs most commonly in the 40–60-year age group (Smeltzer *et al.* 2008).

The presence of a particular Gram-negative bacterium, *Helicobactor pylori*, in the stomach accounts for 70–80% of gastric ulcers (Ford *et al.* 2011). Other factors that are thought to lead to peptic ulcer disease include smoking, alcohol, stress, excessive caffeine intake, prolonged use of aspirin, non-steroidal anti-inflammatory drugs or corticosteroids, and genetic predisposition (Mynatt *et al.* 2009; Nair, 2009a).

Clinical features and complications

Symptoms may vary from mild to severe, depending on the location and degree of ulceration, and can occur intermittently. Common symptoms include:

- epigastric pain that occurs when the stomach is empty and is usually relieved by intake of food, milk or antacids;
- dyspepsia;
- loss of appetite;
- heartburn due to reflux of gastric acid, and belching;
- nausea and vomiting;
- malaena.

Around 20–30% of patients present in the first instance with haemorrhage or perforation in the absence of any preceding symptoms (Smeltzer *et al.*, 2008). These are two of the major complications associated with peptic ulcer disease. Perforation is erosion of the ulcer through the gastric or duodenal wall into the peritoneal cavity, leading to chemical and bacterial peritonitis (Smeltzer *et al.* 2008). These complications are potentially life-threatening and require emergency treatment. Another complication of peptic ulcer disease is pyloric stenosis, in which the pyloric sphincter becomes obstructed due to scarring or stenosis, inhibiting the flow of stomach contents into the duodenum.

Diagnosis

Assessment of the patient with peptic ulcer disease includes:

- the patient's history;
- their presenting symptoms;
- physical observation and examination;
- investigations to aid diagnosis, which include:
  - barium studies;
  - gastroscopy;
  - a full blood count (a low haemoglobin level and haematocrit suggest anaemia);
  - an examination of stool samples for occult blood;
  - a urease breath test and the colorimetric CLO test performed to detect *Helicobactor pylori* in a mucosal specimen obtained by endoscopy (Norton *et al.* 2008).

Treatment

The treatment will be determined by the cause. In the case of ulcers secondary to *Helicobactor pylori* infection, antibiotic therapy using two or three antibiotics (amoxicillin, clarithromycin and metronidazole, for example) along with a proton pump inhibitor such as omeprazole will be prescribed for 10–14 days in an attempt to eradicate the bacteria; this effects a permanent cure in 90% of cases (Norton *et al.* 2008; Ford *et al.* 2011). Proton pump inhibitors and H2 receptor antagonists such as ranitidine are used in the treatment of ulcers that are not associated with *Helicobactor pylori*. Antacids such as calcium carbonate or magnesium salts can be used to treat symptoms such as heartburn and dyspepsia but often provide only temporary relief. Long-term maintenance therapy with medication may be required to prevent recurrence (Smeltzer *et al.* 2008). The management of peptic ulcer disease should also incorporate advice and guidance on relevant lifestyle changes.

Nursing management

Nausea and vomiting can be treated with an antiemetic such as prochlorperazine (Stemetil) or metoclopramide. The patient's response to the medication administered, and the effects and side effects, must be observed, documented and reported to the medical team when necessary.

Complications associated with peptic ulcer disease include haemorrhage, perforation and pyloric stenosis. If any of these complications occur, intravenous access will need to be established and fluid replacement initiated to correct hypovolaemia. In addition, the insertion of a nasogastric tube will allow aspiration to decompress and empty the stomach, and there should be continual monitoring of vital signs and ongoing reassurance and support. Oxygen therapy and monitoring of oxygen saturation levels will be required if there is haemorrhage, and replacement of blood components may become necessary if the haemorrhage is severe. The patient's full blood count and urea and electrolyte levels should be checked. A urinary catheter should be inserted and the urinary output closely observed. Intravenous antibiotic therapy may be required to prevent septic shock where a perforation has occurred. Depending on the type and severity of the complication, the patient may also need to be prepared for endoscopy, as in the case of pyloric stenosis (to dilate the pylorus), or surgery, as in the case of perforation.

In order to reduce the risk of recurrence of peptic ulcer disease, the patient should be advised to stop smoking, reduce their caffeine and alcohol intake and modify their diet to include small regular meals and avoid foods that trigger gastrointestinal symptoms. Medications such as aspirin and non-steroidal anti-inflammatory drugs should be avoided where possible. The patient should endeavour to reduce the level of stress in their life if this is thought to be a contributing factor. Stress-relieving activities such as regular exercise, yoga and meditation should be encouraged.

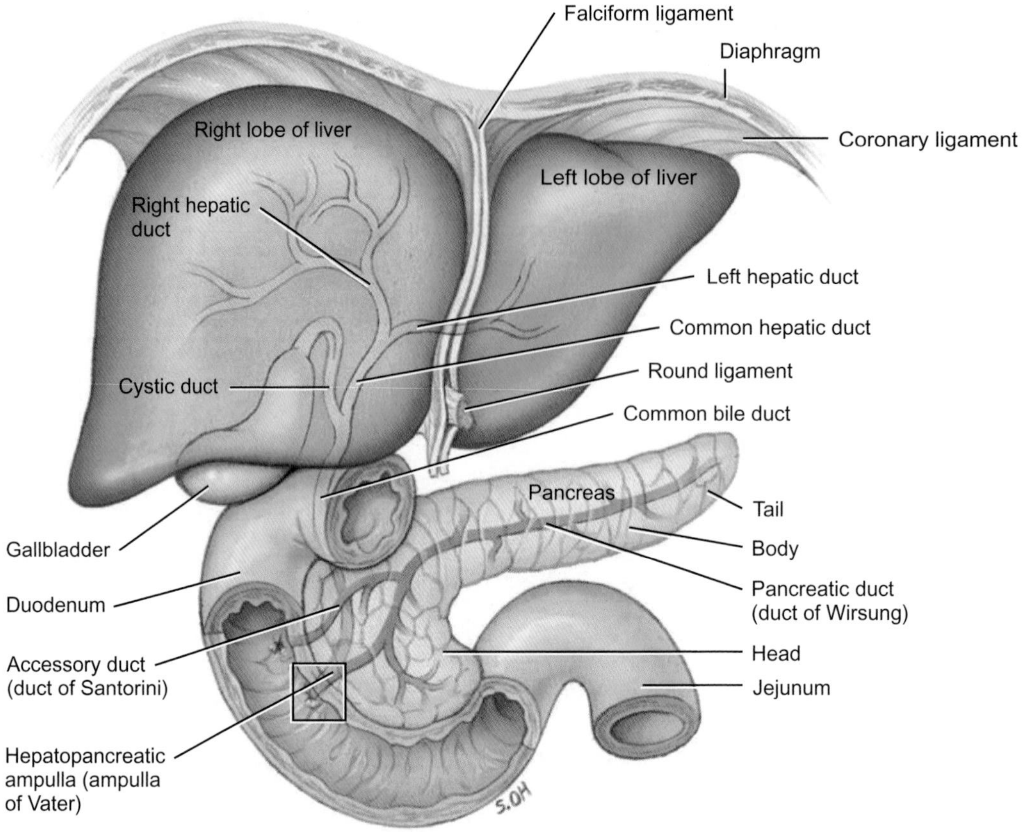

Figure 14.6 The liver. Common sites for peptic ulcer development. Reproduced from Nair, M. & Peate, I. (2013) *Fundamentals of Applied Pathophysiology*, with kind permission from Wiley Blackwell.

The biliary system

The liver

The liver, which is the largest organ in the body and weighs approximately 1.5 kg, is located in the upper right quadrant of the abdominal cavity just below the diaphragm (Figure 14.6). It has numerous important functions (Nair, 2009a), in that it:

- detoxifies noxious substances such as drugs and alcohol;
- creates body heat through metabolism;
- produces bile, which emulsifies dietary fat for absorption;
- contributes to maintaining the blood glucose level;
- produces and stores glycogen;
- manufactures plasma proteins such as albumin and globulins;
- produces clotting factors such as fibrinogen and prothrombin;
- creates the anticoagulant heparin;
- plays a part in the destruction of red blood cells, releasing bilirubin, which is eliminated in the faeces;
- stores iron, copper, fat-soluble vitamins A,D, E and K, and water-soluble vitamin B_{12};
- produces cholesterol, and stores and modifies fats for more efficient utilisation by the cells.

Conditions affecting the liver can be categorised by their underlying aetiology. These categories comprise infections (such as hepatitis A, B, C, D, E and G), autoimmune and chemically induced (e.g. alcohol and/or drugs) conditions, and cirrhosis (primary or secondary). Such conditions tend to be chronic in nature, with varying degrees of severity and progression, and all have the potential to lead to hepatocellular carcinoma and liver failure (Manns *et al.* 2010; O'Shea *et al.* 2010). Where possible, preventive measures should be employed to avoid contracting or developing liver disease in the first instance. Where a liver condition develops, however, early detection is key to optimising management and long-term outcomes for the individual.

Manifestations of liver disease can vary according to the underlying condition, and some patients may be asymptomatic for a while. Some of the common presenting features include a dull ache in the right upper quadrant, jaundice (discoloration of the skin and sclerae due to an accumulation of bilirubin in the skin), fatigue, weight loss, anorexia, anaemia, oedema, hepatosplenomegaly (an enlarged liver and spleen), clotting disorders, ascites (a collection of fluid in the peritoneal cavity), dyspepsia, altered bowel function, gastric or oesophageal varices, vitamin deficiency and portal hypertension (increased pressure in the portal vein).

Diagnosis

The following are used in diagnosis:

- the patient's history;
- physical observation and examination;
- signs and symptoms;
- investigations, including:
  - full blood count;
  - urea and electrolyte levels;
  - liver enzymes (which may be elevated);
  - prothrombin time (which may be abnormal);
  - serum albumin (which may be low);
  - possibly, specific screening for infectious and/or autoimmune sources of hepatitis;
  - stool examination;
  - abdominal ultrasound;
  - a computed tomography (CT) scan;
  - an MRI scan;
  - a liver biopsy (used to confirm the diagnosis and the nature and extent of the disease process).

Treatment

Therapies used may include:

- antiviral treatment, as in the case of infective hepatitis (Ghany *et al.* 2009), and corticosteroids;
- immunosuppressants in the case of autoimmune causes (Manns *et al.* 2010), and the pharmacological management of alcohol or drug misuse in addition to advice on abstaining from alcohol in the case of chemically induced disease (O'Shea *et al.* 2010);
- a liver transplant in advanced disease;
- in the case of irreversible liver disease, perhaps largely palliative treatment focusing on symptomatic relief, maintaining the individual's dignity and comfort and involving the family where possible.

Nursing management

Nursing management is largely supportive and is determined by the specific underlying cause and the individual's symptoms. It is important to consult with a dietitian to develop an individualised dietary plan that will optimise the individual's nutritional intake and status. For example, regular small meals with adequate protein and calories, reduced salt intake and the replacement of deficient vitamins can help to offset the liver's reduced capacity for fat and glycogen storage, and prevent muscle wasting (O'Shea *et al.* 2010). Relief of symptoms such as pain, pruritis (itching), nausea and oedema is integral to maintaining the individual's comfort. The individual's condition and response to all treatments should be documented and reported accordingly.

The gallbladder

The gallbladder is located beneath the right lobe of the liver. It is pear-shaped and measures approximately 7.5–10 cm in length (Figure 14.6). Its function is to store and concentrate bile, which is manufactured by the liver. Bile is released from the gallbladder via the cystic and common bile ducts into the duodenum in response to the hormone cholecystokinin, whose release is triggered by the ingestion of fatty foods. Bile is responsible for the breakdown of fat (Nair, 2009a).

Cholecystitis (inflammation) and cholelithiasis (gallstones) are the two main conditions that affect the gallbladder. Presenting symptoms include abdominal pain in the right upper quadrant, particularly following the ingestion of fatty foods, nausea, pyrexia and rigors. The pain associated with these conditions is described as colicky and occurs as a result of the gallbladder contracting in an attempt to eject bile that is obstructed by the presence of gallstones.

Diagnosis

Diagnosis will involve:

- the patient's history;
- the presenting symptoms;
- a physical observation and examination;
- investigations, including:
  - a full blood count (which may reveal an elevated white cell count, indicating inflammation);
  - liver function tests (which may reveal elevated levels of biliary enzymes and bilirubin);
  - an abdominal ultrasound;
  - a CT and/or MRI scan.

Treatment

Treatment of cholecystitis or cholelithiasis typically involves antibiotic therapy and surgical removal of the gallbladder. Cholecystectomy, conventionally an 'open' surgical procedure, is now typically performed using a laparoscopic ('keyhole') technique. The removal of gallstones is carried out using a procedure known as endoscopic retrograde cholangiopancreatography (ERCP). This is involves passing an endoscope through the mouth, oesophagus and stomach into the duodenum.

Nursing management

The principles of nursing care include identifying potential problems, physical and psychological preparation of the patient for surgery and postoperative recovery, and the early detection and prompt management of postoperative complications. The specific pre- and postoperative care of a patient with a digestive disorder was addressed earlier in the chapter.

Visit **www.wileyfundamentalseries.com/medicalnursing** and read **Reflective Question 14.1** to think more about this topic.

The pancreas

The pancreas is located behind the stomach and extends from the loop of the duodenum towards the spleen (Figure 14.6). It is approximately 12–15 cm long and 2.5 cm thick (Colbert *et al.* 2009; Nair

2009a). Its primary function in the digestive system is to aid the digestion of carbohydrates, proteins and fats by secreting digestive enzymes into the duodenum via the pancreatic duct.

Pancreatic conditions tend to occur primarily as a result of damage to the pancreatic duct by stones, tumours or trauma, releasing pancreatic enzymes that autodigest the duct tissue. These escaping enzymes, in addition to possible bacterial infection, can also leak into the bloodstream; this results in the potential for this to become a multisystem condition, affecting other sites, for example the lungs, which can be fatal. Pancreatitis can be acute or chronic in nature. Presenting symptoms include epigastric pain radiating to the back, nausea, vomiting and abdominal distension and rigidity. In addition to these symptoms, individuals with chronic pancreatitis may also present with weight loss, pain on eating and steatorrhoea (Norton *et al.* 2008).

Diagnosis

The diagnosis is made by considering:

- observation of the patient and the history;
- a physical examination;
- the presenting symptoms;
- investigations, which may include:
  - a full blood count;
  - C-reactive protein level;
  - abdominal and chest X-rays;
  - an abdominal ultrasound scan;
  - a CT scan;
  - an MRI scan;
  - an ERCP.

Treatment

This may include:

- intravenous fluid management in the initial phase;
- nasogastric aspiration to relieve nausea, vomiting, abdominal distension and paralytic ileus;
- prohibition of oral intake to prevent pancreatic enzymes being secreted;
- pain relief as a priority;
- antibiotic therapy if there is infection;
- oral hypoglycaemic drugs;
- palliative measures.

Nursing management

It is imperative to note that individuals with pancreatitis can deteriorate very quickly. Frequent monitoring of the patient's condition and prompt management of any complications that may arise are paramount. Key priorities of nursing care should include management of fluid and electrolyte balance, relief of pain and discomfort, optimising respiratory function, improving nutritional status, and psychological support (Norton *et al.* 2008).

Irritable bowel disease

IBD is used to describe inflammatory conditions of the bowel, including Crohn's disease, ulcerative colitis and diverticulitis. IBD is a chronic disorder characterised by an altered bowel pattern, abdominal pain and discomfort associated with defaecation (National Institute for Health and Clinical Excellence [NICE] 2008). Other signs and symptoms may include severe diarrhoea, the presence of blood, pus or mucus in the bowel movements, nausea, vomiting, poor appetite and weight loss. IBD is typically episodic in nature, with the individual experiencing exacerbations and remissions of the disorder.

Potential contributing factors that have been suggested include food intolerance or hypersensitivity, gastrointestinal infection, autoimmune, genetic and environmental factors, and stress.

Diagnosis

The diagnosis is made by considering:

- the patient's history;
- the presenting symptoms;
- physical observation and examination;
- investigations, which include:
  - endoscopic investigation (sigmoidoscopy or colonoscopy);
  - possibly barium studies;
  - a full blood count;
  - vitamin B_{12} level;
  - C-reactive protein level;
  - stool samples for occult blood.

Treatment

Treatment may include the following:

- Drug therapies typically employed include corticosteroids, immunosuppressants (for autoimmune causes), local and systemic anti-inflammatories, antibiotic therapy and probiotic therapy.
- Depending on the symptoms, laxatives or antidiarrhoeal agents can be used.
- Antispasmodics and pain relief are used to promote comfort (NICE 2008).

In severe cases, surgical intervention may be required, which may, in some cases, result in the formation of a stoma (World Gastroenterology Organisation 2009). Dietary and lifestyle advice and psychological support are imperative in the care of individuals with IBD.

Nursing management

One of the key priorities of nursing management of the individual with IBD is psychological support and education. Given the debilitating and enduring nature of IBD, it has the potential to impact on many aspects of the individual's lifestyle, including their family, work and social activities. This can in turn result in the onset of depression. It is therefore essential to establish a trusting rapport with the individual and to provide sufficient opportunity for them to voice any fears or concerns in relation to these areas. In addition, providing the individual with details of appropriate organisations that can offer ongoing support and help may prove useful in the long-term management of the condition.

A key priority of nursing management is close monitoring of bowel pattern, fluid balance to detect any dehydration, particularly in the presence of diarrhoea, urea and electrolyte levels, nutritional intake, weight and vital signs. A low-residue diet may be indicated during exacerbations, but it is important to encourage the individual to include sufficient fibre, protein and calories in their diet during remissions as well. In cases of extreme diarrhoea, parenteral nutrition may be required until the diarrhoea subsides. Vitamin and mineral supplements may also be indicated.

In an acute phase of the condition, the individual should be encouraged to rest, and assistance with daily activities such as personal hygiene needs may be needed. In order to preserve dignity, the individual with severe diarrhoea should where possible ideally be nursed in a single en suite room; otherwise, close proximity to the bathroom should be ensured.

Close observation of the individual's condition to detect signs of potential complications is imperative. Complications that can arise include perforation and peritonitis, fistula development, bowel obstruction and toxic megacolon. There is also an increased predisposition to the development of colorectal cancer among individuals with IBD compared with the general population (NICE 2011).

Visit www.wileyfundamentalseries.com/medicalnursing and read Reflective Question 14.2 to think more about this topic.

Appendicitis

The appendix is a rudimentary, blind-ending tube located at the caecum that has no function in the human digestive system. Its walls contain lymphatic tissue, and its inner lining secretes mucus that flows into the caecum. Appendicitis, which is inflammation of the appendix, occurs when the lumen becomes obstructed with materials such as faecaliths (small, hardened lumps of faeces), undigested food particles (e.g. seeds or nuts) and lymphoid tissue. This inflammation results in the presenting symptoms associated with appendicitis.

Symptoms

Commonly presenting symptoms include pyrexia, nausea and vomiting, general abdominal discomfort that localises to the right iliac fossa as the condition progresses, and rebound abdominal tenderness, particularly at the junction known as McBurney's point (midway between the umbilicus and the anterior spine of the ilium; Young Johnson 2008). Less common symptoms such as constipation, diarrhoea or urinary symptoms may also be present.

Diagnosis

Diagnosis involves:

- the patient's history;
- the presenting symptoms;
- physical observation and examination;
- investigations, including:
  - a full blood count (to detect an elevated white cell count indicating the presence of infection);
  - urinalysis (to detect urinary tract infection and/or pregnancy in the case of women of child-bearing age);
  - an abdominal X-ray;
  - an abdominal ultrasound.

Treatment

The treatment of appendicitis is surgical removal of the appendix (appendectomy) and antibiotic treatment. There are two surgical approaches: conventional 'open' surgery and laparoscopic surgery. If left untreated, the inflamed appendix may rupture, spilling infection into the peritoneal cavity and resulting in peritonitis and possible septic shock. Possible signs and symptoms of peritonitis include abdominal distension and board-like rigidity, paralytic ileus, nausea and vomiting, pyrexia, tachycardia and hypotension. This is a life-threatening condition that warrants early detection and prompt intervention.

Nursing management

The principles of nursing care include identifying potential problems, physical and psychological preparation of the patient for surgery and postoperative recovery, and early detection and prompt management of postoperative complications. The specific pre- and postoperative care of a patient with a digestive disorder was addressed earlier in the chapter.

Bariatric surgery

Bariatric surgery is a relatively new approach to the management of obesity used in cases where professionally advised weight-reducing diets and exercise programmes have not proven successful. Surgical approaches such as gastric banding and gastric bypass help weight loss by reducing the size of the individual's stomach and therefore the amount of food that the individual can ingest at any given time (Nair 2009b). Although this type of surgery is now available, it is important to emphasise that conservative measures such as lifestyle modifications and pharmacological approaches are available and should, where possible, be considered in the first instance.

Obesity

The World Health Organization (2011) defines overweight and obesity as 'an abnormal or excessive fat accumulation that present a risk to health'. Overweight refers to increased body weight when measured against the individual's height and when the body mass index (BMI) – a calculation of an individual's body fat based on their weight and height measurements – is between 25 and 29.9 kg/m^2 (Nair 2009b). Obesity is said to exist when the BMI exceeds 30 kg/m^2 (World Health Organization 2011). A BMI of 40 kg/m^2 indicates extreme obesity. These conditions predispose individuals to an increased risk of a variety of health issues including hypertension, heart disease, respiratory disease, diabetes mellitus, vascular disease, varicose veins, cerebrovascular accidents and bowel cancer (Nair 2009b; NHS Information Centre for Health and Social Care 2011), all of which increase morbidity, mortality and healthcare costs. Obesity levels are now high and continue to rise globally, particularly in urban settings (Barron *et al.* 2009; NHS Information Centre for Health and Social Care 2011; World Health Organization 2011).

Overview of bariatric surgery

Bariatric surgery generally falls into three categories: restrictive surgery such as gastric banding; primary restrictive techniques with a malabsorptive component such as gastric bypass; and malabsorptive approaches involving various anatomical diversions of the gastrointestinal tract, with the aim of shortening the functional small intestine so the absorption of nutrients is minimised (Kulick & Bovee 2009). In conjunction with psychological support, all of these surgical techniques help with significant weight loss, but they can also produce nutritional and metabolic complications such as protein–calorie malnutrition and deficiencies of various nutrients (Kulick & Bovee, 2009).

Nursing management

The principles of nursing care include the identifying potential problems, physical and psychological preparation of the patient for surgery and postoperative recovery, and early detection and prompt management of postoperative complications. The specific pre- and postoperative care of a patient with a digestive condition was addressed earlier in this chapter. It is important to ensure that the appropriate healthcare personnel, such as the dietitian, are involved in all stages of patient care delivery.

Conclusion

Cancer, constipation, diarrhoea, peptic ulcer disease, hepatitis, cirrhosis, pancreatitis, cholecystitis and appendicitis are common disorders of the digestive system. Careful assessment is essential for aiding accurate diagnosis, providing appropriate nursing care and ensuring a safe recovery and the prevention of complications. Key factors in assessment include observing the patient's general appearance, taking a medical and surgical history, noting the symptoms, and recording vital signs and the results of investigations. When caring for patients with digestive disorders, the main factors to address are communication, vital signs, nutrition, hydration, elimination, pain relief, preparation for investigations, mobility and psychosocial support.

Now visit the companion website and test yourself on this chapter:
www.wileyfundamentalseries.com/medicalnursing

References

Barber, P. & Robertson, D. (2009) *Essentials of Pharmacology for Nurses*. Oxford: Oxford University Press.

Barron, C., Comiskey, C. & Saris, J. (2009) Prevalence rates and comparisons of obesity rates in Ireland. *British Journal of Nursing*, **18**(13): 799–803.

Colbert, B., Ankney, J., Lee, K., Steggall, M. & Dingle, M. (2009) *Anatomy and Physiology for Nursing and Health Professionals*. Harlow: Pearson.

Ford, A.C., Delaney, B., Forman, D. & Moayyedi, P. (2011) *Eradication therapy for peptic ulcer disease in Helicobacter pylori positive patients*. Cochrane Library, (1):CD003840.

Ghany, M.G., Strader, D.B., Thomas, D.L. & Seeff, L.B. (2009) Diagnosis, management, and treatment of hepatitis C: an update. *Hepatology*, **49**(4):1335–74.

Kulick, D. & Bovee, V. (2009) Obesity and bariatric surgery. In: Hark, L. & Morrison, G. (eds), *Medical Nutrition and Disease: A Case-Based Approach*, 4th edn (pp. 39–57). Chichester: Wiley Blackwell.

Manns, M.P., Czaja, A.J., Gorham, J.D. *et al.* (2010) Diagnosis and management of autoimmune hepatitis. *Hepatology*, **51**(6):2193–213.

Mynatt, R.P., Davis, G.A. & Romanelli, F. (2009) Peptic ulcer disease: clinically relevant causes and treatments. *Orthopedics*, **32**(2):104–7.

Nair, M. (2009a) The gastrointestinal system and associated disorders. In: Nair, M. & Peate, I. (eds), Fundament*als of Applied Pathophysiology: An Essential Guide for Nursing Students* (pp. 272–97). Chichester: Wiley Blackwell.

Nair, M. (2009b) *Nutrition and Associated Disorders*. In: Nair, M. & Peate, I. (eds), *Fundamentals of Applied Pathophysiology: An Essential Guide for Nursing Students* (pp. 298–317). Chichester: Wiley Blackwell.

National Cancer Registry of Ireland (2009). *Cancer in Ireland 1994–2007*. Cork: National Cancer Registry of Ireland.

National Institute for Health and Clinical Excellence (2008) *Irritable Bowel Syndrome in Adults: Diagnosis and Management of Irritable Bowel Syndrome in Primary Care*. Clinical Guideline No. 61. London: NICE.

National Institute for Health and Clinical Excellence (2011) *Colonoscopic Surveillance for Prevention of Colorectal Cancer in People with Ulcerative Colitis, Crohn's Disease or Adenomas*. Clinical Guideline No. 118. London: NICE.

NHS Information Centre for Health and Social Care (2011) *Statistics on Obesity, Physical Activity and Diet: England, 2011* (Version 1). Leeds: NHS Information Centre for Health and Social Care, Lifestyle Statistics.

Norton, C., William, J., Taylor, C., Nunwa, A.M. & Whayman, K. (eds) (2008) *Oxford Handbook of Gastrointestinal Nursing*. Oxford: Oxford University Press.

O'Shea, R.S., Dasarathy, S. & McCullough, A.J. (2010) Alcoholic liver disease. *Hepatology*, **51**(1):307–28.

Smeltzer, S.C., Bare, B.G., Hinkle, J.L. & Cheever, K.H. (2008) *Brunner and Suddarth's Textbook of Medical-Surgical Nursing*, 11th edn. Philadelphia: Lippincott, Williams & Wilkins/Wolters Kluwer Health.

Smith, G. & Watson, R. (2005) *Gastrointestinal Nursing*. Oxford: Blackwell Science.

Westby M., Bullock I., Gray W., Lardner-Browne C. & Rashid R. (2005) *Perioperative Fasting in Adults and Children*. London: Royal College of Nursing.

World Gastroenterology Organisation (2009) *World Gastroenterology Organisation Global Guideline: Irritable bowel syndrome*. A Global Perspective. Munich (Germany). April 20. Retrieved 21st June 2011 from http://www.worldgastroenterology.org/assets/downloads/en/pdf/guidelines/20_irritable_bowel_syndrome.pdf.

World Health Organization (2011) *Obesity*. Retrieved 21 June 2011 from http://www.who.int/topics/obesity/en/.

Young Johnson, J. (2008) *Handbook for Brunner and Suddarth's Textbook of Medical-Surgical Nursing*, 11th edn. Philadelphia: Lippincott, Williams & Wilkins/Wolters Kluwer Health.

15

Nursing care of conditions related to the urinary system

Margaret McCann[1], Ciara White[2] and Louisa Fleure[3]

[1]*Trinity College Dublin, Dublin, Ireland*
[2]*Beaumont Hospital, Dublin, Ireland*
[3]*Guy's Hospital, London, UK*

Contents

Introduction	263
Anatomy and physiology	263
Conditions of the prostate	270
Kidney cancer	275
Bladder cancer	278
Urinary tract infections	280
Acute kidney injury	284
Chronic kidney disease	288
Renal replacement therapy	293
Conclusion	297
References	297

Learning outcomes

Having read this chapter, you will be able to:

- Describe the anatomy and physiology of the urinary system
- Outline the medical and nursing management of common urological and nephrology disorders
- Identify the different types of renal replacement therapy

Fundamentals of Medical-Surgical Nursing: A Systems Approach, First Edition. Edited by Anne-Marie Brady, Catherine McCabe, and Margaret McCann.

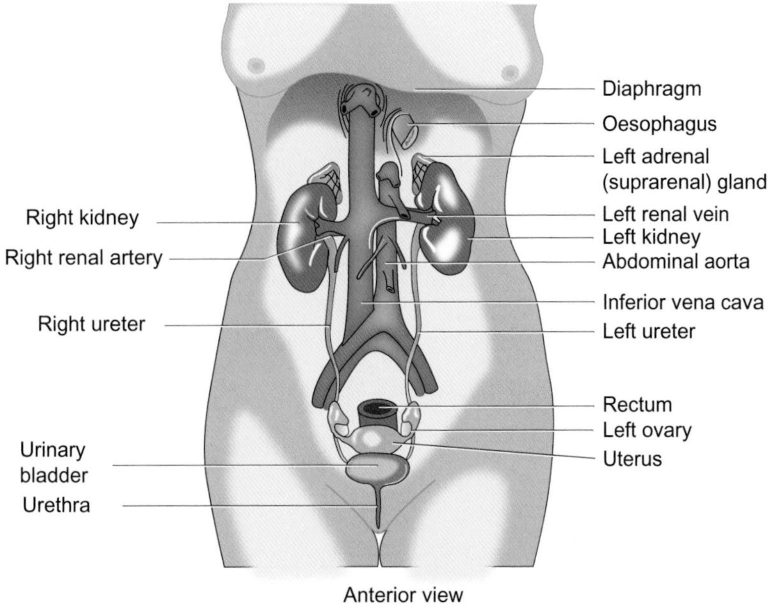

Figure 15.1 The renal system. Reproduced from Nair, M. & Peate, I. (2009) *Fundamentals of Applied Pathophysiology*, with kind permission from Wiley Blackwell.

Introduction

This chapter will address the nursing management of nephrological and urological conditions. Urology is the surgical and medical treatment of conditions of the female and male urinary systems, including the male reproductive system, while nephrology is concerned with medical diseases of the kidney. The nursing management of patients undergoing urological surgery is challenging as such procedures can have a negative impact on patients' body image and sexuality, which can adversely affect their psychosocial well-being.

Anatomy and physiology

The urinary system has a fundamental role in the filtration and disposal of waste products produced naturally within the body (Figure 15.1).

The kidney

Macroscopic structure

The kidneys are bean-shaped organs, approximately 11 cm long, 6 cm wide and 3 cm thick, that lie in the retroperitoneal space between the 12th thoracic and third lumbar vertebrae. The left kidney sits slightly behind the spleen, whereas the right kidney sits behind the liver and is slightly lower than the left. The hilus, a fissure in the central portion of the kidney, is where the blood vessels and ureters enter and leave. The arterial blood supply enters via the renal artery. Each kidney is enclosed in a tough fibrous capsule and is supported and protected by fat tissue.

The interior of each kidney has an outer portion called the cortex and inner portion termed the medulla. Within the renal medulla, there are approximately 5–18 cone-shaped structures known as renal pyramids. The papillae are formed by the free ends of the pyramids, which open into the renal

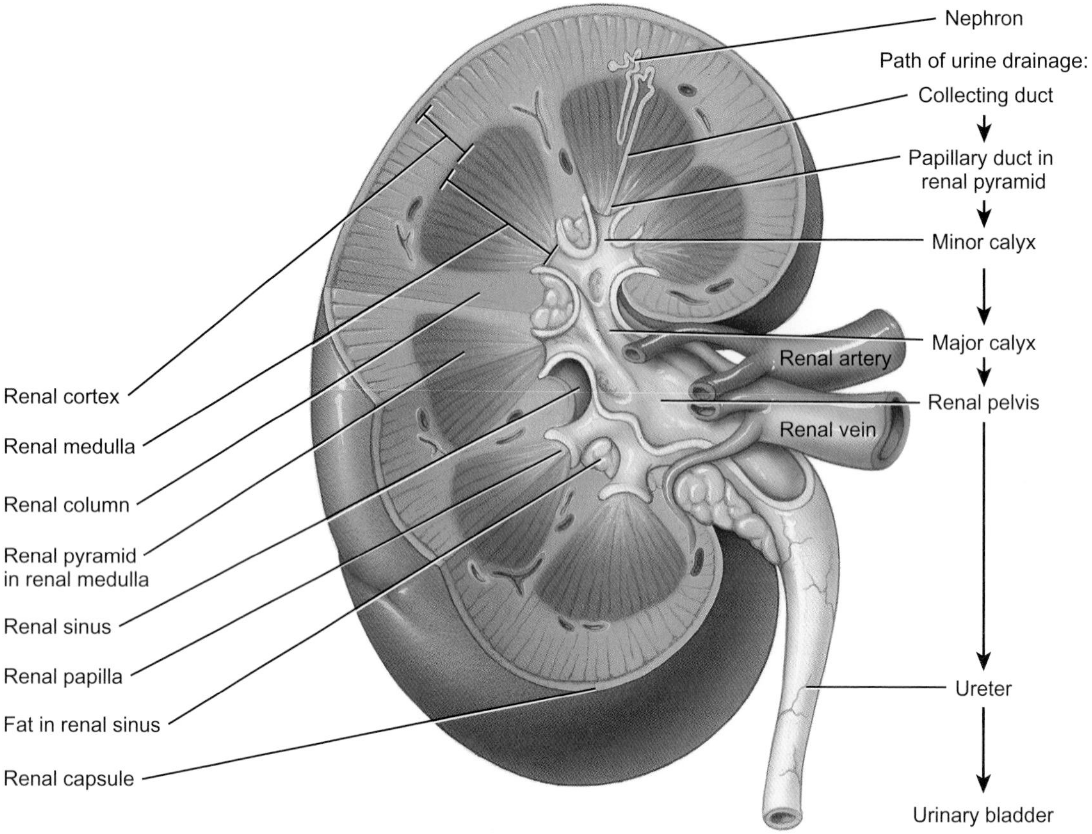

Figure 15.2 The external layers of the kidney. Reproduced from Nair, M. & Peate, I. (2009) *Fundamentals of Applied Pathophysiology*, with kind permission from Wiley Blackwell.

pelvis. The renal pelvis is made up of calyces, receives the urine that has been formed and acts as a reservoir before urine is passed to the bladder via the ureters (Figure 15.2).

Microscopic structure

The functional unit of the kidney is the nephron (Figure 15.3), which consists of:

- the renal corpuscle – which is where blood plasma is filtered and comprises:
  - the glomerulus (the capillary network);
  - the Bowman's or glomerular capsule (a double-walled epithelial cup);
- the renal tubule:
  - the proximal convoluted tubule;
  - the loop of Henle;
  - the distal convoluted tubule.

Each kidney contains approximately 1.2 million nephrons. The glomerulus is a unique, high-pressure capillary filtration system that is located between the afferent and efferent arterioles and lies within Bowman's capsule. As blood flows through the body, it picks up waste products such as urea and creatinine and excesses of substances such as potassium and phosphate, carrying them to the glomerulus via the renal arteries. The glomerulus retains larger substances that the body needs, for example blood cells and protein molecules, and allows smaller molecules to pass through its membrane, so eliminating waste products.

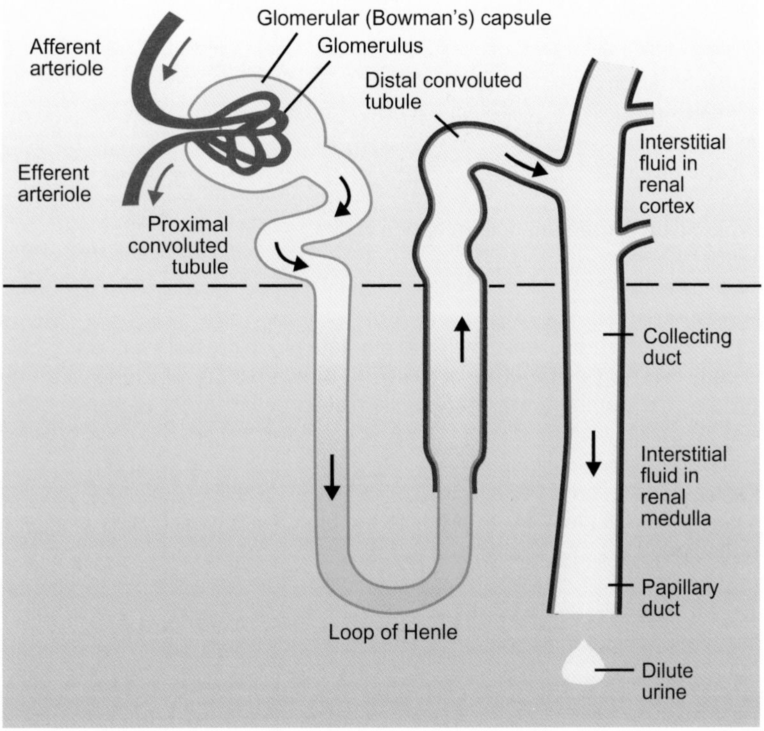

Figure 15.3 The nephron. Reproduced from Nair, M. & Peate, I. (2009) *Fundamentals of Applied Pathophysiology*, with kind permission from Wiley Blackwell.

Filtration produces a plasma-like fluid called filtrate, which leaves the glomerulus and enters the tubules and collecting ducts, where useful substances are reabsorbed. The low-pressure reabsorptive system of the peritubular capillary network, which surrounds the tubular parts of the nephron, arises from the efferent arteriole. The clean filtered blood flows back to the body via the renal veins.

Functions of the kidney

The kidneys carry out a number of functions (Box 15.1).

Micturition

The kidneys process approximately 180 L of filtrate daily. Of this, only 1–2 L is actually voided from the body as urine following tubular reabsorption. Urine is conveyed from the pelvis of each kidney to the bladder via the ureters. The bladder is a muscular sac that acts as a reservoir for urine before it is expelled from the body via the urethra. Bladder capacity varies from 500 to 750 mL. The male urethra is a shared pathway for both urine and semen, and is surrounded by the prostate gland where the urethra joins the bladder. The prostate gland is susceptible to hyperplasia, which, because of its proximity to the urethra, can lead to urinary problems.

Micturition – the act of passing urine – is a complex physiological process that is controlled by a number of neurological mechanisms. The nerve supply to the bladder is both sensory and motor. When the bladder contains approximately 300–400 mL of urine, nerve fibres situated in the bladder wall, which are sensitive to stretch, are stimulated. In healthy humans, the process of urination is under voluntary control, whereas in infants, some elderly individuals and those with neurological injury, urination may occur as an involuntary reflex.

Box 15.1 Functions of the kidney

- It produces urine through:
  - Glomerular filtration
  - Tubular reabsorption
  - Tubular secretion
- It removes waste products
- It regulates:
  - Blood volume by conserving or eliminating water
  - Electrolyte balance
  - Acid–base balance
  - Blood pressure
- It produces the hormone renin, which helps to regulate blood pressure and water balance (Box 15.2)
- It produces and secretes calcitriol (the active form of vitamin D), which helps to maintain healthy bones by increasing the amount of dietary calcium absorbed from the digestive tract and deposited in the bones
- It produces erythropoietin:
  - This is secreted in response to hypoxia
  - It stimulates the bone marrow to produce red blood cells, which carry oxygen in the blood to cells in the body

Box 15.2 The renin–angiotensin–aldosterone system

- Renin is secreted directly into the circulatory system when the blood volume and blood pressure decrease
- Renin converts angiotensinogen (produced by the liver) to angiotensin I
- Angiotensin I is converted to angiotensin II by angiotensin-converting enzyme
- Angiotensin II:
  - Causes vasoconstriction of the arterioles, which helps to increase blood pressure
  - Stimulates secretion of the hormone aldosterone from the adrenal cortex, increasing reabsorption of water and sodium by the tubules, and thus increasing blood volume

The prostate

The prostate is a gland that lies underneath the bladder in men and surrounds the urethra. It is usually the size and shape of a walnut, although it increases in size as men get older. The prostate is part of the male reproductive system and secretes a fluid that is added to sperm during ejaculation. The prostate also secretes prostate-specific antigen (PSA), which is thought to help liquefy the semen after ejaculation.

The prostate is divided into zones. The **peripheral zone** can be felt by a finger inserted into the rectum (digital rectal examination [DRE]) and is the area where most prostate cancers originate. The **transitional zone** surrounds the proximal urethra and is the area that enlarges as men get older (in benign prostatic hyperplasia [BPH]), which can lead to urinary problems. The **central zone** surrounds the seminal vesicles and ejaculatory ducts.

Urinary tract stones

Urinary stones (urinary calculi) are a major cause of morbidity and have an impact on the well-being of patients due to associated renal colic (pain), obstruction of the urinary tract, urinary tract infections

Box 15.3 Classification of urinary stones (European Association of Urology 2012)

Urinary stones are classified in terms of:

- Stone size
- Stone location
- The X-ray characteristics of the stone
- The aetiology of stone formation
- The stone's composition (as there can be different chemical compositions)
- The risk group for recurrent stone formation

(UTIs) and damage to the renal parenchymal. Urinary stones are not just confined to the kidney (renal calculi), but can be found anywhere within the urinary system. The classification of urinary stones is outlined in Box 15.3.

Urinary stones are more common in males than females. A global difference can also be seen, with higher rates of stone formation in the Western world, possibly due to a higher intake of refined carbohydrates, salt and animal protein, with a low intake of fluid and crude fibre. Factors that contribute to stone formation include:

- idiopathic;
- diet;
- metabolic anomalies;
- heredity;
- urinary stasis;
- chronic infection.

The signs and symptoms of stones can include:

- pain (the presentation of which can be linked to the site of the calculi):
  - pelviureteric junction: mild to severe deep flank pain without radiation to the groin, which occurs secondary to distension of the renal capsule;
  - ureter: abrupt, severe, colicky pain in the flank radiating to the testicles or vulvar area; intense nausea and vomiting may also be present;
  - bladder stones are usually asymptomatic;
  - patients possibly writhing in pain, pacing about and being unable to lie still;
- pallor and diaphoresis;
- nausea and vomiting;
- lower urinary tract symptoms; for example, dysuria, suprapubic discomfort, urgency and strangury are associated with bladder and vesicoureteric stones;
- fever, which if present may indicate infection;
- haematuria, usually microscopic.

Management

Patients presenting with suspected urinary stones may undergo the following investigations (European Association of Urology 2012):

- Imaging studies:
  - An X-ray of the kidney, ureters and bladder (KUB) – 60% of stones are radio-opaque
  - Non-contrast computed tomography (CT)

- Ultrasound
- An intravenous pyelogram/urogram

- Urinalysis – blood, protein, nitrites and pH level
- Serum urea, creatinine, uric acid, ionised calcium, sodium and potassium values
- A full blood count
- C-reactive protein level
- An evaluation of stone metabolic parameters for patients at high risk of recurrence.

Initial management options for newly diagnosed patients with ureteral stones smaller than 10 mm in diameter whose symptoms are controlled are observation with periodic evaluation ('watchful waiting'). The management of patients with urinary stones is outlined in Boxes 15.4 and 15.5.

Box 15.4 Management of patients with urinary stones

- Pain:
  - Assess the severity, location and radiation
  - Administer:
    - a non-steroidal anti-inflammatory drug, e.g. diclofenac sodium
    - an opiate
    - an anti-emetic, if needed
- Medication:
  - Medical expulsion therapy: alpha-blockers and calcium antagonists relax the smooth muscles of the ureters, increasing the chance of passing stone spontaneously
- Monitor:
  - Signs of infection (pyrexia)
  - Renal function:
    - urinalysis, haematuria and the presence of leucocytes
    - urine for culture and sensitivity
    - 24-hour urine collection for calculi
    - decreased output could indicate urinary obstruction or dehydration
    - serum urea and creatinine levels
  - The position of the stone
  - Hydronephrosis (distension and dilatation of the renal pelvis and calyces due to obstruction to urine flow from the kidney)
- Ensure a fluid intake of 2–2.5 L – the patient may require intravenous fluids
- Dietary advice (dependent on stone analysis):
  - Ensure a balanced diet, rich in vegetables and fibre
  - Avoid excessive consumption of vitamin supplements
  - Have a normal calcium content (1000–1200 mg/day) unless otherwise directed
  - Limit sodium chloride content (to 4–5 g/day)
  - Limit animal protein content (to 0.8–1.0 g/kg per day)
  - Calcium supplements are not recommended
- Indications for stone removal:
  - Persistent obstruction to urinary flow
  - Failure of stone progression
  - Increasing or unremitting pain
  - Infection
- The choice of technique to remove the stone depends on:
  - Stone size
  - The nature and location of the stone

- First-line treatment (stones >10 mm, persisting pain and/or obstruction):
  - Shock-wave lithotripsy, leading to stone fragmentation – suitable for stones in the renal pelvis and upper ureter
  - Ureteroscopy
  - Percutaneous antegrade ureteroscopy (only in selected cases; used for large stones in the upper ureters)
  - Percutaneous nephrolithotomy, for stones in the renal calyx
- Routine stenting as part of shock-wave lithotripsy treatment is not recommended (European Association of Urology 2012)
- Stenting in uncomplicated ureteroscopy is common; stents are removed 1–2 weeks after the procedure
- Surgical management (where other options have failed or are unlikely to succeed):
  - Laparoscopic or open stone surgery
  - Pyelolithotomy – removal of stones from the renal pelvis
  - Nephrectomy – the kidney is virtually destroyed, with <10% of renal function remaining
- Discharge advice:
  - Stress the importance of high fluid intake
  - Emphasise that the patient should follow the dietitian's advice
  - The patient should monitor for signs of UTI and report them to the GP

Box 15.5 Specific nursing management for urinary stone removal procedures

Shock-wave lithotripsy

- No aspirin for 7 days before surgery
- Stop warfarin and put the patient on heparin instead; this should be stopped 6 hours prior to the procedure
- Analgesia before, during (as it limits pain-induced movements) and after surgery
- After the procedure, monitor the urine for haematuria
- Ensure a high fluid intake
- Give the patient 2–3 days' rest between treatments, with a maximum of three treatments
- Take a follow-up X-ray at 4–6 weeks

Ureteroscopy

- Prepare the patient for a general anaesthetic
- Give short-term prophylactic antibiotics (European Association of Urology 2012)
- After the procedure:
  - Monitor:
    - — urinary output and degree of haematuria
    - — infection (pyrexia)
    - — signs of perforation of the ureters (severe pain and tenderness)
    - — paralytic ileus
  - Administer prescribed analgesia
  - Ensure a high fluid intake
  - Strain the urine for stone fragments
  - Take a KUB X-ray

(Continued)

Percutaneous nephrolithotomy

- The procedure can take place without the need for a nephrostomy tube or ureteral stent
- A general anaesthetic will be administered
- After the procedure:
  - In cases where a nephrostomy tube has been left in the tract (to facilitate drainage of blood and urine, and reduce the risk of an intrarenal haematoma):
    - monitor drainage
    - removal is usually on day 2 postoperatively
  - Ureteral stenting using a JJ stent is common practice
  - Monitor:
    - breathing for complications, e.g. pneumothorax
    - the urinary catheter, urinary output and degree of haematuria
    - infection (pyrexia)
  - Administer intravenous therapy
  - Resume the diet and oral fluids (with a high fluid intake), usually on day 1 postoperatively
  - Discharge advice for the patient:
    - allow 1–2 weeks of convalescence
    - haematuria may be present but is not a cause for concern
    - contact the GP if haematuria persists or becomes heavier
    - keep the nephrostomy tube site covered with a clean dressing until it has sealed over
    - avoid driving until able to do emergency braking
    - attend an outpatient appointment after 6 weeks

Conditions of the prostate

There are a number of conditions associated with the prostate, including:

- prostatitis (inflammation of the prostate gland), which is generally managed by the GP;
- enlargement of the prostate gland:
  - BPH;
  - cancer of the prostate gland.

Benign prostatic hyperplasia

BPH describes an increase in the number of cells in the prostate and is a normal consequence of ageing. When the prostate enlarges, it may press on the urethra, causing it to narrow. Symptoms of an enlarged prostate include:

- difficulty starting to pass urine (hesitancy);
- a weak urinary stream;
- straining or taking a long time to pass urine;
- a feeling that the bladder is not completely empty after voiding;
- dribbling urine after voiding (terminal dribbling);
- a need to pass urine more frequently;
- waking in the night to pass urine more frequently than usual (nocturia);
- the feeling of needing to pass urine quickly without much warning (urgency);
- acute urinary retention:
  - a sudden inability to pass urine;
  - related to a history of BPH or clot/haematuria;
  - may require hospitalisation, catheterisation and often surgery.

About 40% of men over the age of 50 and 75% of men in their 70s have urinary symptoms that may be caused by an enlarged prostate (Prostate Cancer Charity 2009). Investigations for BPH include:

- assessment of symptoms, using tools such as the International Prostate Symptom Score (see http://www.urospec.com/uro/Forms/ipss.pdf and http://www.cpcn.org/ipss.pdf);
- DRE:
  - assesses the size of the prostate;
  - assesses whether any malignant features are palpable;
- renal function:
  - urinalysis;
  - serum urea and creatinine levels;
- PSA – reasons for a raised PSA include cancer, infection, inflammation or enlargement of the prostate;
- ultrasound of the bladder, prostate and kidneys;
- measurement of:
  - flow rate;
  - post-voiding residual volume.

Management

Mild or moderate BPH may involve educating men on the need for periodic monitoring and lifestyle changes, which include:

- an appropriate fluid input (1.5–2 L/day);
- avoidance of fizzy drinks, caffeine and alcohol, which may have a diuretic and irritant effect;
- a reduction in evening fluid intake (to decrease nocturia).

Medical management includes:

- alpha-adrenergic blocking agents (alpha-blockers) to relax the prostatic smooth muscle, which helps to improve urinary flow and bladder emptying;
- 5-alpha reductase inhibitors to reduce the level of dihydrotestosterone, which is responsible for prostatic growth; this reduces the size of the prostate, which may in turn relieve the symptoms;
- surgery if the symptoms are severe.

Different types of surgery are available, all of which aim to relieve the physical obstruction to the urethra. In the vast majority of cases, surgery is performed endoscopically via the penis. The most common endoscopic procedures are transurethral resection of the prostate (TURP) and holmium laser enucleation of the prostate (HoLEP). A thin tube containing a light and a camera is introduced into the urethra, and the prostatic tissue is removed using a heated loop (TURP) or a laser (HoLEP). Both procedures are usually carried out under epidural or spinal anaesthesia, but they may be performed under general anaesthetic. The nursing management of patients undergoing TURP is outlined in Table 15.1.

Prostate cancer

Prostate cancer is the most common cancer in men in the UK and Ireland, with 37,000 men diagnosed each year. Its incidence increases with age, and progression is usually slow. For many men, it may not cause any problems or symptoms during their lifetime; for some, however, it is more aggressive and requires treatment to prevent, delay or contain its spread outside the prostate gland. Around 10,000 men in the UK will die each year from prostate cancer (Prostate Cancer Charity 2011). Risk factors include age, ethnic origin and heredity. Prostate cancer may be:

- localised (confined to the prostate);
- locally advanced (spreading to the area just outside the prostate gland, but not to other parts of the body);
- advanced (with spread from the prostate gland to other parts of the body).

Table 15.1 Nursing management of patients undergoing TURP

Preoperative care	Postoperative care	Discharge advice

Educate patients on:
• The procedure;
• Its complications, e.g. risk of retrograde ejaculation, bleeding and UTI
Stop anticoagulants as per hospital protocol
Commence venous thromboprophylaxis
Nil by mouth
	Monitor for:
	• Pain, and administer analgesia
	• Transurethral resection syndrome:
	  ◦ Rare
	  ◦ Occurs when irrigating fluid is absorbed during surgery
	  ◦ Causes low serum sodium levels and results in breathing problems, sickness, confusion and seizures
	• Signs of excess bleeding (degree of haematuria)
	• Signs of urinary retention due to clot formation:
	  ◦ Decreased urinary output
	  ◦ Abdominal distension
	  ◦ Palpable bladder
	  ◦ Increase in pain
	Administer intravenous fluids until the patient is drinking freely
	Catheter care is part of routine personal hygiene
	Continuous bladder irrigation until the urine is clear of clots (Figure 15.4)
	Bladder washout when urinary retention occurs
	Remove catheter and observe urinary output
	Avoid constipation and straining during defecation
		Takes up to 8 weeks to see a symptomatic improvement
		Teach the patient pelvic floor exercises
		Urine may be bloodstained, particularly for 2 weeks postoperatively
		Drink 1.5–2 L of fluid daily (with minimal caffeine-based drinks)
		Avoid heavy lifting for 2 weeks
		Resume gentle exercise and increase this as able
		Sex can be resumed whenever the patient feels comfortable
		Patient may experience erectile dysfunction postoperatively; this should be reported to the surgical team at the follow-up visit
		Many men will experience retrograde ejaculation following surgery

Prostate cancer is diagnosed and staged using a variety of methods and tools, including:

- a clinical examination, including a DRE;
- measurement of PSA;
- a biopsy of the prostate;
- transrectal ultrasonography, CT, magnetic resonance imaging (MRI) and bone scans.

Management

There are a variety of treatments for prostate cancer (Table 15.2), which aim to completely eradicate or control the cancer. The choice of treatment depends on:

- the stage and grade of the cancer;
- the side effects of treatment;
- any comorbidities;
- the patient's preference.

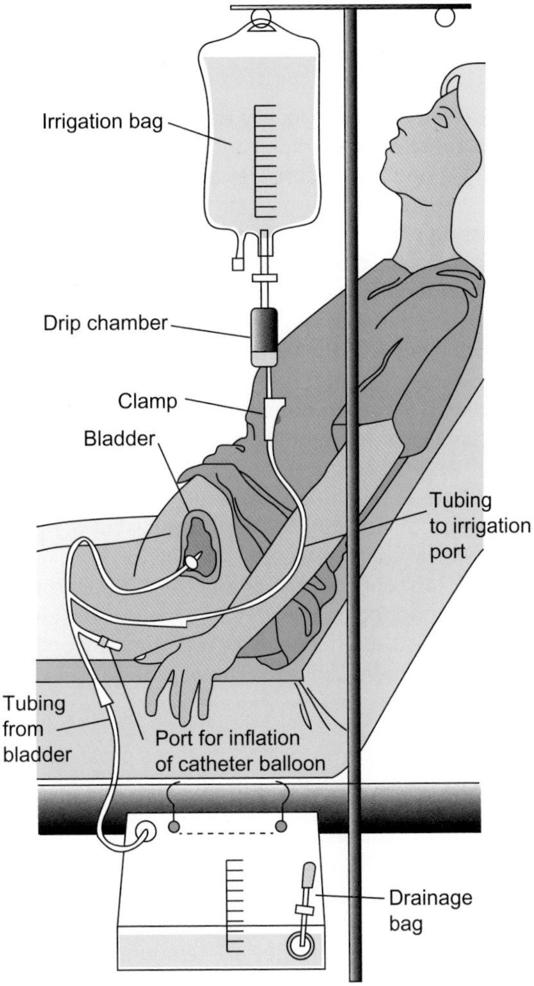

Figure 15.4 Continuous bladder irrigation. Reproduced from Taylor *et al.* (2005) *Fundamentals of Nursing: The Art and Science of Nursing Care*, with kind permission of Lippincott Williams &Wilkins

Table 15.2 Treatment for prostate cancer

Treatment	Information
Active surveillance	Localised, low-risk cancer Slow growing and less aggressive cancers are closely monitored using: • PSA levels • DRE • Repeat biopsies Aim to avoid or delay unnecessary treatment and its side effects

(*Continued*)

Table 15.2 (*Continued*)

Treatment	Information
Radical prostatectomy	Localised and some locally advanced prostate cancer The entire prostate gland and seminal vesicles are removed by: ● An open procedure (retropubic or perineal) ● Laparoscopic surgery (by hand or robot-assisted) **Nursing care** General anaesthetic The urethra is re-sutured to the bladder around an indwelling urinary catheter; this acts as a conduit from the bladder and as a 'stent' around which healing of the urethra and bladder neck occurs The urinary catheter is left in place (for a few days up to 2 weeks) and is removed during an outpatient appointment Sutures/clips are removed 7–14 days postoperatively Discharge advice: ● Care of the urinary catheter ● Risk of incontinence after removal of the catheter ● Pelvic floor exercises ● Treatment options for erectile dysfunction ● Monitoring of PSA levels – increased levels may indicate recurrence of disease and the need for radiotherapy or hormone therapy ● The patient can return to work 6–8 weeks after an open procedure and 2–6 weeks after keyhole surgery
External beam radiotherapy	Localised and some locally advanced prostate cancer May be combined with hormone therapy or brachytherapy
Brachytherapy	May be high dose-rate or low dose-rate Involves implantation of radioactive seeds into the prostate via needles through the perineum With low dose-rate treatment, the seeds are permanent, whereas in high dose-rate treatment, they are temporary
Other focal therapies	High-intensity focused ultrasound may be used – the National Institute for Health and Clinical Excellence (2008a) recommends that this should be as part of a clinical trial
Watchful waiting	Offered to men who are not suitable for radical curative treatment Patients are monitored and later treated with hormone deprivation therapy if and when their cancer becomes symptomatic
Hormone deprivation therapy	Most prostate cancers are androgen-dependent – hormone deprivation therapy using antiandrogens, luteinising hormone-releasing hormone agonists or a combination of the two can delay the cancer's growth and spread for some time Will not cure prostate cancer; it is used in metastatic disease, or in high-risk localised disease if curative options are not advised
Treatments after hormone deprivation therapy	Prostate cancer will become resistant to hormone deprivation therapy The cancer will become more active Other systemic therapies such as chemotherapy may be considered at this point

For further information, see http://www.prostate-cancer.org.uk and http://www.macmillan.org.uk.

Nursing management depends on:

- the patient's personal needs;
- the stage, grade and extent of the disease;
- the treatment choices that the patient makes.

A diagnosis of cancer can be devastating. Many men and their families will need specialist support, whether the diagnosis represents an aggressive life-limiting disease or a need to adapt to life-long monitoring and the resultant stress that this may bring. In localised disease, men may make treatment choices based on side effects and personal preferences.

Most treatments affect continence and potency, and adaptation to such radical changes in body image may need expert practical and emotional support (National Institute for Health and Clinical Excellence [NICE] 2008a). Erectile dysfunction can be managed with phosphodiesterase inhibitors, intracavernosal injections of alprostadil or a vacuum constriction device. Continence issues can be resolved with pelvic floor exercises, medication or surgery depending on the cause.

The most common site for the spread of prostate cancer is bone. Bone metastases can cause pain, fractures and, if the spine is involved, spinal cord compression. This is a medical emergency, and men with bone metastases should be counselled about the signs, symptoms and action to take. Prescribing hormone deprivation therapy can impact greatly on a man's sexuality, mood and body image. It is essential that men are counselled about the side effects of hormone deprivation therapy, along with lifestyle advice to prevent longer term complications, including metabolic syndrome and osteoporosis.

Kidney cancer

Kidney cancer accounts for 2.5% of all cancers in adults and is rarely seen under the age of 40; it is most likely to occur after the age of 55. It strikes almost twice as many men as women (European Network of Cancer Registries 2001).

Renal cell carcinoma accounts for 90% of all kidney cancers in adults and is usually unilateral (one-sided). Metastatic spread may be local to the renal veins, or to lymph nodes, bone, liver and lung. The prognosis depends on the differentiation of the tumour and the presence or absence of metastatic spread. The cause of kidney cancer is unknown, but risk factors include:

- cigarette smoking;
- obesity;
- occupational exposure to asbestos, cadmium, lead, phosphate and petroleum;
- a family history of renal cell carcinoma, especially in siblings;
- renal disease and hypertension.

Management

Kidney cancer is difficult to diagnose in the early stages as there is no screening test; indeed, it may not present until it has spread to adjacent organs. Signs and symptoms usually appear after the tumour has grown or the cancer has spread and include:

- haematuria;
- an abdominal mass;
- persistent fever of unknown origin;
- unexplained pain in the flank or lower back;
- persistent fatigue;
- oedema of the legs and ankles;
- unexplained weight loss.

Investigations include:

- abdominal ultrasound;
- a CT scan;
- an MRI scan;

- a renal biopsy;
- urinalysis (for haematuria);
- a full blood count (for anaemia);
- liver function tests.

Depending on the stage of the tumour, the treatment of choice is nephron-sparing surgery, in which the tumour is resected from the kidney. An open partial nephrectomy is the preferred surgical option. This may not be feasible for all patients due to local advanced tumour growth – it may be technically impossible or there may have been a significant deterioration in the patient's health. In these circumstances, the gold standard of treatment remains a radical nephrectomy, which involves removal of the kidney, the ureters and the portion of the bladder connected to the ureters. The preferred route for a radical nephrectomy is the laparoscopic route, although an open nephrectomy may also be used.

Kidney cancer is resistant to most chemotherapy and radiotherapy. Immunotherapy is used in its management, with interferon-alpha being the gold standard of treatment, although interleukin-2 can also be used.

Nephrectomy

A nephrectomy is the surgical removal of the kidney, performed via an open or laparoscopic route. An open approach has inherent operative and postoperative complications; in contrast, the advantages associated with the laparoscopy include less pain, a shorter hospital stay and a quicker return to work. The nursing management is outlined in Box 15.6. Indications for a nephrectomy include:

- benign tumours (rare);
- kidney cancer;
- uncontrollable renal haemorrhage, for example severe blunt renal trauma or complications of renal biopsy;
- multiple cysts;
- renal calculi;
- malignant hypertension (bilateral and rare);
- removal of a health kidney for transplantation (living donor).

Box 15.6 Nursing management of patients before and after nephrectomy

Preoperative care

- Stop cigarette smoking
- Physiotherapy assessment
- Elimination – a baseline assessment of renal function, urinalysis and the pattern and characteristics of the urinary output
- Educate the patient on the following postoperative care:
  - Breathing and coughing exercises
  - Use of an incentive spirometer
  - Splinting of the wound
  - Pain control
  - Urinary catheter
  - Wound incision line – for both open and laparoscopic procedures
  - The possible presence of a wound drain with an open procedure
  - Leg exercises and use of antithrombosis stockings and anticoagulants
  - Fasting, intravenous therapy, oral fluids and then a light diet

Postoperative care

- Monitor:
  - Respiration
  - Colour

  - Level of consciousness and appearance
  - Pulse oximetry for oxygen saturation levels
  - Signs of respiratory complications, e.g. spontaneous pneumothorax or atelectasis (changes in respiration and oxygen saturation levels)
- Administer prescribed oxygen
- Place in a semi-Fowler's position
- Ensure regular use of an incentive spirometer
- Use pillows to splint the wound when conducting breathing and coughing exercises
- Monitor for signs of hypovolaemic shock due to haemorrhage:
  - Vital signs
  - Colour
  - Skin
  - Wound dressing (check that no blood has seeped round to the back)
  - Wound drainage
- Monitor pain:
  - Assess the level of pain (open versus laparoscopic): following a open nephrectomy, the patient will have a large surgical wound (with or without a wound drain), and the pain will be more intense than in patients whose procedure was carried out via a laparoscopic approach
  - With laparoscopic procedures, shoulder pain and a bloated abdomen may occur and can be alleviated by pain medication and mobilisation
- Administer analgesia (PCA) and assess its effectiveness
- Monitor:
  - Urinary output, and record this on the fluid balance chart
  - The colour and odour of the urine
  - The administration of prophylactic intravenous antibiotics prior to removal of the urinary catheter
  - The postoperative voiding pattern
  - Renal function, e.g. serum creatinine level
  - Bowel sounds
  - Possible paralytic ileus
- Commence oral fluids followed by a light diet
- Prevent constipation:
  - Early mobilisation
  - A high-fibre diet and oral fluids
- The wound:
  - Monitor for signs of infection
  - Remove the wound drain (if present), usually at 48–72 hours
  - Remove sutures/staples (if present) at 7–10 days – the patient can return to the outpatients department or attend a community healthcare provider for this
- Discharge advice:
  - Monitor urinary output and signs of UTI
  - Ensure a fluid intake of 2 L/day
  - Care of the incision site(s)
  - Follow-up care in relation to renal function
  - Avoid strenuous exercises in the initial recovery phase
  - Avoid lifting weights for 6–8 weeks
  - As the patient has only one functioning kidney, they are advised to avoid contact sports in the future
  - Details of medication and its impact on kidney function
  - For renal cancer:
    - — cancer support groups
    - — follow-up treatment and care

Bladder cancer

Bladder cancer is the seventh most common cancer in the UK and is more common in males than females. It can occur between 50 and 70 years of age. There are two forms of bladder cancer:

- Non-muscle invasive cancer, formerly known as superficial cancer, affects the inner lining of the bladder wall, with the cancer confined to the bladder mucosa and submucosa. This form of cancer tends to recur.
- Muscle-invasive cancer spreads into the muscle wall.

Bladder cancer spreads by direct invasion through the bladder wall into adjacent organs such as the prostate, vagina and rectum. The lymphatic system is another route for tumours to spread, initially to the local pelvic nodes, and then to the para-aortic nodes and circulatory system, giving rise to metastases in the liver, lungs and bones. The cancer can also involve the ureteric orifices, leading to unilateral or bilateral hydronephrosis and renal failure. Risk factors include:

- cigarette smoking;
- occupational exposure to chemicals such as dyes, paints, textiles and rubber;
- radiotherapy, which can cause secondary bladder cancer, as seen with gynaecological cancers;
- chronic UTIs and urinary tract calculi, which can result in chronic cystitis, this in turn predisposing to squamous cell carcinoma;
- drugs such as cyclophosphamide.

The signs and symptoms depend on the site of the tumour and the presence of metastatic spread and include the following:

- Haematuria:
  - This is the first sign in 80% of cases, and may be the only sign.
  - It can be painless and intermittent, resulting in many patients ignoring this symptom.
- Irritative urinary symptoms – frequency, urgency and dysuria.
- Pain in the flank or lower back.
- Cystitis.
- Malaise and weight loss.
- Anaemia.
- Pyrexia of unknown origin.
- A late presentation, such as with flank or lower back pain, or lower limb oedema.
  - A suprapubic mass, which usually indicates that this condition is in an advanced stage.

Management

Investigations include:

- urine samples for cytology to detect the presence of abnormal cells; however, its use in the diagnosis of bladder cancer is controversial due to its lack of sensitivity;
- a midstream urine sample for culture for sensitivity;
- a full blood count (for anaemia);
- a full biochemistry screen (for renal function);
- liver function tests;
- a KUB X-ray and intravenous urogram;
- cystoscopy and examination under anaesthetic;
- biopsy and histological examination;
- a CT scan;
- an MRI scan;
- pelvic ultrasound;
- a bone scan;
- an internal examination of the rectum in men, and the rectum and vagina in women; both are close to the bladder and are palpated for any thickening or lumps.

Treatment is determined by the type, stage and grade of the cancer; 83% of cases require some form of surgical intervention. Treatment incorporates the following:

- Non-muscle invasive cancer:
  - Transurethral resection of the bladder tumour.
  - Adjunct intravesical chemotherapy.
  - Adjunct intravesical immunotherapy with BCG vaccine (as both induction and maintenance).
  - The choice of further therapy depends on the patient's risk of tumour recurrence and/or progression.
  - Regular cystoscopies may be necessary, their frequency determined by the risk of recurrence or progression.
- Muscle invasive cancer:
  - Cystoscopy, transurethral resection, chemotherapy and radiotherapy.
  - Chemotherapy.
  - Partial or total (radical) cystectomy as the preferred curative treatment
  - If the tumour is inoperable, patients will commence palliative therapy without surgical intervention. Radiotherapy can be given instead of surgery to avoid removal of bladder.

Cystectomy and urinary diversion

Radical cystectomy involves:

- in males, removal of the bladder plus prostate, upper part of the urethra, seminal vesicles and lymphatics;
- in females, removal of the bladder plus part of the urethra, the uterus, fallopian tubes, ovaries, anterior vagina and pelvis, with lymphadenectomy.

An open, laparoscopic or robot-assisted laparoscopic approach can be used. The most common approach continues to be an open procedure, although laparoscopic and robot-assisted laparoscopic approaches are becoming more evident. All approaches require the formation of a urinary diversion.

There are several types of urinary diversion associated with cystectomy. **Urostomy** (ileal conduit) is the most common diversion. In this, the ureters are implanted into a 10–15 cm segment of the ileum that has been resected from the small intestine with its mesentery (and thus its blood supply) intact. The distal end of the loop is brought to the abdominal surface as a stoma and has the same appearance as an ileostomy, with a small spout.

Continent urinary diversion is a more difficult procedure. A pouch is made in the abdomen using a piece of bowel that has been resected. The ureters are attached to this piece of bowel and the urine empties into the pouch. The end of the bowel is brought out onto the surface of the abdomen to create a stoma. Patients are required to self-catheterise on a regular basis (4–5 times a day) and do not have to wear a urostomy bag. Patients should not let the pouch get full as this can cause urine to leak. Creating this urinary diversion is not without its difficulties, and some patients may need to return for corrective surgery;

Bladder reconstruction is only suitable for those patients whose cancer has a low risk of recurrence, if the urethra has not been affected by the cancer and if there is no evidence of bowel disease.

Management

Patients diagnosed with bladder cancer may be discharged home with a view to readmission at a later date for a cystectomy and creation of a urinary diversion. During this period, patients will be advised on how to prepare themselves both physical and psychologically for this invasive surgery. This preparation involves:

- a preadmission review by the dietitian;
- identification of what services need to be put in place when patients are ready for discharge;

- the need for preoperative physiotherapy;
- smoking cessation;
- psychological preparation:
  - level of understanding, the fact that this is a life-altering procedure, body image, sexual concerns and involvement of the family;
  - the ability to self-care.

Patients undergoing a urinary diversion with the formation of an ileal conduit need to accept and care for a stoma (urostomy) that opens onto the abdominal wall. Following this surgery, many patients fear rejection and abandonment by their partners or, if they are single, believe they will never have a physical relationship again (Gemmill *et al.* 2010).

Preoperative and postoperative nursing management is outlined in Boxes 15.7 and 15.8.

Urinary tract infections

Urinary tract infection refers to infections that occurs at any segment along the urinary tract and is one of the most common infections encountered in the community, with over 84% of such infections linked to women (Hooton 2012). Lower urinary tract infections involve the bladder (cystitis) and the urethra (urethritis), while upper urinary tract infections involve the kidney (pyelonephritis). Pyelonephritis is a bacterial infection of the renal pelvis, tubules and interstitial tissue of one or both kidneys. UTIs can be classified as uncomplicated or complicated cystitis or pyelonephritis.

Uncomplicated UTIs

Uncomplicated UTIs are generally treated in a primary care setting and are seen in non-pregnant, premenopausal women with no history of an abnormal urinary tract. Risk factors (Hooton 2012) include:

- sexual intercourse (which causes microorganisms to move along the urethra into the bladder);
- the use of spermicides;
- a previous UTI;
- a new sexual partner;
- a family history of UTI.

Signs and symptoms of uncomplicated cystitis include:

- dysuria;
- frequency;
- urgency;
- strangury (painful and frequent voiding of small volumes of urine);
- haematuria;
- suprapubic pain.

Signs and symptoms of acute uncomplicated pyelonephritis include:

- fever >38°C;
- chills;
- flank pain that is either constant or colicky in nature;
- costovertebral angle tenderness;
- nausea, vomiting or anorexia;
- sometimes symptoms of cystitis;
- in aged patients, non-specific symptoms such as lethargy, anorexia, low-grade fever, confusion and incontinence.

Box 15.7 Preoperative nursing management of patients undergoing cystectomy and urinary diversion

- Identify psychological concerns:
  - Cancer – death and prognosis
  - Altered body image – stoma, scars, external appliance and altered body habits
  - Sexuality
  - Attitudes of loved ones and society
- Educate patients on:
  - The surgical procedure
  - Preparations for surgery
  - The stoma – describe the physical appearance using diagrams, videos and written information
  - Stents inserted into the stoma to protect the anastomosis between the ureter and intestine
  - Ostomy and related equipment
  - Wearing of a bag
  - Daily activities – there is no need to alter the clothing, and the patient can continue to bathe or shower
- Visits by:
  - The stoma nurse
  - A person who has had a similar experience
  - Support groups
- Involve significant others
- When selecting the stoma site, avoid the following (as the patient may be unable to visualise or reach the site, or there may be leakage and bag difficulties):
  - The rib cage
  - The waist line
  - Bony prominences
  - Umbilicus
  - The hip bones
  - Scars or operation incision lines
  - Groin creases
  - Skin folds
  - Prostheses
  - Breasts
- Stoma site:
  - Usually on the abdominal wall below the waist, on the right-hand side
  - Planned with the patient so that the site does not interfere with standing, lying or sitting
  - Marked with inedible ink
- The skin is tested with adhesive for any allergies
- Bowel preparation – this is not always necessary and is determined by the surgeon's preference
- Preoperative advice from the physiotherapist and dietitian

Box 15.8 Postoperative nursing management of patients following cystectomy and urinary diversion

- Monitor:
  - Respiration
  - Colour
  - Level of consciousness and appearance
  - Pulse oximetry for oxygen saturation levels
  - Pain level
  - The stoma – check that the urostomy bag allows clear visualisation of the stoma; there should be a valve system to prevent reflux over the stoma
- Place the patient in the semi-Fowler's position
- Administer prescribed oxygen and patient-controlled analgesia, and assess its effectiveness
- Physiotherapy and early mobilisation
- Regular use of an incentive spirometer, with breathing and coughing exercises
- Monitor for signs of hypovolaemic shock due to haemorrhage
- Stoma:
  - Should be pink to red in colour and moist
  - Dark red or blue grey in colour could indicate ischaemic changes
  - Should be flush with the skin
  - Monitor:
    - colour and appearance – check 2-hourly for the first 24 hours, and then 4-hourly for 48–72 hours
    - signs of prolapse, retraction or separation of the peristomal skin from the stoma
    - degree of oedema present (this gradually decreases over 6–8 weeks)
    - whether the appliance fits with oedema present – as the oedema decreases, the stoma will need to be remeasured and the aperture in the stoma appliance reduced accordingly
  - Ureteric stents are removed at 10–14 days (they may fall out into the pouch)
  - Sutures are dissolvable
  - Persistent redness, broken skin or complaints of discomfort or an allergic reaction should be investigated and rapidly treated
  - Get patients to look at the stoma as soon as possible as this assists them in adjusting to their altered body image
  - The pouch should be changed as needed, usually 3 days postoperatively
  - Frequent empting prevents leakage of urine onto the incision
  - Urostomy appliances can be changed every 2–3 days
- Changing the appliance:
  - Remove gently to prevent trauma to the surrounding skin
  - Gently wash skin with soap and water, and dry the area
  - Ensure the new appliance has been applied correctly
- Monitor the urine:
  - Output, which should be recorded on the fluid balance chart
  - The presence of mucus; this originates from the segment of bowel used as the conduit and may continue indefinitely
  - Decreased output maybe be due to leakage (causing peritonitis), obstruction by mucus or oedema, dehydration or renal failure

- Educate the patient on ostomy self-care skills:
  - Emptying the appliance and attaching it to straight drainage
  - Care of the stoma and assessment of the normal appearance
  - Measuring the stoma and adjusting the size of the appliance
  - Skin care
  - Odour control:
    - — noxious odours can occur as a result of poor hygiene, alkaline urine, normal breakdown of urine (ammonia), concentration of urine because of insufficient fluid intake, and ingestion of certain types of foods such as eggs
    - — deodorant tablets can be placed in the pouch
    - — reused pouches should be washed thoroughly with soap and lukewarm water, and then soaked in dilute white vinegar or a commercial deodorant product for 20–30 minutes
  - Outline the complications
  - Give dietary guidelines
  - Explore potential problems
  - The stoma nurse will provide further education on stoma care
- Monitor bowel function:
  - Bowel sounds
  - Possible paralytic ileus
- Commence oral fluids followed by a light diet
- The wound:
  - Monitor for signs of infection
  - Remove the wound drain (if present), usually at 48–72 hours
  - Remove sutures/staples after 7–10 days
- Psychological care:
  - Aim to promote a healthy body image
  - Positive encouragement
  - Acceptance of the stoma
  - Contact with the stoma nurse
  - Support groups
  - Family support and involvement in care
- Discharge advice:
  - Preparation for the first month at home
  - Transfer of skills to the home situation
  - Community resources
  - Where to obtain supplies
  - Activity levels and exercise
  - Sexuality
  - Outpatient appointments
  - The stoma nurse's contact details
  - Support groups

Investigations in uncomplicated UTIs include:

- urinalysis using dipsticks that test for leucocyte esterase (an enzyme released by leucocytes) and nitrites;
- urine culture and sensitivity, which is undertaken in women with acute or recurrent pyelonephritis, recurrent cystitis or unresolved symptoms following a course of antimicrobial therapy;
- urological evaluations in women with severe pyelonephritis.

Management

Uncomplicated cystitis rarely progresses to pyelonephritis. A short course of an oral antimicrobial regimen, ranging from a single dose to a 5-day regimen, is recommended as first-line treatment.

Acute uncomplicated pyelonephritis can be treated with antimicrobial regimens including ciprofloxacin for 7 days or trimethoprim–sulfamethoxazole for 14 days. Women should be admitted if their pyelonephritis is severe, oral medication is not tolerated or there is haemodynamic instability (Hooton 2012).

Those women who have had three or more recurrent UTIs in the previous 12 months may require antimicrobial prophylaxis and education on strategies that may be useful in the prevention of recurrent uncomplicated UTIs (Box 15.9).

Complicated UTI

Complicated cystitis and pyelonephritis are UTIs associated with functional, metabolic or anatomical conditions that may increase the possibility of treatment failure or serious outcomes (Hooton 2012). Complicated pyelonephritis can lead to progressive infection and repeated inflammation causing fibrosis and scarring. As a result, renal tissue is permanently destroyed, the kidney becomes contracted and non-functioning, and renal failure may occur. The signs and symptoms are similar to those of acute pyelonephritis, although the condition may be asymptomatic unless an acute exacerbation occurs. Risk factors for complicated UTIs include:

- urinary tract obstruction;
- instrumentation;
- voiding dysfunction;
- metabolic abnormalities;
- pregnancy and immunosuppression.

Investigations involve:

- urine culture and sensitivity;
- CT of the abdomen and pelvis;
- an ultrasound scan.

Management

Episodes of complicated UTI often require hospitalisation, and the treatment strategies are determined by the severity of the illness. The nursing management of patients with complicated UTIs is outlined in Box 15.10. Once the patient has been admitted, parenteral antimicrobial regimens are commenced, with the dosage changed to oral when the patient's condition improves.

Acute kidney injury

Acute kidney injury (AKI), also known as acute renal failure, is a sudden and severe reduction in previously normal renal function that results in a failure to maintain fluid, electrolyte and acid–base

Box 15.9 Strategies to prevent recurrent uncomplicated UTI

- Encourage an oral fluid intake of 3 L/day as this dilutes the urine, increases the volume of urine, lessens irritation and burning sensations, and provides a continuous flow of urine to minimise stasis
- Encourage frequent voiding every 2–3 hours; the patient should completely empty the bladder and not delay urination
- Cranberry juice decreases the frequency of UTI, possibly due to inhibiting bacterial adherence to the mucosa
- Toilet hygiene, wiping from the front to the back, prevents the introduction of microorganisms from the bowel
- Advise the patient to avoid douching
- The patient should wear cotton underwear, avoid tight-fitting underwear and change the underwear daily; this helps to prevent an increase in temperature and accumulation of moisture
- Showers should be taken instead of baths
- Advise patients to avoid the use of perfumed bathing products such as bubble bath, soaps, shower gels, perfumes and perfumed sanitary towels as these can cause irritation and inflammation
- Topical oestrogen can be beneficial for postmenopausal women as it normalises the vaginal flora and reduces the risk of recurrent UTIs
- Provide information related to sexual activity:
  - Personal hygiene for a woman pre- and post sexual activity
  - Personal hygiene for a male partner before sexual activity
  - If spermicides are used, change to another method of contraception for prevention of infection as spermicides alter the vaginal flora, favouring colonisation with uropathogens
  - Void the bladder immediately after sexual activity
  - Increase fluid intake after sexual activity
  - Take prophylactic antibiotics after sexual activity
- Phenazopyridine (Pyridium) is an analgesic agent that can be prescribed for urinary symptoms (burning sensation)
- Educate patients:
  - Patients need to take the antimicrobial regimen as prescribed
  - They should recognise the symptoms of UTI and the need for early medical attention

homoeostasis; it commonly occurs over a number of days. AKI is treatable and often reversible unless there is underlying renal dysfunction. It is associated with a high mortality rate of more than 50%, with the risk depending on the patient's comorbidities (Yaqub & Molitoris 2009). The causes of AKI may be classified into three main groups:

- **Pre-renal causes** result in a loss of kidney perfusion:
  - reduced circulating blood volume, for example from haemorrhage;
  - reduced cardiac output, as with cardiac arrest;
  - extracellular depletion, for example a large gastrointestinal fluid loss;
  - increased peripheral vascular resistance, for instance renal artery thrombosis or embolism.
- **Intrinsic renal** causes are those in which renal function is impaired by damage to the microscopic structure of the kidney including the tubules, interstitium, glomeruli or capillaries. Nephrotoxic substances are a common contributor to the development of intrarenal AKI, such as:
  - drugs – aminoglycoside antibiotics such as gentamicin and non-steroidal anti-inflammatory drugs such as diclofenac;
  - exogenous chemicals – radiographic contrast agents or heavy metals;
  - endogenous toxins – Gram-negative bacteria, for example *Streptococcus*, and myoglobin.
- **Postrenal causes** are generally attributed to an obstruction of the urinary system, as with prostatic hyperplasia or renal calculi.

Box 15.10 Nursing management of patients with complicated UTIs

- Monitor level of pain:
  - Administer prescribed analgesia and antispasmodic agents
- Educate the patient and family on:
  - Disease progression
  - Treatment
  - Measurement of urinary output
  - The need for increased oral fluids
- Monitor for signs of sepsis:
  - Vital signs (pyrexia, tachycardia and hypotension)
  - Chills or rigor
- If the patient is pyrexic:
  - Ensure a well-ventilated environment
  - Remove blankets and provide cold drinks
  - Administer prescribed antipyretics and monitor the response
- Administer antibiotics (but ensure that urine has been obtained for culture and sensitivity prior to the first antibiotic dose)
- Monitor urinary output
- Maintain an accurate fluid balance record
- Monitor for nausea and vomiting, and administer any prescribed antiemetics
- Administer prescribed intravenous fluids
- Encourage oral fluids when tolerated (3 L/day)
- Encourage the patient to drink cranberry juice if appropriate
- If there is a decrease in activity due to the pain, encourage early mobilisation when the pain has been controlled
- Give discharge advice on:
  - The signs and symptoms of UTI (cystitis and pyelonephritis)
  - The need for early medical treatment
  - Antibiotics – the course of therapy and compliance with it
  - Attendance at outpatients for renal follow-up
  - Monitoring of urinary output
  - An oral fluid intake of 3 L/day
  - Include information on strategies to prevent UTIs, as outlined in Box 15.9

Classification of AKI

Over the last decade, a number of attempts have been made to classify AKI. The RIFLE classification system was developed by the Acute Dialysis Quality Initiative panel in 2004 and amended by the Acute Kidney Injury Network (Mehta *et al.* 2007).

In 2012, the Kidney Disease Improving Global Outcomes (KDIGO) international guideline group published a definition and staging classification system that has harmonised previous definitions and classifications; it is anticipated that the KDIGO definition and classification system will be adopted globally. Similar to other classification systems, the KDIGO (2012) distinguishes the stages of renal dysfunction by changes in serum creatinine or urine output. The clinical course of AKI proceeds through four phases:

- The **initiating** stage begins with the renal insult and lasts hours to days. Patients begin to develop signs and symptoms of renal impairment (Box 15.11).
- The **oliguric** stage lasts for 5–15 days (but may persist for weeks), and in this stage, renal healing occurs and tubular cells regenerate.

Box 15.11 Signs and symptoms of AKI

- Urinary output:
  - Oliguria (<400 mL/24 hours)
  - Anuria (<100 mL/24 hours)
  - Haematuria
- Hyperkalaemia:
  - Paraesthesia – a tingling sensation
  - Muscular cramps (in the legs and abdomen)
  - Paralysis
  - Muscle weakness
  - Arrhythmias as a potassium level greater than 7 mmol/L is incompatible with normal cardiac function
- Acidosis:
  - Kussmaul respiration (deep rapid breathing)
  - Weakness
  - Drowsiness
  - Coma
- Fluid overload:
  - Peripheral oedema, e.g. ankle oedema
  - Pulmonary oedema, leading to breathlessness and frothy sputum
  - Weight gain
  - Headache due to hypertension
- Uraemia:
  - Nausea, vomiting and anorexia
  - Headache, apathy, drowsiness, decreased responsiveness, confusion, twitching, coma, irritability or unconsciousness
  - Malaise

- The **diuretic** stage lasts for 1–2 weeks. In this stage, a self-limiting diuresis occurs because renal tubular patency has been restored but the nephrons' ability to concentrate urine has not recovered.
- The **recovery** stage lasts for months to 1 year, completing the healing process.

Management

The goal of treatment is to restore the patient's biochemical balance and prevent the progression of injury by treating the underlying cause. Investigations include:

- serum creatinine and urea levels;
- serum electrolyte levels;
- arterial blood gases;
- a full blood count;
- urinalysis;
- urine for culture and sensitivity, and estimated glomerular filtrate rate (eGFR);
- a KUB X-ray;
- an intravenous pyelogram;
- an ultrasound scan;
- a CT scan;
- a renal biopsy;
- a renal angiogram.

The management of patients is outlined in Box 15.12.

Nurses must provide holistic care when managing patients with AKI, continually monitoring their progress. The care of patients with AKI may involve a large multidisciplinary team and take place in an intensive care setting; however, many patients are nursed on a general ward and require close monitoring by and support from the nursing staff (Box 15.13).

Chronic kidney disease

Chronic kidney disease (CKD) is caused by progressive disease of both kidneys whereby there is irreversible damage to the nephrons. This eventually leads to the retention of waste products, fluid and electrolyte imbalances, metabolic acidosis, anaemia, hypertension and decalcification of bone tissue. Causes of CKD include:

- diabetes mellitus;
- glomerulonephritis;
- adult polycystic kidney disease.

Investigations include:

- dipstick urinalysis;
- urine culture and sensitivity;
- protein/creatinine ratio;
- abdominal X-ray;
- kidney ultrasound;
- possibly a CT or kidney biopsy to establish or confirm a diagnosis and assist in developing a treatment plan.

Serum creatinine level is a traditional marker of kidney function. However, this measurement alone can be insensitive as it is affected by the production of creatinine, largely from muscle, as well as by kidney excretion. Renal function may be significantly impaired before serum creatinine is raised. Predictive equations, which estimate the rate of filtration of the glomeruli (eGFR) taking into account the influence of factors such as age, gender and race, have become a much more widely used measure for estimating the severity of CKD. NICE has published guidelines on the identification and managements of adults with CKD that identifies six stages of severity based on eGFR measurements (NICE 2008b) (Table 15.3).

Irrespective of the cause, CKD usually develops slowly with few signs or symptoms in the early stages. Patients may still be passing normal volumes of urine, and many do not identify that they have an issue until their kidney function has decreased to less than 25% of normal capacity (CKD stage 4). The rate of deterioration of kidney function is individual and variable, and can range from more than 10 years to only a few months. Eventually, patients may reach end-stage renal disease, in which the eGFR is less than 15 mL/min per 1.73 m^2, and renal replacement therapy (RRT) in the form of dialysis or a transplant is required to maintain life (Figure 15.5). At this stage, patients may have a variety of systemic manifestations due to the severe loss of kidney function (Table 15.4).

Management

The management of patients with CKD includes treatment of the underlying cause in order to retard the progression of the disease, along with the development of a therapeutic management plan (Box 15.14).

Box 15.12 Medical management of patients with AKI

Hyperkalaemia

- Temporary measures:
  - Administration of a glucose and insulin infusion, which moves potassium ions back into the intracellular compartment
  - Nebulised albuterol sulphate
  - Sodium bicarbonate (intravenously) only in the presence of acidosis; this also moves potassium into the cells
- Oral or rectal potassium exchange agents, e.g. calcium resonium
- Calcium gluconate (intravenously), which antagonises the cardiac depressant effect of potassium, although it has a constipating effect
- Elimination of potassium and potassium-sparing diuretics or medications
- Dietary restrictions
- Renal replacement therapy may be indicated if potassium levels continue to rise and fail to respond to medical treatment

Metabolic acidosis

- Intravenous infusion of sodium bicarbonate
- Renal replacement therapy may be indicated if treatment is not successful

Uraemia

- Accumulation of metabolic waste products
- Renal replacement therapy may be indicated if patients become symptomatic

Volume overload

- Careful fluid replacement
- Renal replacement therapy may be indicated if conservative therapy fails to maintain fluid and electrolyte balance

Other

- Treat the cause of the AKI

Box 15.13 Nursing management of patients with AKI

- Consider patients' anxieties – reassure patients and explain the treatment strategies
- Record an intake and output chart
- Monitor for fluid overload, which is associated with:
  - Raised central venous pressure readings
  - Hypertension and headache
  - Tachycardia
  - Weight gain
  - Peripheral oedema
  - Pulmonary oedema
  - Pulse oximetry
  - Cyanosis
- Administer prescribed oxygen therapy
- Restrict fluid to 500 mL/24 hours plus the previous day's output to account for insensible losses through respiration, sweating, etc.
- A urinary catheter may be inserted initially; monitor the patient hourly and remove the catheter as soon as possible
- Take a midstream urine sample and ward urinalysis
- Instigate oral hygiene
- Monitor laboratory measurements for hyperkalaemia, acidosis and uraemia:
  - Ensure appropriate management of electrolyte imbalances and uraemia
  - Administer the prescribed medication
- Refer the patient to a dietitian for a nutritional assessment:
  - Aim for a total energy intake of 20–30 kcal/kg per day for any stage of AKI
  - If the patient is not on renal replacement therapy:
    - ensure a low-potassium, low-sodium, low-phosphate intake
    - increase carbohydrate intake
    - give a protein intake of 0.8–1.0 g/kg per day (but only if the patient is not critically ill and is not receiving renal replacement therapy)
  - The protein intake if the patient is critically ill and on renal replacement therapy should be:
    - 1.0–1.5 g/kg per day if the patient is receiving intermittent renal replacement therapy
    - a maximum of 1.7 g/kg per day if the patient is on continuous renal replacement therapy
- Consider bowel care (as potassium exchange resin exchange can cause constipation)
- Monitor blood sugar levels as hyperglycaemia is common, owing to insulin resistance
- In the diuretic phase:
  - Discontinue dietary and fluid restrictions
  - Increase oral fluid intake and monitor for dehydration
  - Ensure strict monitoring of fluid intake and output
  - Educate patients and their families on monitoring urinary output and increasing oral intake
- On discharge, educate patients on:
  - The disease process
  - Signs of:
    - UTI and the importance of prompt treatment
    - a decrease in renal function
    - general infection, with the implication it has for newly recovered kidney function
  - Monitoring of urinary output
  - Attendance at outpatient appointments for assessment of renal function
  - Medications
  - Oral fluids and diet

Table 15.3 Staging of CKD

Stage of CKD	eGFR (mL/min per 1.73 m^2)	Description
1	>90	Normal or increased GFR, with other evidence of kidney damage
2	60–89	A slight decrease in GFR, with other evidence of kidney damage
3a	45–59	A moderate decrease in GFR, with or without other evidence of kidney damage
3b	30–44	A moderate decrease in GFR, with or without other evidence of kidney damage
4	15–29	A severe decrease in GFR, with or without other evidence of kidney damage
5	<15	Established renal failure – dialysis or transplantation may be required

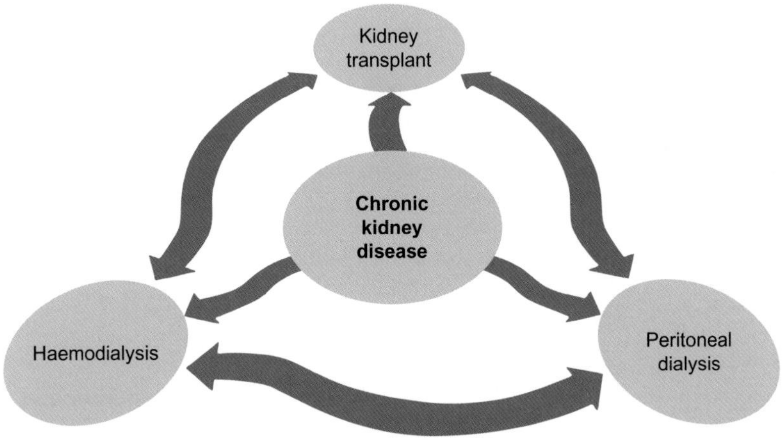

Figure 15.5 CKD and renal replacement options. Reproduced with kind permission of Beaumont Hospital, Ireland.

Table 15.4 Physiological manifestations of end-stage kidney disease

System	Clinical manifestation
Skin	Pallor Grey–bronze skin colour Ecchymoses Purpura Dry, flaky skin Pruritus
Cardiovascular	Volume overload Hypertension Pitting oedema Raised jugular ventricular pressure Left ventricular hypertrophy Uraemic pericarditis Pericardial effusion
Pulmonary	Pulmonary oedema Crackles Tachypnoea Pleuritic pain
Neurological	Fatigue Confusion Inability to concentrate Peripheral and autonomic neuropathy Tremors Restless legs Seizures
Gastrointestinal	Odour of ammonia on the breath Hiccups Anorexia Nausea and vomiting Malnutrition Gastrointestinal bleeding
Haematological	Anaemia Leucocyte and immune system dysfunction Platelet dysfunction
Reproductive	Amenorrhoea Infertility Testicular atrophy Loss of libido
Musculoskeletal	Muscle cramps Loss of muscle strength Renal osteodystrophy Bone pain Fractures

Box 15.14 Management of patients with CKD

- Referral to a dietitian to:
  - Adjust dietary and fluid intake
    - — maintain fluid and electrolyte balance
    - — reduce the retention of nitrogenous waste
  - Dietary proteins may be limited to avoid proteins high in essential amino acids (e.g. eggs, meat, fish and poultry)
  - Dietary potassium is restricted
- The following may be prescribed:
  - Potassium exchange resins if hyperkalaemia persists
  - Antihypertensive drugs
  - Synthetic injectable forms of erythropoietin
- Kidney function of less than 15% requires RRT in order to maintain life:
  - Haemodialysis
  - Peritoneal dialysis
  - Pre-emptive transplantation
  - Cadaveric or living donor kidney transplantation
- Nursing management, including the education and preparation of patients and families at all stages of CKD, aiming to:
  - Help patients develop methods to cope with:
    - — the constraints of available treatments
    - — the possibility of other complications associated with renal failure
  - Place patients at the centre of their care
  - Keep patients fully informed of all available treatment options

Renal replacement therapy

RRT (Box 15.15) affect all aspects of patients' and their families' lives. Therefore, when selecting a treatment modality for patients, their lifestyle, social environment and personality should be considered as well as their clinical condition. Nurses must educate patients on various issues: pre-emptive and early kidney transplantation; the basics of both haemodialysis and peritoneal dialysis; the range of environmental, procedural and scheduling options available to patients undergoing either type of dialysis; and the circumstances in which palliative care should be considered as an alternative to RRT.

Box 15.15 RRT

Dialysis:

- Lowers serum levels of metabolic waste products
- Corrects abnormal electrolyte and fluid balances

Haemodialysis (Figure 15.6):

- Blood is removed from the patient, via a vascular access system, passed through an artificial kidney called a dialyser, which is a synthetic, semi-permeable membrane, and returned to the patient
- Using the principles of diffusion, osmosis and ultrafiltration, toxins and excess water are removed from the blood
- Examples of vascular access include an arteriovenous fistula (Figure 15.7), an arteriovenous graft and a double-lumen central line
- Patients are treated three times a week for 3–4 hours in a dialysis centre or carry out the procedure in their own homes

Peritoneal dialysis (PD):

- The peritoneal membrane acts as a semi-permeable membrane
- A permanent catheter (e.g. a Tenckhcoff catheter) is inserted into the peritoneal cavity
- 2–3 L of warmed sterile dialysate fluid are introduced into the peritoneal cavity, a process called the fill, which takes about 20 minutes; the fluid stays in the cavity for several hours (known as the dwell)
- During the dwell time, through a process of diffusion, osmosis and ultrafiltration, excess fluid and solutes move from the vascular system across the peritoneal membrane into the dialysis fluid in the peritoneal cavity
- Drainage by gravity typically takes another 20 minutes
- The process of draining and filling the peritoneal cavity is called an exchange; this is usually performed four or five times daily, 7 days a week
- Two common forms of PD, both of which are carried out in patients' home, are:
  - Continuous ambulatory peritoneal dialysis (CAPD; Figure 15.8) – this enables patients to move freely and continue with their normal daily activities because it requires no machinery and no restraints
  - Continuous cycler-assisted peritoneal dialysis (CCPD) – this uses a machine called a cycler and performs several exchanges during the night while patients sleep

Renal transplantation (Figure 15.9):

- Is the treatment of choice
- May not be suitable for all patients with end-stage renal disease
- Types of transplant include pre-emptive, cadaver and living donor
- Transplant recipients will remain on medication, including immunosuppressant therapy, for the lifespan of their transplanted kidney

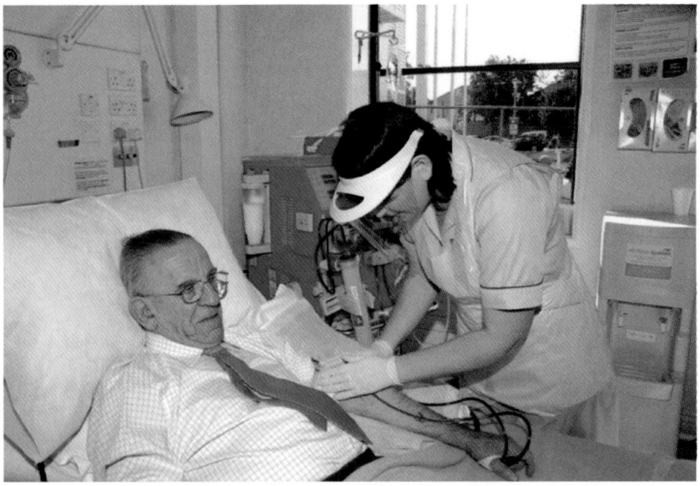

Figure 15.6 Haemodialysis. Reproduced with kind permission of Beaumont Hospital, Ireland.

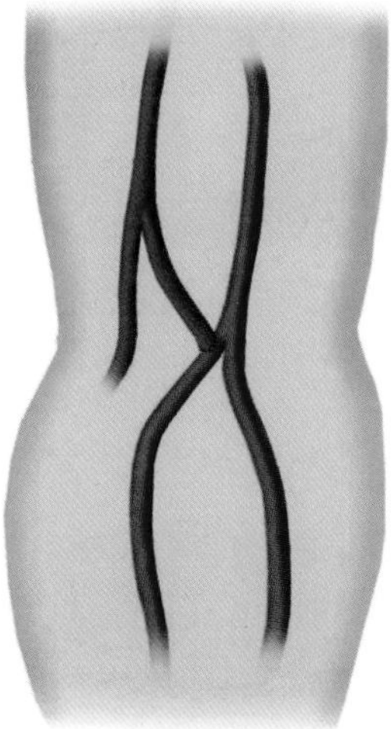

Figure 15.7 Arteriovenous fistula. Reproduced with kind permission of Beaumont Hospital, Ireland.

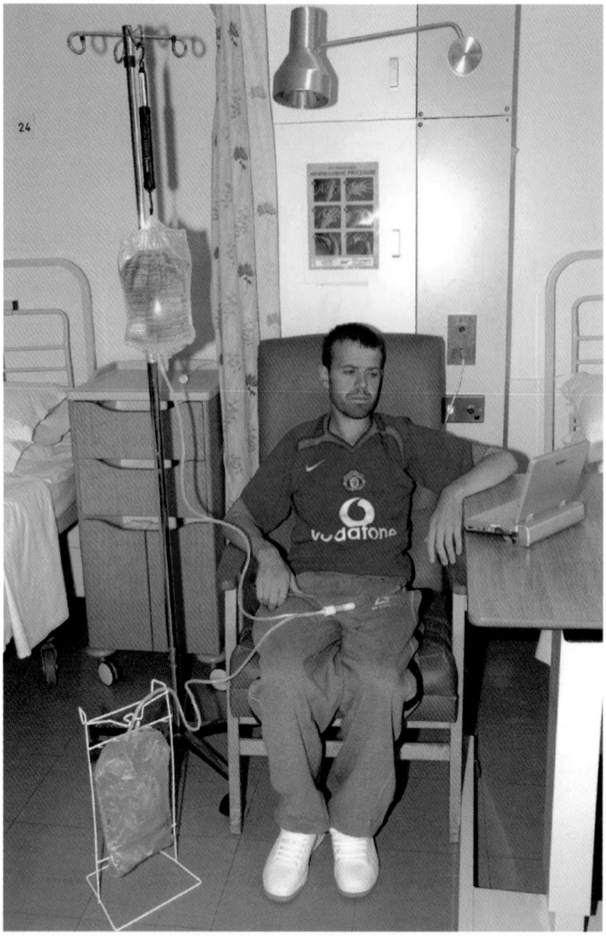

Figure 15.8 Peritoneal dialysis. Reproduced with kind permission of Beaumont Hospital, Ireland.

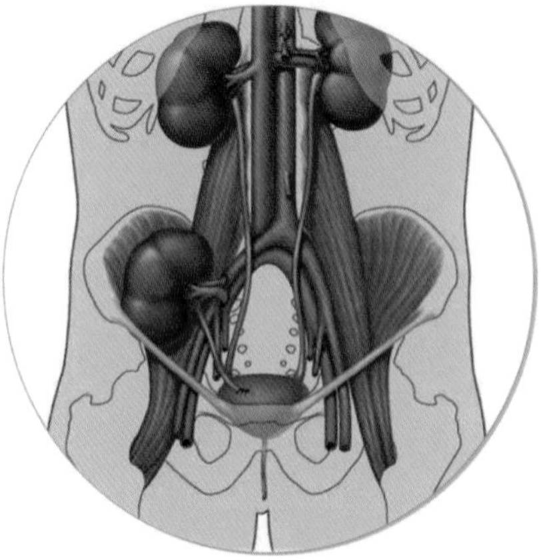

Figure 15.9 Renal transplant. Reproduced with kind permission of Beaumont Hospital, Ireland.

Conclusion

This chapter has outlined some of the conditions that are commonly seen in clinical areas in urology and nephrology. It also provides a snapshot of the nursing management that patients with these conditions require. Additional resources should be used to enhance your knowledge and understanding of these conditions and their associated nursing care.

Visit www.wileyfundamentalseries.com/medicalnursing and read Reflective Questions 15.1 and 15.2 to think more about this topic.

Now visit the companion website and test yourself on this chapter:
www.wileyfundamentalseries.com/medicalnursing

References

European Association of Urology (2012) *Guidelines on Urolithiasis*. Retrieved 21st September 2011 from http://www.uroweb.org.

European Network of Cancer Registries (2001) *Eurocim version 4.0*. European incidence database V2.3, 730 entity dictionary, Lyon

Gemmill, R., Sun, V., Ferrell, B., Krouse, RS., & Grant, M. (2010) Going with the flow: quality of life outcomes of cancer survivors with urinary diversion. *Journal of Wound Ostomy and Continence Nursing*, **37**(1):65–72.

Hooton, T. (2012) Uncomplicated urinary tract infections. *New England Journal of Medicine*, **366**(11):1028–37.

Kidney Disease International Global Outcomes (2012) Clinical practice guidelines for acute kidney injury. *International Society of Nephrology Journal*, **2**(S1):1–138.

Mehta, R., Kellum J., Shah S. *et al*. and the Acute Kidney Injury Network (2007) Acute Kidney Injury Network: Report of an Initiative to Improve Outcomes in Acute Kidney Injury. *Critical Care*, **11**(2):R31.

National Institute for Health and Clinical Excellence (2008a) *Prostate Cancer: Diagnosis and Treatment*. Clinical Guideline No. 58. Retrieved 27th May 2012 from http://www.nice.org.uk/nicemedia/live/11924/39687/39687.pdf.

National Institute for Health and Clinical Excellence (2008b) *Early Identification and Management of Chronic Kidney Disease in Adults in Primary and Secondary Care*. Clinical Guideline No. 73. Retrieved 20th February 2012 from http://www.nice.org.uk/nicemedia/pdf.CG073NICEGuideline.pdf.

Prostate Cancer Charity (2009). *Enlarged Prostate: A Guide for Men Concerned About Benign Prostatic Hyperplasia*. Retrieved 27th February 2012 from http://www.prostatecancer.org.uk/media/41599/bph.pdf.

Prostate Cancer Charity (2011) *Prostate Cancer*. Retrieved 27th February 2012 from http://www.prostate-cancer.org.uk/information/prostate-cancer.

Yaqub, M.S. & Molitoris, B.A. (2009) Acute kidney injury. In: Lerma, E., Berns, J. & Nissenson, A. (eds), *Current Diagnosis and Treatment: Nephrology and Hypertension* (pp. 89–98). McGraw Hill: New York.

16

Nursing care of conditions related to the endocrine system

David Chaney[1] and Anna Clarke[2]

[1]School of Nursing, University of Ulster, Derry~Londonderry, Northern Ireland, UK
[2]Diabetes Federation of Ireland, Dublin, Ireland

Contents

Introduction 299
The endocrine system 299
The hypothalamus and pituitary gland 299
The thyroid gland 303
The adrenal glands 308
The pancreas 314
Conclusion 324
References 325

Learning outcomes

Having read this chapter, you will be able to:

- Identify the main components of the endocrine system
- Discuss the function of the endocrine system
- Describe the medical and nursing management of patients diagnosed with common endocrine disorders

Fundamentals of Medical-Surgical Nursing: A Systems Approach, First Edition. Edited by Anne-Marie Brady, Catherine McCabe, and Margaret McCann.

Introduction

In this chapter, you will learn about different parts of the endocrine system and the conditions that can occur when the endocrine glands do not function, or function inappropriately. The chapter focuses on the most common endocrine conditions that patients experience and is designed as an introduction, which should be supported by further exploration of the current literature.

The endocrine system

The endocrine and nervous systems together coordinate the functions of all the body systems. The nervous system controls homeostasis via nerve impulses, while the endocrine system releases messenger molecules, which bring about changes in metabolic activities. The science underlying the structure and function of the endocrine glands and the diagnosis and treatment of disorders of the endocrine system is called endocrinology.

The glands in the body are of two types: exocrine and endocrine. Exocrine glands secrete their products directly through ducts into body cavities, into the lumen of an organ or onto the outer surface of the body, as when sebaceous glands in the skin secrete oil onto the skin surface. Endocrine glands secrete hormones into the extracellular space; these then diffuse into the circulatory system and are carried to the target organ, as with gonadotrophs that are produced in the pituitary gland and stimulate the secretion of sex hormones from the testes in males and ovaries in females. Hormones have powerful effects but only affect targeted cells, which may be in multiple organs; insulin, for instance, which is produced in the pancreas, stimulates the transport of sugar from the blood into the cells and stimulates the synthesis of glycogen in the liver and triglycerides (triacylglycerols) in adipose tissue. Figure 16.1 displays the location of the endocrine organs within the body.

The hypothalamus and pituitary gland

The hypothalamus, situated inferior to the thalamus, is the integrating link between the nervous and endocrine systems (Figure 16.2). It receives inputs from all parts of the brain and sensory signals from all organs of the body. Cells in the hypothalamus synthesise nine different hormones, which act on either the anterior or posterior pituitary gland located just beneath it; these are either inhibiting or releasing hormones:

- corticotropin-releasing hormone;
- thyrotropin-releasing hormone;
- somatotropin-releasing hormone;
- growth-inhibiting hormone;
- gonadotropin-releasing hormone;
- prolactin-releasing hormone;
- prolactin-inhibiting hormone;
- melanocyte-releasing hormone;
- melanocyte inhibiting hormone.

The pituitary gland is pea-shaped and lies in the sella turcica of the sphenoid bone. It is subdivided into anterior and posterior lobes. Five principal types of anterior pituitary cell (secretory cells) produce seven major hormones (Table 16.1).

The posterior lobe of the pituitary does not synthesise hormones, but it stores and releases two hormones:

- oxytocin;
- antidiuretic hormone (ADH).

During the delivery of a baby, oxytocin enhances contraction of the smooth muscles of the uterus, and after delivery it stimulates milk ejection from the mammary glands in response to the stimulus

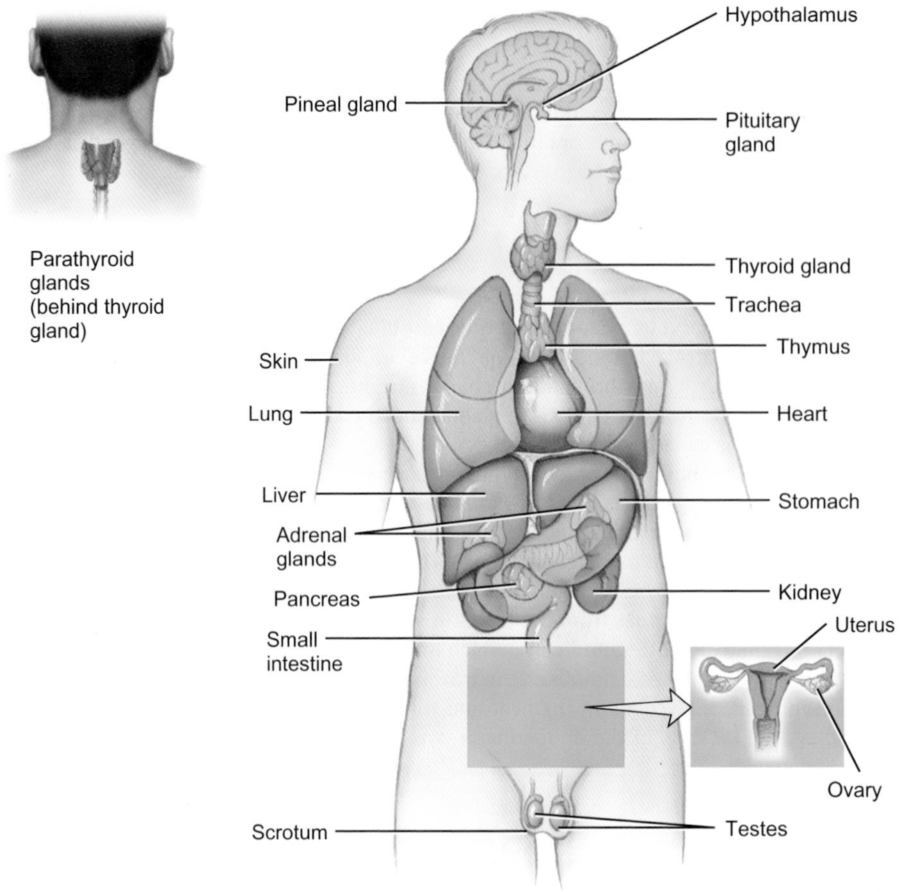

Figure 16.1 The location of the endocrine organs. Reproduced from Tortora, G.J., Derrickson, B. (2011) *Principles of Anatomy and Physiology*, with kind permission of Wiley Blackwell.

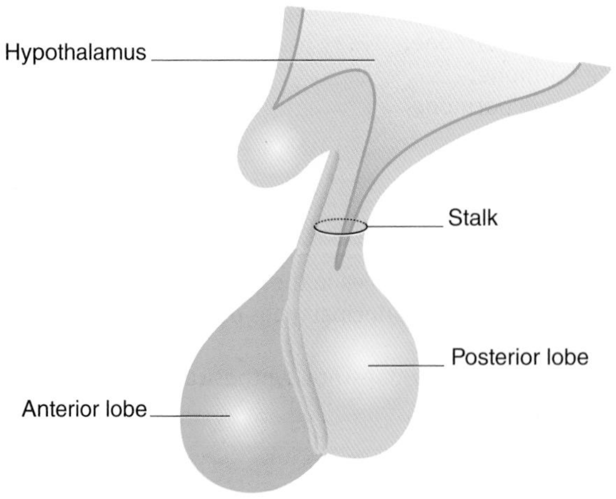

Figure 16.2 The hypothalamus and pituitary gland. Reproduced from Tortora, G.J., Derrickson, B. (2011) *Principles of Anatomy and Physiology*, with kind permission of Wiley Blackwell.

Table 16.1 Anterior pituitary secretary cells

Secretory cell	Hormone produced	Target gland	Effect	Hyposecretion	Hypersecretion
Somatotrophs	Human growth hormone	All body cells	Promote body growth Regulate aspects of metabolism	Dwarfism: • During the growth years • Occurs unless diagnosed early and treated with growth hormone	Gigantism, during the growth years Acromegaly, i.e. thickening of the bones of the face, hands and feet, which occurs during adulthood
Thyrotrophs	Thyroid-stimulating hormone	Thyroid gland	Promote activity of the thyroid gland		Graves' disease
Gonadotrophs	Follicle-stimulating hormone Luteinising hormone	Gonads	Growth of the reproductive system	Sterility	
Lactotrophs	Prolactin	Mammary glands	Milk production in suitably prepared mammary glands		Galactorrhoea (inappropriate lactation) Amenorrhoea (females) Impotence (males)
Corticotrophs	Adrenocorticotropic hormone	Adrenal gland	Secretion of glucocorticoids		Cushing's syndrome
	Melanocyte-stimulating hormone	Skin	Promote skin pigmentation		

provided by a sucking infant. ADH conserves body water and increases blood pressure by reducing the loss of water in the urine and by reducing sweating.

Disorders of the pituitary gland

Diabetes insipidus

Hyposecretion of ADH leads to a condition known as diabetes insipidus (DI). There are two main types of diabetes insipidus:

- **Neurogenic diabetes insipidus** is caused by brain tumours, head trauma or brain surgery that damages the posterior pituitary gland.
- **Nephrogenic diabetes insipidus** is the inability of the renal tubules to sense the presence of ADH and can be hereditary or result from renal failure.

Diabetes insipidus results in:

- increased urinary output, to as much as 20 L per day;
- increased thirst (polydipsia) and dehydration;
- hypernatraemia and hyperosmolality, evidenced by a low specific gravity on urinalysis.

If it has been caused by trauma, symptoms of diabetes insipidus generally appear within 3–6 days. This condition may be short-lived if the cause (e.g. raised intracranial pressure) is resolved; however, the condition may also be chronic and is then generally treated with a nasal spray such as desmopressin acetate.

Syndrome of inappropriate ADH hypersecretion

The syndrome of inappropriate ADH hypersecretion (SIADH) is a condition in which the pituitary gland produces too much ADH. SIADH causes aldosterone to be suppressed, increasing renal excretion of sodium and leading to the retention of fluid within the cells. Patients present with:

- water retention;
- hyponatraemia;
- decreased urinary output with concentrated urine;
- hypo-osmolality;
- neurological manifestations such as headaches or confusion;
- generally a normal serum creatinine level, acid–base balance, adrenal function and thyroid function.

SIADH is caused by the production of ADH by a malignant tumour (e.g. carcinoma of the lung or pancreas), but transient forms of SIADH may also be caused by pituitary surgery, head injury or barbiturate abuse. Treatment includes the following:

- where possible, address the underlying causes;
- fluid is restricted (to 1200–1800 mL per day) to increase serum sodium levels. This should be continued until the cause of SIADH has been identified and, where possible, eradicated;
- if the symptoms are severe, furosemide and intravenous half-strength normal saline can be used to decrease the circulatory volume and prevent sodium excretion;
- demeclocycline, a tetracycline antibiotic with the side effect of inducing excessive urination and inhibiting vasopressin action, may be beneficial in chronic situations and helps to maintain an adequate fluid balance;
- vasopressin antagonists may also be prescribed and are the most beneficial medications for patients with SIADH and cardiac failure;
- monitoring of sodium levels and correction of hyponatraemia must be undertaken with caution in order to prevent cerebral osmotic demyelination.

Nursing care should revolve around educating patients on the need to maintain a strict fluid balance.

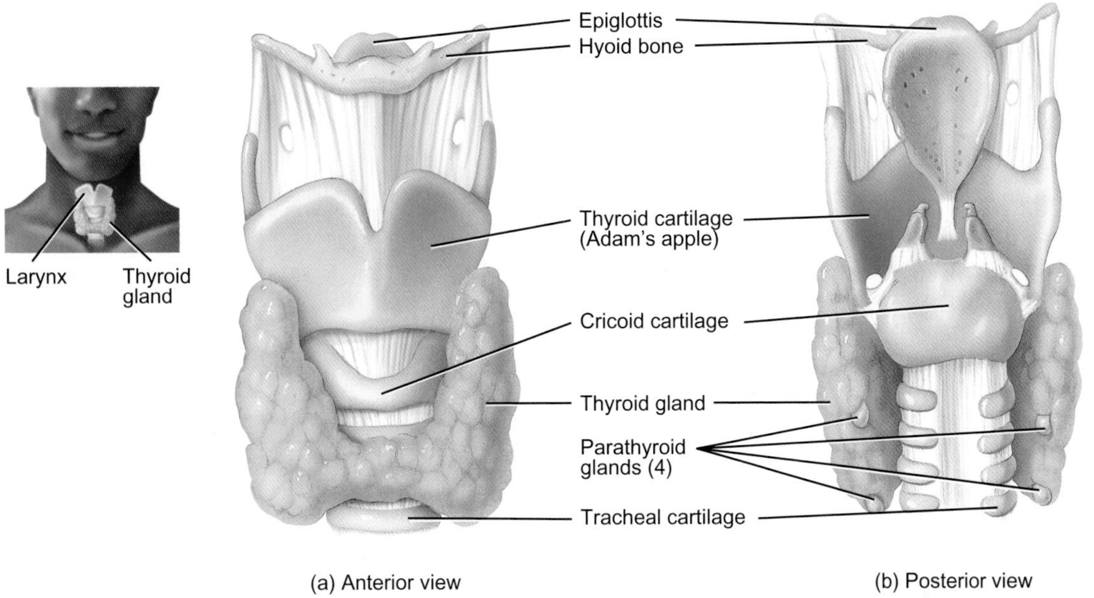

Figure 16.3 The position of the thyroid and parathyroid glands. Reproduced from Tortora, G.J., Derrickson, B. (2011) *Principles of Anatomy and Physiology*, with kind permission of Wiley Blackwell.

The thyroid gland

The butterfly-shaped thyroid gland is located just inferior to the larynx (voice box). The right and left lateral lobes are situated on either side of the trachea, with their connecting isthmus lying anterior to the trachea. The gland weighs about 30 g, has a very rich blood supply (80–120 mL of blood per minute), and can become enlarged (goitre), with or without excess or deficient thyroid hormone production (Figure 16.3).

The thyroid gland is made up of thyroid follicles, the walls of which are composed of follicular cells (Figure 16.4). When inactive, the follicular cells are low cuboidal or squamous in nature, but under the influence of thyroid-stimulating hormone (TSH), they become cuboidal and produce thyroid hormones. These are named after the number of atoms of iodine they contain: thyroxine (T_4) and triiodothyronine (T_3). T_4 is produced in greater quantities, but T_3 is several times more potent. The thyroid hormones regulate:

- oxygen use and basal metabolic rate (the rate of oxygen consumption at rest);
- cellular metabolism;
- growth and development.

Their production is controlled by negative feedback and the amount of circulating iodine. Hyposecretion during fetal life or infancy results in cretinism, a failure of the body and the brain to grow. Testing of newborns ensures that thyroid dysfunction is diagnosed early and treated with replacement therapy for life; screening normally occurs 5–7 days after birth by means of a simple heel prick test, with blood being analysed for both T_4 and TSH.

Disorders of the thyroid gland

Hypothyroidism

Hypothyroidism affects 1% of the adult population and is six times more common in women than men (1 in 50 women and 1 in 300 men).

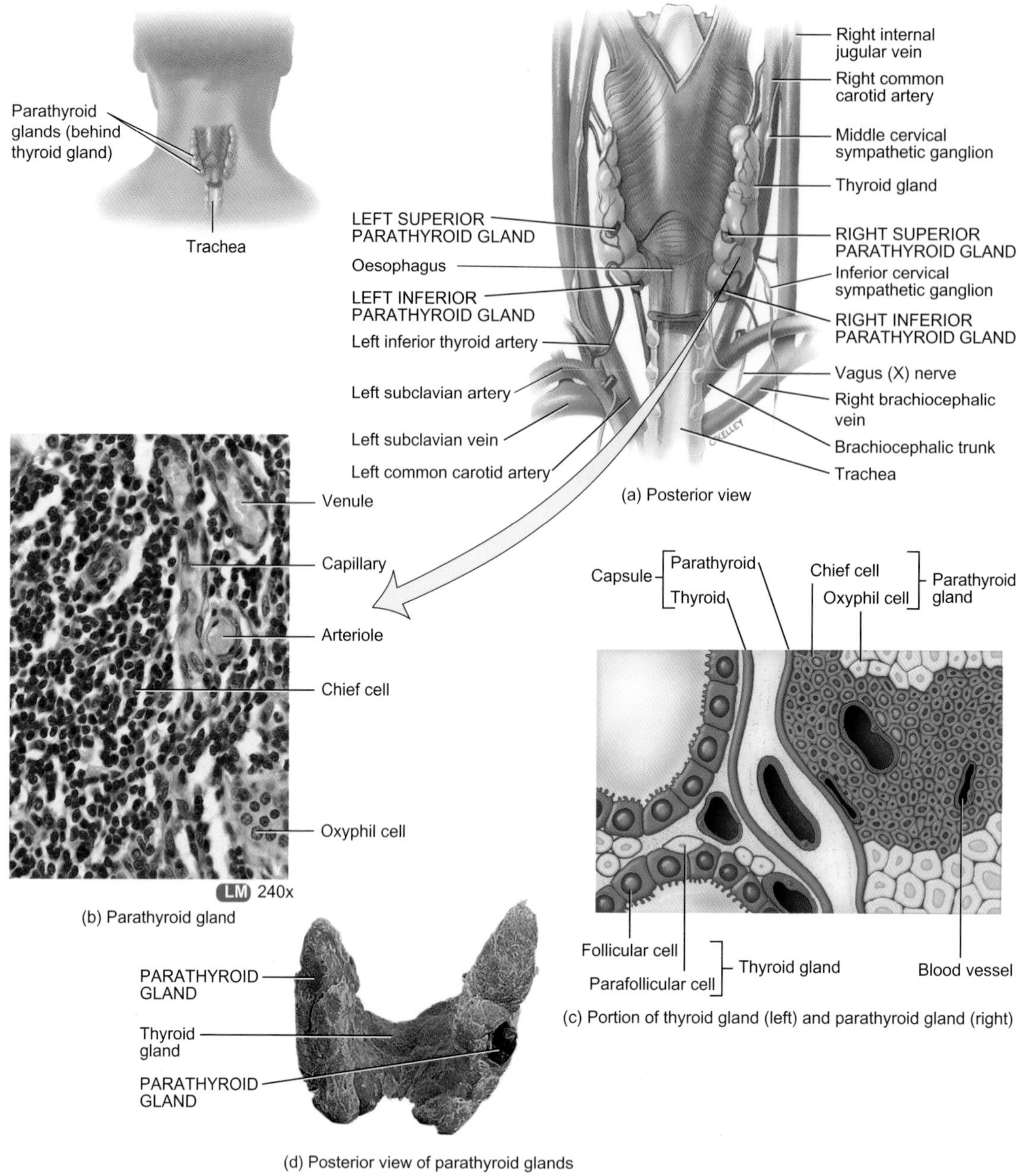

Figure 16.4 The location, blood supply and histology of the parathyroid glands. Reproduced from Tortora, G.J., Derrickson, B. (2011) *Principles of Anatomy and Physiology*, with kind permission of Wiley Blackwell.

Box 16.1 Causes of primary and secondary hypothyroidism

Primary hypothyroidism
Autoimmune destruction of the thyroid gland
Other autoimmune conditions, e.g.:
- Type 1 diabetes
- Addison's disease
- Pernicious anaemia

Following treatment for hyperthyroidism
Congenital hypothyroidism – absence of a thyroid gland after birth, which occurs at a rate of approximately 1 in 3000 live births
Iodine deficiency

Secondary hypothyroidism
Pituitary failure
Hypothalamic failure
After pituitary surgery

Hypothyroidism may be classified as primary or secondary (Box 16.1). Primary hypothyroidism accounts for up to 95% of cases in adults.

Insufficient quantities of T_4 are produced by the thyroid gland in hypothyroidism; low levels of T_4 are also associated with high levels of TSH. The onset of the symptoms is generally slow, and often tiredness and lethargy are mistaken for the effects of normal ageing, resulting in a prolonged period before seeking medical assistance. The patient may present with:

- myxoedema (non-pitting oedema) affecting the hands, feet and eyelids, with facial swelling and puffiness;
- an inability to think quickly;
- constant tiredness;
- weight gain;
- sensitivity to the cold;
- constipation, which may give rise to faecal impaction;
- coarse, brittle hair;
- a decreased glomerular filtration rate;
- anovulatory cycles or severe menorrhagia.

Management

Diagnosing is by means of a thyroid function test. Hypothyroidism is confirmed by a low plasma level of T_4 (<5 pmol/L) and a raised TSH level (>20 mU/L). The measurement of T_3 as a diagnostic tool for hypothyroidism is not recommended as it is considered unreliable and may lead to a missed diagnosis.

Treatment is by means of oral replacement therapy of thyroid hormones. Low-dose T_4 (25–50 µg daily) is initially commenced, gradually increasing in increments of 25–50 µg on a monthly basis until the serum TSH level is normal. Patients are educated on the management of hypothyroidism (Box 16.2).

Nurses should be aware that T_4 interacts with several other medications, such as anticoagulants, oral hypoglycaemic agents and insulin, with a possible need to adjust the medications in these situations. In addition, approximately 40% of patients with angina are unable to tolerate full T_4 replacement therapy even with the addition of beta-blockers or vasodilators. Such patients may need to be referred for coronary angioplasty or coronary bypass grafting before they can tolerate full T_4 replacement. Patients taking T_4 replacement therapy are reviewed annually in order to assess the effectiveness of their treatment and provide them with the opportunity to express any concerns they may have.

Box 16.2 Patient education on the management of hypothyroidism

Educate patients on:

- Their condition
- The reason why replacement therapy must be life-long
- The need to take the medication in the morning, as a single dose on an empty stomach
- The importance of not missing a dose
- The fact that symptomatic relief is achieved in about 2–4 weeks
- That it may take 6 weeks before normal TSH levels are achieved
- The potential for overreplacement
- Signs of hyperthyroidism:
  - Anxiety
  - Restlessness
  - Palpitations
  - Diarrhoea

Failure to ensure patients' adequate understanding may result in poor adherence to medication or increased anxiety levels

Hyperthyroidism

It is possible for the thyroid gland to produce too much T_3 and T_4; this may be caused by a number of conditions, such as:

- Graves' disease;
- toxic multinodular goitre;
- a thyroid neoplasm.

Graves' disease

Graves' disease occurs between 20 and 40 years of age and is seven times more likely to present in women than in men. This condition may be the result of an autoimmune process and is characterised by a triad of thyrotoxicosis, exophthalmos (protruding eyeballs) and infiltrative dermopathy (thick, scaly skin lesions, which may appear like an orange-peel texture).

The symptoms are those listed for hyperthyroidism in Table 16.2 below, including the distinctive triad described above. The diagnosis is normally established by a thyroid function text, with results demonstrating elevated T_3 and T_4 levels and low levels of TSH.

Toxic multinodular goitre

This form of hyperthyroidism is caused by a tumour and is characterised by a number of small nodules that are discrete and function independently. These nodules secrete excessive amounts of thyroid hormones, resulting in symptoms associated with hyperthyroidism. The aetiology is not fully understood; however, genetic mutation of the follicle cells has been suggested as one possible cause. This condition is not associated with the eye or skin pathology as seen in Graves' disease.

Thyroid neoplasm

Thyroid neoplasms, such as follicular adenomas, may cause hypersecretion from the thyroid gland. Thyroid neoplasms take on a wide variety of morphological patterns, although follicular adenoma tends to present as a benign encapsulated mass of follicles. The most common malignant neoplasm found within the thyroid gland is the papillary carcinoma. This slow-growing neoplasm is normally found in

Table 16.2 Effects of hypothyroidism and hyperthyroidism on the body

Body system	Hyposecretion of T_4 and T_3	Hypersecretion of T_4 and T_3
Cardiovascular	Reduced cardiac output Bradycardia	Increased cardiac output Tachycardia
Metabolic	Decreased metabolism Weight gain	Increased metabolism Weight loss
Neuromuscular	Weakness Sluggish reflexes	Tremor Hyperactive reflexes
Mental/emotional	Sluggish mental processes Apathetic personality	Restlessness Irritability and emotional instability
Gastrointestinal	Constipation	Diarrhoea
General	Cold, dry skin	Warm, moist skin

countries where the dietary intake of iodine is either sufficient or excessive. The prognosis following treatment for papillary carcinoma is very good.

Effects of hyperthyroidism

Hypersecretion of T_3 and T_4 may be referred to as thyrotoxicosis or more commonly as hyperthyroidism. Table 16.2 outlines the effects that hypothyroidism and hyperthyroidism have on different systems of the body.

Management

Hyperthyroidism is confirmed by the presence of elevated levels of T_3 and T_4. Patients suspected of having thyroid nodules or neoplasms may undergo a thyroid scan or magnetic resonance imaging scan for full evaluation. There are three main treatment options (Box 16.3). A number of potential complications are associated with thyroid surgery (Table 16.3).

Thyroid crisis (thyroid storm)

Thyroid crisis occurs as the result of a rapid increase in metabolic rate resulting in excessive thyroid hormone production; it is a medical emergency and is considered life-threatening. Thyroid crisis is associated with undiagnosed hyperthyroidism, but is rare due to effective diagnosis and treatment. Signs and symptoms include:

- hyperthermia (39–41°C);
- tachycardia;
- hypertension;
- abdominal pain;
- gastrointestinal disturbances;
- restlessness;
- agitation;
- seizures.

It is vital that patients are treated urgently as any delay may result in increased mortality. Treatment for thyroid crisis comprises fluid replacement, management of electrolyte imbalance, cooling, avoidance of aspirin as it may increase free thyroid hormone levels, stabilisation of cardiovascular function and reduction of the synthesis and production of thyroid hormones.

Box 16.3 Treatment options for hyperthyroidism

Medication

- Anti-thyroid medications, e.g. carbimazole or methimazole
- Reduces the synthesis of new T_3 and T_4
- Symptoms may take a number of weeks to reduce due to existing stores of thyroid hormone within the gland

Radioactive iodine therapy

- Radioactive iodine (^{131}I) is given
- The thyroid absorbs the radioactive iodine
- This destroys thyroid cells, resulting in the production of lower levels of thyroid hormones
- It is administered orally
- This is an outpatient procedure
- The treatment effect may take as long as 6–8 weeks
- It is not suitable for pregnant women as radioactive iodine crosses the placenta, affecting the development of the fetal thyroid gland
- It is not always possible to control how much of the thyroid gland is destroyed, so patients may go on to develop hypothyroidism as a result of treatment

Surgery

One of six procedures may be undertaken:

- Partial thyroid lobectomy – removal of the upper or lower portion of one lobe
- Thyroid lobectomy – removal of one entire lobe
- Thyroid lobectomy with isthmusectomy – removal of one lobe and the isthmus
- Subtotal thyroidectomy – removal of one lobe, the isthmus and most of the other lobe
- Total thyroidectomy – removal of the entire gland
- Radical total thyroidectomy – removal of the entire gland and cervical lymphatic nodes

The adrenal glands

There are two adrenal glands, one lying superior to each kidney; the right is triangular in shape, the left semilunar (Figure 16.5a). Each gland has two distinct structures: the adrenal cortex and the adrenal medulla (Figure 16.5b). The adrenal cortex is subdivided into three zones (Figure 16.6 and Table 16.4).

Disorders of the adrenal glands

Addison's disease (chronic adrenocortical insufficiency)

Addison's disease is a chronic endocrine disorder resulting from complete destruction or dysfunction of the adrenal cortex. The adrenal cortex no longer produces aldosterone, glucocorticoids or adrenal androgens. The condition is generally found in adults under 60 years of age. Causes include:

- autoimmune processes;
- adrenal haemorrhage;
- tuberculosis;
- adrenoleukodystrophy.

Table 16.3 Complications and nursing care of patients after thyroid surgery

Complications	Nursing interventions
Haemorrhage	The thyroid gland is situated within an abundant supply of blood vessels Surgical intervention for haemorrhage occurs in approximately 0.1–1.5% of patients Normal postoperative observations are required Monitor for signs of haemorrhage in the postoperative period Haemorrhage is likely to occur between 6 and 12 hours post-surgery Assess anterior and posterior dressings as this is where blood tends to accumulate If there is evidence of haemorrhage, surgical intervention should be sought immediately
Respiratory distress	Occurs as a result of: ● Haemorrhage ● Oedema, causing compression of the trachea ● Laryngeal spasms due to hormone imbalance Assess: ● Respiratory rate, depth and rhythm ● The patient's colour ● Oxygen saturation level Any signs of distress should be acted upon immediately
Laryngeal nerve injury	Is due to: ● Incision clamping ● Stretching of the nerve ● Local compression due to oedema, haematoma or electrocoagulation during surgery Assess quality of voice and the swallow reflex, and report any concerns to the medical team Some weakness of the vocal chords may occur, but these should resolve within 6 weeks
Tetany	The parathyroid gland is located in close proximity to the thyroid There is a risk of injury or accidental removal of the parathyroid gland This results in calcium deficiency after surgery, with signs and symptoms of: ● Tingling of the toes, fingers and lips ● Muscular twitches ● Positive Chvostek's and Trousseau's signs Calcium gluconate should always be available locally and administered immediately intravenously, if necessary
Wound infection	There is potential for wound infection The most likely causative organisms are staphylococcal or streptococcal bacteria Wound infection is rare after thyroid surgery (0.3–0.8%) Monitor: ● Temperature ● The wound site for signs of infection, such as the presence of an odorous discharge

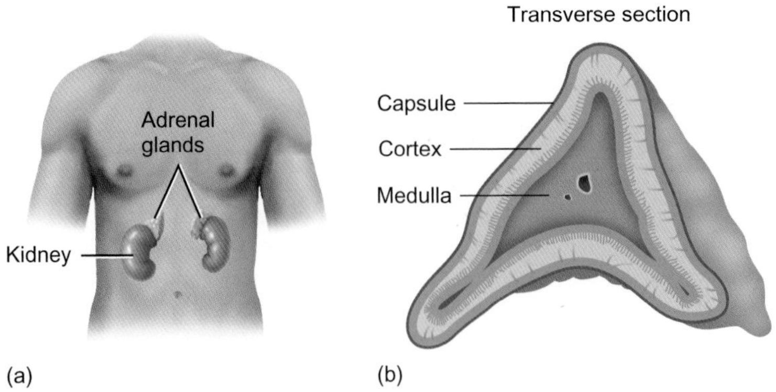

Figure 16.5 The position (a) and structure (b) of the adrenal glands. Reproduced from Tortora, G.J., Derrickson, B. (2011) *Principles of Anatomy and Physiology*, with kind permission of Wiley Blackwell.

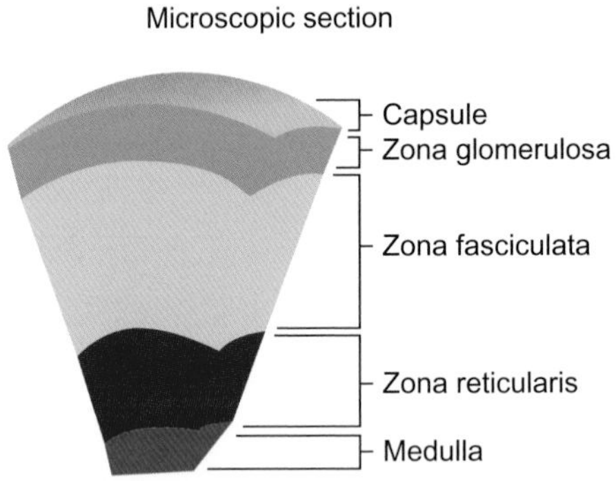

Figure 16.6 A cross-section of the adrenal cortex. Reproduced from Tortora, G.J., Derrickson, B. (2011) *Principles of Anatomy and Physiology*, with kind permission of Wiley Blackwell.

The onset of the disease is slow, symptoms often remaining absent until 90% of cortical function has been lost. Symptoms include:

- lethargy;
- muscle weakness;
- weight loss;
- hypotension;
- hypoglycaemia;
- hyponatraemia;
- hyperkalaemia;
- hyperpigmentation, which is most obvious on exposed areas of skin.

Management

Management is focused on replacing both corticosteroids and mineralocorticoids. Patients are encouraged to increase the sodium in their diet and take hydrocortisone and fludrocortisone orally. Patients should carry a medical alert card stating their diagnosis, details of their medication and their maintenance dosage. They should be aware that this dosage may need to be increased during times of unusual stress, and they must be provided with contact details of where to obtain advice in the event of such situations occurring.

Table 16.4 The three zones of the adrenal cortex

Zone	Type of cell	Hormone produced	Effect	Hyposecretion	Hypersecretion
Zona glomerulosa	Cells are arranged in arched loops	Mineralocorticoids – aldosterone	Controls water and electrolyte balance	Addison's disease: • Decreased sodium • Increased potassium • Muscle wasting • Excessive pigmentation	Aldosteronism: • Increased sodium • Decreased potassium
Zona fasciculata	Cells are arranged in long straight cords	Glucocorticoids: • Cortisol • Cortisone • Corticosterone	Prepare body for flight Raise blood sugar through gluconeogenesis Aid fat, protein and carbohydrate metabolism Suppress the immune system		Cushing's syndrome: • Redistribution of fat • Thin limbs • Flushed moon face and buffalo hump • Hyperglycaemia • Osteoporosis • Recurrent infection • Friable skin
Zona reticularis	Cells arranged in branching cords	Androgens	Prepubertal growth In males, exert masculinising effects	Reduced sex drive (both sexes)	Masculine effects

Addison's crisis

This is a life-threatening condition that results from an acute destruction of the adrenal cortex (by surgery or trauma) or an abrupt withdrawal of long-term corticosteroid therapy. The condition may manifest with:

- any of the symptoms of Addison's disease;
- severe vomiting, dehydration and diarrhoea leading to circulatory collapse;
- abdominal pain;
- high fever;
- hypotension;
- tachycardia.

Treatment must commence immediately, requiring skilful management of fluid replacement in conjunction with the administration of glucocorticoids, until an appropriate fluid balance has been restored and the symptoms have been negated.

Patients on corticosteroids

Corticosteroids are used extensively for:

- adrenal insufficiency;
- suppressing inflammation;
- suppressing autoimmune reactions;
- controlling allergic reactions;
- reducing the rejection process in transplantation.

The anti-inflammatory and anti-allergy actions of corticosteroids make them an effective treatment method for conditions such as rheumatoid arthritis and systemic lupus erythematosus. Corticosteroids may also be used in the management of other chronic conditions, such as asthma and multiple sclerosis. As with all medications, the use of corticosteroids is not without consequence as they have numerous side effects and drug interactions that need to be considered (Table 16.5).

Cushing's syndrome

Cushing's syndrome is a chronic disorder characterised by an excessive production of cortical hormones. It is more common in women than men and is usually diagnosed between the ages of 30 and 50 years, although it can occur at any age. Cushing's syndrome has various causes (Box 16.4). Signs and symptoms include:

- rapid weight gain, particularly of the trunk and face;
- hirsutism (facial hair growth), especially in women;
- an irregular or absent menstrual cycle;
- fat pads along the collar bone;
- hyperhidrosis (excessive sweating);
- thinning of the skin;
- the appearance of purple lines over the abdomen, thighs or buttocks (as a result of weakening and rupture of the deeper layers of skin).

Management

Cushing's syndrome caused by a pituitary tumour is generally treated by means of long-term medication in conjunction with surgery or radiation. Medication may also be used for patients with inoperable malignant tumours of the pituitary or adrenal glands. Where the cause of Cushing's syndrome has been established as an adrenal cortical tumour, the treatment of choice is an adrenalectomy. Usually, only one adrenal gland is removed; however, in the presence of an adrenocorticotropic hormone-producing tumour, bilateral adrenalectomy may be performed. Specific aspects of nursing care that need to be considered for patients undergoing an adrenalectomy are outlined in Box 16.5.

Table 16.5 Nursing care of patients on long-term corticosteroid therapy

Potential complication	Nursing action
Cardiovascular Hypertension Thrombophlebitis Thromboembolism Accelerated atherosclerosis	Monitor blood pressure for signs of hypertension Assess for a positive Homans' sign (indicating a deep vein thrombosis) Educate patients on: • Avoiding positions and situations that restrict blood flow (e.g. crossing the legs or prolonged sitting in the same position) • Foot and leg exercises • Low sodium intake • A low saturated fat diet
Immunological Increased risk of infection	Assess for signs of infection (bacterial and fungal) and inflammation Encourage: • Patients to avoid exposure to others with known infections or colds • Hand-washing and good hygiene practices
Eye changes Glaucoma Corneal lesions	Encourage yearly eye examinations Refer patients to an ophthalmologist if changes in visual acuity are detected
Musculoskeletal Muscle wasting Poor wound healing Osteoporosis: • Vertebral compression fractures • Pathological fractures of the long bones • Aseptic necrosis of head of femur	Refer to a dietitian Encourage a diet high in protein, calcium and vitamin D Calcium and vitamin D supplementation, if indicated Take measures to avoid falls and other trauma Use caution when moving and turning patients Encourage postmenopausal women on corticosteroids to consider bone mineral density testing and treatment, if indicated Instruct the patient to rise slowly from the bed or chair in cases of postural hypotension Promote regular physical activity
Metabolic Alterations in glucose metabolism Steroid withdrawal syndrome	Monitor blood glucose levels In the event of steroid-induced diabetes, refer to the diabetes nurse for education and management Report signs of adrenal insufficiency Monitor fluid and electrolyte balance Administer fluids and electrolytes as prescribed Educate patients on: • The importance of taking corticosteroids as prescribed without abruptly stopping therapy • Obtaining and wearing a medical identification bracelet • Notifying all healthcare providers (e.g. the dentist) about the need for corticosteroid therapy
Changes in appearance Moon face Weight gain Acne Thinning of the skin Tendency to bruise easily	Encourage a low-calorie, low-sodium diet Assure patients that most changes in appearance are temporary and will disappear if and when corticosteroid therapy is no longer necessary Monitor skin changes Instruct on active bruising avoidance, e.g. the use of stockings to prevent injury to the shins in affected individuals

Box 16.4 Causes of Cushing's syndrome

- Iatrogenic (the most common) – from long-term use of pharmacological glucocorticoid preparations
- Pituitary adenoma – a hypersecretion of adrenocorticotropic hormone occurs, referred to as Cushing's disease
- Ectopic tumours – adrenocorticotropic hormone-secreting tumours, e.g. small cell lung cancer
- Adrenal causes:
  - Excessive production of cortisol
  - Benign or malignant tumour

Box 16.5 Specific preoperative and postoperative care following an adrenalectomy

Preoperative care

- Dietary consultation:
  - Stress the importance of a diet high in vitamins and proteins, which are necessary for tissue repair and wound healing
  - If hypokalaemia exists, include foods high in potassium
  - Glucocorticoid excess increases catabolism
- Ensure medical and surgical asepsis when providing care and treatments (as cortisol excess increases the risk of infection)
- Monitor electrolyte and glucose levels – any imbalances should be corrected before surgery
- Educate patients on:
  - Coughing techniques
  - Deep-breathing exercises
  - Changing positions in bed
  - These activities are particularly important for patients at risk of infection

Postoperative care

- Results in adrenal insufficiency
- Addison's crisis and hypovolaemic shock may occur
- Cortisol is given on the day of surgery and in the postoperative period to replace inadequate hormone levels
- Assess:
  - Body temperature
  - White blood cell levels
  - Wound drainage
- Use aseptic technique as impaired wound healing increases the risk of infection

The pancreas

The pancreas is composed of both endocrine and exocrine tissue. Figure 16.7 depicts the location of the pancreas in relation to the liver and gallbladder.

Scattered around the pancreas are 1–2 million tiny islets of Langerhans, which are made up of four types of hormone-secreting cell:

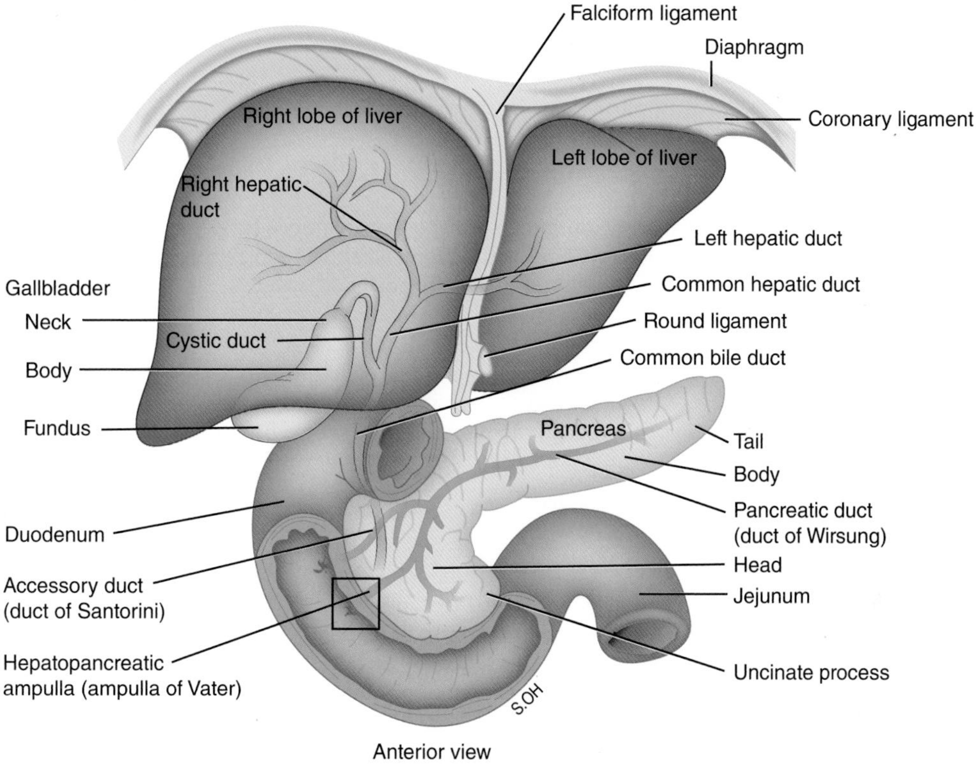

Figure 16.7 View of the liver, gallbladder and pancreas. Reproduced from Tortora, G.J., Derrickson, B. (2011) *Principles of Anatomy and Physiology*, with kind permission of Wiley Blackwell.

- **Alpha or A** cells secrete glucagon to raise the blood sugar level.
- **Beta cells** secrete insulin to lower the blood sugar level.
- **Delta or D** cells secrete somatostatin to slow the absorption of nutrients from the gut and inhibit insulin release.
- **F cells** secrete pancreatic polypeptide to control the secretion of digestive enzymes and contraction of the gallbladder.

All of these hormones are directly related to maintenance of blood sugar levels, with hyposecretion or hypersecretion resulting in a group of disorders known as diabetes mellitus.

Disorders of the pancreas

Diabetes mellitus

Diabetes mellitus refers to the group of disorders that have one common sign – an elevation in blood glucose level (hyperglycaemia). As hyperglycaemia increases:

- glucose spills out into the urine (glucosuria), causing
- osmotic diuresis (not correctable in the loop of Henle), which leads to
- excessive urine production (polyuria) and
- excessive thirst (polydipsia).

Box 16.6 Diagnosis of diabetes mellitus (American Diabetes Association 2011)

- Fasting plasma glucose ≥7.0 mmol/L
- Fasting is defined as no caloric intake for at least 8 hours

Or

- 2-hour plasma glucose ≥11.1 mmol/L during an oral glucose tolerance test
- The test should be performed as described by the World Health Organization, using a glucose load containing the equivalent of 75 g anhydrous glucose dissolved in water

Or

- In a patient with classic symptoms of hyperglycaemia or hyperglycaemic crisis, a random plasma glucose ≥11.1 mmol/L
- NB: In the absence of unequivocal hyperglycaemia, the result should be confirmed by repeat testing

Diabetes is normally classified as either type 1 or type 2. Box 16.6 outlines the current diagnostic criteria for diabetes mellitus. The most common form of diabetes is type 2, which is normally associated with diagnosis above the age of 40 years. Type 1 diabetes accounts for approximately 10% of diagnosed diabetes and is normally associated with individuals diagnosed below the age of 30 years (National Institute for Health and Clinical Excellence [NICE] 2009). Although type 1 and type 2 diabetes are both associated with a relative or absolute lack of insulin, the two conditions have very different disease patterns and are therefore managed differently.

Type 1 diabetes mellitus

Type 1 diabetes is one of the most common chronic conditions affecting children and adolescents in the UK. Life expectancy is reduced by approximately 15 years when compared with that of healthy individuals of the same age (DIAMOND Project Group 2006; NICE 2009).

Type 1 diabetes is an autoimmune disorder resulting from T cell-mediated destruction of the beta-cells in over 90% of cases. The remaining 10% of cases are referred to as idiopathic diabetes, often classified as type 1B diabetes mellitus. The exact aetiology of this autoimmune process is not completely understood, with environmental, toxic, nutritional, viral and infective factors all being implicated. Genetic susceptibility to type 1 diabetes is associated in particular with human leucocyte antigen genes.

Beta-cell destruction leads to a near-total insulin deficiency, resulting in the development of hyperglycaemia. In the absence of insulin, the body is unable to utilise the glucose present within the bloodstream:

- This prompts the liver to release further stores of glucose in an effort to maintain normal cell function and homeostasis.
- The results in a further increase in hyperglycaemia.
- In an effort to sustain energy levels and maintain normal function, the body utilises both muscle and fat stores.
- This results in lethargy and weight loss.
- High levels of circulating glucose lead to osmotic diuresis.
- This in turn leads to polyuria, polydipsia, dehydration, severe electrolyte imbalance and coma (if untreated).
- Increased circulating levels of fatty acids lead to hyperlipidaemia (a risk factor for atherosclerosis).
- Fat metabolism results in the production of ketones, an acidic by-product, which are toxic to the body at high levels.

- If left untreated, this leads to diabetic ketoacidosis (DKA), a life-threatening condition that is the leading cause of mortality and morbidity in children and young people with type 1 diabetes. Approximately 25% of children and young people with new-onset diabetes present in DKA (NICE 2004).

The estimated prevalence of type 1 diabetes in the UK is 1 in 700–1000 children, suggesting a current population of 25,000 children and young people under the age of 25 years diagnosed with type 1 diabetes (Department of Health 2007). In Ireland, there are an estimated 3500 children and adolescents with type 1 diabetes (Diabetes Federation of Ireland 2011). The incidence of type 1 diabetes is increasing at an average rate of approximately 3% per year, with the greatest rise noted in those under 4 years old (International Diabetes Federation 2011).

Type 2 diabetes mellitus

Type 2 diabetes develops as a consequence of insulin resistance, reduced insulin production and utilisation, and has been associated with poor lifestyle choices and obesity. Type 2 diabetes tends not to be associated with autoimmunity; however, recent evidence suggests that type 2 diabetes in the young may be as a result of both insulin resistance and autoimmunity.

Type 2 diabetes develops over years and is the progression from normal glucose tolerance to abnormal glucose tolerance (postprandial blood glucose levels increasing first) and eventual fasting hyperglycaemia. The aim of treatment is to control:

- hyperglycaemia, thought to be the determinant of microvascular complications, such as renal and retinal complications;
- hyperlipidaemia, related to insulin resistance, which results in raised low-density lipoprotein (LDL) cholesterol, reduced high-density lipoprotein (HDL) cholesterol, and raised levels of triglycerides and fibrinogen (a thrombotic agent);
- hypertension, more common in people with diabetes and varying between different ethnic, racial and social groups.

The care of patients with type 2 diabetes has been shaped by findings from the UK Prospective Diabetes Study (1998). This landmark 20-year study of 5102 people newly diagnosed with type 2 diabetes showed that the complications of type 2 diabetes, previously regarded as inevitable, could be reduced by improving blood glucose and/or blood pressure control. As all people with type 2 diabetes are at high risk of cardiovascular events, the control of cholesterol attains equal importance. Table 16.6 presents the differing nature of type 1 and type 2 diabetes mellitus.

Management

The primary goal of diabetes care is the maintenance of optimal glycaemic control while ensuring good physical and psychological well-being, as well as normal growth and development (NICE 2004). Patients are required to undertake a complex daily regimen:

- insulin injections (two to four per day);
- blood glucose monitoring (at least before meals and before bed);
- a healthy diet;
- regular exercise.

Diabetes management requires:

- goal-setting;
- dietary and exercise modifications;
- medications;
- self-monitoring of blood glucose;
- monitoring for complications.

Appropriate goal-setting

Patients must be engaged in their own diabetes management, referred to as diabetes self-management. They are involved in their own goal-setting, and receive appropriate support to assist them in making

Table 16.6 Characteristics of type 1 and type 2 diabetes mellitus

Characteristics	Type 1	Type 2
Risk factors	Genetic + Exposure to environmental factors + Exposure to trigger factors	Poor diet Overweight Sedentary lifestyle Genetics ≥40 years of age High-risk ethnic group Previous altered blood glucose metabolism, e.g. gestational diabetes Certain medications
Nature of the illness	An autoimmune condition – beta-cells are destroyed, resulting in an absolute deficiency of insulin	Both insulin inefficiency and insulin deficiency must be present, i.e.: • Inadequate beta-cell insulin production • Peripheral body cells resisting insulin
Symptoms – some overlapping	Fast onset of: • Extremely high blood sugar levels • Weight loss • Hunger • Fatigue • Thirst • Frequent urination	Medium to long onset of: • Dry mouth • Thirst • Nocturia • Fatigue, especially after a meal • Recurrent, difficult to treat infections The patient may have no symptoms The condition is diagnosed on presentation: • In a routine health check • With symptoms of a complication of diabetes
Onset	Quick onset – within a few weeks or months	Slow onset over years
Treatment	Daily self-management of insulin – balancing the effects of food intake and/or exercise on blood sugar levels Multiple injections of insulin or infusion through an insulin pump	Daily self-management of food intake Exercise Medication to enhance insulin usage or/and insulin production May need to use insulin injections
Age of onset	Early childhood or teenage years Can occur at any age	Adults, but can occur at any age
Prevalence in Ireland	16,000–18,000 persons	160,000–180,000 persons

Table 16.6 (*Continued*)

Characteristics	Type 1	Type 2
Complications	Short-term complications give rise to acute emergencies such as: • DKA • Hypoglycaemia (as a side effect of medical management) Long-term exposure to low blood sugar levels can cause hypoglycaemic unawareness Long-term exposure to high blood sugar levels causes micro- and macrovascular changes	May have following complications at diagnosis from damage to the large and small blood vessels, resulting in: • Retinopathy/blindness • Cardiac disease • Kidney disease • Amputation • Gastroparesis • Earlier mortality
Preventable	No	Yes, by as much as 58%, by: • A healthy diet • Keeping the weight under control
Reversible	No	No But easily managed by losing excessive weight and with a healthy diet

lifestyle changes and medical decisions to manage their health. Educating patients on the 'ABC' of diabetes is a common starting point:

- 'A':
  - **A_{1c}** – a glycated haemoglobin (HbA_{1c}) test, a laboratory measurement of the average blood sugar level over the previous 12 weeks, is carried out.
  - The target level should be between 50 and 60 mmol depending on the patient's age and comorbidity.
- 'B':
  - Maintain the **blood pressure** lower than 130/80 mmHg.
  - In the ≥65-year age group with comorbidity, a target of 140/80 mmHg may be appropriate to avoid the risk of nocturnal hypotension.
  - The nursing care of high-risk individuals should include instructions on getting up to a standing position slowly.
- 'C':
  - Total **cholesterol** <4.5 mmol/L.
  - LDL cholesterol <2.5 mmol/L.
  - HDL cholesterol >1.0 mmol/L in males, >1.2 mmol/L in females.
  - Triglycerides <2.0 mmol/L.
  - To reduce the risk of cardiovascular disease, the European Society of Cardiology *et al.* (2007) have set targets for patients with diabetes that are lower than those for the general population.
  - Nurses have an important role in motivating and supporting patients to make lifestyle modifications in order to reach these targets.

There are several nursing interventions that can be made:

- Instruct patients on basic food types and their effect on blood sugar levels.
- Assist in:
  - meal planning to normalise blood sugar levels and meet weight loss targets, if appropriate;
  - designing a personalised physical activity plan.

- Help patients to achieve mastery in glucose testing and insulin administration, if appropriate.
- Advise on the need for diabetes reviews, and stress the importance of regular medical follow-up.
- Instruct patients on good foot care and hygiene to minimise complications.

Dietary modifications

Eighty per cent of people diagnosed with type 2 diabetes are overweight, so dietary advice must include normal healthy eating guidelines and portion size control. It is difficult to determine a diet for all patients, but general guidelines are outlined below.

Only 10% of daily food intake should come from **saturated fats**, i.e. fats that are solid in their natural state, such as animal fats. Simple rules include the following:

- Remove visible fat from meat.
- Reduce fat when cooking by grilling or poaching foods.
- Choose low-fat varieties of daily products such as milk, cheese and yogurt.
- Opt to have poultry on 1 or 2 days a week instead of meat.
- Choose fish on other days.
- Reduce the intake of processed foods such as sausages, puddings and burgers.
- Foods that are 'manufactured' tend to have saturated fats added, as is seen with packets and jars, cans, etc.

Liquid fats are less harmful (except when used in cooking or processing), but should be kept to a minimum.

Refined sugars should be controlled. Nearly all foods contain natural sugar in some form or other; for example, milk contains lactose and fruit contains fructose. A slow absorption of natural sugars into the bloodstream prevents quick increases in blood sugar levels, allowing the insulin present to work more effectively:

- Natural sugars are more complex than processed sugars and take longer to break down in the body.
- Some natural sugars require more energy to break them down, making them less harmful. For example, an apple contains around the same amount of sugar as a biscuit, but it requires more energy to break this down, with the sugar becoming available to the body much more slowly.

There is no place for foods that are labelled as '**suitable for diabetics**', which are low sugar but mostly have additional fats in them. A better alternative is healthy choices or foods labelled as 'diet' on the supermarket shelves. Some pharmacists continue to sell chocolate suitable for diabetics, but a person with diabetes cannot eat unlimited amounts because of the increased fat content and the laxative effect. Indeed, a small amount or regular, good-quality chocolate is less expensive and also preferable. General guidelines for **alcohol** are:

- women: 14 standard drinks per week;
- men: 21 standard drinks per week.

Patients taking insulin or oral hypoglycaemic medication that may cause low blood sugar levels should be advised to alternate their drinks so that some sugar is consumed to prevent hypoglycaemia. To lower their blood pressure, patients may be advised to eat less **salt**:

- Do not add salt to foods.
- Reduce foods that have salt added, for example processed foods.
- Reduce or avoid high-salt foods such as bacon and crisps.

Exercise modification

The benefits of regular exercise for those diagnosed with diabetes (Michaliszyn *et al.* 2009) include:

- increased insulin sensitivity;
- reduced weight gain;

- improved psychological health;
- a reduced risk of cardiovascular disease.

Recommendations for patients with type 1 diabetes are the same as for the general population. The universal recommendations with regard to physical activity are as follows:

- Accumulate at least 30 minutes of moderate intensity physical activity on most days of the week.
- A total of 30 minutes spread over the entire day is equally beneficial to one 30-minute walk.
- Activities of daily living such as housework and using the stairs are valuable in increasing physical activity.

Medications for type 1 diabetes

The aim of insulin therapy in type 1 diabetes is:

- to provide sufficient basal insulin for a 24-hour period;
- to deliver boluses of rapid-acting insulin matched to the carbohydrate content of meals or snacks throughout the day.

Insulin therapy has changed dramatically since it was first used in 1922, with many different insulin products and insulin regimens now being used throughout the world. In the past 10 years, there has been a move to new analogue insulin in the hope that this will lead to improved diabetes care and better outcomes in diabetes. Analogue insulin has a different molecular structure from that of human or animal insulin, leading to a different profile of action when administered subcutaneously (NICE 2004). Insulin therapy needs to be delivered as part of a package of care including diabetes education, specific dietary support, practical instruction and ongoing support for living with diabetes.

Medications for type 2 diabetes

People with type 2 diabetes will generally be taking medication to control hypertension and hyperlipidaemia, and may also be on oral hypoglycaemic agents. The first-line oral hypoglycaemic agents:

- are biguanides, which increase the effectiveness of insulin (e.g. metformin [Glucophage]);
- are introduced when dietary and exercise modifications are unable to achieve appropriate glycaemic control.

Second-line (dual) therapy may then be introduced:

- Failure to achieve glycaemic control using biguanides and lifestyle modifications necessitates the addition of a second drug class.
- Glitazones and dipeptidyl peptidase-4 (DPP-4) inhibitors are the choice for second-line therapy.
- Older sulphonylureas (e.g. gliclazide [Diamicron MR]) are less commonly used; they encourage the pancreas to produce more insulin and are used in non-obese people or when metformin is not well tolerated. Alternative options for these patients or patients with irregular daily blood glucose patterns are the second-generation sulphonureas known as insulin secretagogues (e.g. nateglinide [Starlix]).

There are several alternative medical options:

- Glitazones makes available insulin work more effectively (e.g. rosiglitazone [Avandia]).
- Glucagon-like peptide-1 (GLP-1) receptor agonists delay the breakdown of insulin; they are only available as injectables (e.g. exenatide [Byetta]).
- DPP-4 inhibitors delay the breakdown of insulin and are given orally (e.g. sitagliptin [Januvia]).
- Prandial glucose regulators stimulate extra insulin production when sugar is taken; however, the effects do not last very long and it is only taken with meals (e.g. repaglinide [NovoNorm]).
- Alpha-glucosidase inhibitors help to slow the break-up of food in the digestive system; side effects can include stomach upsets and problems with wind (e.g. acarbose [Glucobay]).

Insulin therapy becomes necessary when other medications fail to achieve adequate control, or when the presence of liver or renal dysfunction contraindicates their usage.

Appropriate self-monitoring of blood glucose

Home blood glucose monitoring (HBGM) is a good educational tool for people with diabetes and may be necessary to prevent acute complications (hypoglycaemia and hyperglycaemia). Not all people with type 2 diabetes will benefit from HBGM, so consideration must be given to the daily stress and inconvenience for the individual compared with the potential benefits. When a person is undertaking HBGM, they should be aware of their target values and what to do when these are not achieved. The target levels for fasting or preprandial capillary plasma glucose should be values below 6.0 mmol/L, or postprandial capillary plasma glucose should be below 8.0 mmol/L, depending on age and comorbidity (Harkins 2008).

Complications

The complications of diabetes may be described as either emergency or long term. The emergency complications of diabetes are classified as:

- hypoglycaemia;
- DKA;
- hyperosmolar hyperglycaemic syndrome (HHS).

Long-term complications include:

- diabetic retinopathy;
- nephropathy;
- neuropathy:
- cardiovascular disease (i.e. myocardial infarction and cerebral vascular accident).

Hypoglycaemia is considered to be any blood glucose level below 4 mmol/L and may be:

- mild – patients experience symptoms and self-treat their low blood glucose levels;
- moderate – patients need help to treat their low blood glucose;
- severe – patients are unconscious or unable to treat their low blood glucose and require a third party to do this for them.

Boxes 16.7 and 16.8 detail the symptoms and treatment of hypoglycaemia.

DKA is a complex disordered metabolic state characterised by hyperglycaemia, acidosis and ketonaemia. It usually occurs as a consequence of absolute or relative insulin deficiency that is accompanied by an increase in counterregulatory hormones (i.e. glucagon, cortisol, growth hormone and epinephrine). This type of hormonal imbalance enhances hepatic gluconeogenesis and glycogenolysis, resulting in severe hyperglycaemia.

Enhanced lipolysis increases serum free fatty acids that are then metabolised as an alternative energy source in the process of ketogenesis, which results in the accumulation of large quantities of ketone bodies and subsequent metabolic acidosis. Ketones include acetone, 3-beta-hydroxybutyrate and acetoacetate. The predominant ketone in DKA is 3-beta-hydroxybutyrate (NHS Diabetes 2010a).

Hyperosmolar hyperglycaemic syndrome (HHS) is one of the most serious acute metabolic complications of type 2 diabetes. The main difference between HHS and DKA is the absence of a build up of

Box 16.7 Symptoms of hypoglycaemia

Autonomic signs/symptoms	Neuroglycopenic symptoms
Pallor	Loss of concentration
A sense of anxiety	Blurred vision
Sweating	Aggressive behaviour
Tremor	Lack of cooperation or confusion
Palpitations (tachycardia)	Seizures
	Transient neurological deficits
	Reduced level of consciousness

keto-acids in the bloodstream, with a more severe fluid loss in HHS, many patients showing a fluid deficit of up to 9 L. As HHS is associated with type 2 diabetes, it is suggested that the presence of small amounts of endogenous insulin inhibits the breakdown of fats, preventing ketosis.

Diabetes is the leading cause of blindness in people of working age in the UK and Ireland. **Diabetic retinopathy** is a complication of diabetes that affects the blood vessels in the retina. Diabetes causes the retinal capillaries to become blocked, resulting in an inhibition of sight. If retinopathy is identified early by retinal screening and treated appropriately, blindness can be prevented in 90% of those at risk.

Box 16.8 Treatment for hypoglycaemia (adapted from NHS Diabetes 2010b)

Mild hypoglycaemia
(Adults who are conscious, orientated and able to swallow)

Step 1

- Immediate action:
- Give 15 g fast-acting carbohydrate using one of the following:
    - 100 mL of Lucozade
    - 150 mL of any non-diet drink
    - 150 mL of pure fruit juice
    - 3–5 glucose tablets
    - 3–4 regular sweets, e.g. jelly babies
- Wait 10–15 minutes for the sugar to be absorbed into the bloodstream
- If, after 10 minutes, the blood sugar is:
    - Still <4 mmol/L, a sugary option from the above list should be given again
    - > 4 mmol/L, proceed with Step 2

Step 2

- The actions outlined in Step 1 must be followed by a slow-acting carbohydrate snack, which may be any one of the following:
    - A roll/sandwich
    - A portion of fruit
    - A cereal bar
    - Two plain biscuits
    - A meal if it is due

Moderate hypoglycaemia
(Adults who are conscious but confused, disorientated, unable to cooperate or aggressive, or have an unsteady gait, but are able to swallow)

- If the patient is capable and cooperative, follow the treatment outlined for mild hypoglycaemia
- If the patient is not capable and/or is uncooperative but is able to swallow, give either:
    - 1.5–2 tubes of Glucogel or Dextrogel squeezed into the mouth between the teeth and gums; if this is ineffective give:
    - Glucagon 1 mg intramuscularly (although this may be less effective in patients who are prescribed sulphonylurea therapy)
- Monitor the blood glucose level after 15 minutes – if it is still <4.0 mmol/L, repeat the treatment (up to three times)
- If the blood glucose level remains <4.0 mmol/L after 45 minutes (or three cycles of initial treatment), consider intravenous 10% glucose infusion at 100 mL per hour
- Once the blood glucose is >4.0 mmol/L and the patient has recovered, follow Step 2 for mild hypoglycaemia

DO NOT omit an insulin injection if it is due (although a dose review may be required)

- NB: Patients given glucagon require a larger portion of long-acting carbohydrate to replenish their glycogen stores (double the amount suggested above)
- Ensure regular capillary blood glucose level monitoring is continued for 24–48 hours, whether at home or in hospital. Give hypoglycaemia education or refer the patient to a diabetes specialist nurse

(Continued)

Severe hypoglycaemia
(Adults who are unconscious and/or having seizures and/or are very aggressive)

- Check the:
  - Airway
  - Breathing
  - Circulation
- Call an ambulance, or if in hospital seek medical help immediately
- If in hospital, the following three options are all appropriate (adhering to local hospital policy):
  - Glucagon 1 mg intramuscularly (although it may be less effective in patients prescribed sulphonylurea therapy). Glucagon may take up to 15 minutes to take effect. It mobilises glycogen from the liver and will not work if given repeatedly or in starved patients with no glycogen stores, or those with severe liver disease. If this is the situation or if prolonged treatment is required, intravenous glucose is better
  - If intravenous access is available, give 75 mL of 20% glucose (over 12 minutes):
    - — repeat the capillary blood glucose measurement 10 minutes later
    - — if the blood glucose is <4.0 mmol/L, repeat the treatment
  - If intravenous access is available, give 150 mL of 10% glucose (over 12 minutes):
    - — repeat the capillary blood glucose measurement 10 minutes later;
    - — if the blood glucose is <4.0 mmol/L, repeat the treatment
- Once the blood glucose is >4.0 mmol/L and the patient has recovered, follow Step 2 for mild hypoglycaemia
- Ensure regular capillary blood glucose level monitoring is continued for 24–48 hours, whether at home or in hospital
- Give hypoglycaemia education or refer the patient to a diabetes specialist nurse

Neuropathy is nerve damage. There are three different types of neuropathy: sensory, autonomic and motor. Each type will affect the body in different ways, for example loss of feeling, erectile dysfunction or disrupted movement.

Nephropathy is kidney damage and is a microvascular complication associated with diabetes mellitus. This condition mainly affects the glomerulus of the kidney, leading to basement membrane thickening and expansion of the mesangium, which results in a declining glomerular filtration rate and ultimately renal failure. No protein can usually leak through the renal glomeruli; however, long-term high blood sugar and/or high blood pressure causes stresses in the walls of the glomeruli, allowing progressively larger protein molecules to pass through. All people with diabetes from puberty are routinely prescribed renoprotective antihypertensive agents. Nurses have a responsibility to help patients understand the importance of taking this medication, even when they are not hypertensive.

Angiopathy is disease of the blood vessels (arteries, veins and capillaries). Long-term exposure to high blood sugars causes inflammation of the blood vessels and contributes to the build-up of fatty plaques within them. Microangiopathy occurs when smaller blood vessel walls become weak and thick, for example in retinopathy. Macroangiopathy occurs when fat and blood clots build up in larger blood vessels, adhere to the walls and impede the blood flow; this is seen in, for example, cardiovascular disease.

Gestational diabetes is diabetes that is diagnosed in pregnancy and disappears immediately after delivery. It is due to changes in glucose metabolism during pregnancy as a direct result of the antagonistic effect of pregnancy hormones.

Conclusion

This chapter has endeavoured to provide readers with a basic knowledge of many common disorders of the endocrine system. It addresses the challenges nurses encounter when caring for patients with complex endocrine disorders and provides an overview of relevant nursing management. The chapter should not be considered sufficient in itself and should be used in conjunction with other published material in order to ensure further development of knowledge gained.

Visit www.wileyfundamentalseries.com/medicalnursing and read Reflective Questions 16.1 and 16.2 to think more about this topic.

Now visit the companion website and test yourself on this chapter:
www.wileyfundamentalseries.com/medicalnursing

References

American Diabetes Association (2011) Standards of medical care in diabetes. *Diabetes Care*, **34**(Suppl. 1):S11–61.

Department of Health, Diabetes Policy Team (2007) *Making Every Young Person with Diabetes Matter*. London: Department of Health.

Diabetes Federation of Ireland (2011) *Diabetes in Ireland*. Retrieved 5th July 2011 from http://www.diabetesaction.ie/diabetes-in-ireland.

DIAMOND Project Group (2006) Incidence and trends of childhood diabetes worldwide 1990–1999. *Diabetic Medicine*, **23**:857–66.

European Society of Cardiology and Other Societies on Cardiovascular Disease Prevention in Clinical Practice (2007) *European Guidelines on Cardiovascular Disease Prevention in Clinical Practice*. ESC, Sophia Antipolis Cedex.

Harkins, V. (2008) *A Practical Guide to Integrated Type 2 Diabetes Care*. Kildare: Health Service Executive.

International Diabetes Federation (2011) *World Atlas of Diabetes*. Retrieved December 2011 from http://www.eatlas.idf.org.

Michaliszyn, F.S., Shaibi, G.Q., Quinn, L. *et al.* (2009) Physical fitness, dietary intake and metabolic control in adolescents with type 1 diabetes. *Pediatric Diabetes*, **10**:389–94.

National Institute for Clinical Excellence (2004) *Type 1 Diabetes: Diagnosis and Management of Type 1 Diabetes in Children, Young People and Adults*. Clinical Guideline No. 15. London: NICE.

National Institute for Health and Clinical Excellence (2009) *Diabetes Update*. London: NICE.

NHS Diabetes (2010a) *Joint British Diabetes Societies Inpatient Care Group Guidance on the Management of Diabetic Ketoacidosis*. London: NHS Diabetes.

NHS Diabetes (2010b) *The Hospital Management of Hypoglycaemia in Adults*. London: NHS Diabetes.

UK Prospective Diabetes Study Group (1998) Tight blood pressure control and risk of macrovascular and microvascular complications in type 2 diabetes: UKPDS 38. *British Medical Journal*, **317**:703–13.

17

Nursing care of conditions related to the neurological system

Elaine Pierce[1] and Mary E. Braine[2]

[1]London South Bank University, London, UK
[2]College of Health and Social Care, University of Salford, Manchester, UK

Contents

Introduction	327
Anatomy and physiology	327
Investigations	337
Nursing assessment of the neurological system	338
Traumatic brain injury and raised ICP	340
Intracranial tumours	343
Cerebrovascular disorders	347
Epilepsy	349
Infections of the neurological system	353
Multiple sclerosis	355
Motor neuron disease	356
Parkinson's disease	358
Alzheimer's disease	359
Conclusion	362
References	363

Learning outcomes

Having read this chapter, you will be able to:

- Describe the anatomy and physiology of the neurological system
- Discuss the components of a neurological assessment
- List important investigations required to diagnose neurological conditions
- Outline the medical and nursing management of common neurological disorders

Fundamentals of Medical-Surgical Nursing: A Systems Approach, First Edition. Edited by Anne-Marie Brady, Catherine McCabe, and Margaret McCann.

Introduction

The nervous system is one of the most complex body systems, controlling and integrating all other body systems. An understanding of this complex system underpins many aspects of patient care. This chapter includes an overview of the anatomy and physiology of the central and peripheral nervous systems and appropriate management plans for key neurological disorders.

Anatomy and physiology

This system receives and processes information and initiates actions through an intricate network of specialised cells called neurons (nerves). It regulates, controls and coordinates the actions and activities of all body systems, thereby maintaining homeostasis. The nervous system has two parts:

- the central nervous system (CNS) – the brain and spinal cord;
- the peripheral nervous system (PNS) – the cranial and spinal neurons.

The PNS refers to neurons outside the CNS and consists of the somatic and autonomic nervous systems, which can be subdivided into sympathetic and parasympathetic (Figure 17.1).

Cells

The cells of the neurological system are:

- the neuroglia (glia), which support, nourish and protect the neurons (Table 17.1);
- the neurons (nerves), a given neuron communicating with and being connected to other neurons and cells in the body (Table 17.2 and Figure 17.2).

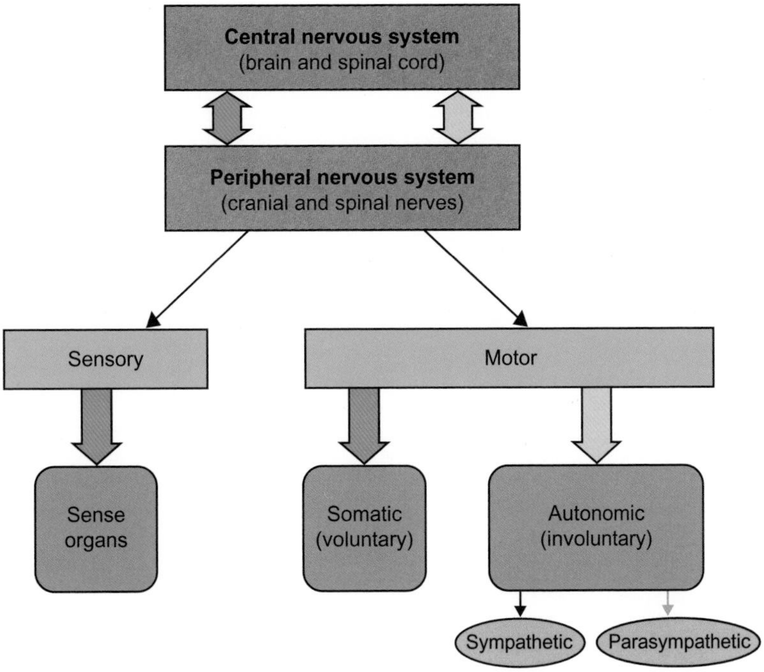

Figure 17.1 Divisions of the human nervous system. Reproduced from Nair, M. & Peate, I. (2009) *Fundamentals of Applied Pathophysiology*, with kind permission from Wiley Blackwell.

Table 17.1 Neuroglia

Neuroglia	Description	Function	Location
Polydendrocytes	Recently discovered	Are the stem cells of the CNS Generate both glia and neurons	CNS
Macroglia	Astrocytes: • Are star-shaped • Have many processes • Are the biggest, most numerous glia • Can be reactive • Are known as astroglia when clumped together	Fill the spaces between the neurons (supportive role) Regulate extracellular chemicals and ions Transport glucose and other substances from the blood Reactive astrocytes together with microglia respond to injury	CNS
	Oligodendroglia: • The cytoplasm and nucleus are more dense than in astrocytes • Have smaller and fewer processes than astrocytes	Provide support to axons Produce myelin/myelin sheath to insulate the axons	CNS and PNS
	Schwann cells – the equivalent of oligodendrocytes in the PNS	As above Also facilitate neuronal regeneration after injury	PNS
Microglia	Are small round cells Have many processes and little cytoplasm Are resting or active/reactive	Have a phagocytic macrophage function in response to injury or invasion of pathogens	CNS
Ependymal cells	Line the ventricles and central canal of the spinal cord	Are involved with the directional flow of cerebrospinal fluid, which facilitates the transport of nutrients and removal of waste	CNS

Table 17.2 Neuronal components

Component of neuron	Description	Function
Cell body (perikaryon)	Is the enlarged portion of the nerve cell from which the dendrites and axon extend Is greyish in colour	The nucleus produces all neurotransmitters, hormones and proteins
Dendrites	Are hair-like structures or processes Extend from the cell body The ends have synaptic knobs	Conduct incoming signals Synaptic knobs form connections with adjacent neurons
Axon (nerve fibre)	Extends from the cell body The length varies (millimetre to metre) Has processes or branches at its end	Conducts outgoing signals
Schwann cell	See Table 17.1	
Myelin sheath	A fat-like sheath Is composed of a complex mix of protein and phospholipids (fat) Is white in colour	Surrounds and protects the axon Acts as an insulator Increases the rate of impulse transmission
Nodes of Ranvier	Gaps occurring at regular intervals in the myelin sheath that surrounds the axon	Assist impulse transmission through repolarisation and depolarisation of the nerve membrane Allow entry of nutrients Allow exit of waste
Synapse	The small gap between the axon of one cell and the dendrite of another	Releases neurotransmitters, such as acetylcholine or dopamine

Impulses or action potentials are received by the dendrites and cell bodies of one neuron and transmitted in a firing pattern, via the axon, to the next neuron. Action potentials are responsible for the release of neurotransmitters at the synapse. Axons can be myelinated or unmyelinated.

The different types, locations and functions of neurons are outlined in Table 17.3. Neuronal cell bodies, found in groups in the CNS called nuclei, make up the grey matter. Elsewhere in the body, these groups are called ganglia. The axons of the cell groups form the white matter.

The brain

The brain consists of over 100 billion neurons, accounts for 2% of body mass and in adults weighs approximately 1.3–1.5 kg. The main divisions of the brain are outlined in Figure 17.3 and Table 17.4.

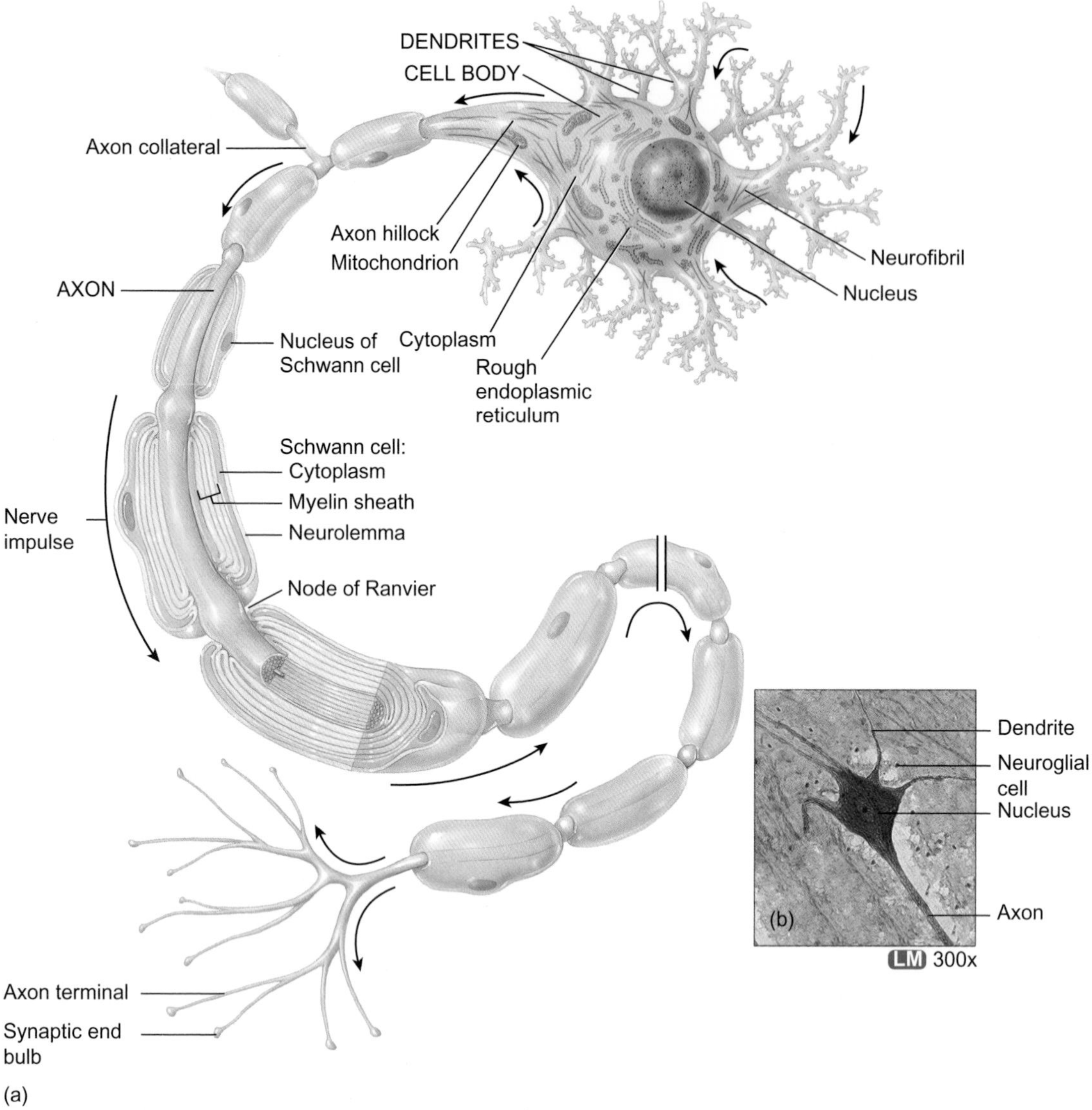

Figure 17.2 (a) Parts of a neuron. (b) Motor neuron. LM, light microscope. Reproduced from Tortora, G.J., Derrickson, B. (2011) *Principles of Anatomy and Physiology*, with kind permission of Wiley Blackwell.

Table 17.3 Types of neuron

Type	Location	Function
Motor (efferent)	CNS and PNS Originate in the brainstem and spinal cord	Are controlled by the motor areas of the brainstem and the cerebral cortex, and influenced by the basal ganglia and cerebellum Transmit impulses from the CNS to muscles and glands within the body
Sensory (afferent)	PNS and CNS Originate in the sensory organs	Transmit impulses from the sensory organs and other parts to the CNS These are processed by relay nuclei, including the thalamus, before being analysed by the cortex
Mixed	PNS and CNS Include most large nerves, e.g. the brachial and spinal nerves	Consist of both sensory and motor nerves
Relay	CNS	Transmit impulses generated by stimuli to other neurons within the CNS

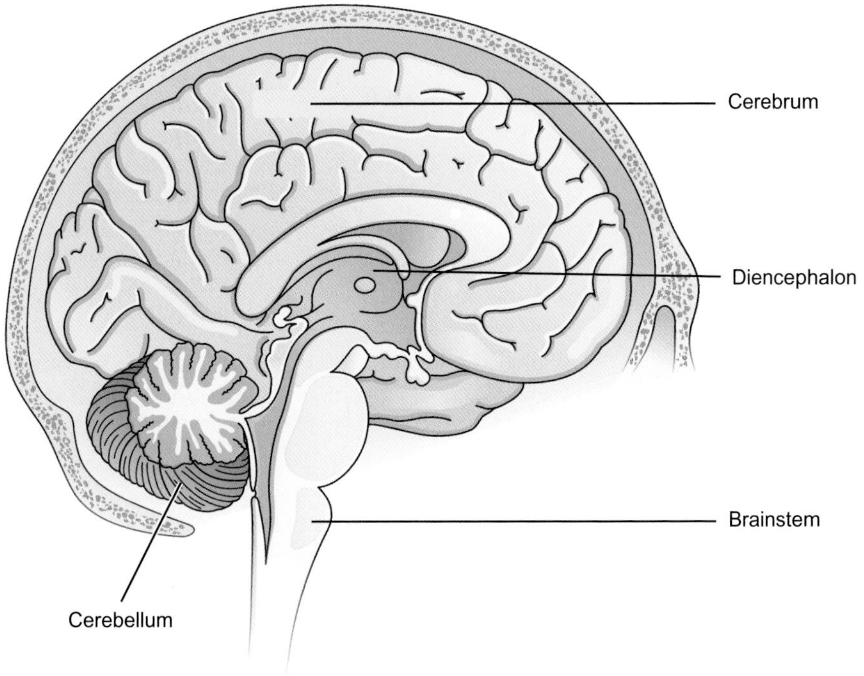

Figure 17.3 The four main parts of the human brain. Reproduced from Nair, M. & Peate, I. (2009) *Fundamentals of Applied Pathophysiology*, with kind permission from Wiley Blackwell.

Table 17.4 The brain

<table>
<tr><th>Main division</th><th colspan="2">Function</th></tr>
<tr><td rowspan="5">Cerebrum
The largest division
Is divided into the right and left cerebral hemispheres
The two hemispheres:
• Are 'twins'
• Are connected by the corpus callosum
• Receive sensory (afferent) impulses
• Initiate motor (efferent) impulses
• Are made up of grey matter (outside) and white matter (inside)
• Are subdivided into four further lobes
The left lobe of the cerebrum sends and receives information from the right side of the body
The right lobe sends and receives information from the left side of the body
Contains the basal ganglia</td><td>Lobe</td><td>Function</td></tr>
<tr><td>Frontal</td><td>Controls fine movements and smell
Is the centre for abstract thinking and judgement
In the left hemisphere, incorporates the language centre for expressive and motor speech</td></tr>
<tr><td>Parietal</td><td>Coordinates sensory information (spatial orientation and perception)
Deals with:
• Pain
• Form
• Temperature
• Shape
• Texture
• Pressure
• Position
Has some memory function (in the receptive aspects of language)</td></tr>
<tr><td>Temporal</td><td>Responsible for:
• Dreams
• Memory
• Emotions
• Learning
Centre for auditory function (processing auditory information)</td></tr>
<tr><td>Occipital</td><td>Responsible for vision and the recognition of objects</td></tr>
<tr><td>Cerebellum
The second largest division
Is found below the cerebrum
Is composed of two hemispheres
Has an outer cortex of grey matter
Receives and sends impulses via the brainstem
Incoming information is received from the cortex via the pons
Outgoing information goes to the cortex via the thalamus</td><td colspan="2">Balance
Muscle tension
Fine motor control
Eye movement
Equilibrium of the trunk
Spinal nerve reflexes
Posture and balance of the limbs</td></tr>
</table>

Table 17.4 (*Continued*)

Main division	Function	
Diencephalon Located between the cerebrum and the midbrain Contains two important structures: • Thalamus • Hypothalamus	**Structure**	**Function**
	Thalamus: • An egg-shaped mass of grey matter • Divided into right and left parts	Is the main synaptic relay centre and processes motor information; acts as the 'gatekeeper' to the cerebral cortex Receives and relays sensory information to and from the cerebral cortex
	Hypothalamus: • A collection of ganglia • Is located below the thalamus • Is closely associated with the pituitary gland	Senses change in body temperature Regulates sympathetic and parasympathetic nervous systems Controls the pituitary gland Regulates appetite Is part of the arousal/alerting mechanism
Brainstem Consists of: • Medulla oblongata • Pons • Midbrain (mesencephalon of cerebral peduncles) The medulla is the most important All functions of the brainstem are associated with cranial nerves III–XII	**Structure**	**Function**
	Medulla and pons Medulla	Breathing, respiration Heart rate, blood pressure, vomiting, coughing, swallowing, hiccupping, sneezing
	Midbrain and pons	Reflex centres for the pupils and eye movements

Blood supply

The main arteries supplying the brain (Figure 17.4) are:

- two internal carotid arteries;
- two vertebral arteries, which join to become the basilar artery.

Both set of arteries give rise to the arteries that form the circle of Willis (Figure 17.5).

The coverings of the brain and spinal cord

The brain and spinal cord are covered by three membranes (the meninges):

- the dura mater – the thick outer fibrous membrane, which has two layers and contains large venous sinuses;
- the arachnoid mater – the middle thin avascular membrane, which is covered with mesothelial cells and has arachnoid villi or granulations that project into the venous sinuses and veins;
- the pia mater – the thin inner fibrous membrane, which is attached to the surface of the brain and the spinal cord. It is connected to the arachnoid mater by delicate fibrous trabeculae.

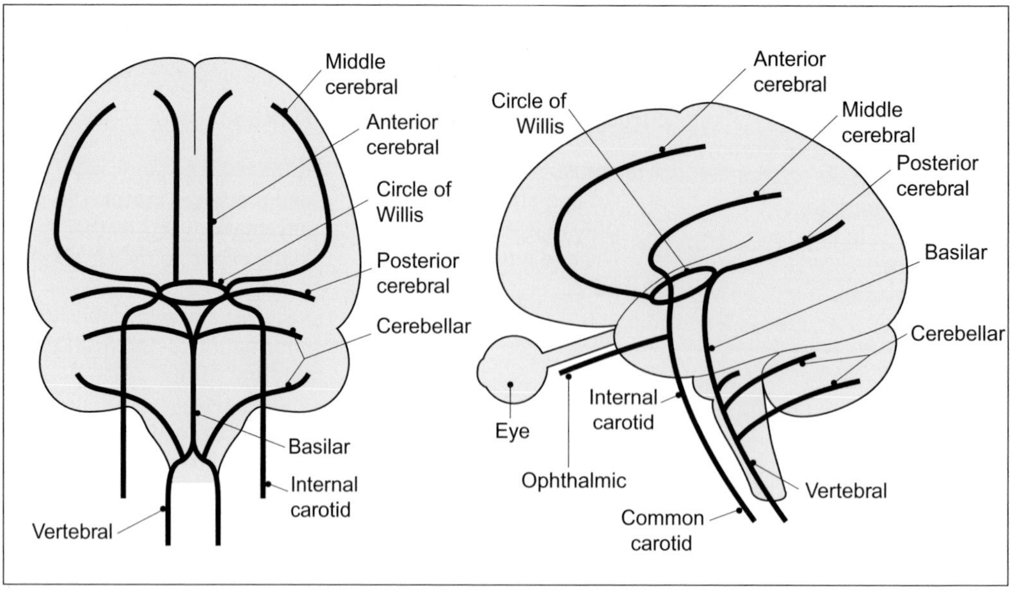

Figure 17.4 The arteries supplying the brain. Reproduced from Wilkinson & Lennox (2005) *Essential Neurology*, with kind permission of Wiley Blackwell.

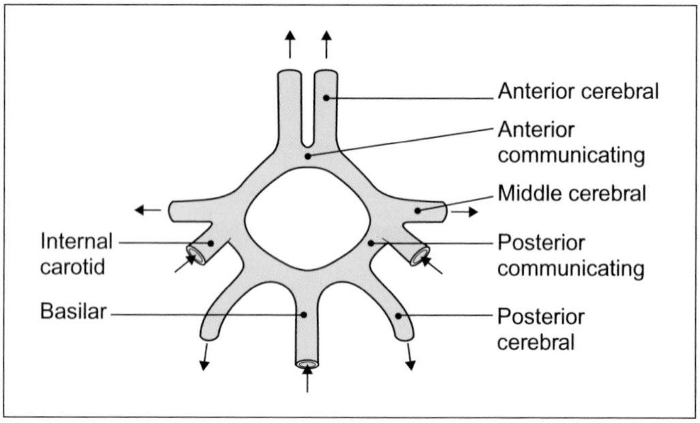

Figure 17.5 The circle of Willis. Reproduced from Wilkinson & Lennox (2005) *Essential Neurology*, with kind permission of Wiley Blackwell.

Cerebrospinal fluid

About 400–500 mL of cerebrospinal fluid (CSF) is produced each day by the specialised ependymal cells in the choroid plexus of the brain. The CSF is clear and colourless and flows in the subarachnoid space (between the arachnoid and the pia) in a unidirectional flow. Its functions are to:

- remove waste and potentially noxious substances such as drugs;
- lubricate the meninges and provide frictionless movement of the brain;
- cushion and protect against impact injury.

The blood–brain/CSF barrier

The blood–brain barrier (BBB) and the CSF barrier act to regulate the exchange of substances entering the brain in order to maintain optimum levels of, for example, glucose, proteins and electrolytes for normal brain activities. The function of the endothelial cells is to filter and restrict the diffusion and permeation of molecules in order to protect the brain against harmful toxins and metabolites. Although neurologically protective, it can, however, be a hindrance as it allows, for example, the entry of small or fatty (lipid) molecules such as some viruses and toxins (carbon monoxide), and limits the entry of larger molecules like therapeutic drugs (e.g. antibiotics and antiepileptic medication).

The spinal cord

The spinal cord is a continuation of the medulla oblongata and extends to the lower back or about two-thirds down the vertebral column, which protects it. The vertebral column is made up of 33 vertebrae (7 cervical, 12 thoracic, 5 lumbar, 5 sacral and 4 coccygeal, although the sacral and coccygeal vertebrae are fused). There are 31 pairs of spinal nerves (their names relating to where they enter or exit the vertebrae), which transmit impulses to and from various parts of the body (Figure 17.6).

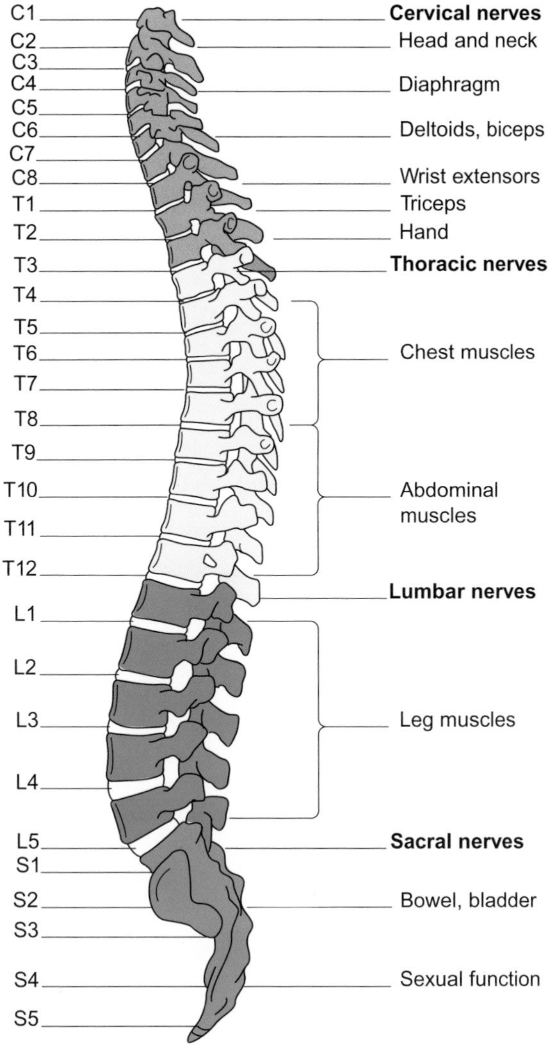

Figure 17.6 The spinal nerves and their areas of innervations. Reproduced from Woodward & Mestecky (2011) *Neuroscience Nursing: Evidence Based Practice*, with kind permission of Wiley Blackwell.

The cranial neurons

There are 12 pairs of cranial nerves (I–XII), the majority of their functions relating to structures within the head and neck; however, the functions of three cranial nerves extend beyond these areas (Table 17.5).

Table 17.5 Cranial nerves (type and function)

Number	Name	Motor (M) or sensory (S)	Function
I	Olfactory	S	Sense of smell
II	Optic	S	Sensory function of the retina
*III	Oculomotor	Mainly M with some S	Most eye movements Pupillary constriction
*IV	Trochlear		Downward and inward eye movements
*VI	Abducens		Lateral eye movements
V	Trigeminal (has three branches): • Ophthalmic • Maxillary • Mandibular	M, S	Cornea Face Mouth Jaw
VII	Facial	M, S	Facial muscles Lacrimal glands Salivary glands Taste
VIII	Known as: • Acoustic • Auditory, or • Vestibulocochlear	M, S	Hearing Equilibrium Balance Body position Orientation to space
IX	Glossopharyngeal	M, S	Coordination of swallowing Sensation in the pharynx Taste Salivation
X	Vagus	M, S	Controls swallowing, phonation and movement of the soft palate and uvula Sensation of the mucosa of the pharynx, soft palate, tonsils, viscera of the thorax and abdomen Smooth muscles of the thorax and abdomen
XI	Spinal accessory	M, S	Sternocleidomastoid muscles Upper trapezius Palate and pharyngeal muscles
XII	Hypoglossal	M, S	Tongue movement in swallowing and speech

*These three neurons are usually grouped together because they are concerned with eye movement.

Investigations

Following physical and neurological examinations, a number of diagnostic tests may be ordered to investigate any abnormal findings. The least invasive procedures are normally carried out first, proceeding to more invasive investigations. These investigations can be anxiety-provoking for both patients and their families. Nurses need to provide:

- emotional support to patients by educating them on the procedure;
- relevant nursing care before, during and after the procedure.

Radiological examinations

Radiological examinations include the following:

- Skull and spine X-rays, used to identify:
  - fractures;
  - displacement of the vertebrae;
  - spinal curves;
  - tissue displacement.
- Computed tomography (CT) scans:
  - which may require an injection of contrast medium prior to the scan to provide anatomical clarity;
  - however, no additional nursing preparation is needed; close observation is not required unless patients' consciousness is impaired.
- Magnetic resonance imaging (MRI):
  - identify any contraindications such as medical or electronic devices (e.g. pacemakers, cochlear implants and metal pins);
  - remove jewellery, hairclips and any metal objects as they interfere with the magnetic field of the MRI scanner;
  - patients need to remain still during the scanning process, which may take up to 20 minutes.

Cerebral blood flow tests

These can be non-invasive or invasive procedures, and are used to visualise blood vessels in the brain and neck. In CT angiography (CTA) and magnetic resonance angiography (MRA):

- MRA is performed with or without the injection of contrast medium;
- CTA involves the injection of contrast medium via a peripheral cannula followed by a series of images of the cerebral vessels being taken.

Cerebral angiography is an invasive procedure, undertaken with or without sedation, that involves the injection of contrast medium usually via catheterisation of the femoral artery. Patients may need to be nil by mouth for a period of time before the procedure. Specific nursing considerations include:

- regular neurological observations including vital signs, both before and after the procedure;
- assessment of the puncture site for haemorrhage and haematoma;
- bed rest, usually for 4 hours after the procedure.

Neurophysiology tests

Neurophysiology tests such as nerve conduction studies, electromyograms (EMGs), evoked potentials (EPs) and electroencephalograms (EEGs) are usually performed by clinical neurophysiologists:

- EMG and nerve conduction studies test the integrity and functioning of the skeletal muscles and large myelinated nerve fibres in the arms and legs.

- EPs measure the brain's response to particular stimuli; for example, visually evoked potentials measure the visual pathway from the retina to the occipital cortex.
- EEGs are used to measure the electrical activity of the brain.
- Lumbar puncture:
  - is used to measure CSF pressure and obtain a sample of CSF by inserting a spinal needle into the subarachnoid space of the spinal canal, usually between the L3–L4 or L4–L5 vertebrae, once a local anaesthetic has taken effect;
  - is normally performed at the patient's bed, with the patient lying on their left side with their knees drawn up to their chest;
  - involves observations being recorded after the procedure;
  - involves patients being encouraged to rest and drink plenty of fluids.
- A muscle biopsy is indicated if the integrity of the muscle unit is disrupted.

Nursing assessment of the neurological system

Glasgow Coma Scale

The Glasgow Coma Scale (GCS; Teasdale and Jennett 1974) is an assessment instrument that is extensively used before and after patients arrive at hospital, and provides an indication of the initial severity of trauma to the brain and its subsequent changes over time.

Damage to or a lesion in the cerebral hemisphere impairs its function so that it is unable to respond to afferent stimuli. Damage in the brainstem not only affects the structures there, but also limits or stops the access of afferent neurons to the cerebral hemispheres. Impaired pupillary reactions to light and pupillary dilatation may indicate damage or a lesion in the midbrain. The GCS assessment (Figure 17.7) provides a framework for eliciting information on the following:

Neurological Observation Chart																			
Glasgow Coma Scale	Eye opening	Open spontaneously (4)	•																(C) = Eyes closed due to swelling
		Open to speech (3)		•	•														
		Open to pain (2)				•	•												
		Closed (1)						•	•	•									
	Verbal response	Orientated (5)																	(T) = intubated
		Confused (4)	•	•	•														
		Inappropriate words (3)				•	•												
		Incomprehensible sounds (2)						•	•										
		No verbal response (1)								•									
		Obeys commands (6)	•	•															
	Motor response	Localises to pain (5)			•														Record best arm response
		Flexion withdrawal (4)				•	•												
		Abnormal flexion (3)						•											
		Extension to pain (2)							•										
		No movement (1)								•									
		Total (out of 15)	14	13	12	9	9	6	5	3									

Figure 17.7 Documentation of the GCS. Reproduced from Woodward & Mestecky (2011) *Neuroscience Nursing: Evidence Based Practice*, with kind permission of Wiley Blackwell.

- Eye opening
- Verbal response
- Best motor response

} Derived from a score in the ranges 1–4 (eye), 1–5 (verbal) and 1–6 (motor), known as the Glasgow Coma Score (total 15)

- Vital functions, such as respiration, blood pressure, temperature and pulse
- Pupil size
- Pupillary reactivity.

The Glasgow Coma Score

The score is used as an indication of neurological status and to monitor any changes effectively. The maximum score of 15 indicates that patients are fully conscious, alert and responsive. The minimum score of 3 indicates comatose and unresponsive patients. Scores may be affected for other reasons:

- The eyes may be closed due to severe swelling.
- The verbal and motor responses may be absent or reduced as a result of:
  - intubation;
  - muscle relaxants;
  - sedation.

Vital signs

Abnormal vital signs indicate problems in the pons and/or medulla. An increase in temperature, pulse, respiration and blood pressure denotes autonomic dysregulation. The initial measurements of respiration, blood pressure, temperature and pulse will form the baseline for monitoring and assessing deterioration or improvement. For head-injured patients, the National Institute for Health and Excellence [NICE] (2007) recommend:

- half-hourly observations if the Glasgow Coma Score is less than 15;
- once the Glasgow Coma Score reaches 15 or above, half-hourly observations for 2 hours;
- followed by hourly observations for 4 hours;
- and thereafter 2-hourly observations;
- but should patients with a Glasgow Coma Score of 15 deteriorate at any time after the initial 2-hour period, observations should revert to half-hourly and follow the above pattern again.

A similar or modified version of this approach could be used for other neurological conditions or after anaesthesia or neurosurgery, depending on local policy. Staff using the GCS should be adequately trained and have the necessary skills and experience to recognise changes. Individual components of the assessment should be adequately described and communicated, both verbally and in writing. For example, patients with a total score of 13 (4 for eye-opening, 4 for verbal response and 5 for motor response) should be reported as E4, V4 and M5 (NICE 2007).

The rate, depth and pattern of respiration should be closely observed. Shallow, rapid respirations, low blood pressure and tachycardia may result from a reduced circulating volume following surgery or injury. If patients require oxygen, their oxygen saturation should be maintained to avoid hypoxia, which leads to reduced cerebral blood flow (CBF). If blood flow to any part of the brain is reduced, the following can occur:

- ischaemia;
- a reversible loss of function;
- if it is prolonged and/or severe, infarction and irreversible cell death.

Ischaemic brain damage with swelling results from a combination of hypotension and hypoxia.

A 1°C increase in temperature increases the cerebral metabolic rate by 10%, which can affect neurological recovery. Pyrexia may denote infection from surgical and/or non-surgical sources. Reducing the body temperature in traumatic brain-injured patients significantly lowers raised intracranial pressure (ICP). Raised ICP can have deleterious effects; however, **any** changes in temperature should be reported and monitored.

Traumatic brain injury and raised ICP

Traumatic brain injury (TBI) or head injury refers to any injury to the scalp, skull (cranium or facial bones) or brain that disrupts the function of the brain, patients' life and the lives of their families and caregivers. TBI is a leading cause of mortality and morbidity in young people, and is a major ethical and social burden with regard to long-term disability and social economic costs. TBI can be classified according to the mechanism of injury (how it occurred):

- An open (penetrating) head injury occurs when the outer layer of the meninges is breached (e.g. by a knife or bullet).
- A closed head injury is one that occurs without the integrity of the skull being compromised.

TBI can also be divided into:

- the primary injury (induced by a mechanical force):
  - acceleration injury – the head is struck by a moving object;
  - deceleration injury – the head hits a stationary object;
  - acceleration–deceleration injury – the head hits an object and the brain 'rebounds' within the skull;
  - injuries to the brain including concussion, contusion and diffuse axonal injury;
  - intracranial haemorrhage, including haematomas; this can be extradural, subdural or intracerebral;
  - injuries to the skull (including fractures);
- secondary injuries:
  - occurring after the initial injury as a result of progression events, which affect the perfusion and oxygenation of the brain cells;
  - most commonly occurring as a result of brain swelling, with an increase in ICP (Box 17.1);
  - if the raised ICP is left untreated, a decrease in cerebral perfusion leads to ischaemia;
  - the ability to cope with an increase in ICP differing from person to person and ultimately being dependent on the compliance of the brain tissue.

The leading causes of TBI are falls, road traffic accidents and assaults. Three age groups are at highest risk of TBI, those aged:

- 1–4 years;
- 15–24 years (with TBIs being more common in males than females);
- over 70–75 years.

Management

A CT scan of the brain is the main diagnostic test for any person with a suspected intracranial injury. In the early assessment, the mnemonic ABCDE is used to prioritise the initial treatment (Box 17.2).

Box 17.1 Symptoms of raised ICP

- Altered mental status
- A progressive deterioration in consciousness
- Nausea and vomiting, usually in the morning, with an accompanying headache
- A headache that is often worse on waking in the morning (due to lying flat and the ICP typically increasing at night), and worse on coughing or moving the head
- Restlessness, weakness and incoordination
- Pupillary changes, including irregularity, i.e. changes in pupil size or dilatation in one eye with impaired reactivity to light, a sluggish pupillary reaction to direct light or no response
- Other late signs include 'Cushing's response' (hypertension, a widening pulse pressure, bradycardia and irregular respiration)
- Papilloedema (optic disc swelling) and fundal haemorrhage

The classification of TBIs is important in determining treatment and rehabilitation plans and for patient outcomes, including prognosis and long-term disability. TBIs are graded according to their severity (Table 17.6), based on several parameters including:

- duration of loss of consciousness (LOC);
- level of consciousness, as per the GCS, at the time of the injury;
- the length of time (after the injury) that the patient remains in a post-traumatic amnesic state, which is a period of confusion and disorientation after emergence from coma.

Box 17.2 The ABCDE

Airway – intubation may be required for patients with severe TBI (Glasgow Coma Score <8)
Breathing – maintain oxygenation and normocapnia
Circulation:

- Measure the heart rate and blood pressure
- Treat hypotension, aiming for a target mean arterial pressure (MAP) of over 80 mmHg

Disability – GCS assessment to detect changes in level of consciousness, and to assess the severity of the injury
Exposure and environment – look for signs of injury, e.g. scalp wounds

Table 17.6 TBI grading

Grade of TBI	GCS score	Duration of post-traumatic amnesia	Length of LOC	Morbidity
Mild • Referred to as concussion • Frequently missed or not diagnosed	13–15	<1 hour	<30 minutes	May not result in mild consequences Post-concussive syndrome: • Short-term memory problems • Concentration difficulties
Moderate	9–13 Lethargic or stuporous	30 minutes to 24 hours	1–24 hours	May have focal neurological deficits Can display a wide spectrum of physical, cognitive and behavioural impairments
Severe	3–8 Comatose Unable to open the eyes or follow commands	Severe: 1–7 days Very severe: 1–4 weeks Extremely severe: >4 weeks	>24 hours	Permanent neurological sequelae Functional disability

Data from Teasdale and Jennett (1974), Jennett and Teasdale (1981) and Greenwald *et al.* (2003).

Individualised multidisciplinary care that is initiated early and continued throughout the patient's journey is critical in maximising recovery and reducing long-term disability. Physical disabilities are varied, depending on the severity and area of injury. Patients may experience:

- language and swallowing problems;
- impaired mobility and coordination;
- visual and sleep disturbances;
- a number of cognitive, behavioural and emotional difficulties.

These difficulties can negatively impact on patients establishing productive and satisfying lifestyles, and can affect family members and caregivers, causing caregiver burden, distress and a sense of loss (Braine 2011). Care for patients after a TBI should start as early as possible and includes:

- individualised rehabilitation interventions aimed at promoting functional recovery;
- the prevention and treatment of secondary complications;
- control of CBF, which is the focus of care strategies and forms the basis of patient management.

Patients who sustain a moderate or severe TBI require close monitoring, as well as medical management strategies aimed at minimising secondary injury. This may require patients to be cared for in intensive care units where they can be closely observed and systematically monitored. Table 17.7 provides detailed information on the nursing management of patients with a TBI and raised ICP.

In cases of severe TBI, disorders of consciousness can arise and present one of the most challenging conditions of the human brain (Table 17.8). Table 17.9 lists non-physical problems associated with TBI.

Table 17.7 Nursing management of patients with a TBI and raised ICP

Nursing intervention	Rationale
GCS Monitor neurological status using the GCS – a GCS score ≤8/15: • Is indicative of coma • Requires patients to be intubated and ventilated immediately Observe and control any seizure activity	The GCS is the gold standard tool for assessing LOC In sedated, ventilated patients with no ICP monitor, regular pupil checks are crucial as pupillary changes may be the only sign of further neurological deterioration Seizure activity will increase cerebral metabolic rate for oxygen and exacerbate cerebral hypoxia
Respiratory status Observe and monitor respiratory gases and status May be mechanically ventilated to control the partial pressure of oxygen (PO_2) and carbon dioxide (PCO_2) to within set parameters, avoiding hypoxia and hypercapnia Monitor and record pulse oximetry Administered prescribed oxygen	Blood oxygen levels regulate CBF Hypoxia – an arterial partial pressure of oxygen (PaO_2) ≤60 mmHg (8 kPa) – will impair autoregulation and increase CBF Hypercapnia ($PaCO_2$ >45 mmHg, or approximately 6 kPa), a potent cerebral vasodilator, can increase CBF and ICP and impair cerebral perfusion
Cardiovascular status Maintain MAP sufficiently to maintain a cerebral perfusion pressure (CPP) >70 mmHg Aim to achieve a target MAP of 90 mmHg until ICP monitoring has been established	Hypotension is associated with decreased CPP Maintaining CPP and MAP (at >70–80 mmHg) reduces mortality and morbidity rates (NICE 2007)

Table 17.7 (*Continued*)

Nursing intervention	Rationale
Fluid status Maintain fluid levels to ensure hydration Avoid overhydration and dextrose solutions Monitor and maintain normal blood glucose levels	Overhydration and dextrose solutions can exacerbate cerebral oedema and increase ICP The brain uses glucose for energy so hypoglycaemia will cause neurons to die A high blood glucose level increases cerebral metabolism and oedema, increasing ICP
Nutritional status Maintain nutritional support May require an enteral feeding regimen (nasogastric or percutaneous endoscopic gastrostomy)	Cerebral trauma induces a state of hypermetabolism and hypercatabolism A high-energy, high-protein diet avoids the effects of protein catabolism and loss of lean body mass
Temperature Monitor core temperature Maintain normothermia (36–36.5°C)	Hyperthermia increases brain oxygen and glucose demand, increasing CBF and CPP With each 1°C increase in temperature, cerebral metabolic rate for oxygen increases by 6–9%, and ICP subsequently rises
Mobility Nurse in a head-up position of 30° Maintain the head and neck in a neutral position Minimise physical activity and cluster care activities	A 30° head-up position promotes cerebral venous drainage, optimises CPP and can reduce ICP Positioning patients at more than 90° at the hip when in bed can increase intra-abdominal pressure Minimising movement will prevent increased metabolic demand
Elimination Maintain a normal urine output (0.5 mL/kg per hour) Monitor bowel movements Avoid constipation	Neuroendocrine disturbances can result in diabetes insipidus, leading to severe dehydration and increasing the risk of ischaemia Constipation increases intra-abdominal pressure, increasing intrathoracic pressure and increasing ICP
Families/carers Assess families and carers for coping strategies Involve them in care, as appropriate Prepare them for the potential outcomes of the injury Collaborate with other support services, e.g. a chaplain or support organisations	

Intracranial tumours

Intracranial tumours are tumours arising within the cranium; their causes are mostly unknown and their origin can be primary or secondary (spreading from the lung, breast, kidney, colon or skin melanoma).

Brain tumours are usually named after the area where they grow; for example, a tumour of the meninges is called a meningioma, and Table 17.10 outlines other examples. Intracranial tumours are

Table 17.8 Disorders of consciousness

Disorder of consciousness	Awareness	Sleep/wake cycle	Motor function
Coma State of unresponsiveness; complete lack of arousal and awareness	No awareness of self or surroundings	None	No purposeful movement No ability to localise to noxious stimuli
Vegetative state Wakefulness without awareness Persistent vegetative state – vegetative state with a duration >1 month	No awareness of self or surroundings	Yes (evident on EEG) Eye-opening and closing	No purposeful movement
Minimal consciousness state Post-coma unresponsiveness or minimally responsive state	Partial – inconsistent	Yes Eye-opening and closing	Inconsistent; can show repeated purposeful movement
Locked-in syndrome Pseudocoma, not a disorder of consciousness but an impairment of voluntary motor function	Yes	Yes	No motor movement Incompletely locked-in patients are able to produce eye movement

Data from Royal College of Physicians (2003), Laureys & Boly (2008) and Monti *et al.* 2010).

Table 17.9 Non-physical problems associated with TBI

Cognitive	Emotional	Behavioural
Memory Poor attention and concentration Lack of insight and awareness Impaired problem-solving Poor initiation	Emotionally labile Depression Manic features Anxiety	Disinhibition Impulsivity Apathy Restlessness Agitation Aggression and anger outbursts on a 'short fuse' Personality changes – 'not the same person'

classified in terms of their growth rate and are graded accordingly (the more rapidly the tumour grows, the higher the grade), and also classified by whether they are benign or malignant (low-grade tumours tending to be benign and high-grade tumours tending to be malignant). Tumours can also be referred to as:

- space-occupying lesions;
- localised or focal – a clear distinction between the brain tissue and the tumour can be seen on a scan or during surgery;
- diffuse – with no clarity between the tumour and the tissue.

There are often exceptions to the general rules for brain tumours; for example, benign tumours are sometimes treated with radiotherapy and chemotherapy. Irrespective of whether a tumour is benign or malignant, it can be life-threatening or cause serious deficits depending on its location. One such

Table 17.10 Examples of CNS tumours

Tumour name	Where it develops from	Rate of growth	Benign (B) or malignant (M)	Spread	Who is affected
Examples of gliomas					
Astrocytomas including glioblastoma multiforme (GBM) • The most common type • Graded 1 to 4, e.g. GBM grade 4, anaplastic astrocytoma grade 3	Astrocytes	Slow or fast High or low grade	M	To other parts of the brain	Adults Children
Oligodendrogliomas • Often found in the frontal and temporal lobes	Oligodendrocytes	Slow or fast	M	Within the CNS via the CSF	Mostly adults Can occur in children
Acoustic neuromas					
May grow for a long time before being diagnosed Associated with the genetic condition neurofibromatosis type 2 If genetic, is more likely to occur in younger people Can be bilateral May develop meningiomas	Acoustic nerve	Slow growing	B	Do not spread	Mainly older people
Haemangioblastomas					
Can grow in the brainstem Difficult to treat Can be part of another syndrome called von Hippel–Lindau syndrome (which runs in families)	Grow from blood vessel cells	Slow growing	Behave differently in different people	Do not spread	Can affect any age, but mainly occur in middle-aged adults
Pituitary tumours					
Or pituitary adenomas	Pituitary gland tissue	Slow growing	B	Do not spread	Mainly adults

(Continued)

Table 17.10 (*Continued*)

Tumour name	Where it develops from	Rate of growth	Benign (B) or malignant (M)	Spread	Who is affected
Primitive neuroectodermal tumours					
The most common type is the medulloblastoma Grow in the cerebellum	Develop from cells left over from early development in the womb that become cancerous	Fast growing	M	Within the CNS via the CSF	Children and young adults
Primary cerebral lymphomas					
Can originate elsewhere Most are a type called diffuse large B cell non-Hodgkin's lymphoma	Lymphocytes	Fast growing	M	One or more tumours may occur in the CNS	Affect anyone with poor immunity due to AIDS or medications after organ transplant
Meningiomas					
Atypical meningiomas: • Grow more aggressively than normal meningiomas • Grow into the brain tissue • Recur after surgery	Meninges	Slow growing	Usually benign		More common in older people and in women
Germ cell tumours					
Commonly occur in the pineal and suprasellar areas	Primitive developing cells in the embryo that develop into the reproductive system	Slow or fast growing	B or M	Dependent on cell type	Young adults
Spinal cord					
Meningiomas and neurofibromas: • Are most common in adults • Grow outside the spinal cord Astrocytomas and ependymomas: • Astrocytomas are most common in children; ependymomas are most common in adults • Grow in the spinal cord tissue					

area is the brainstem, which controls the vital signs, so any pressure from a tumour, for example on the respiratory centre, could result in a respiratory arrest. It is often not possible to remove tumours from delicate areas as this may cause more disability or even death. High doses of radiotherapy are also not recommended if these will cause more damage to the surrounding area.

Management

Management involves:

- a full history and examination;
- blood tests; for example, germ cell tumours produce chemicals that can be detected in the blood;
- CT and MRI scans of the brain;
- surgery – biopsy or partial or complete removal;
- laboratory tests:
  - haematoxylin and eosin staining;
  - immunohistochemical staining (to determine the type and proliferation of the tumour cells);
- radiotherapy;
- chemotherapy.

Some very slow-growing benign tumours are less likely to recur or spread after complete removal and may not need chemotherapy or radiotherapy post-surgery. Malignant tumours tend to recur and may spread to other parts of the brain or spinal cord even if, macroscopically, they seem to have been completely removed; they may thus require radiotherapy and/or chemotherapy to slow their growth and/or to try and prevent a recurrence.

The diagnosis of a brain tumour could signal the start of a long period of uncertainty, anger, guilt and fear for those involved. Patients may have neurological and cognitive deterioration, which they and their families and carers have to cope with before and/or after surgery. In addition, disorders of consciousness (see Table 17.8) can arise, especially after surgery. Patients may also experience side effects from chemotherapy and following radiotherapy, including:

- loss of pituitary function;
- diminished intellectual function;
- hydrocephalus;
- cerebral necrosis.

The key elements of nursing management are the same as for patients with a TBI and/or raised ICP (see Table 17.7). In addition:

- physical and cognitive abilities need to be assessed;
- an individualised rehabilitation programme should be started as early as possible.

Cerebrovascular disorders

A stroke is a sudden decrease in blood flow to a localised area of the brain, characterised by a gradual or rapid onset of neurological deficits due to compromised CBF. It is a medical emergency, requiring rapid treatment in order to prevent avoidable death and long-term disability. It is the third most common cause of death worldwide. An estimated 20–30% of people who have had a stroke will die within 1 month. Few stroke victims will make a full recovery as most are left with some form of disability. Risk factors include:

- certain diseases, such as diabetes mellitus or heart disease;
- lifestyle habits, for example smoking and a sedentary lifestyle;
- dietary factors, such as saturated fats and high alcohol consumption;
- race , higher incidences being seen in Asian and African-Caribbean individuals;
- gender, strokes being more common in men than women;
- age, as the incidence of stroke increases dramatically over the age of 55 years.

The main types of stroke are ischaemic and haemorrhagic. Ischaemic stroke:

- is a sudden vascular occlusion resulting in reduced blood oxygen supply to the brain cells;
- occurs in 85% of all strokes;
- leads to irreversible brain damage and the death of brain cells, known as infarction;
- is most commonly caused by atherosclerosis, which leads to stenosis of the blood vessels; thrombosis is a less likely cause.

Haemorrhagic stroke:

- is seen in 20% of strokes;
- may be due to:
    - intracerebral haemorrhage;
    - subarachnoid haemorrhage;
- both of these being caused by a rupturing of cerebral blood vessels producing haemorrhage (bleeding) into the brain.

Transient ischaemic attacks (TIAs), also known as minor or mini-strokes, occur when stroke symptoms resolve within 24 hours and are a warning that a further stroke may occur.

The neurological deficits vary according to the cerebral artery involved, the size and area of the brain affected, and the length of time the blood flow is decreased or stopped. Signs and symptoms include:

- a sudden onset;
- a focal nature;
- usually a one-sided deficit;
- hemiplegia (paralysis on one side of the body); as the motor pathways cross (decussate) at the junction of the medulla and spinal cord, loss or impairment of sensorimotor functions occurs on the side of the body opposite to the side of the brain that is damaged;
- a stroke in the right hemisphere of the brain manifested by deficits in the left side of the body, and vice versa.

Management

Early assessment and diagnosis is critical if early and effective management decisions are to be implemented. This is especially important for those patients with thrombotic strokes as a small window of opportunity exists in which thrombolytic treatment (to break up the thrombosis or emboli) can be administered. The earlier thrombolysis is started, the greater the benefits. CT scans of the brain play a crucial role in the diagnosis of acute stroke.

Diagnosis begins with a complete history and careful physical assessment, including a thorough neurological examination. One way of identifying suspected acute stroke patients is the FAST stroke identification tool (Box 17.3), a quick score based on three specific symptoms of stroke; if any one of the three symptoms is positive, patients should seek urgent medical attention.

Box 17.3 FAST Assessment (Department of Health 2009)

Facial weakness:

- Can the person smile?
- Has their mouth or eye drooped?

Arm weakness:

- Can the person raise both arms?

Speech problems:

- Can the person speak clearly and understand what you say?

An important component in the management of TIAs and ischaemic stroke is to minimise the high risk of recurrent stroke; treatment will therefore include antithrombotic regimens such as antiplatelet therapy (e.g. aspirin) and anticoagulants (e.g. warfarin). The nursing management of a stroke is outlined in Table 17.11.

Epilepsy

Epilepsy affects up to 50 million people of all ages, races, and ethnic backgrounds worldwide. It is not one condition but a diverse group of disorders, all having in common the presence of at least one

Table 17.11 Nursing management of patients following stroke

Nursing interventions	Rationale
Neurological status Use the GCS and/or National Institutes of Health Stroke Scale (NIHSSS)	The NIHSS, a systematic assessment tool, provides a quantitative measure of stroke-related neurological deficit Neurological examination serves as a baseline for assessment of neurological improvement or worsening
Physiological monitoring Monitor the vital signs – maintain blood pressure within specified limits observing for severe hypertension (systolic blood pressure >200 mmHg) or relative hypotension (systolic blood pressure <110 mmHg) Maintain a normal blood sugar level (4–11 mmol/L) (Royal College of Physicians 2008)	Vital signs and neurological status may fluctuate rapidly immediately after a stroke 78% of acute stroke patients are hyperglycaemic on admission High blood sugars can cause further damage to the neurons in the brain; this is associated with an increased risk of death and more severe disability (Royal College of Physicians 2008)
Respiratory status Assess respiratory status Monitor and record pulse oximetry, and maintain oxygen saturations levels above 95% Administered prescribed oxygen	Oxygen saturation <95% should be treated with oxygen therapy (Royal College of Physicians 2008) Blood oxygen levels regulate CBF
Temperature Monitor core temperature	Hyperthermia increases brain oxygen and glucose demand, thus increasing CBF and CP
Mobility Mobilise the patient as soon as possible (their condition permitting) Maintain correct and careful handling and positioning of the limbs Refer early to physiotherapy Administer antispasmodics Splinting and passive range of movement exercises	Prevents potential complications arising from reduced mobility, e.g. deep vein thrombosis Prevents complications associated with incorrect positioning: • Spasticity • Shoulder (glenohumeral) subluxation • Pressure sores • Contractures Optimises muscle function and recovery Helps patients to learn to deal with their disabilities Ensures correct and appropriate use of devices, e.g. walking aids and sticks Prevents spasticity, which may interfere with the patient's rehabilitation and recovery *(Continued)*

Table 17.11 (*Continued*)

Nursing interventions	Rationale
Communication Early identification of communication difficulties Referral to speech and language therapist Patients are screened for visual problems Expression of pain management Assessment and management of post-stroke pain	Ensures an appropriate communication strategy is identified and implemented Stroke patients with visual deficits have an increased risk of falling Post-stroke neuropathic pain is common; this is caused by central or peripheral nerve damage Hemiplegic shoulder pain occurs in approximately 24% of stroke patients and is associated with poor upper limb recovery
Nutritional status Patient will remain nil by mouth until after a swallow assessment by an appropriately trained healthcare professional, e.g. a speech and language therapist An enteral feeding regimen is used if the patient is unable to swallow safely (nasogastric or percutaneous endoscopic gastrostomy) Assess nutritional status using a recognised assessment tool, e.g. the Malnutrition Universal Screening Tool	Assesses appropriateness of oral feeding and minimises complications associated with dysphagia, e.g. aspiration pneumonia Dysphagia is common Maximises nutritional intake; enables early nutritional management to be identified and implemented
Elimination Assess for incontinence Monitor fluid intake and output volumes and frequency Monitor bowel movements	Incontinence is common Assesses: • Minimal and maximal bladder volumes • The length of time between voidings of urine Enables appropriate bladder training programmes to be instigated
Psychological support Observe for signs of anxiety and depression Refer to an appropriately trained professional for assessment Assess for post-stroke fatigue Help patients and their families adjust to their disability Provide patient education, advice and support	Anxiety may be associated with post-traumatic stress disorder Depression is common and can inhibit engagement with the rehabilitation process Fatigue is common, adversely impacting on quality of life and recovery
Families/carers Provide advice and support about being a carer Include caregivers in the discussions Provide information about benefits, stroke support groups, family support workers and specialist services	Care-giving can be both stressful and distressful, resulting in emotional, physical and social disruption

seizure. It is a chronic disorder characterised by an abnormal recurring, excessive and self-terminating electrical discharge from the neurons in the brain. It is this electrical discharge that can be recorded with EEG scalp electrodes. This abnormal neuronal activity may involve all or part of the brain and disturbs skeletal motor function, sensation, autonomic function of the viscera, behaviour and/or consciousness.

Epilepsy may be:

- idiopathic (no identifiable cause), with multiple episodes diagnosed as a seizure disorder;
- secondary to conditions affecting the brain or other organs, for example drug and alcohol overdose and withdrawal, meningitis and cerebral bleeding.

Signs of seizures are dependent on the brain location of the epileptogenic focus and the extent and pattern of the epileptic discharge. Typical signs include:

- temporary changes in mental status and LOC;
- abnormal sensory changes;
- abnormal movements.

There are currently over 30 different types of epilepsy, with no agreed definitive classification system. Most systems rely heavily on descriptions of the seizures. Three main categories can be identified: focal or partial seizures, generalised seizures and unclassified seizures (Box 17.4).

Tonic-clonic and absence seizures are the most common forms of generalised seizure activity, with tonic-clonic seizures following a typical pattern (Table 17.12). Status epilepticus occurs when patients' seizure activity is continuous and they do not regain consciousness between seizures. Prompt treatment is required to prevent irreversible neurological damage and preserve life.

Box 17.4 Classification of epilepsy

Partial or focal seizures

- The hyperactive activity of the epileptogenic focus remains localised, causing partial or focal seizures
- They involve an area in one of the cerebral hemisphere at the onset
- All types of partial seizures can spread, resulting in secondarily generalised tonic-clonic seizures
- Typically, a portion of the motor cortex is affected, causing recurrent muscle contractions
- Partial seizures can be further subdivided into:
  - Simple partial seizures, without impaired consciousness
  - Complex partial seizures, with impaired consciousness
  - Partial seizures evolving into secondary generalised seizures

Generalised seizures

- Abnormal activity begins simultaneously in both hemispheres of the brain, resulting in impaired consciousness
- They can be further subdivided into six major categories:
  - Generalised tonic-clonic seizures, also known as 'grand mal' seizures
  - Tonic seizures
  - Clonic seizures
  - Myoclonic seizures
  - Atonic seizures
  - Absence seizures, also known as 'petit mal'
    - — sudden brief cessations of all motor activity accompanied by a blank stare and unresponsiveness
    - — last only 5–10 seconds
    - — vary from occasional episodes to several hundred per day
    - — are more common in children than adults

Unclassified epilepsies

- Seizures that cannot be clearly classified into one of the existing categories until further information permits diagnosis

Table 17.12 Tonic-clonic seizure pattern

Phase	Description
Aura (a warning)	A vague sense of uneasiness or an abnormal gustatory, visual, auditory or visceral sensation (e.g. a metallic taste in the mouth or a smell of burning rubber) Seizures can occur without warning
Tonic phase	Sudden LOC Tonic muscle contractions Loss of postural control, so if standing, patients will fall to the floor Rigid muscles, with the arms and legs extended Clamping down of the jaw; the tongue may get caught between the teeth and be bitten Incontinence may occur Respiration may stop and cyanosis develop The phase lasts 10–20 seconds and may persist for up to a minute
Clonic phase	Alternating contraction and relaxation of the muscles Phase varies in duration
Postictal period or phase	Patients remain unconscious and unresponsive to stimuli Gradually regain consciousness May be confused and disoriented Often amnesic of the seizure and the events just prior to the seizure activity

Psychogenic non-epileptic seizures (PNES) or psychogenic syncopes:

- are events that resemble epileptic seizures and are relatively common;
- are not associated with abnormal EEG discharges;
- are presumed to be caused by a psychological disorder;
- are often mistaken for epileptic seizures;
- if misdiagnosed, can lead to inappropriate treatment with antiepileptic drugs (AEDs) and can be life-threatening.

Management

Diagnosis is based on a number of sources and should only be confirmed by a specialist in the field of epilepsy. Misdiagnosis rates of 20–31% are reported by the All-Party Parliamentary Group on Epilepsy (2007). The distinction between epilepsy and non-epileptic seizures is complex, so patients should be referred for a neurological assessment if either PNES or psychogenic syncope is suspected. Typical investigations that are conducted to support a diagnosis are illustrated in Box 17.5. AEDs, also known as anticonvulsant medications, aim to:

- reduce or control the seizure activity;
- prevent irreversible complications (e.g. cerebral and cardiovascular changes) as a result of seizures.

The choice of AEDs is dependent upon the type of seizure and any side effects that patients may experience. In some cases, brain surgery is an option and aims to remove the epileptogenic focus. Other treatment options include:

Box 17.5 Investigations used to diagnosis epilepsy

- A clinical history from the patient or an eye-witnesses to the attack, along with a physical examination
- Diagnostic testing to determine any treatable causes and precipitating factors, e.g. a skull X-ray, MRI or CT scan
- An electroencephalogram to help localise the epileptogenic focus and confirm the diagnosis
- Other tests may include:
  - A lumbar puncture to assess spinal fluid for CNS infections
  - Blood tests, e.g. for plasma electrolytes, glucose and calcium, to rule out other causes

- stereotactic radiotherapy (gamma knife surgery), aimed at destroying the abnormal brain cells;
- neurostimulation therapy, for example deep brain stimulation and vagus nerve stimulation, designed to prevent seizures by sending regular small pulses of electrical energy to the brain via the vagus nerve.

Patients with epilepsy may require hospitalisation for seizure monitoring, for management or to confirm a diagnosis. Immediate care during a seizure will depend upon the type of seizure but generally involves:

- providing a safe environment, aiming to protect patients from any injury;
- securing the airway:
  - loosening clothing around the neck;
  - positioning patients in the recovery position (after the clonic phase);
  - assessing cardiac and respiratory function;
  - suction if excessive salivation has occurred;
  - administration of oxygen therapy;
- intravenous access for AEDs to be administered (especially in status epilepticus);
- documenting an account of the seizure:
  - any aura;
  - behavioural/motor activity;
  - LOC;
  - incontinence;
  - the time the seizure commenced;
  - the length of time of the entire seizure;
  - the period elapsed since the last seizure.

Timely information, training and support aimed at assisting patients and their families to accept, understand and psychosocially adjust to their diagnosis is an important nursing intervention. Monitor patients for toxic signs of AEDs and stress the importance of compliance with the prescribed medication regimen.

Infections of the neurological system

The brain and spinal cord are extremely well protected by the skull, the vertebral column, the BBB and the CSF barrier; however, infections of the CNS ranging from mild to fatal do occur:

- Meningitis (infection of the meninges):
  - is primarily caused by viruses;
  - is life-threatening if bacterial in nature (although it is less common);
  - is rarely caused by spirochaetes and fungi.
- Encephalitis (infection of the brain substance) is mainly caused by viruses such as herpes simplex virus (the most common).

- Human immunodeficiency virus:
  - causes mild meningitis;
  - in full-blown acquired immune deficiency syndrome may cause subacute encephalitis.
- Brain abscesses:
  - are usually defined, localised lesions;
  - occur singularly or in multiples;
  - occur after surgery, trauma, extending osteomyelitis or ear infections.
- Rabies, a fatal infection, enters the PNS following a bite from an infected animal and migrates to the CNS.
- Rubella and measles are linked to a rare complication called subacute sclerosing panencephalitis, which is fatal and may only manifest 10 years after uncomplicated measles.
- Spongiform encephalopathies such as Creutzfeldt–Jakob disease (CJD) and variant CJD are progressive neurodegenerative diseases resulting in death.
- *Clostridium tetani* (which causes tetanus) blocks inhibitory mediators at the nerve synapses, resulting in intense muscle spasm and causing injury to the tissues and eventually death.
- *Clostridium botulinum* blocks the release of acetylcholine, resulting in flaccid paralysis and death from respiratory or cardiac failure.

Management

For most neurological infections, biochemical and microbiological tests, especially on the CSF and blood, can yield important information to assist diagnosis. CSF is obtained via a lumbar puncture, and its colour may also be indicative of the diagnosis (Table 17.13). Difficulties may be experienced in culturing pathogens such as bacteria if patients have received antibiotics prior to the lumbar puncture. A lumbar puncture is not without risk to patients; if the ICP is significantly raised, as may be the case with an abscess, a lumbar puncture may result in fatal cerebellar coning. CT scans and brain biopsies may be undertaken in, for example, brain abscesses, encephalitis and rabies. For some infections, antibiotics and immunisation have markedly reduced the risk of contacting infections such as meningitis and tetanus. Other drugs, such as aciclovir for viral encephalitis, have similar effects.

Patients may be extremely ill, requiring basic nursing care in addition to constant monitoring. The early detection and prevention of neurological deterioration and life-threatening complications is a priority. Nursing management includes the following:

- Monitor neurological function, vital signs and GCS score.
- Use isolation or barrier nursing (if required):
  - Seek advice from the infection prevention and control team.
  - Follow local policy.
  - Address patients' emotional well-being (mental health, safety).
  - Identify the mode of transmission (airborne, faecal/oral route).
  - Assess the risk of spread (to other patients and health workers).
- Provide information and prophylaxis (treatment and screening) to close family and carers, for example to eliminate the nasopharyngeal carriage of organisms.

Table 17.13 Diagnosing infections of CNS: the colour of the CSF

Possible diagnosis	CSF colour
Viral meningitis Chronic meningitis	Slight opalescence
Acute bacterial meningitis	Markedly turbid or cloudy
Traumatic lumbar puncture Subarachnoid haemorrhage	Bloodstained
Tuberculosis meningitis	A spider's web clot appearance due to the high protein content of the CSF

Multiple sclerosis

Multiple sclerosis (MS), also known as disseminated sclerosis, affects an estimated 2.5 million people globally. It is the most common cause of severe disability in young people in the UK.

MS is an autoimmune disease that attacks the CNS, resulting in damage to the myelin sheath and the formation of localised areas of inflammation called 'plaques'. The exact cause remains unknown and the condition is incurable. It is thought that there is damage to the BBB, resulting in cells entering the CNS and triggering an immune response in there. This immune response is thought to be triggered by a prior viral infection or environmental exposure in childhood in a genetically susceptible person:

- The onset is usually between 20 and 40 years of age.
- It peaks around the age of 25.
- MS is more common in women than men.

There are four main types of MS:

- relapsing-remitting, the most common type of MS, which accounts for approximately 80% of cases of MS;
- primary progressive;
- secondary progressive;
- progressive-relapsing.

The signs and symptoms are determined by where in the CNS the demyelination plaques occur, and can vary in character, number and duration:

- sensory impairment;
- transient muscle weakness;
- fatigue, which is the most disabling symptom;
- sleep disorders;
- visual changes (diplopia and visual loss);
- cognitive impairment.

MS is characterised by:

- periods of exacerbation or 'relapse':
  - signs and symptoms that are highly pronounced;
  - lasting for days, weeks, or months;
- periods of remission:
  - a period of relapse followed by a period when the damaged myelin sheath undergoes remyelination;
  - the symptoms thus improving.

In the early stages, MS is commonly a relapsing and remitting disease; over time, however, the myelin sheath becomes unable to repair itself completely during the remission period and patients are left with residual deficits. Repeated healing and inflammation can lead to scarring (gliosis) and loss of axons. Axonal and neuronal degeneration is evident on MRI scanning as black holes. As the disease progresses, remissions become shorter and fewer, and patients become more physically disabled.

Management

Diagnosis is based on the following:

- A clinical history and examination are necessary. A common feature of MS is blurred vision due to optic neuritis, caused by demyelination of the nerve fibres.
- MRI scans may reveal white areas within the white matter.

Table 17.14 Medical therapies used in MS

Therapies	Examples
Disease-modifying therapies: • Reduce the number of exacerbations (relapses) by reducing the production of interferon gamma, thought to be involved in the formation of demyelination plaques • Reduce antibody/lymphocyte activity • Prevent specific inflammatory events leading to the development of lesions	Interferon-beta-1a and interferon beta-1b are the drugs of choice in relapsing-remitting MS, and are given intramuscularly Glatiramer acetate (Copaxone), given subcutaneously Natalizumab (Tysabri), given intravenously
Disease-suppressing therapies: • Are given in the early inflammatory phase (in relapses) • Suppress the immune response	Immunosuppressant drugs, e.g. azathioprine
Corticosteroids – hastens recovery from a relapse	Methylprednisolone – a high dose given intravenously or orally
Medications for the treatment of signs and symptoms	Muscle relaxants (e.g. baclofen and dantrolene) to relieve muscle spasms and spasticity; in severe cases, botulinum toxin may be injected into specific sites Antidepressant drugs for depression Urinary frequency and urgency may be treated with anticholinergic drugs Amantadine for fatigue

- Lumbar puncture may reveal the presence of oligoclonal bands in the CSF, reflecting proteins synthesised within the CNS during the immune response (which is found in 95% of patients with established MS).
- Evoked response testing (visual, auditory and somatosensory) may show delayed conduction (slowing of the nerve messages).

The management varies according to the acuity of exacerbations (relapses) and the presenting signs and symptoms. It involves the treatment of acute relapses, disease modification and symptom management, all of which require an interdisciplinary individualistic approach. Although there is no cure for MS, a number of medical therapies are available, which may slow the progression of the disease and help to manage some of its symptoms (Table 17.14).

The goal and focus of nursing care are to retain as much independence and function as possible, to control symptoms and to reduce potential complications. Supportive and symptomatic care may help to minimise patients' disability and also help to achieve optimal levels of physical and psychological adjustment. As the disease often affects young adults, the psychosocial and economic effect can be devastating. Many nursing care interventions relate to the inability to perform activities of daily living and to problems arising from musculoskeletal changes or altered nerve conduction.

Motor neuron disease

Motor neuron disease (MND) is a devastating and progressive life-limiting disease leading to advancing paralysis and eventual death, with the intellect remaining intact throughout. Sensory neurons, bladder

Table 17.15 Types of MND

Type	Description
Amyotrophic lateral sclerosis (ALS)	The most common form Referred to as classic MND Patient may experience: • Muscle wasting • Fasciculation • Speech and swallowing problems • Muscle spasms
Progressive muscular atrophy (PMA)	Less common and tends to progress more slowly than ALS Patients may go on to develop ALS
Progressive bulbar palsy	Mainly affects the muscles in the tongue, throat and face Causes difficulties with speech, swallowing, coughing and clearing the throat Emotional lability – individuals laugh or cry for no apparent reason
Primary lateral sclerosis	Very rare Patients experience spasticity, but no muscle wasting or fasciculations

and bowel function, emotional feelings and sexual desire generally remain intact. Some individuals may laugh or cry at inappropriate moments and have subtle cognitive changes, and a rare subtype may be associated with dementia (Chawla *et al.* 2012). The upper motor neurons (in the brain) and/or the lower motor neurons (in the brainstem, spinal cord, arms, legs and torso) may be affected. The neurons become damaged and eventually stop working, resulting in weakness, wasting and atrophying of the muscles supplied by these neurons.

The incidence of MND annually is 2 in 100,000 (GPs seeing only one or two cases during their entire career). More men than women are affected, with the onset of symptoms after the age of 40 years (most commonly between 50 and 70 years) (McDermott & Shaw 2008).

There are different types of MND (Table 17.15). The disease initially affects the hands, feet or mouth and throat, depending on the type of MND. Although the signs and symptoms of the different types may differ at the start, they tend to overlap as the disease progresses, so that in the final stages there is very little or no differentiation between all types of MND.

Management

There is no definitive test to diagnose MND, the diagnosis being based on:

- a full and thorough history and neurological examination;
- interpretation of the clinical signs and symptoms;
- investigations to exclude other causes.

There may initially be limited signs, or alternatively the symptoms may be those of other treatable conditions whose signs and symptoms mimic MND (McDermott & Shaw 2008). Tests that can be used to exclude other conditions include:

- blood tests (to exclude problems such as kidney, liver, thyroid and inflammatory conditions);
- lumbar puncture;
- EMG;
- nerve conduction studies;
- transcranial magnetic stimulation, which measures the activity of the neurons from the brain to the spinal cord;

- MRI;
- muscle biopsy.

The only medication found to be beneficial in MND is riluzole. The effect is modest, prolonging life by only 3–4 months. Non-invasive ventilation, initially used overnight during sleep and in the later stages also during the day, has been found to be associated with an extended median survival rate of about 7 months in patients with good bulbar function (McDermott & Shaw 2008). Patients use a mask and a small portable ventilator system (usually involving bilateral positive airway pressure).

Nursing care involves implementing measures to ensure the best quality of life for patients and using measures to compensate for the progressive loss of bodily functions. Among other approaches, treatment should include:

- collaboration and close working with the multidisciplinary team;
- respiratory care;
- implementation of the patient's wishes, i.e. information on healthcare advocates and advanced directives being made available;
- hospice care for later stages of the disease, which can be introduced gradually in the form of respite care for the family and carers.

Parkinson's disease

Parkinson's disease is a common, slowly progressive neurodegenerative disorder that affects older adults. It usually develops after the age of 60 years and is more common in men than in women. There are approximately 120,000 people in the UK and over 8000 in Ireland with Parkinson's disease (Parkinson Disease Society 2008; Parkinson's Association of Ireland 2011). Its prevalence is expected to increase in the future. Parkinson's disease involves:

- the death of dopamine-releasing neurons;
- the formation of 'Lewy bodies' (small spherical protein deposits that are found in neurons).

There is a progressive development of motor and non-motor symptoms. There is no cure, and in the majority of cases the cause is not known, although there is evidence that both genetics and environmental factors play a role. Parkinson's disease is characterised by:

- motor impairment;
- bradykinesia;
- rigidity;
- repetitive tremor;
- postural instability.

Non-motor symptoms (key determinants of reducing functionality and quality of life) include:

- loss of smell;
- sleep disturbances;
- dysphagia (difficulty swallowing);
- excessive salivation and drooling;
- softening of the voice;
- apathy;
- cognitive decline;
- dementia, which occurs in 80% of patients (Butler *et al.* 2008).

Symptoms may present at any stage but tend to occur in the later stages. The severity of symptoms fluctuates, making them difficult to predict and control. Patients subsequently experience a reduction in motor function. These fluctuations in symptoms can be accompanied by high rates of depression (40–50%; Goetz *et al.* 2002), reduced psychological well-being and caregiver distress. Table 17.16 presents some of the common terminology used in describing the signs and symptoms of Parkinson's disease.

Table 17.16 Terminology to describe the signs and symptoms of Parkinson's disease

Terminology	Description
Bradykinesia	Slowness of movement or difficulty in starting to move
Dyskinesia	Abnormal involuntary movements of the limbs, trunk or face occurring with: • Peak plasma levodopa levels • Fluctuating plasma levodopa levels • Low plasma levodopa levels
Dystonia	Sustained and painful muscle contractions Often affect the neck, trunk and limbs, and result in abnormal postures
'On–off' phenomenon	Severe fluctuations in motor function during levodopa treatment
	'On' – states of good mobility or the patient is asymptomatic when the medication is effective
	'Off' – states of poor mobility or the patient is symptomatic, e.g. bradykinesia, rigidity and/or tremor, as the medication wears off
Freezing	States in which patients suddenly stop and become 'stuck' when walking, talking or performing any movement

Management

The mainstay of treatment for Parkinson's disease is medication, which aims to increase the level of dopamine or mimics its effect by stimulating the area of the brain where dopamine works. Patients are often prescribed a combination of medications to control and manage their symptoms (Box 17.6).

Nurses' assessment needs to include the many symptoms that can accompany Parkinson's disease. The following should be assessed:

- the intensity, frequency and duration of symptoms;
- the distress associated with the symptoms as this enables nurses to understand patients' complete symptom experiences.

This assessment will identify symptoms that need to be targeted and the necessary interventions to address those symptoms. Nurses can then evaluate the effectiveness of these interventions on the targeted symptoms.

Nurses should administer medications at the prescribed time and consider supporting self-medication (in which patients control their own medication) if they are able to ensure a constant therapeutic level of symptom control.

As Parkinson's disease is a chronic, progressive disease, intervention is unlikely to completely eliminate a symptom. However, some symptoms are associated with potential complications, such as freezing, and postural instability is associated with a high risk of falls. Nurses should assess patients for risks such as falling and implement strategies to improve their posture and balance (see Chapter 6 for more detailed information on falls and risk assessment).

Alzheimer's disease

Alzheimer's disease is a progressive disease during which protein (senile) plaques and neurofibrillary tangles develop in the structure of the brain, resulting in the death of cells and synapses. This loss occurs mainly in the cerebral cortex and leads to atrophy of the brain. There is a shortage of

Box 17.6 Pharmacological management of Parkinson's disease

Levodopa therapies:

- Are highly effective
- Are commonly prescribed drugs that are converted to dopamine in the brain

Dopamine agonists:

- Stimulate the dopamine receptors in the brain, in particular the dopamine D2-receptors
- An example is bromocriptine, a ergot-derived dopamine agonist

Non-ergot dopamine agonist (NEDAs):

- Stimulate the dopamine receptors in the brain, in particular the D2- and D3-receptors
- Examples of NEDAs are ropinirole, pramipexole and apomorphine (which cannot be given orally)

Monoamine oxidase type B (MAO-B) inhibitors:

- Block the enzyme MAO-B, which breaks down dopamine in the brain
- An example is selegiline

Catechol-O-methyl transferase inhibitors:

- Block the enzyme that breaks down levodopa, prolonging its effect
- Are used in combination with levodopa; examples are entacapone and tolcapone

acetylcholine, which, apart from functioning as a neurotransmitter, also has a role in memory and learning. Alzheimer's disease is characterised by a gradual decline in:

- mental abilities;
- cognition;
- reasoning;
- exercising judgement;
- spatial and language abilities;
- planning and executing familiar tasks;
- personality and mood.

Alzheimer's disease is the most common cause of dementia (Table 17.17). The progress of Alzheimer's disease and its associated signs and symptoms are individual to the person and may not be manifest in everyone. It is important to remember that:

- each stage of Alzheimer's disease is more devastating not only to the individual, but also to their family and carers;
- an individual with mild cognitive impairment (difficulty remembering or thinking clearly) may not have Alzheimer's disease.

Early diagnosis and intervention is key to evidence-based treatment and care (Prince *et al.* 2011).

Management

There is no specific test for Alzheimer's disease; diagnosis is based on the exclusion of other conditions with similar signs and symptoms. The consultation will first be with the patient's own doctor or GP and then with a specialist such as a neurologist, psychiatrist or care of the elderly specialist. The following are carried out:

- a detailed history and thorough examination;
- blood tests – to exclude infections, nutritional deficiencies, thyroid problems and side effects of medication;

Table 17.17 Stages, signs, symptoms and medication in Alzheimer's disease (adapted from NICE 2011)

Stage of disease	Some common signs and symptoms	Medication/drug treatments
Early/initial	Lapses of memory Problems finding the right words or names Work performance affected Loss of interest Reluctant or hesitant to use own initiative, make decisions or act Difficulties with planning and organising	Donepezil (Aricept) Rivastigmine (Exelon)
Mild/moderate	Obvious memory loss Difficulties with simple tasks and/or instructions Decreased ability to perform mental challenges, e.g. counting backwards from 100 Confusion or agitation – this is called sundowning or sundown syndrome when it is more noticeable in the late afternoon or early evening Verbal outbursts and threatening and/or violent behaviour Purposeless and inappropriate activities (fidgeting, pacing, moving things around) May have periods of irritability, paranoia and anxiety Wandering, getting lost	Galantamine (Reminyl) All of the above for mild and moderate stages
Late/severe	Inability to manage independently Becomes bedridden Loss of intelligible speech Urinary incontinence Faecal incontinence Motor problems such as inability to smile, grimacing instead Requires support to sit up without falling Difficulty holding head up Physical and neurological changes (rigidity, re-emergence of the grasp and sucking reflexes, contractures)	Memantine (Ebixa) Only for moderate to severe stages

- X-rays – to exclude chest infection;
- assessment of memory – to assess both recent and past memories.

Families and carers should be involved in the history-taking as they may be extremely useful in providing information patients may have forgotten. Other tests may include a brain scan (to assess any changes such as atrophy) and a further more detailed memory and thinking skills assessment undertaken by a clinical psychologist.

Alzheimer's disease is profoundly life-changing, and the approach to nursing care should be centred on the individual (Box 17.7 and Box 17.8).

There is currently no cure for Alzheimer's disease, but if the disease is diagnosed early medication may help to improve or stabilise the symptoms. The progression of the condition varies, with some

Box 17.7 Key features of person-centred care (reproduced from Woodward & Mestecky (2011) *Neuroscience Nursing: Evidence Based Practice*, with kind permission of Wiley Blackwell.)

- Looks at care from the perspective of the individual
- Acknowledges each person as a unique individual with a rich history and their own memories, preferences, wishes and needs
- Respects the dignity, autonomy and independence of the person with dementia
- Focuses on the positive rather than the negative
- Focuses on strengths and abilities rather than weaknesses and disabilities
- Promotes well-being
- Ensures care is planned around the individual not around the care system
- Acknowledges that there is usually a reason for a behaviour and views behaviours that challenge others as an expression of feelings and/or a means of communication
- Accepts the reality of the person with dementia and does not insist on bringing them into another reality that can cause them distress

Box 17.8 Key features in the nursing management of patients with Alzheimer's disease

The nurse should:

- Ensure the care plan is tailored to patients' needs
- Regularly assess, evaluate and identify patients' and carers' needs
- Engage and work in partnership with patients and their families and carers
- Be sufficiently knowledgeable to recognise the progression of the disease
- Have the knowledge, skills and time to deal with problems as they occur
- Refer patients and/or families to the relevant agencies that can offer assistance and support

individuals progressing rapidly and others more slowly; but as the condition worsens, care becomes more challenging and intensive. Families and carers should be viewed as equal partners. Where possible, the initial care should be in the individual's home, with respite care periods offered. As the disease progresses, there may be occasions when a stay in hospital will be beneficial, and palliative care should be available if and when required. Additional information on the nursing care of older people with dementia can be found in Chapter 6.

Conclusion

To ensure good practice, staff caring for neurological patients should have the necessary skills and experience especially in the utilisation of tools such as the GCS. The nursing care of conditions related to the neurological system lends itself to the acquisition of valuable diverse skills and knowledge, which are transferable to other disciplines. Nurses have to collaborate with patients and/or their families and carers and the multidisciplinary team according to patients' holistic needs, goals and care requirements.

Visit www.wileyfundamentalseries.com/medicalnursing and read Reflective Questions 17.1–17.5 to think more about this topic.

Now visit the companion website and test yourself on this chapter:
www.wileyfundamentalseries.com/medicalnursing

References

All-Party Parliamentary Group on Epilepsy (2007) *The Human and Economic Cost of Epilepsy in England: Wasted Money, Wasted Lives*. London: APPG on Epilepsy.

Braine, M.E. (2011) The experience of living with a family member with challenging behaviour following acquired brain injury. *Journal of Neuroscience Nursing*, **43**(3):156–64.

Butler, T.C., van den Hout, A., Mathews, F.E. *et al.* (2008) Dementia and survival in Parkinson disease: a 12-year population study. *Neurology*, **70**:1017–22.

Chawla, J., Hoffmann M., Talavera, F. & Verghese J. (2012) *Dementia in Motor Neuron Disease*. Retrieved 22nd February 2012 from http://emedicine.medscape.com/article/1134953-overview.

Department of Health (2009) *Stroke: Act F.A.S.T. Awareness Campaign*. London: Department of Health.

Goetz, C.G., Koller, W.C., Poewe, W. *et al.* (2002) Treatment of depression in idiopathic Parkinson's disease. *Movement Disorders*, **17**(4):S112–19.

Greenwald, B.D., Burnett, D.M. & Miller, M.A. (2003) Congenital and acquired brain injury. Brain injury: epidemiology and pathophysiology. *Archive of Physical Medical Rehabilitation*, **84**(3 Suppl. 1): S3–7.

Jennett, J. & Teasdale, G. (1981) *Management of Head Injuries*. Philadelphia: FA Davies.

Laureys, S. & Boly, M. (2008) The changing spectrum of coma. *Nature Clinical Practice Neurology*, **4**:544–6.

McDermott, C.J. & Shaw, P.J. (2008) Diagnosis and management of motor neurone disease. *BMJ*, **336**:658–62.

Monti, M.M., Laureys, S. & Owen, A.M. (2010) The vegetative state. *BMJ*, **10**(341):c3765

National Institute for Health and Clinical Excellence (2007) *Head Injury: Triage, Assessment, Investigation and Early Management of Head Injury in Infants, Children and Adults*. NICE Clinical Guideline No. 56 (Partial update of NICE Clinical Guideline No. 4). London: NICE.

National Institute for Health and Clinical Excellence (2011) *Alzheimer's Disease – Donepezil, Galantamine, Rivastigmine (Review) and Memantine*. Retrieved 27th September 2011 from http://guidance.nice.org.uk/TA111.

Parkinson's Association of Ireland (2011) *Press Releases for Parkinson's Awareness Campaign*. Retrieved 6th April 2012 from http://www.parkinsons.ie/mediacentre_pressreleases.

Parkinson's Disease Society (2008) *Life with Parkinson's Today – Room for Improvement*. London: Parkinson's Disease Society.

Prince, M., Bryce, R. & Ferri, C. (2011) *The benefits of early diagnosis and intervention*. World Alzheimer Report 2011. Retrieved 22nd February 2012 from http://www.alz.co.uk/research/WorldAlzheimerReport2011.pdf.

Royal College of Physicians (2003) *The Permanent Vegetative State: Guidance on Diagnosis and Management. Report of a Working Party*. London: RCP.

Royal College of Physicians (2008) *Stroke. National Clinical Guidelines for Diagnosis and Initial Management of Acute Stroke and Transient Ischaemic Attack (TIA)*. London: RCP.

Teasdale, G. & Jennett, B. (1974) Assessment of the coma and impaired consciousness. A practical scale. *Lancet*, **2**(7872):81–4.

18

Nursing care of conditions related to the immune system

Michael Coughlan and Mary Nevin

School of Nursing and Midwifery, Trinity College Dublin, Dublin, Ireland

Contents

Introduction 365
The immune system 365
Organ transplant 367
Hypersensitivity disorders 370
Anaphylaxis 370
Autoimmunity 372
Human immunodeficiency virus and acquired immune deficiency syndrome 375
Conclusion 384
References 385

Learning outcomes

Having read this chapter, you will be able to:

- Outline how the immune system protects individuals from infection
- Discuss the potential difficulties faced by patients undergoing an organ transplant
- Describe the different types of hypersensitivity reactions
- Discuss the medical and nursing management of patients with HIV/AIDS

Fundamentals of Medical-Surgical Nursing: A Systems Approach, First Edition. Edited by Anne-Marie Brady, Catherine McCabe, and Margaret McCann.

Box 18.1 Innate and acquired body defences

Innate body defences
- Skin
- Mucous membranes, etc.
- Cellular and chemical defences:
  - Phagocytes
  - Inflammatory response
  - Complement and chemical responses

Acquired body defences
- Lymphatic system and lymphocytes
- Primary and secondary responses to infection
- Organ rejection (in line with the clonal selection theory)

Introduction

The human body is an ideal host for many pathological organisms that live in the environment. These organisms, on invading the body, can cause disease and ultimately death; to prevent this occurring, the human body has developed an immune system that can identify those organisms or cells that are foreign and destroy them. This chapter will present some conditions related to altered immunity and conditions in which the immune system has to be controlled in order to ensure ongoing health.

The immune system

The human body is constantly under siege from a wide variety of microorganisms. Some live in relative harmony on the external or internal body surfaces (e.g. *Staphylococcus epidermidis* on the skin and *Bacteroides* in the bowel), while others such as viruses are constantly attempting to gain access to cells in the body and cause disease. In order to survive, the human body must be protected from all micro-organisms as even commensals will cause disease if they can gain access to sterile cavities such as the bladder or enter through breaks in the skin. Protection of the human body, its cells and its organs is the role of the immune system.

The immune system can be subdivided into two parts (Box 18.1).

Innate body defences

Intact skin acts as a barrier to infective organisms, while resident commensals have a role to play by preventing the build-up of pathogenic organisms. Where natural openings to the body occur, other defences exist to prevent pathogenic organisms entering (Box 18.2).

When pathogenic organisms gain access to the body, the next line of defence is the inflammatory response. This is initiated mainly by granulocytes and monocytes. The effect is to attract phagocytes to the area to destroy the pathogens. Complement may also be activated, and coating these pathogens (opsonisation) facilitates their destruction by neutrophils and monocytes.

Acquired body defences

Humans and higher vertebrates are the only animals that have a system of acquired immunity. This allows the human body to recognise pathogens, develop defences against them and retain a memory of those pathogens. Linked to this ability is the presence of a lymphatic system. This gathers lymph from around the body and filters it through lymph nodes and glands. Any organisms present encounter and are destroyed by T and B lymphocytes and macrophages (monocytes that have left the bloodstream).

Box 18.2 Body defences preventing pathogenic organisms entering the body

Gastrointestinal tract

- The tract is lined from the mouth to the anus with a mucosal membrane that helps to prevent organisms gaining entry
- The mouth:
  - Has glands that produce saliva, which:
    - prevents drying out of the membrane
    - contains lysozyme (an antibacterial enzyme)
    - contains immunoglobulin A (which has an antiviral effect)
  - Contains commensals, which control the number of pathogenic organisms
- The stomach has:
  - An environment that is strongly acidic and in which very few pathogenic organisms can survive
- The bowel contains:
  - Commensal organisms, such as *Bacteroides* and *Escherichia coli*, which help to control the number of pathogenic organisms

Respiratory tract

- This is lined with ciliated mucosa, which restricts the access of microorganisms by trapping them in mucus and wafting them out of the airway

Genitourinary tract

- The flow of urine from the bladder helps to clear away organisms ascending through the urethra
- The vagina has an acidic environment, which militates against pathogenic organisms due to the presence of a bacterium called *Lactobacillus*

T and B lymphocytes are both derived from cells in the bone marrow (see Chapter 19); T cells go to the **t**hymus gland to mature, while B cells mature in the **b**one marrow. During the early stages of maturation, both T and B cells undergo a negative selection that identifies and destroys those B cells that are likely to react with antigens on the surfaces of the body's own cells and organs, thus preventing autoimmunity. Individuals have a unique set of antigens on their cell surface known as human leucocyte antigens (HLAs); these are not affected by that person's immune system.

On the surface of both B and T cells are antigen-specific receptors. When a T or a B cell interacts with a specific antigen, it becomes activated, returns to the lymph tissue to complete its maturation and clone itself. The result is antigen-specific antibodies and T cells.

T cells are involved in cellular immunity. In the thymus gland, they differentiate into different types of T cells:

- Cytotoxic T cells destroy tissue and organisms that they regard as foreign.
- Memory T cells recognise foreign organisms that have previously been encountered and destroy them.
- Helper T cells support the immune response.
- Suppressor T cells control and switch off the immune response.

B cells offer what is called humoral immunity. After contact with an antigen, these B cells form antibodies (immunoglobulin, or Ig). There are five groups of antibodies – IgG, IgM, IgA, IgE and IgD – which destroy antigens that are regarded as foreign. Memory B cells are also formed. These long-lived cells, similar to memory T cells, have the ability to rapidly recognise and respond to previously encountered antigens; thus, individuals have immunity to previously encountered illnesses such as measles.

Organ transplant

Organ transplantation was first successfully undertaken in humans in the 1950s, and since then it has become, to some degree, almost a routine surgical operation. For a successful organ transplant, it is necessary to have as close a HLA match between the donor and the recipient as possible. The poorer the HLA match, the greater likelihood that rejection will occur. Identical twins tend to be the closest HLA matches, often having the same HLA type, and have the least risk of rejection. Siblings have a 1 in 4 possibility of having a close HLA match; after that the chances of a good match become much less with both other family members and unrelated individuals. Individuals waiting for an organ transplant, for example a kidney, may therefore have to wait a number of years for a donor with a close HLA match. Different types of transplants include:

- autograft transplants, in which individuals receive a transplant of their own tissue, for example a skin or bone marrow transplant;
- allograft transplants, between individuals who are not HLA-identical;
- isograft or syngenic transplants, between individuals who are HLA identical, for example monozygotic twins;
- xenograft transplants, between different species, such as between a porcine donor and a human recipient.

The major difficulty faced by individuals receiving an organ transplant, except for individuals who are receiving autograft or isograft transplants, is organ rejection. For patients who receive a kidney transplant, rejection can mean a return to dialysis, but for patients who receive a heart or bone marrow, the outcome can be death. Rejection occurs because the acquired immune system recognises the antigens on the surface of the transplanted organ as foreign and so begins to attack it. Immunosuppressant drugs, such as ciclosporin, help to reduce the risk of rejection by reducing the immune response.

Transplants of bone marrow (see Chapter 19) are different from other tissue transplants in that the bone marrow is the source of the cells that cause organ or tissue rejection. T cells from the transplanted marrow have undergone negative selection for a different set of host tissue antigens, and will therefore now start to attack these new organs. This condition is known as graft-versus-host disease.

Management

Issues that need to be considered when caring for individuals who have received an organ or tissue transplant include:

- increased risk of infection;
- graft rejection;
- psychological issues.

Increased risk of infection

Patients suffering from end-organ failure have increased morbidity, increasing their susceptibility to infection even before the prospect of a transplant. Organ transplantation frequently involves lengthy surgery and damage to the skin's integrity from surgical incisions, increasing the risk of infection. On receiving an organ transplant, patients are exposed to drugs that will suppress their immune system to prevent the livelihood of rejection. These drugs further increase patients' susceptibility to opportunistic infections. Nursing interventions aimed at reducing the risk of infection are outlined in Box 18.3.

Box 18.3 Nursing interventions to prevent infection

- Nurse the patient in a single room, away from other patients with infections
- Those not allowed access to patients are:
  - Individuals with infections
  - Individuals exposed to contagions, e.g. viruses such as chickenpox or measles
  - Young children (as they have greater likelihood of exposure to infections)
- Employ hand hygiene on entering and leaving the patient's room
- Ensure patient hygiene as one of the greatest sources of infection is the patient's own body flora
- Educate patients on hand hygiene after using the toilet and before meals
- Monitor the vital signs for indications of infection
- A rise in temperature may be the first indicator of infection
- Ensure regular oral hygiene:
  - Patients should use a soft, small-headed toothbrush, especially after eating and at night
  - Educate patients to report soreness or ulcers in the mouth
- Aseptic techniques must be used when managing wound dressings or any break in the skin's integrity
- Monitor intravenous (IV) cannulas for signs of inflammation and infection
- Change IV cannulas at least every 72 hours (and in line with local policy)
- Change IV giving sets at least every 48 hours to reduce the risk of bacterial contamination
- Liaise with the dietitian as a good diet is essential to promote wound healing and strengthen the immune system
- Monitor blood tests for signs of an increased white cell count as this may indicate the presence of infection

Graft rejection

There are a number of different forms of graft rejection:

- Hyperacute rejection starts within minutes of transplantation and is a humoral response associated with the presence of antibodies due to a previous exposure to the antigen. This exposure may have been in the form of an earlier transplant or blood transfusion.
- Accelerated rejection occurs within days of the transplant and is a cellular response; previous exposure is responsible for the rapid onset of rejection.
- Acute rejection occurs in the immediate days or weeks following transplantation and results from T cells recognising the non-self antigens on the surface of the newly transplanted tissue or organ and commencing a delayed hypersensitivity reaction.
- Chronic rejection occurs months or even years after organ transplantation; the cause is not completely clear. Elements of acute rejection can be observed with both immune and non-immune factor involvement. There is a deterioration in organ function over a period of time, which can resemble the original onset of organ failure.

Management

In order to prevent graft rejection, it is necessary for all patients receiving an allograft to be prescribed immunosuppressant medications (Table 18.1). Nursing management involves the administration of medicines and educating patients to safely self-administer these medications after their discharge.

Rejection is most common in the days and weeks following transplant. Early identification is essential, to preserve the transplanted organ. Signs of rejection include:

- fever and rigors;
- inflammation around the transplant site;

Table 18.1 Immunosuppressant medications

Generic name	Administration route
Azathioprine	IV or oral
Mycophenolate mofetil	IV or oral
Ciclosporin (cyclosporin)	IV or oral
Basiliximab	IV
Tacrolimus	IV or oral
Sirolimus	Oral
Antithymocyte immunoglobulin	IV
Corticosteroids	IV or oral

IV, intravenous.

- fluid retention;
- weight gain;
- hypertension.

Patients should be educated to recognise these symptoms and report them immediately to healthcare staff. Blood tests should be monitored and, depending on the organ transplanted, should include the white cell count, urea and electrolyte levels and liver function tests.

Treatment may involve adjustments or changes in immunosuppressant medications and their administration. Patients who receive an allograft need to understand that the risk of rejection will always remain and thus the importance of compliance with medication and continued vigilance in relation to the signs and symptoms of rejection.

Psychological issues

Patients may face a number of psychological issues while waiting for and receiving an organ transplant:

- guilt that someone may have to die in order for an organ to become available;
- anxiety regarding organ rejection;
- fear of death.

Nurses can support and help patients in coming to terms with their fears and worries through the application of good communication skills:

- Observe patients' body language as this helps in assessing signs of anxiety and worry.
- Actively listen to patients' fears and worries and offer appropriate support.
- Empower patients through education so that they can make decisions about and be actively involved in their own care.
- Identify and encourage the use of appropriate coping strategies that have been helpful to patients in the past.
- Encourage family members and significant others to support patients and, where appropriate, participate in their care.
- Recognise the need for other support services, such as counselling, to be involved in patients' care.

Box 18.4 Examples of allergens

- Plant pollens
- Dust mite
- Latex
- Certain foods, e.g. milk, peanuts, shellfish and eggs
- Antibiotics, e.g. penicillin and tetracycline
- Venoms, e.g. wasp, honeybee and snake

Preparation for discharge

It is important, before receiving a transplant, that patients understand the benefits of receiving a donated organ, as well as the associated risks, for example infection and rejection. The risk of rejection and infection continues after discharge, so patients need to be educated in relation to:

- ongoing compliance with the immunosuppressive regimen that has been prescribed;
- the increased risk of infection that is associated with these medications, the need to avoid individuals with infections, and the need to report any signs or symptoms of an infection immediately to the GP;
- the signs and symptoms of rejection, and the need to contact the GP if these occur;
- the need to keep outpatient follow-up appointments;
- the need to wear a medical alert bracelet.

Hypersensitivity disorders

The inflammatory and immune response is an integral part both of the mechanism of tissue growth and repair following injury, and of protection against disease. These usually protective mechanisms can sometimes produce detrimental reactions in the body that cause damage to normal tissues. Such reactions are known as hypersensitivity reactions, and they may be immediate or delayed.

Almost any substance can be an allergen for some individuals. These allergens can enter the body through various routes such as inhalation, injection, ingestion or direct contact with the skin (Bryant 2007). Hypersensitivity usually appears on repeated contact with the allergen (Box 18.4). Hypersensitivity reactions can be:

- localised, affecting one body part or a limited area, for example hives, sneezing, abdominal cramps or swelling of the lips;
- systemic, affecting several parts or the entire body, for example acute anaphylaxis or bronchoconstriction.

Hypersensitivity reactions can be divided into five main types. Each type may occur alone or with other types (Table 18.2).

Anaphylaxis

Anaphylaxis is a severe allergic reaction that is of rapid onset and can have a potentially fatal outcome, even with appropriate medical intervention. It affects many organs within seconds or minutes of exposure to the allergen, so prevention is critical (Griffiths 2008). A list of common symptoms associated with anaphylaxis is included in Box 18.5 below.

Treatment involves removing or discontinuing the causative agent and administering drugs such as adrenaline, hydrocortisone and antihistamines. Nurses have a responsibility to recognise the signs and symptoms of anaphylaxis and respond promptly and efficiently.

Table 18.2 Types of hypersensitivity reaction

Type	Alternative names	Mediators	Examples of disorders
I	Immediate, allergic, anaphylactic	IgE	Atopy Anaphylaxis Allergic asthma Hay fever Skin reactions
II	Cytotoxic, antibody dependent	IgG or IgM Complement	Thrombocytopenia Autoimmune haemolytic anaemia Goodpasture's syndrome Myasthenia gravis ABO transfusion incompatibility
III	Immune complex	IgG Complement	Systemic lupus erythematosus Vasculitis Rheumatoid arthritis Serum sickness
IV	Delayed, cell mediated	T cells	Chronic transplant rejection Contact dermatitis Tuberculosis
V	Autoimmune, stimulated	IgG or IgM Complement	Graves' disease

Box 18.5 Symptoms associated with anaphylaxis

- Angio-oedema or swelling
- Hives
- Redness
- Pruritus
- Confusion
- Anxiety
- Wheezing
- Dyspnoea
- Laryngeal oedema
- Hypoxia
- Tachycardia
- Hypotension

Note on patient safety

Allergy identification

The best treatment for anaphylaxis is prevention. It is important that all the patient's known allergies and usual reactions are identified, communicated to all relevant members of the healthcare team and clearly documented in the relevant clinical notes according to local policy.

Autoimmunity

The immune system can usually distinguish 'self' from 'non-self'. Autoimmunity occurs when there is some interruption of the usual control process or when there is an alteration in some body tissue so that it is no longer recognised as 'self' and is thus attacked. This can lead to a variety of autoimmune diseases in which the immune system attacks normal body cells, believing them to be an invading organism.

It is not known what causes an autoimmune response. However, certain individuals are genetically susceptible, and a person's sex also appears to have some role in the development of autoimmunity, with females more likely to develop a number of autoimmune conditions, for example systemic lupus erythematosus (SLE) and Graves' disease. There is no known cure; management involves treatment of the symptoms, along with anti-inflammatory and immunosuppressive medication.

Goodpasture's syndrome

Goodpasture's syndrome is also known as Goodpasture's disease or antiglomerular basement membrane disease. It is a type II hypersensitivity reaction to Goodpasture's antigens on the basement membrane of the glomeruli in the kidneys and on the pulmonary alveoli. Individuals may experience lung and/or kidney problems. As with many autoimmune conditions, the exact cause or triggering agent is not yet known.

Signs and symptoms

The following are seen in Goodpasture's syndrome (Bergs 2005):

- The first symptoms can be vague – fatigue, nausea, skin pallor and anaemia.
- Pulmonary symptoms include dry cough, shortness of breath and pulmonary haemorrhage.
- There is involvement of the kidney with:
  - haematuria and proteinuria;
  - rapid progression to renal failure requiring haemodialysis or a kidney transplant.
- Death can result if the condition is not recognised and treated early.

Management

Treatment involves corticosteroids and immunosuppressive medication to lower the body's normal immune response and reduce the symptoms; however, these treatments cannot reverse permanent kidney damage. Nursing care priorities include:

- monitoring patients' respiratory and renal function for complications of the disease, such as:
  - uncontrolled bleeding;
  - pulmonary failure;
  - fluid overload or deficit;
  - renal failure;
- monitoring patients' response to drug therapy;
- strict adherence to infection control principles – this is vital due to the increased risk of infection with immunosuppressant therapy.

Myasthenia gravis

Myasthenia gravis is an autoimmune neuromuscular disease characterised by weakness and easy fatigability of the voluntary muscles. This occurs due to an antibody attack on the acetylcholine receptors, which interferes with impulse conduction at the neuromuscular junction and results in a reduced ability of the muscles to contract.

Myasthenia gravis is a rare type II hypersensitivity reaction whose cause is not known; at present, there is no cure for it. Women have a higher incidence than men, and the disease can be diagnosed at any age, although it typically occurs between the ages of 20 and 30 years. Myasthenia gravis is diagnosed based on clinical presentation and by testing the person's response to anticholinesterase medication. As myasthenia gravis is a rare disorder, the diagnosis is often delayed or missed. People experience periods of remission and relapse of symptoms.

Signs and symptoms

- In the mild form, there are:
  - disturbances of the ocular muscles:
  - weakness, double vision and a droopy or sleepy appearance of the face.
- Severe symptoms include:
  - difficulties with swallowing and chewing;
  - generalised muscle weakness;
  - fatigue;
  - altered bladder and bowel function;
  - respiratory difficulties.

Management

Treatment involves the use of anticholinesterases and immunosuppressants, which reduce the symptoms and increase the time periods between remissions and relapses. Removal of the thymus gland (thymectomy) may also improve the symptoms. Two major complications may arise due to medication:

- Cholinergic crisis occurs due to overmedication with anticholinesterase drugs.
- Myasthenic crisis occurs if there is undermedication with anticholinesterase drugs.

Both crises lead to an acute worsening of myasthenic symptoms. Patients may experience a sudden inability to clear secretions or breathe adequately, requiring mechanical ventilation and intensive care until medication levels have been controlled. Nursing care priorities include:

- assessing and managing symptoms associated with reduced muscle function and fatigue;
- promoting mobility and self-care (which improves muscle strength);
- encouraging rest during times of weakness and fatigue;
- close observation of respiratory function (as there is a potential for weakening of the diaphragm and intercostal muscles); check for:
  - difficulty breathing;
  - coughing;
  - increased secretions;
  - and provide support where necessary;
- assistance with communication, eye care and nutritional support if patients have difficulty swallowing or have weakness in their eyes or facial muscles;
- close monitoring of patients' responses to drug therapy, enabling an early recognition of myasthenic or cholinergic crises.

SLE

SLE (also referred to as 'lupus') is a chronic progressive inflammatory connective tissue disorder. It is a type III hypersensitivity reaction caused by antibody–immune complex formation that results in widespread damage to the connective tissues; it is characterised by periods of remission and relapse. Typically, multiple body organs and systems are affected at different times (Rooney 2005).

There is no cure for SLE and its cause is unknown; however, genetic and environmental factors appear to play a role. Young women are more likely to be diagnosed with SLE than men (Rooney 2005).

Table 18.3 Signs and symptoms of SLE

System affected	Signs and symptoms
Musculoskeletal	Morning stiffness Joint pain and swelling Muscle weakness Arthritis
Dermatological	Photosensitivity Malar rash (butterfly rash) on the cheeks and bridge of the nose Alopecia
Renal	Proteinuria Haematuria Nephritis
Cardiovascular	Pericarditis Myocarditis Endocarditis Atherosclerosis
Gastrointestinal	Anorexia Nausea Vomiting Abdominal pain Peritonitis
Pulmonary	Pleuritis Pleural effusion Pneumonitis Pulmonary hypertension
Haematological	Anaemia Thrombocytopenia
Neurological	Headaches Seizures Psychosis Depression

Medications prevent flare-ups of symptoms and reduce their severity and duration when they do occur; they include non-steroidal anti-inflammatory drugs, corticosteroids, disease-modifying antirheumatic drugs and immunosuppressants.

Signs and symptoms

The course and severity of SLE vary, so early signs and symptoms, for example fever, fatigue and weight loss, may be non-specific and may mimic those of other disorders. Clinical manifestations of the disease are included in Table 18.3.

Management

Patients may be very well when in remission and have no limitations on their daily activities. During periods of relapse, however, the symptoms may be so severe that patients may have to be admitted to a critical care unit. Nursing interventions at this time are directed towards the assessment and management of individual patient symptoms, which may include acute confusion. The prevention of seizures, maintenance of skin integrity, prevention of infection and monitoring of renal and respiratory function are all priorities. Increased joint pain and fatigue are managed in much the same manner as when caring for patients with acute rheumatoid arthritis (see Chapter 20).

Patient education on autoimmune diseases

Following the diagnosis and stabilisation of their symptoms, the majority of people with autoimmune diseases manage their conditions comfortably at home. Patient education and psychosocial support to promote coping and self-esteem are vital. For patients living with a chronic incurable autoimmune disease, it is important that they and their carers' are educated fully on:

- the condition;
- the medication regimen;
- how to identify potential complications and what to do if they occur;
- lifestyle modifications that should be considered.

Living with the uncertainty of a chronic illness is stressful, and patients should develop a good support system around them.

Human immunodeficiency virus and acquired immune deficiency syndrome

Human immunodeficiency virus (HIV)/acquired immune deficiency syndrome (AIDS) is now in its third decade as a pandemic,. The outbreak appears to have started in the 1970s, although there is evidence of isolated cases of the condition before this time. Today an estimated 33.3 million people are living with HIV/AIDS globally (UNAIDS 2010). In the UK, the number is thought to be approximately 86,500 people, of whom about a quarter do not realise that they are infected (Health Protection Agency 2010).

HIV is a retrovirus, i.e. a virus that uses ribonucleic acid (RNA) to replicate itself. It has an affinity for cells that express a particular glycoprotein called cluster of differentiation 4 (CD4 on their cell surfaces (CD4+ cells). The virus also needs the presence of co-receptors (CCR5 [chemokine C-C motif receptor type 5] and/or CXCR4 [chemokine C-X-C motif receptor type 4]) to allow it to bind to the CD4 receptor. In the absence of these, HIV cannot infect the cell.

Cells that express the CD4 protein include T lymphocytes, monocytes, dendritic cells (cells that present antigens to the T cells) and brain microglia (resident macrophages in the brain and spinal cord). HIV attacks and damages the immune system, leaving individuals susceptible to opportunistic and pathogenic infections. When the immune system is so compromised and is no longer able to defend the body from these infections, the person is said to have AIDS.

There are two strains of HIV: HIV-1 and HIV-2. HIV-1 is the more common form of the virus. HIV-2 was identified in patients with AIDS in West Africa, is predominantly found in that region, and is thought to have first infected humans in the 1940s. It appears to be less infective in the initial stages than HIV-1, but overall the presentation and disease trajectory are clinically the same.

Transmission of HIV

There are three routes by which HIV can be transferred:

- sexual transmission;
- transmission via body fluids including blood and blood products;
- transmission vertically from mother to child.

Sexual transmission

Everyone, whether young or old, who is sexually active is at risk of contracting HIV. Any form of unprotected sexual contact (vaginal, anal or oral) with an infected individual can lead to infection. Anal sex is still regarded as having the highest risk, as the mucosal lining of the anal canal can be easily damaged, increasing the risk of the virus gaining access to the body. Oral sex has the lowest risk but is not risk-free.

Heterosexual, homosexual and bisexual individuals who have unprotected sex are all at risk of contracting HIV. Heterosexual infection is now the most common method of transfer of HIV in the UK (Health Protection Agency 2010). The risk of transmission from male to female is greater than from female to male. Having a sexually transmitted infection increases an individual's susceptibility to contracting HIV by up to five times, and increases the risk of transmitting the disease (Centers for Disease Control and Prevention [CDC] 2010a). In young homosexual men, the incidence of HIV is on the increase, a doubling of new cases having been seen (Health Protection Agency 2008). A number of sexual practices increase an individual's risk of contracting HIV (Box 18.6).

The most effective way of avoiding sexually transmitted HIV is to abstain from all forms of sexual intercourse or to be in a long-term, mutually monogamous relationship with an uninfected partner. The use of latex condoms reduces the risk of contracting HIV and is recommended for vaginal, anal and oral intercourse. Condoms made of polyurethane or other synthetic materials appear to be equally as effective at reducing the risk of HIV transmission but carry a greater risk of breakage. 'Natural' condoms, although effective at preventing pregnancy, are porous and may allow the transmission of HIV. Female condoms have also been shown to be effective in preventing HIV transmission (CDC 2010b).

Transmission via body fluids including blood and blood products

HIV has been isolated from and transmitted via blood, blood products, body fluids (Box 18.7) and transplanted organs. Although the risk of contracting HIV from a blood transfusion or blood products

Box 18.6 Risk behaviours for contracting HIV

- Unprotected vaginal, anal or oral sex with multiple partners or an infected partner
- The presence of a sexually transmitted disease
- Sex for reward (money, drugs, etc.)
- The use of drugs during sex, including alcohol, sexual enhancers and illegal drugs

Box 18.7 Blood and body fluids associated with the transmission of HIV

- Whole blood
- Packed cells
- Human plasma
- Clotting factors
- Seminal fluid
- Vaginal secretions
- Amniotic fluid
- Breast milk
- Saliva
- Synovial fluid

is very low in Western counties, there always is a possibility of this, so all body fluids including blood should be regarded as potentially infected.

Intravenous drug use

Intravenous drug (IVD) use is probably the most effective method of HIV transmission. In Western countries, it is the second most common method of transmission after sexual intercourse (Department of Health and Children 2008). Individuals who are IVD users are usually sexually active, and are at a greater risk of disease transmission unless proper precautions are undertaken. Advice to IVD users should include the following:

- Stop using IVDs.
- Use needle exchange programmes and use a sterile needle when injecting.
- Clean equipment between use.
- Do not share equipment with others.

Occupational infection

A large proportion of the population are infected with HIV but are not aware that they are; standard precautions should therefore be used when caring for all patients (Health Protection Agency 2010). Standard precautions recommend that every patient is treated as if they were HIV-positive, and recommend treating all blood and body fluids as infected. This also includes all bodily waste (except sweat), non-intact skin and mucous membranes. Care should be taken when handling needles and sharps. Several precautions should be taken:

- Never re-sheath needles.
- Never remove needles from disposable syringes.
- The needle and syringe should be disposed of intact.
- Needles should not be purposely bent or broken by hand.
- Used sharps should be disposed of in the appropriate sharps container.
- Sharps containers should never be filled to more than three-quarters.
- In theatre, scalpels and other sharps should be transferred from one user to another in a receiver.

In the case of a sharps injury, local guidelines for reporting and recording the incident should be followed. Management usually includes:

- cleaning the injury site under running water and encouraging bleeding;
- identifying patients who are a potential source of infection;
- informing the appropriate medical staff;
- counselling and baseline testing to identify current HIV status (consent is required for this);
- post-exposure prophylaxis with antiretroviral drugs;
- follow-up checks for HIV at 1, 3, 6 and occasionally 12 months.

Vertical transmission

Vertical transmission is from mother to baby and can occur during birth and also through breast-feeding. The higher the viral load in the mother, the greater the risk. To reduce the risk of infecting the fetus or child, the mother should be started on antiretroviral medication during pregnancy, delivery should be by caesarean section, and the mother should be discouraged from breast-feeding (Public Health Service Task Force 2010).

Stages of HIV/AIDS

Primary infection (acute HIV infection/syndrome)

The first stage begins at the time of infection and lasts until HIV antibodies are present in the blood. During this stage, the virus is rapidly replicating itself, and the individual is infected and highly infectious. There is a 'window period' during the early part of primary infection when the individual will test HIV-negative. After about 2–3 weeks, tests for viral load and virus glycoprotein antibodies can indicate the presence of HIV.

The first indication of infection is usually influenza-like symptoms, which are evident in up to 90% of infected individuals and typically last a number of days. Other symptoms include:

- fever;
- rigors;
- night sweats;
- lymphadenopathy;
- a rash;
- muscle and joint pain and other symptoms associated with the flu.

As the virus replicates, the number of CD4+ cells begins to fall due both to the virus and to antibodies attacking the infected cells. The CD4+ counts at this stage are usually between 0.5 and 1.5×10^9/L. By the time the individual is able to produce sufficient antibodies to fight the infection, the HIV is already well entrenched and a stalemate has been reached between the antibodies and the virus. This is known as the 'viral set point'. The higher the viral set point, the poorer the prognosis in relation to disease progression; at this point, the disease moves into the next stage.

HIV asymptomatic stage (CD4+ count >0.5 × 10^9/L)

This stage begins at the viral set point and can continue for a number of years. The HIV is now a chronic infection, and although the CD4+ levels fall slowly, they remain high enough to fight other infections. Individuals generally feel well, suffer few symptoms and can, without intervention, remain in this stage for about 10 years, depending on the viral set point.

HIV symptomatic stage (CD4+ count 0.499–0.2 × 10^9/L)

As the CD4+ levels fall, individuals succumb to an HIV-related infection or an infection due to lowered immunity. Initially, the symptoms are mild, including:

- oral or vaginal thrush;
- recurrent eruptions of herpes;
- fever;
- weight loss;
- diarrhoea.

During this time the amount of virus in the blood (the viral load) continues to increase while the CD4+ count continues to fall.

AIDS (CD4+ count <0.2 × 10^9/L)

The presence of one or more AIDS-associated illnesses (Box 18.8) will identify that the person has now got AIDS. At this stage, the viral load is high and the CD4+ count is low; individuals are very exposed to contracting opportunistic infections. Once a person has been identified as having AIDS, they remain in this diagnostic stage even if the viral or CD4+ counts improve.

Management of HIV/AIDS

Survival rates for patients with HIV/AIDS improved greatly with the launch of antiretroviral medications in the 1990s. Highly active antiretroviral therapy (HAART) involves the use of a minimum of two or ideally three HIV/AIDS medications, which can:

- increase life expectancy;
- reduce the incidence of HIV related infections;
- improve an individual's quality of life.

Box 18.8 AIDS-associated illnesses

- Candidiasis of the bronchi, trachea or lungs
- Candidiasis, oesophageal
- Cervical cancer, invasive
- Coccidioidomycosis, disseminated or extrapulmonary
- Cryptococcosis, extrapulmonary
- Cryptosporidiosis, chronic intestinal (longer than 1 month's duration)
- Cytomegalovirus disease (other than of the liver, spleen or lymph nodes)
- Cytomegalovirus retinitis (with loss of vision)
- Encephalopathy, HIV-related
- Herpes simplex: chronic ulcer(s) (longer than 1 month's duration); or bronchitis, pneumonitis or oesophagitis
- Histoplasmosis, disseminated or extrapulmonary
- Isosporiasis, chronic intestinal (longer than 1 month's duration)
- Kaposi's sarcoma
- Lymphoma, Burkitt's (or equivalent term)
- Lymphoma, immunoblastic (or equivalent term)
- Lymphoma, primary, of the brain
- *Mycobacterium avium* complex or M. *kansasii*, disseminated or extrapulmonary
- *Mycobacterium tuberculosis*, any site (pulmonary or extrapulmonary)
- *Mycobacterium*, other species or unidentified species, disseminated or extrapulmonary
- *Pneumocystis jiroveci* pneumonia
- Pneumonia, recurrent (more than one episode in a 12-month period)
- Progressive multifocal leucoencephalopathy
- *Salmonella* septicaemia, recurrent
- Toxoplasmosis of the brain
- Wasting syndrome due to HIV

This is achieved through a reduction and suppression of the viral load and maintenance of the CD4+ count. These drugs are, however, toxic and resistance can develop. There is some debate over the optimal time for commencing treatment: current guidelines (Hammer *et al.* 2008) recommend commencing treatment before the CD4+ count falls below 0.35×10^9/L. There are six different groups of HIV antiretroviral medication:

- Nucleoside reverse transcriptase inhibitors, such as abacavir and tenofovir;
- Non-nucleoside reverse transcriptase inhibitors, such as efavirenz and etravirine;
- Protease inhibitors, such as atazanavir and darunavir;
- Integrase inhibitors, such as raltegravir;
- Fusion inhibitors, such as enfuvirtide;
- CCR5 antagonists, such as maraviroc.

The first four groups of drug work by interfering with HIV replication, while the last two interfere with the entry of HIV into the CD4+ cells.

The nursing needs of individuals with HIV/AIDS depend on the degree to which the disease has progressed. With the advent of HAART, disease progression has become much slower, and the severity of some of the opportunistic infections affecting patients with HIV/AIDS has been reduced. The nursing care of patients who have not progressed beyond the asymptomatic stage is similar to that for non-HIV-positive individuals. For patients who have become symptomatic or have developed AIDS, the risk of contracting an opportunistic infection (Table 18.4) becomes greater. Factors that need to be considered when caring for patients who have HIV/AIDS include:

- psychological support;
- body temperature;
- neurological status;
- respiratory status;
- nutritional status;
- fatigue;
- impaired skin integrity.

Table 18.4 Opportunistic infections, conditions and treatment in persons with HIV/AIDS

	Overview	Treatment
Fungal infections		
Pneumocystis jiroveci (formerly *carinii*) pneumonia	Over 75% of HIV/AIDS sufferers develop this infection without prophylactic intervention Insidious onset Clinical features include: • Fever • Cough • Shortness of breath • Tachypnoea • Tachycardia	Co-trimoxazole (IV/oral) Atovaquone (oral) Pentamidine isetionate (IV/nebulised)
Cryptococcus neoformans	Causes meningitis in immunocompromised individuals Clinical features include: • Fever • Headache • Mental changes	Amphotericin B (IV/oral) Flucytosine (IV) Fluconazole (IV/oral)
Candida albicans	Fungal infection Oral and vaginal thrush Oral infections can extend to the oesophagus Clinical features include: • Sore mouth • Loss of taste and appetite • Difficulty swallowing	Fluconazole (IV/oral) Nystatin (suspension/pastilles) Amphotericin B (IV)
Bacterial infections		
Tuberculosis	Results from reactivation of an old infection or exposure to the bacterium Not only confined to the lungs Other organs include the bone marrow, liver and gastrointestinal tract Clinical features include: • Fever • Chills • Cough • Shortness of breath • Weight loss	A combination of anti-tuberculosis drugs including: • Isoniazid (oral) • Rifampicin (oral) • Ethambutol (oral) • Pyrazinamide (Oral)
Mycobacterium avium complex	Disseminated, multiorgan disease Clinical features include: • Fever • Night sweats • Weight loss • Fatigue • Diarrhoea • Abdominal pain	Clarithromycin (oral) Ethambutol (oral) Rifabutin (oral)

Table 18.4 (*Continued*)

	Overview	Treatment
Viral infections		
Cytomegalovirus (CMV)	Common presentation is CMV retinitis; if untreated, it will lead to blindness	Ganciclovir (IV) Valganciclovir (oral) Foscarnet sodium (IV)
Parasitic infections		
Toxoplasma gondii	Usually seen when CD4+ counts fall below 50×10^9/L in previously infected individuals Common feature is focal encephalitis progressing to seizures and coma if untreated Early clinical features include: • Headache • Confusion • Motor weakness	Pyrimethamine + sulfadiazine + leucovorin Co-trimoxazole (oral) Atovaquone (oral)
Cryptosporidium	Clinical features include: • Non-bloody, watery diarrhoea • Fever • Sometimes malabsorption	Patients who have not commenced HAART should be started on it
Opportunistic conditions		
Kaposi's sarcoma	Is an AIDS-defining illness Since the advent of HAART, it is: • Less common • Slower in its progression Can range from localised cutaneous lesions to a widespread multiorgan condition	Antineoplastic drugs may be used to slow progression in rapidly advancing conditions Pain relief

IV, intravenous.

Psychological support

The initial diagnosis of HIV is often a devastating blow for individuals who may not have even suspected that they were infected. This can lead to a grief response, which includes anger, denial, bargaining, depression and acceptance (Kübler-Ross 1973). Patients with HIV/AIDS can also feel socially isolated due to the stigma that is still associated with this condition. This isolation can be further exacerbated if recurrent hospitalisation for treatment is required. Nursing management includes the following:

- Identify social supports that can be used to assist patients and help them manage their condition more effectively.
- Educate and encourage family members and significant others to be involved in the patients' care and support.
- Observe for and recognise stages of grief.
- Identify appropriate coping mechanisms that were helpful in the past.
- Listen to patients' fears and worries and offer support as appropriate.

- Empower patients in relation to their condition. Knowledge allows patients to make choices and become active participants in their own care.
- Educate patients on:
  - HIV/AIDS;
  - virus transmission;
  - how to reduce the risk of spread;
  - compliance with medication and drug side effects.
- Recognise the need for other support services, such as counselling, to be involved in patient care.

Body temperature

Due to the immune-deficient status of individuals with HIV/AIDS, a rise in body temperature may be the only initial indicator that patients have an infection. Nursing management includes the following:

- Monitor the vital signs, in particular temperature, for signs of infection.
- Educate patients on the importance of reporting and seeking medical assistance when a rise in temperature occurs or when chills, rigors or any other symptoms of infection are experienced.
- If the temperature rises to 38°C or above, a full culture and sensitivity screening should be undertaken.
- Administration of antimicrobial medications should be as prescribed.

Neurological status

The neurological status of patients with HIV/AIDS can be affected by encephalopathy as a result of the HIV infection itself or because of any one of a number of other opportunistic infections (Box 18.8). Nursing care involves:

- neurological assessment for levels of consciousness and verbal and motor responses;
- recording any sensory deficits such as changes in peripheral sensation or vision;
- observation for and reporting of any incidence of headaches or seizures that may indicate a change in neurological status;
- provision of appropriate care for the person with a neurological deficit (see Chapter 17).

Respiratory status

Infections of the respiratory tract are common in the advanced stages of HIV/AIDS, patients being at risk of conditions such as *Pneumocystis jiroveci* pneumonia and tuberculosis, as well as other infections. Nursing care includes:

- assessment of the rate and depth of breathing, the presence of cough or sputum, shortness of breath, cyanosis, pain when breathing or the use of accessory muscles;
- obtaining sputum samples for culture and sensitivity;
- encouraging deep breathing and coughing exercises;
- positioning patients to achieve maximum lung expansion, for example in a Fowler's or semi-Fowler's position;
- administration of oxygen and nebulisers, as prescribed;
- tracheal suctioning as appropriate.

Nutritional status

A number of factors can affect the nutritional status of persons with HIV/AIDS, including opportunistic infections and the effects of wasting syndrome, which is an AIDS-defining condition. Nursing care involves:

- nutritional assessment to identify the baseline status and to develop a healthy eating programme;

- educating patients on:
  - reporting episodes of nausea, vomiting, diarrhoea, anorexia, sore mouth or difficulty swallowing, which may be indicators of opportunistic infections;
  - oral assessment and hygiene, to reduce the risk of oral infections;
- monitoring fluid and electrolyte balance, especially during hospitalisation;
- monitoring patients' weight to identify any change that occurs;
- liaising with the nutritional team.

Fatigue

Fatigue is a common complaint of patients suffering from HIV/AIDS and one that is often dismissed or poorly managed. A number of factors can cause or exacerbate fatigue, so it is important not to regard fatigue as simply part of the patient's condition. Nursing care includes:

- assessment of fatigue:
  - identification and/or elimination of potential causes of fatigue;
  - how long has the symptom existed;
  - what factors improve or exacerbate it;
- treatment of underlying causes, for example infection and anaemia;
- encouraging mild exercise and sufficient rest;
- encouraging the use of family and other social supports in coping with this symptom.

Impaired skin integrity

The skin of individuals who suffer from HIV/AIDS is susceptible to damage from opportunistic infections, side effects of treatment and conditions such as Kaposi's sarcoma. In the later stage of the disease, skin problems associated with long-term bed rest can also develop. Nursing care includes:

- assessment for signs of lesions or breaks in the skin's integrity;
- risk assessment for patients on bed rest;
- planning interventions appropriate to the patient's level of risk;
- encouraging mobilising as appropriate;
- keeping the skin clean and dry;
- the use of appropriate moving and handling techniques to avoid damaging the skin through friction or sheering.

Family and patient education

Ideally, families and significant others as well as patients need to be educated about HIV/AIDS. Informational needs will vary, depending on what individuals already know about the condition. This information should include:

- information about HIV/AIDS, routes of transmission, and the disease trajectory and outcome;
- the safe management and disposal of soiled items and body fluids;
- the importance of hygiene and hand-washing;
- avoiding contact with people who have infections, have recently been vaccinated or have come in contact with someone with an infectious disease;
- the risks posed by smoking and excessive alcohol intake;
- not sharing needles or equipment if the individual is an IVD user;
- not sharing personal equipment such as razors.

Family members need to understand the facts about the disease and how it is spread in order to prevent accidental transmission.

Prevention

There is no cure and no effective vaccine for HIV; the aim for all healthcare staff should therefore be prevention. Transmission can be reduced through:

- safer sexual practices;
- not sharing needles;
- the use of needle exchange programmes;
- non-donation of blood by at-risk individuals and groups;
- the use of standard precautions;
- the proper management of sharps.

Conclusion

The human immune system has a major role to play in ensuring that individuals live a healthy, disease-free life. Sometimes, however, the system whose role it is to protect the body falls victim to disease or responds in a way that damages health and can cause illness. This chapter has discussed some of these conditions, their impact on patients and the relevant medical and nursing management.

Visit www.wileyfundamentalseries.com/medicalnursing and read Reflective Questions 18.1 and 18.2 to think more about this topic.

Now visit the companion website and test yourself on this chapter:
www.wileyfundamentalseries.com/medicalnursing

References

Bergs, L. (2005) Goodpasture syndrome. *Critical Care Nurse*, **25**(5):50–8.
Bryant, H. (2007) Anaphylaxis: recognition, treatment and education. *Emergency Nurse*, **15**(2):24–8.
Centers for Disease Control and Prevention (2010a) The Role of STD Detection and Treatment in HIV Prevention, CDC Fact Sheet. Retrieved 7th June 2011 from http://www.cdc.gov/std/hiv/STDFact-STD-HIV.htm.
Centers for Disease Control and Prevention (2010b) Sexually Transmitted Diseases Treatment Guidelines, 2010: Clinical Prevention Guidance. Retrieved 7th June 2011 from http://www.cdc.gov/std/treatment/2010/clinical.htm.
Department of Health and Children (2008) *HIV and AIDS Education and Prevention Plan 2008–2012*. Dublin: Stationery Office.
Griffiths, M. (2008) Emergency treatment of anaphylaxis: implications for nurses. *Primary Health Care*, **8**(2):14–15.
Hammer, S.M., Eron, J.J., Reiss, P. *et al*. (2008) Antiretroviral treatment of adult HIV infection: 2008 recommendations of the international AIDS Society USA Panel. *Journal of the American Medical Association*, **300**(5):555–70.
Health Protection Agency (2008) Sexually Transmitted Infections and Young People in the United Kingdom: 2008 Report. Retrieved 7th June 2011 from http://www.hpa.org.uk/web/HPAwebFile/HPAweb_C/1216022461534..
Health Protection Agency (2010) HIV in the United Kingdom: 2010 Report. 4(47), 26th November 2010. Retrieved 7th June 2011 from http://www.hpa.org.uk/hivuk2010.
Kübler-Ross, E. (1973) *On Death and Dying*. London: Tavistock Routledge.
Public Health Service Task Force (2010) Recommendations for Use of Antiretroviral Drugs in Pregnant HIV-1-Infected Women for Maternal Health and Interventions to Reduce Perinatal HIV Transmission in the United States. Retrieved 16th June 2011 from http://www.aidsinfo.nih.gov/contentfiles/perinatalGL.pdf.
Rooney, J. (2005) Systemic lupus erythematosus: unmasking a great imitator. *Nursing*, **35**(11):54–61.
UNAIDS (2010) Global Report: UNAIDS Report on the Global AIDS Epidemic 2010. Retrieved 7th June 2011 from http://www.unaids.org/documents/20101123_GlobalReport_em.pdf.

19

Nursing care of conditions related to haematological disorders

Mairead Ni Chonghaile[1] and Laura O'Regan[2]

[1]*St James' Hospital, Dublin, Ireland*

[2]*St George's University of London and Kingston University, London, UK*

Contents

Introduction	387
Overview of blood	387
Blood transfusion	395
Investigations	397
Anaemia	402
Polycythaemia	408
Haemophilia	409
Thrombocytopenia	409
Disseminated intravascular coagulation	410
Multiple myeloma	410
Leukaemia	413
Lymphoma	415
Haematopoietic stem cell transplant	417
Conclusion	420
References	421

Learning outcomes

Having read this chapter, you will be able to:

- Outline the normal and altered pathophysiology of the haematology system
- Describe the medical and nursing management of patients with haematological disorders
- Describe nursing care principles governing safe practices in the transfusion of blood and blood products

Fundamentals of Medical-Surgical Nursing: A Systems Approach, First Edition. Edited by Anne-Marie Brady, Catherine McCabe, and Margaret McCann.

Introduction

Nursing knowledge and skills related to the haematological system are also applicable to all areas of medical and surgical nursing. A sound knowledge and understanding of haematology, and how to interpret it, underpins assessment and care planning interventions. This chapter will address normal and abnormal pathophysiology, including the nursing care and treatment of both malignant and non-malignant haematological conditions.

Overview of blood

The haematological system comprises blood, bone marrow and lymph nodes. Blood is considered to be an organ, although it exists in fluid connective tissue and develops from the mesenchyme, a connective tissue in which the blood cells and smaller components are suspended in and surrounded by plasma fluid. The pH of the blood is between 7.35 and 7.45. The total blood volume is estimated at 4–5 L in females and 5–6 L in males, accounting for approximately 8% of the body weight. The composition and function of blood are outlined in Boxes 19.1 and 19.2.

Cellular components

There are three main types of blood cell; erythrocytes (red blood cells [RBCs]), leucocytes (white blood cells [WBCs]) and thrombocytes (platelets). The blood cells originate from a pluripotent stem cell type

Box 19.1 Components of the blood (adapted from Nair & Peate 2009)

Body weight and volume

Whole blood (8%):

- Plasma (55%)
- Blood cells (45%)

Other fluids and tissues (92%)

Formed cells

Plasma:

- Proteins (7%)
- Water (91.5%)
- Other solutes (1.5%)

Blood cells:

- Platelets (150,000–400,000/µL)
- White blood cells (>5000–10,000/µL):
  - Neutrophils (60–70%)
  - Lymphocytes (20–25%)
  - Monocytes (3–8%)
  - Eosinophils (2–4%)
  - Basophils
- Red blood cells (4.8–5.4 million/µL)

Box 19.2 Main functions of blood

- Acts as a transport system, carrying oxygen, blood cells, hormones, enzymes, chemical and minerals
- Obtains nutrients from the alimentary canal, distributing them throughout the body
- Removes waste products, e.g. carbon dioxide from the lungs and excretory waste from the kidneys
- Regulates body heat by distributing the temperature
- Haemostasis (control of bleeding)
- Regulates water and electrolyte balance
- Circulates antibodies, providing a protective immune function

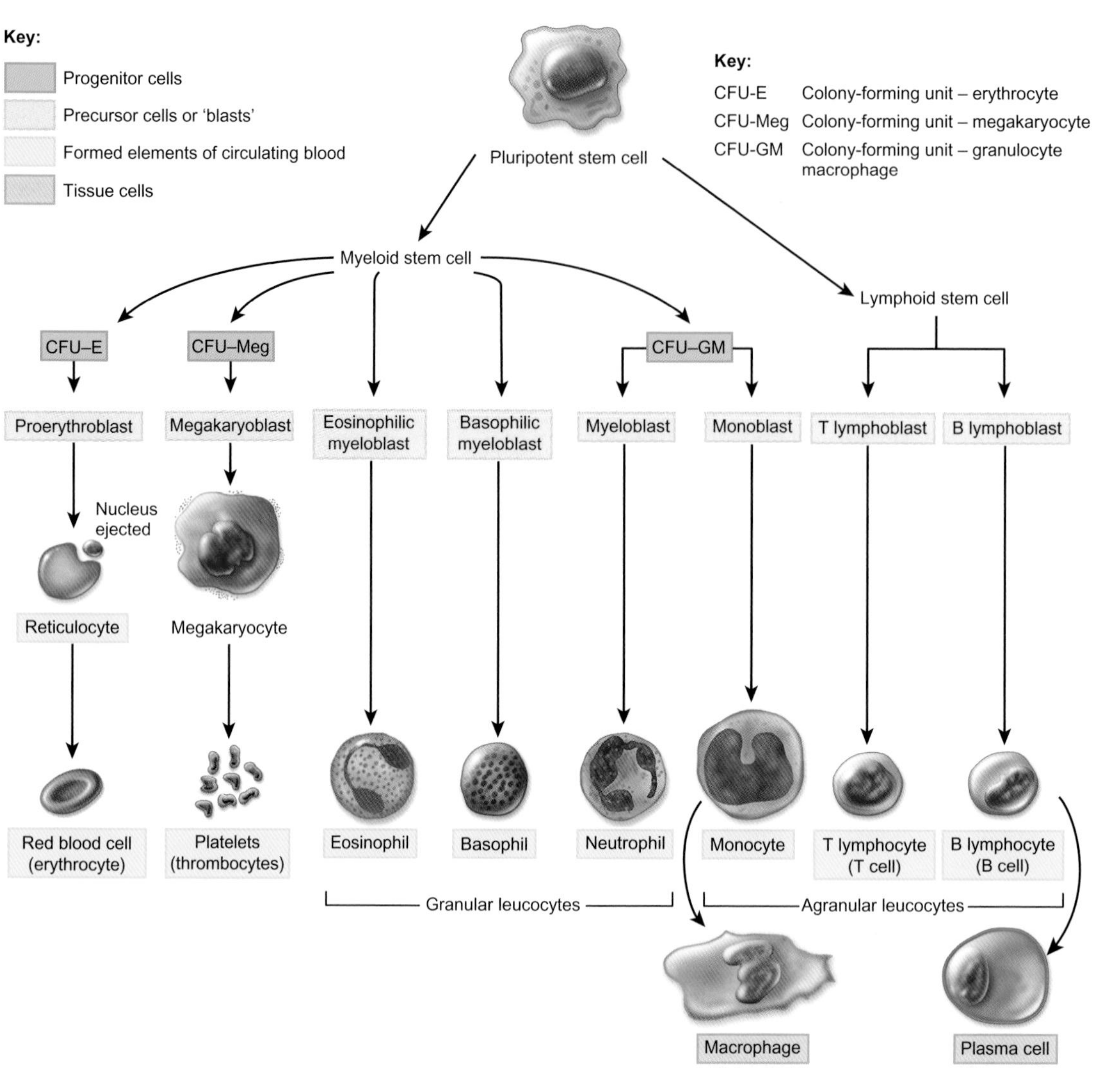

Figure 19.1 The formation of blood cells. Reproduced from Nair, M. & Peate, I. (2009) *Fundamentals of Applied Pathophysiology*, with kind permission from Wiley Blackwell.

synthesised in the bone marrow and found in the iliac crest of the pelvis, the long bones of the humerus and the vertebrae, skull, ribs and sternum. This pluripotent stem cell differentiates into specific blood cell lines. Haemopoiesis (or haematopoiesis) is the term that refers to the formation of specific cell types (Figure 19.1). Many disorders of the haematological system arise from a deviation from normal haemopoiesis, resulting in malformation of blood cells along the developmental line.

Erythrocytes

Normal RBCs are biconcave discs, approximately 8 μm in diameter, whose shape and pliability gives them the flexibility to pass through capillary walls, facilitating gaseous exchange and the carriage of essential oxygen around the body. Mature RBCs contain no nucleus. Reference values for RBCs are outlined in Table 19.1.

Table 19.1 Erythrocyte reference values (adapted from Waugh & Grant 2010)

Measure	Normal values
Erythrocyte count • Number of erythrocytes per litre, or per cubic millilitre (mm^3), of blood	Males: 4.5–6.5 × 10^{12}/L (4.5–6.5 million/mm^3) Females: 3.8–5.8 × 10^{12}/L (3.8–5.8 million/mm^3)
Packed cell volume (PCV, haematocrit) • The proportion of red cells per litre, or per mm^3, of blood	0.40–0.55
Mean cell volume (MCV) • The volume of an average cell, measured in femtolitres ($1\,fL = 1 \times 10^{-15}\,L$)	80–96 fL
Haemoglobin • The weight of haemoglobin in whole blood, measured in g/100 mL blood	Males: 13–18 g/100 mL Females: 11.5–16.5 g/100 mL
Mean corpuscular haemoglobin (MCH) • The average amount of haemoglobin per cell, measured in picograms ($1\,pg = 10^{-12}\,g$)	27–32 pg/cell
Mean corpuscular haemoglobin concentration (MCHC) • The weight of haemoglobin in 100 mL of red cells	30–35 g/100 mL of RBCs

Haemoglobin

Haemoglobin consists of a protein called globin and haem, a pigment containing iron. The haemoglobin molecule, composed of four polypeptide chains, consists of two alpha and two beta chains, and has four atoms of iron, each carrying one molecule of oxygen. Each RBC contains about 280 million haemoglobin molecules.

Haemoglobin accounts for 33% of the weight of the RBC by virtue of its iron content and is responsible for giving blood its characteristic red colour, oxygenated blood being a brighter red colour than deoxygenated blood. When haemoglobin binds with oxygen, it produces oxyhaemoglobin, which makes up the oxygen-carrying capacity of blood. RBCs do not contain any mitochondria and use anaerobic respiration to produce energy, thus conserving the oxygen they are carrying.

In addition to iron, vitamin B_{12}, folic acid, pyridoxine (vitamin B_6) and other factors are required for the healthy synthesis of erythrocytes. Where there is a deficiency during erythropoiesis, a decreased number of erythrocytes are produced and anaemia occurs.

Erythropoiesis

Hypoxia increases erythropoiesis by stimulating the production of erythropoietin in the kidneys, which increases the production of proerythroblasts to enter the blood and the rate of reticulocyte maturation. As a result, the number of erythrocytes and the amount of oxygen uptake increase, reducing the hypoxic state.

The average life span of erythrocytes is 120 days, after which they are destroyed in a process known as haemolysis and are removed by the reticuloendothelial system, particularly in the liver and the spleen. The reticuloendothelial cells produce bilirubin from haemoglobin that is released from the RBCs, and this is excreted in the bile. Iron released from haemoglobin during bilirubin formation is carried in the plasma to the bone marrow, bound to a protein called transferrin and used for the production of new haemoglobin.

Leucocytes

Leucocytes (WBCs) are divided into two groups: granulocytes (60%) and agranulocytes (mononuclear cells; 40%). They are easily differentiated from RBCs as they contain a nucleus, are larger and have the ability to move out of blood vessels, a process called diapedesis.

Granulocytes

Granulocytes are defined by the presence of granules in the cytoplasm. Their diameter is 2–3 times that of RBCs, and their nuclear matter is arranged in lobes, between two and four in number, giving rise to the name polymorphonuclear leucocytes. The number of circulating granulocytes remains constant except in the presence of infection, during which numbers increase (leucocytosis). A decrease from normal values is called leucopenia. Granulocytes are further divided into three groups:

- basophils
- eosinophils
- neutrophils.

Basophils account for approximately 1% of granulocytes, contain lobed nuclei and have a specific immune function as they bring about a reaction to harmful substances. Their cytoplasmic granules contain heparin, histamine and other substances, which cause inflammation. Allergens – antigens that cause an allergy – stimulate the basophils to release the contents of their granules.

Eosinophils account for 2% of granulocytes, contain a B-shaped nuclei and have a specific phagocytic mode of action. They contain enzymes and peroxidase in their granules, which function against parasites. Eosinophil numbers increase during allergic reactions.

Neutrophils account for 60–70% of total circulating WBCs, and their primary function is phagocytosis. Their nuclei are multilobed and their cytoplasm contains lysosomes. They are capable of moving out of the blood vessel in response to foreign material and are present at the site of inflammation within an hour. The number of neutrophils increases in the presence of:

- infection
- leukaemia
- inflammation
- metabolic disorders
- injury to the body
- pregnancy
- myocardial infarction.

Agranulocytes (mononuclear leucocytes)

There are two types of agranulocyte: lymphocytes, accounting for 25%, and monocytes, accounting for 5% of the total number of leucocytes.

Lymphocytes are suspended in lymphatic fluid, which is found in the lymphatic tissues and spleen. Their lifespan is between a few hours and years, and they differ from other WBCs in their mode of action as they are not phagocytic. There are two types of lymphocyte: T and B lymphocytes. T cells are formed in the **t**hymus gland, while B cells originate in the **b**one marrow (see Figure 19.1).

T lymphocytes are involved in graft reactions and in fighting cancer and viruses by direct cell-kill, while B lymphocytes make antibodies in response to antigens in the body. Once this occurs, and assisted by T lymphocytes, B lymphocytes enlarge and divide, producing two types of cell:

- plasma cells
- memory B cells.

Plasma cells release antibodies, or immunoglobulins. Once antibodies have bound to antigens, they are prime targets for helper T lymphocytes, cytotoxic T lymphocytes and macrophages. Antibodies bind to the toxin and activate the complement system, which in turn accelerates the phagocytic response. This process of the combination of B and T lymphocyte production leads to the release of cytokines and is more specifically referred to below in relation to macrophage activity. The cytokines produced are chemical messengers released by specific cells of the immune system that are used by immune cells to communicate with one another. Examples of cytokines include interleukins and interferons.

The **memory B lymphocytes** hold within them the memory of the interaction that has occurred for a variably long period of time afterwards, providing immunity against the same antigens (see Chapter 18).

Monocytes are the largest of the leucocytes and have two modes of action; one is phagocytosis, where as the other mode of action involves their entering the tissues and developing into macrophages. Interleukin-1, which is produced by both types of cell, has a specific function in the inflammatory response and in producing immunity. Interleukin-1 acts on the hypothalamus, increasing the body temperature, stimulates the development of some globulins in the liver and enhances the activation of T lymphocytes.

The monocyte and macrophage system is also referred to as the reticuloendothelial system. A number of macrophages are fixed in particular body locations – as synovial cells, Kupffer cells (in the liver), Langerhans cells (in the skin), alveolar macrophages (in the lungs), sinus (reticular) cells (in the spleen), cells in the lymph nodes and thymus gland, mesangial cells (in the kidney) and osteoblasts (in bone). Macrophages release cytokines, for example interleukin-1, and link the specific with the non-specific immune reaction.

Thrombocytes (platelets)

Platelets lack a nucleus, are disc-shaped particles measuring 2–4 μm in diameter, arise from megakaryocytes in the bone marrow and are regulated by thrombopoietin. Platelets usually circulate for approximately 1 week before being destroyed and have a key role in haemostasis (the control of bleeding).

Blood clotting

There are three phases of haemostasis:

- Phase 1 is vasoconstriction of the injured blood vessel.
- Phase 2 sees the formation of a platelet plug.
- Phase 3 involves the formation of a fibrinogen clot.

The final stage is called fibrinolysis and involves the breakdown of the clot.

Vasoconstriction

The first phase of clotting begins in response to an injury to the blood vessel, causing the vessel to go into spasm and constrict. Thrombocytes produce serotonin, causing the muscles of the vessel wall to constrict and thus decrease the blood flow. Constriction is also brought about by other factors, including the stimulation of pain receptors and the release of thromboxanes by the damaged cell wall.

Platelet plug formation

Platelets adhere to one another, releasing thromboxanes and ADP (adenosine diphosphate), which further promote platelet aggregation. The result is the formation of a primary platelet plug, from which the intrinsic coagulation pathway arises due to breakdown of parts of the platelets and the release of substances into the bloodstream. The extrinsic pathway arises from the release of tissue factors a result of vessel injury. There is an overlap between the two pathways, involving the interaction of a complex series of clotting factors (Figure 19.2).

Fibrinogen clot formation

There are two pathways by which coagulation occurs – the extrinsic and the intrinsic pathway – in collaboration with the various clotting factors listed in Box 19.3. The extrinsic pathway is activated when the vessel is damaged, causing the release of certain clotting factors to work in collaboration with

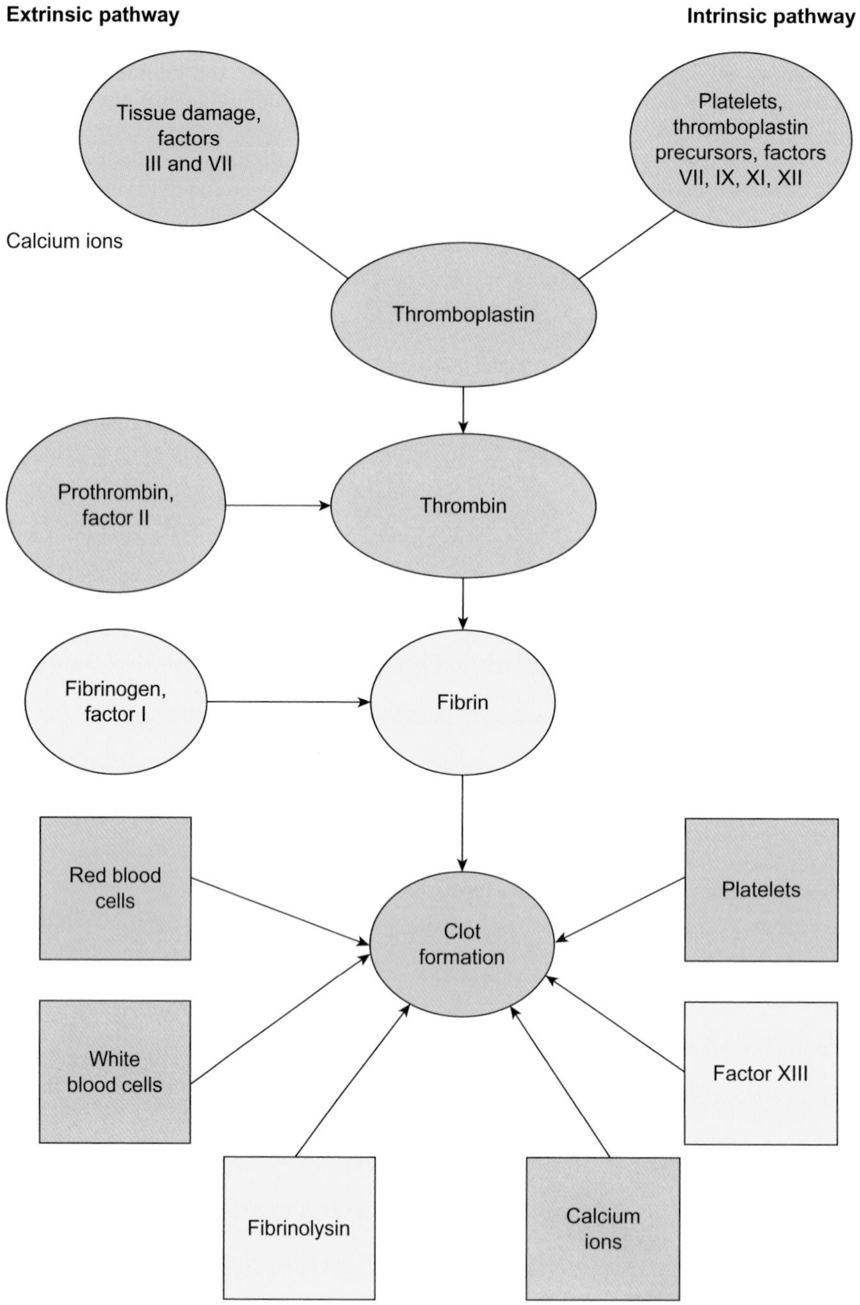

Figure 19.2 The clotting cascade.

calcium to release thromboplastin. As a result of a series of reactions, prothrombin is converted to thrombin, which in turn converts fibrinogen to fibrin. The intrinsic pathway is activated when the collagen lining of the blood vessel is exposed, producing thromboplastin.

The fibrin forms a mesh across the damaged vessel, trapping blood cells and allowing the cut to heal. Clots that form in the body are broken down by the fibrinolytic system, which consists of plasmin and other proteolytic enzymes. As the tissue is repaired, the clots dissolve.

Box 19.3 Clotting factors. Reproduced from Nair, M. & Peate, I. (2009) *Fundamentals of Applied Pathophysiology*, with kind permission from Wiley Blackwell

I	Fibrinogen
II	Prothrombin
III	Thromboplastin
IV	Calcium
V	Proaccelerin, labile factor
VII	Serum prothrombin conversion accelerator
VIII	Antihaemophilic factor
IX	Christmas factor, plasma thrombin component
X	Stuart–Power factor
XI	Plasma thromboplastin antecedent
XII	Hageman factor
XIII	Fibrin-stabilising factor

Blood plasma

Plasma is the straw-coloured, fluid part of blood in which all the cellular components are suspended (Box 19.4); it is made up of 92% water and accounts for 55% of the blood volume.

Blood groups

Antigens are located on the surface of RBCs, while antibodies are found in the circulating plasma. Antibodies are antigen-specific, combining to a certain antigen and causing agglutination, i.e. clumping together, of the cells. The combination of antigens and antibodies can also cause haemolysis, rupturing the blood cells. Blood grouping is derived from the antigens on the surface of RBCs, which make up the ABO and rhesus systems (Table 19.2).

The use of the term 'universal donor' for individuals with group O blood can be misleading as there are two mechanisms by which group O blood can cause a reaction:

- There may be mismatching of groups other than ABO, emphasising that all blood groups should be correctly matched.
- Donors' antibodies can react with recipients' antigens. Type O blood contains anti-A and anti-B antibodies. Therefore, if, for example, type O is transfused to a type A patient, the A antibodies will react against the A antigens on the surface of the type O blood. This is, however, not usually cause for concern due to the dilution of the donor's antibodies in the recipient's blood.

The distribution of blood groups often correlates with different ethnicities, as suggested in Table 19.2.

Rhesus factor

The rhesus factor is an important antigen found on the surface of some RBCs. In the UK, it is estimated that 85% of the population are rhesus-positive (as they have factor D) and the remaining 15% are rhesus-negative (as they do not have factor D). If rhesus-positive blood is given to a rhesus-negative person, agglutination will occur, and there are important implications here for cross-matching. Antibodies against the rhesus antigen occur when there is exposure through a transfusion of blood or by cross-placental transfer of blood that is positive to a rhesus-negative mother.

Box 19.4 Components of plasma

Albumin
- This accounts for 60% of plasma proteins
- It helps to regulate the osmotic pressure of the blood
- Low levels (hypoalbuminaemia) cause movement of fluid into the cellular spaces, resulting in oedema
- Albumin has carrying capacity for fatty acids, drugs and hormones
- Along with fibrinogen, it is held to be responsible for plasma viscosity

Fibrinogen
- Fibrinogen accounts for 4% of plasma proteins

Globulins
- Globulins account for 36% of plasma proteins
- They can be divided into three types:
  - Alpha
  - Beta
  - Gamma
- Alpha/beta globulins:
  - Are produced in the liver
  - Are transport globulins and carry substances such as thyroxin on thyroid-binding globulin, iron on transferrin, and fat-soluble vitamins
- Gamma globulins are produced by B lymphocytes and are known as antibodies or immunoglobulins

Electrolytes
- These are inorganic molecules that separate into ions when dissolved in water
- They have an important function in regulating osmosis, pH balance, muscle contraction and nerve impulses
- The main electrolytes are sodium, potassium, calcium, magnesium, chloride and bicarbonate

Cellular waste
- Plasma forms a transport medium for urea, creatinine and uric acid

Nutrients
- Plasma transports amino acids, glucose, glycerol and fatty acids to the alimentary tract

Hormones
- Hormones are transported in plasma to their target organs, where they exert their function

Gases
- The main gases transported are oxygen and carbon dioxide
- Oxygen combines with haemoglobin to form oxyhaemoglobin
- Carbon dioxide is present as bicarbonate ions in the plasma

Rhesus incompatibility can pose a major problem in pregnancy when fetal blood crosses the placenta; the mother becomes sensitised to the rhesus antigen and produces antibodies, which cross the placenta causing agglutination or a condition called haemolytic disease of the newborn, which can be fatal. There is usually no problem in the first pregnancy as the cross-placental passage of antigens is minimal and occurs in late pregnancy or at birth due to a tear in the placenta; there is little time for the mother to produce antibodies against the antigens. In subsequent pregnancies where the fetus is rhesus-positive, the reaction to a leak of blood across the placenta is more pronounced as the mother is already sensitised to the antigen. In severe cases of haemolytic disease of the newborn, a transfusion through the umbilical cord may be necessary and premature birth may be induced.

Mothers are monitored for antibody levels and given an injection of anti-D antibody after the first birth, miscarriage or abortion, or prior to birth. Its purpose is to inactivate the fetal antigens and prevent sensitisation of the mother and production of antibodies, or further antibody production by the mother.

Blood transfusion

Donated blood is routinely screened for HIV, hepatitis B and C and syphilis. Some countries do not allow blood donation from prospective donors who have lived in the UK between 1980 and 1996, in order to remove the risk of transmission of Creutzfeldt–Jakob disease (CJD). Blood is currently leucodepleted as this reduces the risk of transmission of CJD and other infectious reactions. Box 19.5 provides details on the nursing management of a blood transfusion, while Table 19.3 outlines different blood products.

Table 19.2 Blood grouping (adapted from Nair & Peate 2009)

Blood Group	Frequency in the UK (%)	Antigens	Antibodies	Can donate to	Can receive from
A	42	Antigen A	Anti-B	A, AB	A, O
B	8	Antigen B	Anti-A	B, AB	B, O
AB	3	Antigen A Antigen B	None	AB	A, B, AB, O
O	47	None	Anti-A Anti-B	A, B, AB, O Universal donor, if rhesus negative	O

Box 19.5 Nursing management of a blood transfusion – core principles

Ascertaining the rationale for blood transfusion

- The rationale needs to outweigh the risks
- The reasons for a transfusion are:
  - Life-saving situations (massive blood loss due to trauma)
  - Replacing blood loss due to surgery or a procedure
  - Treatment of conditions that result from bone marrow failure, e.g. anaemia, haemophilia or sickle cell disease
- Check the hospital thresholds for ordering blood (which are set out to minimise blood waste and give optimal treatment to a specific patient group); e.g. the haemoglobin level needs to be below 8 g/L in some haematology day care units
- The clinical abnormality determines the type of transfusion
- In massive blood loss, defined as >1.5 L, an emergency blood alert is sounded immediately by contacting the blood bank
- Each emergency is classified and coded, according to the clinical indication; each has appropriate specific guidelines and blood issuing requirements

(Continued)

Blood sampling

- Safety measures are paramount to good-quality care
- This is the responsibility of registered nurses and phlebotomists
- Ensure the correct labelling of blood samples:
  - Complete all information fields, and check off the patient's name band
  - The sample bottle must be signed by the professional
  - The sample blood bottle label is completed at the patient's bedside by the staff member who takes the blood
- Serious ABO mismatch errors occur at the time of sampling or when the blood is given to the patient due to incorrect identification (Provan *et al.* 2009)

Cross-matching/requesting

- Check local policy guidelines to ensure that the appropriate professional with the correct training and competency completes the cross-match form and requests the blood
- The patient's details, type of blood, amount and time to transfuse (urgency) as well as any specific requirements must be clearly written on the request form
- Special requirements include whether the blood should be negative for cytomegalovirus or have been irradiated prior to issue; this is particularly important for stem cell transplant patients

Prescription

- In the UK and Ireland, blood can be prescribed by suitably trained nurse practitioners or doctors
- It is prescribed on the drug chart under the 'IV medicines' section or on a transfusion prescription record
- The unit of blood or any blood product is checked by two registered nurses or one registered nurse and a doctor
- Yearly competency training in the handling and administering of blood products is a professional requirement

Consent/checking procedure

- Patients must provide consent prior to administration; this must be documented by the prescriber. A separate consent form is not necessary
- Educate patients on:
  - The rationale for transfusion
  - The potential side effects
  - Any possible alternatives
- Provide an information leaflet to patients who regularly receive blood transfusions
- For patients who lack the capacity or are unconscious, the 'best interests' principle is followed in the absence of an advance directive
- Patients need to be cross matched and consented prior to major surgery
- Ascertain whether patients have any religious beliefs that might prelude them from consenting to a blood transfusion, e.g. they are Jehovah Witnesses:
  - Clearly document what, if any, blood product is acceptable for that patient
  - It is recommended that suitable emergency contingency plans be documented in care plans prior to major elective surgery or prior to giving birth. Such plans must be agreed well in advance (at least 3 weeks) by the physician or surgeon with the inclusion of the patients, and if necessary religious ministers and legal representatives

Record-keeping

- Manage the traceability of blood by means of a paper trail
- Blood is not dispatched from the blood blank until it has been checked and registered by trained professionals
- Accompanying paperwork must match the identification and requirements of patients and their prescription
- Regular traceability audits and blood transfusion error audits are required
- Observations must be monitored and reactions reported

Administration

- The care and management of blood transfusions needs to comply with local policy
- Prior to administration:
    - At the bedside, two registered nurses must check the patient's identification against the name band
    - Check the prescription against the paperwork accompanying the blood
    - Check for damage to the packaging and for suspended components or clotting
- Monitor vital signs prior to commencement, every 15 minutes during the first hour and then hourly
- Observe for:
    - Acute and delayed haemolytic reactions
    - Anaphylaxis
    - Acute lung injury
    - Post-transfusion purpura
    - Pyrexia
    - Transfusion-associated graft versus host disease
    - Transfusion-transmitted infection
    - Fluid overload
- Report signs of abnormality to the medical team; the blood will be stopped and the appropriate treatment administered
- Report adverse events or 'near misses' to the:
    - Transfusion manager
    - Risk management team, via the internal incident reporting system
- In the UK and Ireland, problems associated with blood transfusion are reported to:
    - Serious Hazards of Transfusion (SHOT) schemes
    - The risk management incident reporting system
- Further investigation and reporting to SHOT is the responsibility of the blood bank manager and the hospital transfusion committee
- SHOT receives yearly reports of numerous avoidable errors (the most common being administration of the wrong blood to patients)

Transfusion reactions

A number of blood reactions can occur when transfusing blood products (Box 19.6). General signs and symptoms include pyrexia, tachycardia, rigors, urticaria, bone and muscle pain, dyspnoea and gastrointestinal upset.

Investigations

Since the collection of specimens requires an invasive procedure, consent must be sought from patients, who are informed about:

Table 19.3 Blood products (adapted from Dougherty & Lamb 2009)

Transfusion type	ABO/rhesus cross-matching	Administration	Shelf-life storage
RBC transfusions	Yes ABO compatible	A blood-giving set with an integral filter Change 12-hourly Change if giving another fluid type	Shelf life: 35 days at 2–6°C Once out of the fridge, use within 30 minutes Maximum time to complete infusion is 5 hours
Platelets	Rhesus-negative patients under the age of 40 should be given rhesus D-negative platelets Preferably ABO compatible	Platelet-giving set Change for each unit	Shelf-life: 4–5 days at 20–24°C once on the platelet agitator Start 30 minutes after the platelets have left the agitator Give within 30 minutes
Fresh frozen plasma	Yes ABO compatible	Blood-giving set with an integral filter Should be changed every 12 hours Change if giving another fluid type	Storage: up to a year at −30°C Administer as soon as thawed Complete infusion within 4 hours Anaphylaxis is a risk with rapid infusion
Cryoprecipitate	Yes ABO compatible	Blood-giving set with an integral filter Should be changed every 12 hours Change if giving another fluid type	Storage: up to a year at −30°C Administer as soon as thawed Complete infusion within 4 hours Anaphylaxis is a risk with rapid infusion

- the purpose of the test;
- the time frame in which they will know the result;
- how the result will be communicated.

Care of the venepuncture site and specimen collection should adhere to good clinical practice guidance.

Blood tests

Blood tests (Box 19.7) are routinely collected to:

- confirm disease;
- monitor disease;
- regulate therapy or treatment.

Box 19.6 Management of transfusion reactions

- Stop the infusion and contact the medical team
- Check the vital signs
- Check the patient's identity against the paperwork
- Mild fever:
  - Paracetamol
  - Infuse at a slower rate
- Mild allergic reactions:
  - Stop the infusion
  - Give chlorphenamine prior to a slower recommencement of the transfusion
- Suspected ABO incompatibility:
  - Send the unit to the blood bank
  - Set up a saline infusion and initiate early warning scoring
  - Monitor and support urinary output
- Severe allergic reactions (anaphylaxis):
  - Chlorphenamine
  - Bronchodilators
  - Intravenous fluids
  - If necessary, adrenaline, hydrocortisone and dopamine
  - Send the unit to the blood bank
- Suspected bacterial infection:
  - Blood cultures
  - Intravenous antibiotics and oxygen therapy
  - The unit of blood must be investigated
- Fluid overload:
  - Furosemide and oxygen therapy
  - Monitor the patient closely

Bone marrow aspirate/biopsy

Bone marrow aspiration and trephine biopsy are used to diagnose haematological conditions and monitor the success of treatment. A sample is taken by inserting an aspiration needle into the bone marrow. The routine site is the iliac crest, although rarely the sternum can be used, but only for aspiration. The sample is then sent for specific cytogenesis (chromosomal testing), immunophenotyping and molecular analysis. The procedure is performed by suitably trained healthcare professionals.

Nurses are routinely involved with patient care before, during and after the procedure (Box 19.8). Patients who require a bone marrow aspirate or biopsy experience high anxiety. The procedure is painful, and the discomfort can last for 3 days.

Box 19.7 Blood tests

Blood film

- This requires a small sample of blood in EDTA (ethylenediaminetetraacetic acid)
- It can discern various haematological conditions, such as leukaemia

Full blood count (FBC)

- The FBC gives information about RBC, haemoglobin, WBC and platelet levels, including the differential breakdown or percentage of each nucleated cell per cubic millilitre of blood
- It fulfils a role in detecting and monitoring a disease
- It is essential for the surveillance of ongoing treatment
- The FBC also gives the value of the reticulocyte count, the haematocrit or PCV (packed cell volume), and the mean cell volume (MCV)

Haemoglobin

- Haemoglobin is measured during the FBC and expressed in grams per litre

Erythrocyte sedimentation rate

- The erythrocyte sedimentation rate (ESR) measures the rate at which the RBCs fall in columns in a capillary tube
- A raised ESR is indicative of an infection, inflammatory disorder and/or malignancy

Neutrophil count

- Neutrophils are a type of WBC
- They are documented on a differential blood count
- Neutropenia is characterised as a count $<2.0 \times 10^9$/L
- The risk of developing infective complications greatly increases as the count reduces
- Their parameters are as follows:
  - A count of $1.0–1.5 \times 10^9$/L carries no significant risk of infection
  - A count of $0.5–1.0 \times 10^9$/L carries a moderate risk of infection, and the patient can usually be treated as an outpatient
  - A count $<0.5 \times 10^9$/L carries a major risk of infection and necessitates admission and intravenous antibiotic treatment

Coagulation screen

- The screen measures various bleeding times by measuring the activity of certain components of the clotting mechanism:
  - Prothrombin time (PT) – assesses the extrinsic clotting pathway. It is prolonged in patients who are on warfarin therapy, and in patients with liver disorders and disseminated intravascular coagulation (DIC)
  - Activated partial thromboplastin time (APTT) – assesses the intrinsic clotting pathway. It is prolonged in patients receiving heparin and those who have liver disease and DIC
  - International normalised ratio (INR) – measures the PT of patients compared with an international average range

Sickling test

- This is the diagnostic test for sickle cell anaemia

Coomb's test

- A positive Coomb's test or direct antiglobulin test (DAT) indicates the presence of RBC antibodies
- This is the diagnostic tool to detect red cell haemolysis

Reticulocyte count

- This is the percentage of young (1–2-day-old), non-nucleated erythrocytes in the peripheral blood
- Raised or lowered reticulocyte counts are indicative of altered physiological states

Haemoglobin electrophoresis

- This is performed to detect abnormal haemoglobin production
- It is used to diagnose haemoglobinopathies or thalassaemias

Human leucocyte antigen (HLA) typing

- HLA typing is a histocompatibility test to discern gene complexes encoding the cell surface membranes of the immune system
- It ascertains an HLA match for patients being considered for stem cell or bone marrow transplants from a donor
- The degree of likeness of the complexes between the recipient and perspective donor will determine the likelihood of the selection and potential side effects after transplantation

Box 19.8 Nursing management of patients undergoing bone marrow aspiration

- Ensure that:
  - Consent is obtained and information provided on:
    - the rationale for the test
    - what the test entails
    - potential side effects
  - Patients are:
    - offered short-acting sedation (lorazepam or midazolam)
    - given local anaesthetic
    - offered oral analgesia during and following the procedure
- Position patients in the left or right lateral position
- Take observations before and immediately after the procedure and at 15-minute intervals thereafter
- Observe patients throughout, and give further sedation as required
- Observe oxygen saturation levels after the procedure, as the sedative effect can cause hypoxia
- Assist practitioners (specialist nurse or doctor) with collecting and labelling the samples
- Apply a pressure dressing to the site
- Observe the site for haemorrhage, haematoma and infection
- Observe patients for 1–4 hours after the procedure, depending on the amount of drug used and in line with local policy
- Document in the notes the procedure, the samples taken and the patient's condition
- Educate patients on observing the wound site for infection and haemorrhage
- Give the patient an information leaflet, which will also indicate whom to contact should any complication occur
- Inform patients when the results will be available and who will provide this information

Anaemia

Anaemia is derived from the Greek word meaning 'without blood' and refers to a reduction in the number of RBCs and/or the haemoglobin level. Anaemia is not a disease but a laboratory term used to describe this altered physiological state, and is defined as occurring when the haemoglobin level is less than 13.5 g/dL in males or 11.5 g/dL in females.

Various terms are used to classify anaemia. Groupings can be associated with causative factors or the appearance of the RBCs. The causative factors include:

- a decrease in RBC production due to:
  - external deficiencies such as iron deficiency;
  - bone marrow failure;
- excessive haemorrhage;
- an increased demand for RBCs in pregnancy;
- haemolysis;
- malaria.

When anaemia is classified according to the appearance of the cells, the terms 'microcytic', 'macrocytic' and 'normocytic' are used. Chronic anaemia can be associated with other conditions such as lymphoma, leukaemia, HIV and metastatic cancers.

Management

When planning the care of anaemic patients (Table 19.4), it is useful to plan according to the basic needs assessment, putting the first priority on symptoms that can be life-threatening, such as blood loss and hypoxia.

Table 19.4 Nursing management of anaemic patients

	Management
Care of life-threatening complications	Cardiac failure can occur in acute blood loss or where anaemia is experienced in conjunction with other conditions such as chronic obstructive pulmonary disease, cardiogenic shock or chronic pre-existing blood loss Dyspnoea in extreme cases causes collapse and respiratory failure Shock can occur where the condition is acute or untreated In life-threatening situations, early warning scoring needs to be performed; where necessary, patients' level of care and dependency is increased to the level of intensive care monitoring
Diagnosis and monitoring	Recognise signs and symptoms Take routine blood tests and correctly interpret them Assist with investigations
Administration of medication	Administer prescribed medications when dietary supplementation is insufficient Administer blood transfusion as per local policy
Dyspnoea	Nurse the patient in the upright position to maximise lung expansion Use an integrated approach that concurrently manages both anxiety and breathlessness Physical demands will be great due to this symptom; care must be taken to assist patients with activities of daily living while promoting independence

Table 19.4 (*Continued*)

	Management
Blood transfusions	Caution is required with elderly patients to ensure against overload of the circulatory system; blood may need to be given more slowly or spaced over 2 days Monitor fluid balance Administer erythropoietin if prescribed; this may improve quality of life as hospitalisation for blood transfusions will no longer be necessary
Tiredness	Patients can experience tiredness with the slightest exertion Educate patients that tiredness should lessen as the treatment takes effect Assistance should be given as required; periods of rest are encouraged Patients may be debilitated and may need to be on bed rest; maintain the Waterloo score and attend to pressure sore prevention and risk of deep vein thrombosis
Anxiety and depression	Patients may experience light-headedness and confusion due to hypoxia Anaemia may cause altered body image and loss of normal personal body state, which is replaced by a more dependent life-limiting persona This can increase anxiety and bring about feelings of depression Patients need: • Assistance to restore functioning • Reassurance • Monitoring • Understanding of the condition Specific management is required in severe cases
Maintaining a safe environment	Patients are susceptible to falls due to symptoms of anaemia Skin integrity is impaired, and skin is easily damaged so must be monitored carefully Educate patients on the maintenance of body heat and mobilisation Mental attention span is lessened; time off work and assistance in the home may be required A social services referral may be required following assessment
Mouth care	Monitor and record any injuries Patients may experience cracks at the corners of the mouth; instruction on mouth care and maintenance of nutrition is necessary
Nutritional assessment and guidance	Refer to a dietitian Reinforcement of essential foods is required Provide information leaflets
Discharge planning	Ensure patients are safe to go home Educate patients on self-care, recognition of anaemia and medications Where required, dietetic support is ongoing Arrange an outpatient appointment Alternatively, a follow-up appointment can be made with the GP Elderly people or those who struggle with family responsibilities may need social services support in place prior to discharge

Iron deficiency anaemia (microcytic anaemia)

Iron deficiency anaemia, also referred to as microcytic anaemia, in which RBCs are characteristically small, is the most common anaemia in the world. Low levels of iron in the blood result in decreased haemoglobin synthesis and a decrease in oxygen-carrying capacity. Causes include:

- dietary deficiency of iron;
- loss of iron due to haemorrhage;
- poor absorption of iron from the gastrointestinal tract after gastrectomy;
- an increase in demand for iron due to pregnancy and growth.

Iron is required daily for the production of haemoglobin and RBCs. After iron has been ingested, it is bound by transferrin, stored in the liver and readily available for use. When iron is deficient, erythropoiesis initially continues as normal; however, when stores are depleted, increased numbers of microcytic RBCs are produced in place of the normal mature RBCs.

The normal total body iron content is 3 g; approximately 0.5–1 g of iron is absorbed per day through the walls of the intestinal tract, particularly the stomach and small intestine. Iron is found in foods such as meat, fish, eggs, chicken and pulses. In developing countries and social situations where it is difficult to access such foods, the lack of iron in the diet can predispose to iron deficiency anaemia.

The patient's clinical presentation together with a history of known risk factors can lead to a suspicion of iron deficiency anaemia (Table 19.5).

Table 19.5 Diagnosis of iron deficiency anaemia

Investigations based on clinical history and symptoms	Specific signs and symptoms	General signs and symptoms
Haemoglobin below normal limits	Brittle or spoon-shaped nails	Tiredness
Iron studies (ferritin) below normal level	Brittle hair	Anxiety
Elevated reticulocyte count if bleeding	Hypoxia	Dyspnoea
Faecal occult blood on rectal examination	Cracks in the corner of the mouth (cheilosis)	Cyanosis
Gastroscopy to detect a source of bleeding	Atrophy of the papillae on the tongue	Collapse due to light-headedness
Sigmoidoscopy	Dyspnoea or breathlessness	Poor peripheral circulation and sensitivity to the cold
Colonoscopy	Loss of appetite due to mouth sores as above	Skin integrity impaired
Radiology	Craving to eat clay, starch or coal (pica)	Hypothermia
Ultrasound of the abdomen	Dysphagia and glossitis with the formation of a pharyngeal web, called Paterson–Kelly syndrome (also known as Plummer–Vinson syndrome)	Depression

Management

Nursing management is outlined in Table 19.4. Medications for iron deficiency anaemia include the following:

- Oral supplementation is given as iron sulphate 200 mg, three times a day with food for up to 6 months as required.
- As constipation is a side effect, stool softeners may need to be given.
- Alternative oral preparations may need to be considered if abdominal side effects are too limiting.
- Intramuscular iron supplements are given in malabsorption disorders or when there is poor compliance; these need to be given in a 'Z–track' manner to prevent tracking and discoloration of the skin.

Macrocytic anaemia

Macrocytic or megaloblastic anaemia is characterised by large stem cells or macrocytes. This occurs due to defective deoxynucleic acid (DNA) synthesis, leading to an ineffective and lower production of RBCs in the bone marrow. The RBCs that are produced are abnormally shaped, large and tend to have a reduced lifespan. Causes of macrocytic anaemia include:

- folate deficiency;
- vitamin B_{12} deficiency;
- prolonged exposure to certain therapies;
- alcohol abuse.

Vitamin B_{12} deficiency

This is the most common cause of macrocytic anaemia and results from a deficiency of vitamin B_{12}. Vitamin B_{12} is found in meat and dairy products, cannot be synthesised in the human gut and is often added to cereals to fortify them. It is essential for the synthesis of DNA, with deficiency causing impaired cellular production of RBCs. Vitamin B_{12} is absorbed from the intestine in the presence of the intrinsic factor (IF), which is produced by the gastric mucosa. Lack of vitamin B_{12} and folic acid alters the structure of the IF, disrupts the production of RBCs and affects the functioning of the nervous system.

Pernicious anaemia is an autoimmune condition in which the body's antibodies target the gastric parietal cells and the IF. The exact mechanism of action is not clearly understood. It is speculated that it occurs in association with other autoimmune conditions and can be linked to hereditary factors such as blood group A in middle-aged females.

Vitamin B_{12} deficiency due to low intake can be attributed to:

- total or partial gastrectomy or gastrojejunostomy;
- gastric lesions;
- stomach cancer;
- alcohol abuse;
- malabsorption due to inflammatory bowel conditions such as Crohn's disease.

Signs and symptoms can take up to 2 years to present in patients with chronic inflammatory conditions or following gastric surgery. Apart from the general symptoms of anaemia, the clinical picture relates to damage to other bodily functions and includes:

- varying degrees of jaundice due to an increased breakdown of abnormal RBCs in the liver;
- degenerative neurological changes such as peripheral neuropathy and central changes that can be irreversible:
  - as vitamin B_{12} is necessary for the maintenance of myelin (the myelin sheath) that surrounds the nerves;
  - showing varying degrees of neurological disturbances when insufficiencies occur;

Box 19.9 Management of patients with vitamin B_{12} deficiency

- As per the nursing management of anaemic patients (see Table 19.4)
- Treat as an outpatient or where necessary as an inpatient
- Monthly injections of cyanocobalamin are needed for patients who lack IF:
  - These can cause anaphylactic reactions so patients should be observed for at least 30 minutes after administration
- As this is not a curable condition, treatment is life-long
- Administer blood transfusions as necessary
- Provide care and support for jaundice and neurological dysfunction
- Arrange follow-up care with the GP or nurse practitioner in the community

  - with an initial presentation of poor vision, unsteady gait, ataxia and loss of sympathetic nervous system function affecting elimination and sexual functioning;
  - untreated neurological symptoms, which can be fatal.
- uncontrolled elimination or diarrhoea;
- impaired balance and perception of self in space;
- smooth tongue.

The nursing management is outlined in Box 19.9.

Normocytic anaemia

Normocytic anaemia refers to conditions in which RBCs are relatively normal in size and haemoglobin content but there are an insufficient number of cells. Three main conditions fall under this categorisation:

- Aplastic anaemia
- Sickle cell anaemia
- Haemolytic anaemia.

Aplastic anaemia

If left untreated, aplastic anaemia is a rare yet life-threatening condition. There is a significant decrease in blood cell production in the bone marrow, which leads to a deficiency of RBCs, WBCs and platelets. Fat cells proliferate to replace the stem cells. When all three cells lines are deficient, patients are said to be pancytopenic. Up to 30% of aplastic anaemia is thought to be caused by:

- chemical compounds such as benzene;
- cytotoxic medications, for example busulfan;
- other medications like chloramphenicol and antiepileptic drugs;
- ionising radiation, either therapeutic or non-therapeutic;
- viral infections, for example hepatitis;
- bone marrow infiltration in diseases such as myeloma, or by metastases.

The remaining 70% of causes are said to be idiopathic (i.e. as having no detectable cause). Symptoms are insidious; 1–2 months can elapse following exposure to a causative factor prior to its onset. Classical symptoms of anaemia are present in addition to possible infections and bleeding. It may not be obvious on taking the history that there has been an exposure to a causative factor.

The diagnosis is usually made from a laboratory analysis and the clinical features. A full blood count and blood film will reveal pancytopenia; however, a bone marrow aspirate is the only way to achieve a definitive diagnosis. Management is outlined in Box 19.10.

Box 19.10 Management of aplastic anaemia

Medical treatment

- Urgent hospital admission
- Treatment of the presenting symptoms with:
  - Blood transfusion
  - Platelets
  - Intravenous antibiotics
- Stem cell or bone marrow transplant:
  - Assess for:
    - human leucocyte antigen matching
    - medical fitness
  - Admit to hospital for at least 4 weeks to enable regeneration of the bone marrow
  - If successful, this can bring about a cure for aplastic anaemia
- Regular blood test screening for non-transplanted patients
- Medications:
  - Corticosteroids (methylprednisolone)
  - Ciclosporin, given alone or with antithymocyte or antilymphocyte globulin; these suppress the immune cells responsible for destroying the bone marrow
  - Stimulating growth factors for the regeneration of blood components
  - May be administered on either an inpatient or outpatient basis, as the patient's condition dictates
  - Potential side effects are life-threatening due to bone marrow depression
  - This course of treatment is used for moderate aplastic anaemia or for those not eligible for stem cell or bone marrow transplant

Nursing care

- Administer blood transfusion and anti-infection therapy
- For patients on corticosteroids:
  - Monitor blood sugars
  - Daily urinalysis – if glucose is detected, check the blood glucose for secondary diabetes mellitus; insulin may be required if the result is positive
  - Blood pressure monitoring
  - Give information on side effects, e.g. mood changes
  - Administer in the morning to avoid sleep disturbance
- Educate patients on:
  - Treatments, medications and their side effects
  - Prevention of infection
  - Dietary support and maintenance of good supplies of essential nutrients for blood cell regeneration
- Ongoing management for non-transplanted patients, including education to detect for signs of pancytopenia
- Monitoring of transplant patients for up to 2 years, observing for any graft versus host reaction
- Regular bone marrow aspiration to ascertain disease status

Sickle cell anaemia

Sickle cell anaemia is a hereditary chronic haemolytic anaemia. Sickle cell trait and sickle cell disease are found in individuals of African-Caribbean, Middle Eastern, East European, Indian and Pakistani origin. It is thought that the sickle cell trait helps to provide protection against contracting malaria in these countries.

Sickle cell conditions are characterised by the presence of abnormal haemoglobin molecules (HbS), which result from the replacement of one amino acid molecule (valine) with another amino acid (glutamic acid). In the heterozygous variant, the person inherits the abnormal haemoglobin HbS gene from one parent and the normal HbA gene from the other parent. This person will inherit the HbSA sickle cell trait and may not be aware of this abnormality unless tested for it or exposed to hypoxic conditions, at which time the individual will become symptomatic. The trait will be passed onto the next generation. In a homozygous variant, the abnormal haemoglobin is inherited from both parents and the person will suffer from sickle cell anaemia. When the abnormal haemoglobin molecule is deoxygenated, it causes the RBCs to adopt a sickle-like shape.

The significance of the stiff, sickle-like shape, which occurs in stressful or environmentally cold conditions, is that it is fixed, unlike that of normal RBCs, whose concave shape can alter, enabling them to pass into the thin capillaries in all conditions. Sickled cells become trapped and obstruct the blood flow causing ischaemia (lack of blood supply), which in turn results in pain, often of a severe nature. Once the sickled RBCs have been reoxygenated, they regain their normal shape. However, when a person encounters repeated crises, known as sickle cell crises, the ability of RBCs to return to their normal shape diminishes as the elasticity of the cell walls weakens, leading to haemolysis.

The mechanism by which sickle cell crises occurs is unclear, but a crisis can last from several hours to several weeks. Certain conditions and trigger factors are known to precipitate a crisis, including:

- hypoxia, such as at high altitude or during strenuous exercise;
- anaesthesia;
- infection;
- pregnancy;
- dehydration;
- cold climatic conditions;
- excessive alcohol;
- emotional stress.

Symptoms include:

- pain and swelling of the occluded blood vessels, such as in the abdominal cavity, or stasis in the vessels of the hands and feet;
- pulmonary hypertension;
- tachycardia;
- association with infection, particularly of a bony nature;
- elevated platelet and WBC counts that contribute to the vessel occlusion;
- haematuria;
- persistent erection of the penis.

The nursing management of sickle cell anaemia is shown in Table 19.6.

Polycythaemia

Polycythaemia is a condition characterised by an abnormally higher than normal level of haemoglobin and carries with it a high risk of clotting. The condition can be primary or secondary. Primary polycythaemia is due to a mutation in the stem cells to produce excessive numbers of RBCs; secondary polycythaemia is due to hypoxia at high altitudes or overuse of erythropoietin. Regular venesection (removal of blood from the circulation) is the treatment of choice.

Table 19.6 Nursing management of patients with sickle cell anaemia

Parameter	Nursing management
Pain management	Patients experience moderate to severe pain Assess pain using a pain assessment tool Medications: • Mild to moderate pain – anti-inflammatory drugs • Severe pain – opiates Bed rest Oxygen therapy
Blood transfusion	As per local policy
Vital signs	Record these 4-hourly Treat infection promptly
Fluid balance	Intravenous therapy may be indicated to promote blood flow
Counselling	Designated haematology units may have sickle cell specialists who can provide families with genetic counselling
Discharge advice	Educate the patient on: • What triggers a crisis • What to do • Whom to contact when the situation occurs
Pregnancy	Specialist pregnancy care for sickle cell patients, in collaboration with the haematology team

Haemophilia

Haemophilia is an inherited disorder that results from a life-long deficiency of clotting factors (factor VIII; haemophilia A) or Christmas factor (factor IX; haemophilia B). Treatment involves replacement of the clotting factors and specialist haematological monitoring and intervention.

Thrombocytopenia

Thrombocytopenia is a reduced platelet count resulting from excessive bleeding or an inability of the bone marrow to produce a normal number of platelets.

Types of thrombocytopenia

- **Idiopathic thrombocytopenic purpura** (ITP; acute or chronic) is an autoimmune disorder in which the body makes antibodies, mediated by B lymphocytes, that destroy platelets. Acute ITP is more common in children, whereas the chronic form is associated with adults.
- **Thrombotic thrombocytopenic purpura** occurs when small blood clots form throughout the body; a large number of platelets are used up in this, reducing the count in the peripheral circulation.
- **Haemolytic-uraemic syndrome** is characterised by reduction in both platelet and RBC levels. It can be a side effect of ciclosporin therapy or result from *Escherichia coli* infection.

Box 19.11 Management of thrombocytopenia

- Platelet transfusion
- Steroid treatment
- Splenectomy may be indicated
- Treat secondary causes
- Monitor:
  - Sites that are bleeding
  - Vital signs to allow early recognition of a worsening condition
- Regular mouth care – to maintain oral hygiene due to bleeding tendencies
- Management of dehydration and fluid balance
- Educate patients on observing for and preventing bleeding at home
- Avoid:
  - Constipation, by encouraging dietary fibre
  - Aspirin, as it can interfere with platelet function

The causes of thrombocytopenia are:

- chemotherapy;
- radiotherapy;
- infection;
- increased body heat;
- pernicious anaemia;
- systemic lupus erythematosus;
- HIV infection;
- heparin-induced thrombocytopenia.

The signs and symptoms include:

- unexpected bleeding;
- petechiae;
- gastrointestinal bleeding;
- joint pain;
- epistaxis;
- heavy menstrual bleeding.

Box 19.11 outlines the management of thrombocytopenia

Disseminated intravascular coagulation

Disseminated intravascular coagulation is a serious life-threatening condition that results from simultaneous overactivation of the coagulation system and fibrinolytic pathways. This leads to a dual effect of widespread clotting with a propensity for bleeding. The causative factors include transfusion reactions, leukaemia and cytotoxic treatment. It requires intensive monitoring and specialist haematological input. A balance needs to be achieved between replacing clotting factors, by means of infusing cryoprecipitate and fresh frozen plasma, and anticoagulating patients with heparin.

Multiple myeloma

Multiple myeloma is rare and accounts for 10% of all haematological malignancies. It is characterised by an abnormal and unregulated proliferation of plasma cells, which develop from B lymphocytes. The incidence is higher in those over the age of 40 years, and the condition is common in men and twice as common in the African-Caribbean population. The bone marrow becomes infiltrated with myeloma, causing pancytopenia, and there is life-limiting bone damage and skeletal destruction. The cause of multiple myeloma is unknown. However, there is increased risk:

- in patients who have relatives with *BRCA1* and *BRCA2* gene mutations;
- with previous exposure to radiation, rubber, wood, chemicals and textiles.

There is evidence of high levels of abnormal proteins in the blood and urine, which can cause renal failure. Increased blood viscosity can cause clotting, while abnormal proteins surrounding the organs and blood vessels can cause amyloidosis. There is also a reduction in immunoglobulins, increasing the risk of infection. The signs and symptoms include:

- bone pain and fractures of unknown origin;
- spinal cord compression;
- unexplained pancytopenia and associated symptoms;
- infection;
- renal failure (see Chapter 15);
- amyloidosis;
- hypercalaemia.

Multiple myeloma is not curable but a number of effective treatments are available that can delay the progression of the disease for a number of years and provide supportive therapy and improved quality of life. The medical and nursing management are outline in Boxes 19.12 and 19.13.

Box 19.12 Medical management of multiple myeloma

First-line treatment
- Chemotherapy with combination regimens including the use of cyclophosphamide, thalidomide and steroids is given for 6–8 cycles

Relapse
- Autologous stem cell transplantation is often offered at the first relapse
- The patient may have a number of autologous transplants, with varying degrees of success
- Recent therapies at second relapse include Velcade and lenalidomide, the full efficacy of which is under investigation

Bone involvement
- Radiotherapy is given as a supportive therapy to treat bone lesions; it can be a palliative measure
- Bisphosphonates can be used to treat bone destruction
- Surgical intervention, e.g. verteplasty (vertebroplasty), may be required to treat pathological fractures or stabilise bones

Other treatments
- Erythropoietin
- Management of:
  - Pancytopenia
  - Infection
  - Renal failure

Box 19.13 Nursing priorities in patients with multiple myeloma

Spinal cord compression
- This is an oncological emergency; patients can either collapse or have severe sensorimotor impairment and require prompt medical management

Pain management
- Initiate pain assessment and ongoing management of pain
- The patient may require:
  - Drug therapy
  - Supportive approaches through the use of mobilisation aids
  - Referral to the palliative care team early in the illness journey for management of pain and control of symptoms

Maintenance of a safe environment
- The patient is often elderly with impaired mobility, which requires referral to the physiotherapy and occupational therapy departments for suitable equipment
- Bone fractures and lesions put these patients in a high-risk category for falls and pressure sores

Prevention and management of renal failure
- The patient may present with renal failure, which must be treated
- Ongoing disease and its management can cause renal failure
- Fluid balance monitoring and electrolyte assessment is important
- Education on the need for adequate fluid intake is required prior to discharge

Pancytopenia
- Low RBC and platelet counts are usually treated with transfusions; administration is as per local hospital guidelines

Infection
- Ascertain the microbiology results
- Administer antibiotic therapy
- Educate patients on how to protect themselves from contracting infections and adhere to a good nutritional diet

Hypercalcaemia
- This results from bone destruction and the release of excessive amounts of calcium into the blood
- Observe the patient for confusion
- Administer pamidronate
- Gentle mobilisation reduces the release of calcium

Physiological and psychological support
- Ongoing support from a specialist centre is needed due to the range of problems that patients experience
- Refer the patient to social services, financial support and patient support groups, all of which can assist patients to deal with the longevity of the disease

Discharge planning
- Involve the palliative care team and community specialists
- The level of mobility will be assessed and suitable aids provided
- Organise appropriate home care
- Family support is important to support patients at home and assist with transport to hospital for monitoring

Table 19.7 Classification of leukaemia

Cell line	Acute	Chronic
Lymphoid	Acute lymphoblastic leukaemia (ALL)	Chronic lymphocytic leukaemia (CLL)
Myeloid	Acute myeloid leukaemia (AML)	Chronic myeloid leukaemia (CML)

Leukaemia

Leukaemia is the name for cancer of the blood. The abnormality occurs in the bone marrow where all blood cells are made, resulting in an overproduction of highly abnormal WBCs. There are several types of leukaemia, depending on which type of cell is affected (Table 19.7). The remaining healthy cells in the bone marrow have less space in which to develop, meaning that fewer RBCs and platelets are produced. The incidence ranges from 8 to 12 per 100,000 of the population, increasing with age. About 90% of all leukaemias are diagnosed in adults.

Acute leukaemia is characterised by a rapid increase in the number of immature blood cells, leaving the bone marrow unable to produce healthy blood cells. Immediate treatment is required due to the rapid progression and accumulation of the malignant cells, which spill over into the bloodstream and spread to other organs of the body.

The excessive build-up of relatively mature, but still abnormal, WBCs characterises chronic leukaemia. Cells are produced at a higher rate than normal cells, resulting in many abnormal WBCs being seen in the blood. Chronic leukaemia may be monitored for some time before there is any need for treatment; it can take months or years to progress, mostly occurs in older people but can theoretically occur in any age group.

Acute lymphoblastic leukaemia

In acute lymphoblastic leukaemia (ALL), immature WBCs (lymphoblasts) grow too quickly, the bone marrow becomes crowded, and the blood cannot develop properly. ALL diminishes the body's ability to fight infection.

Acute myeloid leukaemia

In acute myeloid leukaemia (AML), the immature myeloid cells are cancerous and the proliferation of abnormal WBCs is uncontrollable, causing an abundance of blast cells to be present. These crowd out the bone marrow and prevent the normal growth of WBCs, RBCs and platelets.

Chronic lymphocytic leukaemia

This is a cancer of the lymphoid cells (lymphocytes). Lymphocytes usually die off naturally at the end of their lifespan, in chronic lymphocytic leukaemia (CLL) these cells live on even when they are no longer useful in fighting infection. They build up in the bone marrow until there is no space for normal blood cells to develop.

CLL is the most common leukaemia in the Western world, and the chance of developing it increases with age. Most individuals are over 65 years old at the time of diagnosis, it rarely occurs in people under the age of 30, and it does not affect children. It is more common in men than women.

Chronic myeloid leukaemia

Chronic myeloid leukaemia (CML) is a cancer of granulocytes, leading to a hyperproliferation of immature abnormal granulocytes in the bloodstream. This type of leukaemia can occur at any age but is common in middle-aged and older people.

Box 19.14 Signs and symptoms of leukaemia

- Tiredness, breathlessness and pale skin (due to anaemia)
- Fever (pyrexia)
- Infections that do not clear
- Abnormal bruising or bleeding
- A petechial rash
- Bone and joint pain (due to overcrowding of the bone marrow)
- Swollen lymph nodes
- Abdominal discomfort (due to an enlarged spleen)
- Loss of appetite and weight loss
- Swollen gums
- Swollen testicles
- Headaches and vision problems
- Itchy skin
- Night sweats and fevers

Causes of leukaemia

The exact causes of leukaemia are unknown, but risk factors include:

- increasing age;
- smoking;
- exposure to high doses of radiation;
- radon gas;
- benzene;
- previous treatment for cancer;
- Down's syndrome;
- blood disorders such as Fanconi anaemia, myelodysplastic syndromes and myeloproliferative disorders.

Symptoms are vague and vary depending on the type of leukaemia and how advanced it is. There may be no symptoms in the early stages, especially with chronic leukaemia, or they may be mild at first and then worsen (Box 19.14). Chronic leukaemia usually presents with enlarged lymph glands (in the neck, underarms and groins).

Diagnosis

The following investigations are performed for leukaemia:

- Physical examination
- Full blood count
- Blood film
- Bone marrow aspirate and biopsy
- Analysis of abnormal cells found in the blood and bone marrow (cytogenetics and immunophenotyping)
- Computed tomography (CT)
- Magnetic resonance imaging (MRI)
- Ultrasound scans
- Lumbar puncture (in ALL).

Management

Treatment is determined by the type of leukaemia; it involves chemotherapy being delivered in a cyclical manner in order to maximise its therapeutic effect and maintain remission. The aim of chemotherapy is to induce remission and eliminate the hidden leukaemic cell population. Patients are treated according to national and international agreed protocols and, where possible, entered onto trial protocols.

In AML, patients receive four or five courses of chemotherapy, each lasting 5–10 days, followed by a 2–3-week period of profound myelosuppression. The drugs used include:

- cytarabine
- daunorubicin
- idarubicin
- thioguanine
- mitoxantrone
- etoposide
- amsacrine.

The treatment of ALL is divided into three phases – induction of remission, consolidation and maintenance – and can last for 2–3 years. Regimens vary according to age and local policy, and combine immunosuppressive and chemotherapeutic agents.

In CML, the use of tyrosine kinase inhibitors (imatinib, disatinib and nolitinib) has revolutionised the treatment and prognosis of this group of patients.

Lymphoma

Lymphoma is a disease that affects the lymphocytes, which become malignant, grow and multiply uncontrollably, and may not die off when and how they ought to. Lymphomas are divided into two major categories:

- Hodgkin's disease has a unique pattern of spread through the body.
- Non-Hodgkin's lymphoma (NHL) makes up all other lymphomas and is more common than Hodgkin's disease.

Worldwide, about 301,000 new cases of NHL occur each year. NHL is the seventh most common cancer and in some countries ranks even higher. About 95% of new cases occur in adults, with an average age at diagnosis of approximately 65 years. The risk of developing NHL increases with age. Risk factors include genetic abnormalities and viral infections, but the most closely associated risk factors are:

- primary (inherited) immune deficiency diseases, for example:
  - severe combined immunodeficiency syndrome;
  - Wiskott–Aldrich syndrome;
  - ataxia–telangiectasia (Louis–Bar syndrome);
- acquired immunosuppression:
  - viral infections;
  - after organ transplant.

Although the link between exposure to pesticides and organic solvents and NHL has been studied, no conclusive evidence pointing to a definite cause and effect relationship has been found.

The signs and symptoms of lymphoma are similar to those of leukaemia and include:

- painless swelling of the lymph glands in the neck, under the arms or in the groin;
- loss of appetite and weight loss;
- fever;
- excessive sweating at night;

Table 19.8 Diagnostic tests

Blood tests	Full blood count Erythrocyte sedimentation rate Liver and kidney function Lactate dehydrogenase level Uric acid
Imaging	Chest X-ray CT scan Ultrasound MRI scan Positron emission tomography
Biopsy/cytology	Biopsy of any suspicious lesions (the most important diagnostic test), usually lymph nodes (surgical biopsy being the preferred method) Fine-needle aspiration Bone marrow aspiration and/or biopsy Lumbar puncture (spinal tap)
Molecular analysis	Immunophenotyping Genotyping

- itchiness all over the body;
- a feeling of weakness;
- breathlessness with swelling of the face and neck.

The initial assessment includes a full physical examination, special attention being paid to all lymph node-bearing regions and Waldeyer's ring (the ring of tissues formed by the tonsils and their connecting lymphatic tissue). Nurses can help patients through the diagnosis and disease evaluation period by providing reassurance, support and information on the disease and the diagnostic tests (Table 19.8).

Staging of lymphoma

Stage 1 lymphoma involves a single lymph node or lymph node region; stage 2 involves two or more lymph node regions on the same side of the diaphragm; stage 3 involves lymph node regions on both sides of the diaphragm; and stage 4 shows disseminated involvement. Figure 19.3 provides an overview of the Ann Arbor staging system. Lymph node regions are defined as the area around localised lymph nodes (e.g. the groin, armpits and neck).

Classification of lymphoma

The classification of lymphoma determines the most appropriate treatment, based on the origin of the lymphoma. NHL is classified according to:

- the tissue's morphology (its form and structure);
- the tissue's histology (its minute structure and organisation);
- the clinical course of the disease;
- the signs and symptoms;
- immunophenotyping;

NHL can be categorised as:

- indolent – low-grade, slow-growing lymphomas;
- aggressive – high-grade, fast-growing lymphomas.

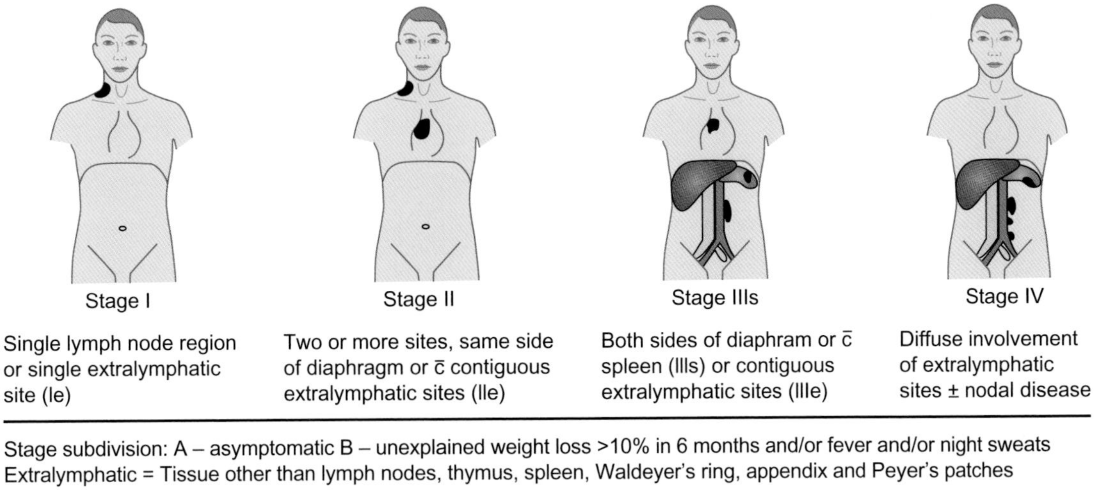

Stage I
Single lymph node region or single extralymphatic site (Ie)
Stage II
Two or more sites, same side of diaphragm or c̄ contiguous extralymphatic sites (IIe)
Stage IIIs
Both sides of diaphram or c̄ spleen (IIIs) or contiguous extralymphatic sites (IIIe)
Stage IV
Diffuse involvement of extralymphatic sites ± nodal disease
Stage subdivision: A – asymptomatic B – unexplained weight loss >10% in 6 months and/or fever and/or night sweats
Extralymphatic = Tissue other than lymph nodes, thymus, spleen, Waldeyer's ring, appendix and Peyer's patches

Figure 19.3 Ann Arbour staging for lymphoma.

Management

Chemotherapy is commonly used and may be given as a single agent or in combination with other drugs. This treatment, which is tailored to patients' specific disease needs, may be combined with radiotherapy or monoclonal antibody therapy. Single-agent chemotherapy regimens (e.g. chlorambucil or fludarabine) are easily administered and generally well tolerated. Combination chemotherapy regimens involve the use of two or more drugs and are often associated with greater side effects. Standard combination regimens include:

- CHOP – cyclophosphamide, hydroxydaunorubicin (doxorubicin), oncovin (vincristine) and prednisone;
- CVP (also known as COP) – cyclophosphamide, oncovin (vincristine) and prednisone.

Lymphomas may become resistant to chemotherapy, so many different regimens, including experimental drugs, can be used. Consideration should be given to the logistics of receiving chemotherapy, such as who will take patients to the clinic, whether adequate transportation is available and whether patients will need to take time off work. The nursing management of leukaemia and lymphoma is outlined in Box 19.15.

Haematopoietic stem cell transplant

A haematopoietic stem cell transplant (HSCT) is used to eliminate an underlying disease and restore haematopoietic and immune function. There are two types of stem cell transplant:

- In **autologous transplantation**, stem cells are collected from patients and frozen until required. The cells are then reinfused after high-dose chemotherapy has been administered.
- In **allogeneic transplantation**, stem cells are collected from a carefully matched related or unrelated donor and administered to patients following high-dose chemotherapy and/or radiotherapy.

Autologous transplantation is most common but is not suitable for patients who are unable to produce sufficient stem cells themselves or who have relapsed following a previous autologous transplant. There is a risk of relapse due to residual lymphoma cells in the transplant.

Box 19.15 Nursing management of leukaemia and lymphoma

Prevention of infection

- Hand-washing
- Protective isolation while neutropenic
- Prophylactic antibiotics and antifungal agents
- 4-hourly vital signs while neutropenic
- Blood cultures when pyrexial
- Antipyretics (e.g. paracetamol)
- Monitoring for signs of infection
- Granulocyte colony-stimulating factor therapy to reduce the length of neutropenia
- Dietary restrictions, e.g. no unpasteurised foods
- Patient education:
    - Avoid unnecessary crowds and people who may have an infection
    - Contact the healthcare team if symptoms of infection develop
    - Avoid spicy food, caffeine, alcohol, sugar and hot drinks
    - Wear loose cotton clothing
    - Layer clothing and bedding for easy temperature adjustment
    - Use sprays and moist wipes to cool the skin

Fatigue/anaemia

- If anaemic, use:
    - Blood transfusions
    - Drug therapy (e.g. erythropoietin)
- Patient education:
    - Eat a healthy, well-balanced diet
    - Take regular gentle exercise
    - Have adequate rest
    - Avoid caffeine just before bedtime

Bleeding/thrombocytopenia

- Severe risk of bleeding if the platelet count is below $10–20 \times 10^9$/L
- Platelet transfusion
- Replacement of clotting factors, if required
- Patient education:
    - Avoid cuts, bruises and falls
    - Take care when:
        - — blowing your nose
        - — shaving
        - — cleaning your teeth

Fertility

- Sperm banking
- Oocyte/embryo cryopreservation (if time allows)

Psychosocial care

- Anxiety
- Information needs
- Education on the illness and the side effects of treatment

Nausea/vomiting

- Give an antiemetic before and after chemotherapy and/or radiotherapy
- Arrange a prescription for nausea control at home
- Try serotonin receptor antagonists
- Patient education:
  - Drink plenty of fluids before, during and after therapy
  - Eat frequent small meals and snacks
  - Adapt meals and drinks according to symptoms
  - Consider complementary therapy (e.g. relaxation techniques and aromatherapy)

Hair loss

- Refer to a hospital wig services or wig supplier experienced in fitting people with cancer
- Patient education:
  - Visit a wig supplier before all hair is lost to ensure a good colour, texture and style match
  - Alternatively, use hats, hair bands, scarves and bandanas

Sore throat/mouth (mucositis)

- Monitor for signs of infection:
  - Pink or red bleeding lesions
  - Dry mucosa or tongue
  - Painful, white patches
- Adequate pain management
- Regular oral assessment and mouth care
- Patient education:
  - Use a soft toothbrush and brush the teeth (and tongue) gently after every meal
  - Avoid mouthwashes containing alcohol; salt water or baking soda may be used instead
  - Rinse the mouth with water as often as needed
  - Avoid irritating acidic and spicy foods
  - Drink plenty of fluids

Allogeneic transplantation is associated with a high rate of transplant-related mortality and morbidity due to infections, organ-related problems, graft versus host disease and sometimes graft failure.

Both procedures can be physically and emotionally difficult, so patients often require support and counselling. Patients are hospitalised for a few weeks while the bone marrow and blood cell count returns to normal. The risk of infection during this period is high, so patients may be placed under reverse isolation, and special precautions are taken to reduce infection. Complications are outlined in Box 19.16.

Sources of cells for HSCT are:

- bone marrow, which is aspirated from the posterior iliac crests under general anaesthesia, marrow volumes of 800–1200 mL usually being taken;
- peripheral blood stem cells, obtained following the administration of granulocyte colony-stimulating factor and collected by apheresis;
- umbilical cord blood cells, which are collected from the umbilical cord at birth.

Box 19.16 Complications of HSCT

Early complications

- Infections (bacterial, fungal, viral)
- Haemorrhage
- Anaemia
- Nausea and vomiting
- Acute graft versus host disease
- Graft failure
- Diarrhoea
- Acute organ toxicity:
  - Haemorrhagic cystitis
  - Interstitial pneumonitis
  - Veno-occlusive disease
  - Cardiac failure
  - Acute respiratory distress syndrome
  - Acute renal failure
- Mucositis
- Alopecia

Late complications

- Infections, especially varicella-zoster virus and encapsulated bacteria
- Chronic pulmonary disease
- Autoimmune disorders
- Immunodeficiency
- Cataracts
- Endocrine dysfunction
- Chronic graft versus host disease:
  - Arthritis
  - Malabsorption
  - Hepatitis
  - Scleroderma
  - Sicca syndrome
  - Lichen planus
  - Pulmonary disease
  - Serous effusions
- Infertility
- Growth retardation in children
- Secondary malignancies
- Disease recurrence or relapse
- Skeletal disorders
- Cardiac disorders
- Iron overload

Conclusion

As blood is essential for the body to function, it is imperative that nurses have a knowledge and understanding of the normal parameters of haematology and the pathophysiology of haematological disorders. An in-depth scientific knowledge provides a sound basis for the nursing care of haematology patients not only in a haematology setting, but also in medical and surgical care settings.

Visit www.wileyfundamentalseries.com/medicalnursing and read Reflective Questions 19.1 and 19.2 to think more about this topic.

Now visit the companion website and test yourself on this chapter:
www.wileyfundamentalseries.com/medicalnursing

References

Dougherty, L. & Lamb, J. (2009) *Intravenous Therapy in Nursing Practice*, 2nd ed. Oxford: Blackwell Publishing.

Nair, M. & Peate, I. (2009) *Applied Pathophysiology. An Essential Guide for Nursing Students*. Oxford: Wiley Blackwell.

Provan, D., Singer, C.R., Baglin, T. & Dokal, I. (2009) *Oxford Handbook of Clinical Haematology*, 3rd ed. Oxford: Oxford Medical Publications.

Waugh, A. & Grant, A. (2010) *Ross and Wilson's Anatomy and Physiology in Health and Illness*, 11th ed. Edinburgh: Churchill Livingstone/Elsevier.

20

Nursing care of conditions related to the musculoskeletal system

Sonya Clarke[1] and Julia Kneale[2]

[1]*School of Nursing and Midwifery, Queen's University Belfast, Belfast, Northern Ireland, UK*
[2]*School of Nursing and Caring Sciences, Faculty of Health, University of Central Lancashire, Preston, Lancashire, UK*

Contents

Introduction	423
Anatomy and physiology	423
Osteoarthritis	430
Osteomyelitis	434
Rheumatoid arthritis	435
Fracture injuries	437
Osteoporosis	441
Neurovascular assessment and plaster care	444
Bone metastases	445
Conclusion	446
References	446

Learning outcomes

Having read this chapter, you will be able to:

- Identify key features and elements of the skeletal system
- Explain the difference between osteoarthritis and rheumatoid arthritis
- Outline the medical and nursing management of common musculoskeletal disorders
- Recognise the clinical signs and symptoms of a fracture and explain different methods of stabilising a fracture
- Understand the specific orthopaedic care of a patient with a hip fracture

Fundamentals of Medical-Surgical Nursing: A Systems Approach, First Edition. Edited by Anne-Marie Brady, Catherine McCabe, and Margaret McCann.

Introduction

Orthopaedic and trauma care is a dynamic and constantly evolving area of practice, with patients increasingly being seen in settings other than the traditional ward and clinic areas, and an increased focus on shared care, day case interventions and community-based care. This chapter provides an outline of the skeletal anatomy and an overview of common conditions related to the musculoskeletal system, including osteoarthritis, osteomyelitis, rheumatoid arthritis, fracture injuries, osteoporosis, femoral neck fracture and bone metastases. An 'A-Z glossary of common orthopaedically related terms' (available at http://orthoinfo.aaos.org/glossary.cfm) may assist the reader in understanding this chapter.

Anatomy and physiology

The musculoskeletal system is composed of bones, joints, muscles, tendons and ligaments. The skeletal system provides form for the body, protects the vital organs and acts as a framework to attach the muscles to that is also designed to permit motion of the body (Figure 20.1). The skeleton consists of 206 bones that are divided into the 'axial' and the 'appendicular' skeleton, with the spine viewed as having cervical, thoracic, lumbar, sacral and coccygeal sections (Figure 20.2).

At birth, the spine is one concave primary curve, which remains in the thoracic, sacral and coccygeal bones (Figure 20.3). The upper extremity includes the shoulder girdle, arm, elbow, forearm, wrist and hand. The lower extremity similarly comprises the hip, thigh, knee, leg and foot.

Bone

In essence, the bones protect and shape the body; the two types of bone tissue are compact (cortical/hard) and spongy (cancellous/soft) bone. The components of a typical long bone are depicted in Figure 20.4. The function of the bones include giving the body a framework, providing attachment sites

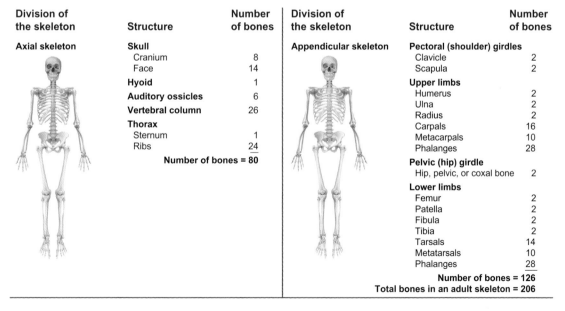

Division of the skeleton	Structure	Number of bones
Axial skeleton	**Skull**	
	Cranium	8
	Face	14
	Hyoid	1
	Auditory ossicles	6
	Vertebral column	26
	Thorax	
	Sternum	1
	Ribs	24
	Number of bones = 80	

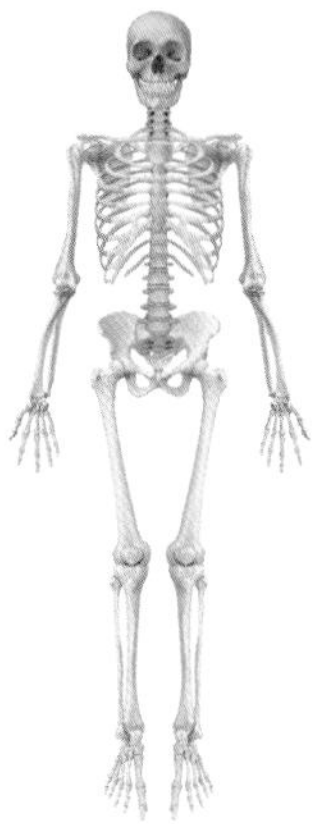

Division of the skeleton	Structure	Number of bones
Appendicular skeleton	**Pectoral (shoulder) girdles**	
	Clavicle	2
	Scapula	2
	Upper limbs	
	Humerus	2
	Ulna	2
	Radius	2
	Carpals	16
	Metacarpals	10
	Phalanges	28
	Pelvic (hip) girdle	
	Hip, pelvic, or coxal bone	2
	Lower limbs	
	Femur	2
	Patella	2
	Fibula	2
	Tibia	2
	Tarsals	14
	Metatarsals	10
	Phalanges	28
	Number of bones = 126	
	Total bones in an adult skeleton = 206	

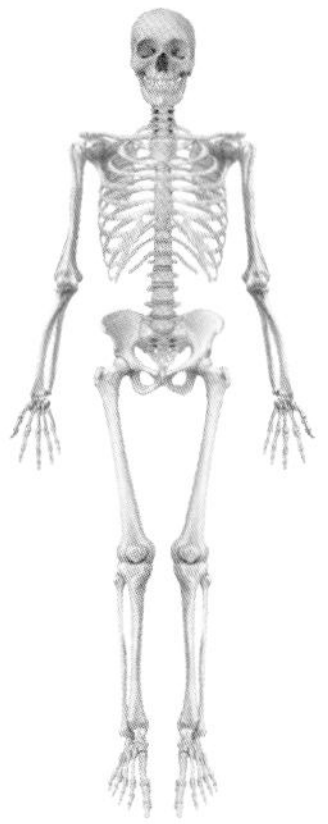

Figure 20.1 The bones of the adult skeletal system. Reproduced from Tortora, G.J. & Derrickson, B. (2011) *Principles of Anatomy & Physiology; Organization, Support and Movement, and Control Systems of the Human Body* (13th edition) Volume 2, John Wiley & Sons Ltd.

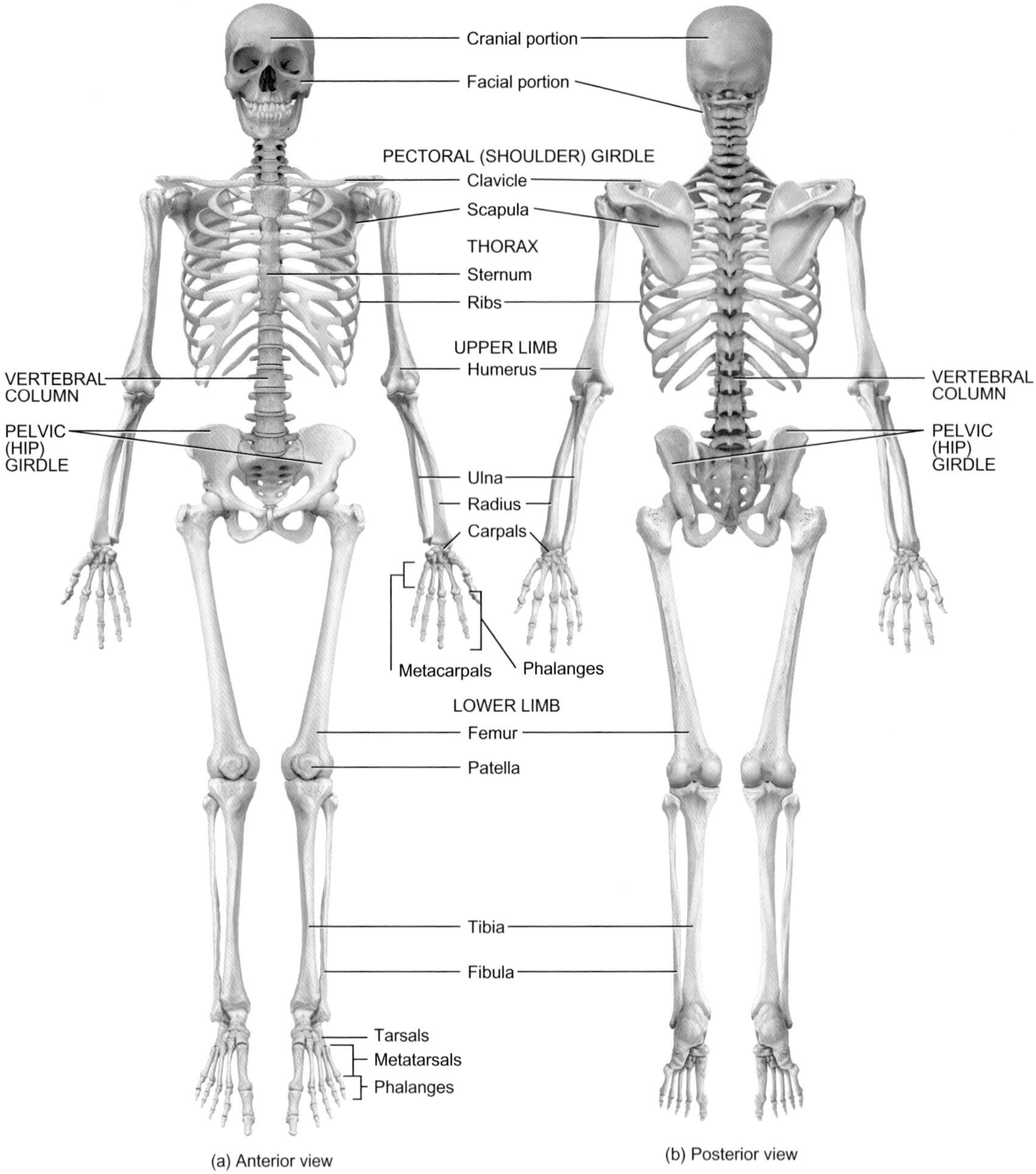

Figure 20.2 Divisions of the skeletal system (with the axial skeleton indicated in blue). Reproduced from Tortora, G.J. & Derrickson, B. (2011) *Principles of Anatomy & Physiology; Organization, Support and Movement, and Control Systems of the Human Body* (13th edition) Volume 2, John Wiley & Sons Ltd.

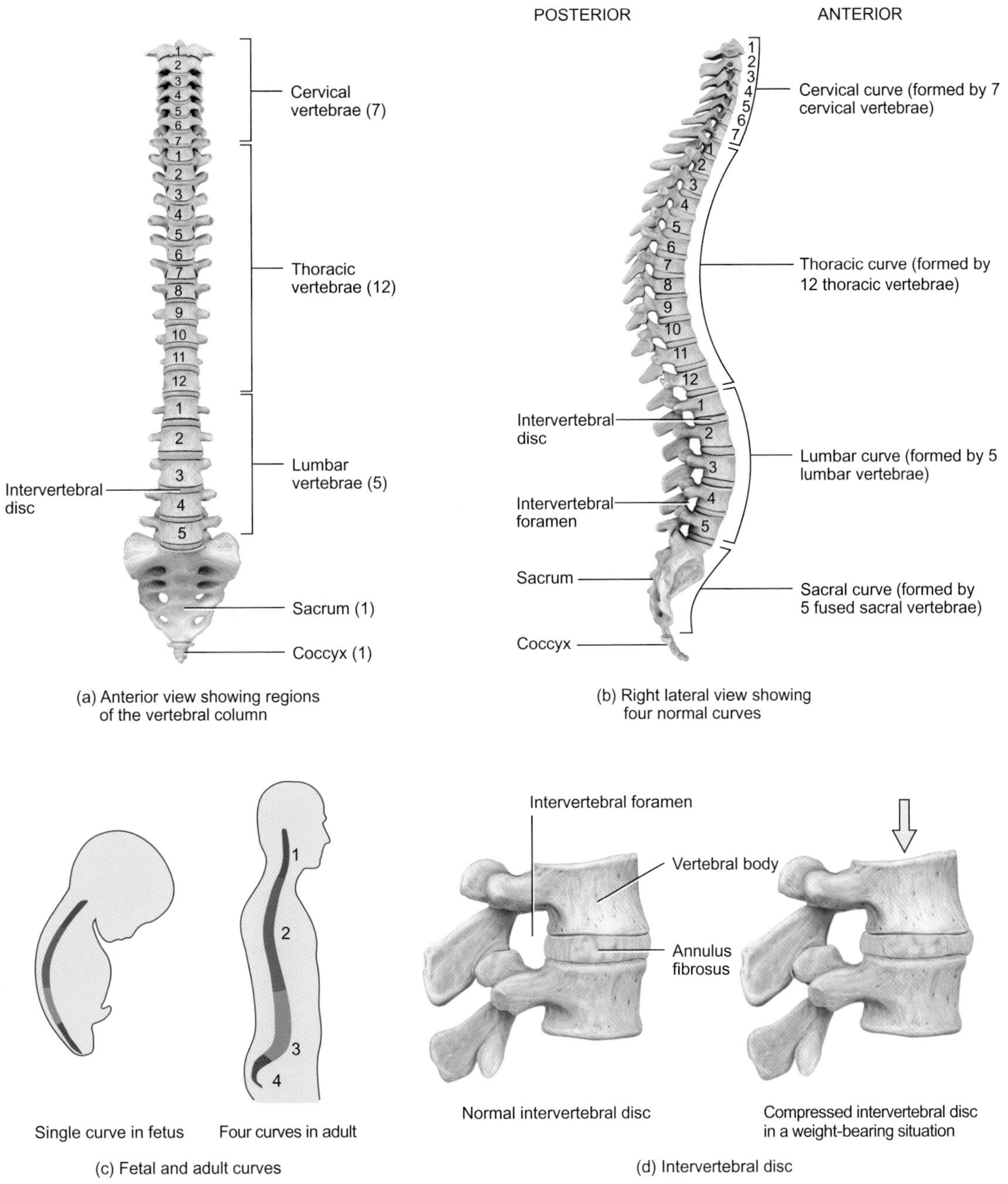

Figure 20.3 The vertebral column. Reproduced from Tortora, G.J. & Derrickson, B. (2011) *Principles of Anatomy & Physiology; Organization, Support and Movement, and Control Systems of the Human Body* (13th edition) Volume 2, John Wiley & Sons Ltd.

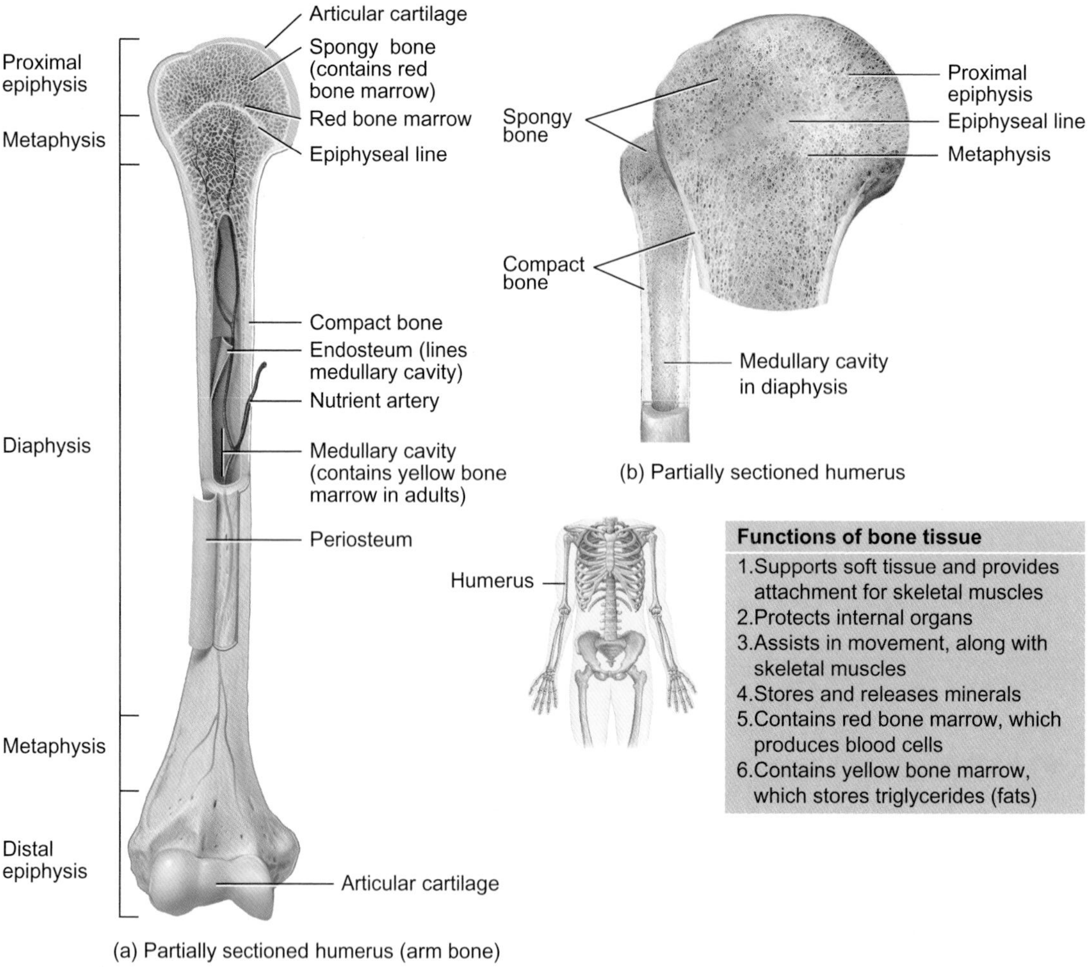

Figure 20.4 Parts of a long bone. Reproduced from Tortora, G.J. & Derrickson, B. (2011) *Principles of Anatomy & Physiology; Organization, Support and Movement, and Control Systems of the Human Body* (13th edition) Volume 2, John Wiley & Sons Ltd.

for muscle and tendons, allowing movement of the body as a whole and of parts of the body by forming joints that are moved by muscles, being involved in haemopoeisis, and providing a storage site for minerals (calcium phosphate) and a reservoir for blood calcium. Box 20.1 outlines types and examples of bones, showing how their characteristic structure and location relates to their overall function.

Muscle

The bones are unable to move the body on their own, so the muscles provide movement and also generate heat. The motion of the skeletal system arises from the contraction and relaxation of the skeletal muscles. Four major muscle groups of the body include the muscles of the head and neck, the trunk, the upper extremity and the lower extremity. The principal anterior superficial skeletal muscles are depicted in Figure 20.5. The muscles constitute approximately 23% of the body weight in females and 40% in males.

There are three types of muscular tissue: smooth (located in the walls of the hollow visceral organs), cardiac (located in the walls of the heart) and skeletal, which occurs in the muscles attached to the

Box 20.1 Types of bones and their structure

- **Long bones** consist of a shaft and two extremities; examples are the femur, tibia and fibula
  - Long bones are from a diaphysis (shaft) and two epiphyses (extremities). The periosteum is a vascular membrane composed of two layers, an outer tough and fibrous layer, with an inner layer containing cells that build bone (osteoblasts) and cells that reabsorb bone (osteoclasts).
- Short, irregular, flat and **sesamoid bones** are diverse in shape and size and have no extremities; examples are the carpals (short), vertebrae and some skull bones (flat), sternum, ribs and most skull bones (irregular), and patella (sesamoid)
  - Sesamoid bones a relatively thin outer layer of compact bone, and also contain cancellous (spongy) bone packed with red marrow, which is enclosed by periosteum. The exception to this is the inner layer of the cranial bones, where it is replaced by dura matter (the outermost of the three layers of the meninges surrounding the brain and spinal cord)

skeleton. The skeletal muscle fibres are striated in appearance and are under voluntary control (Figure 20.6).

By sustained contraction or alternating contraction and relaxation, muscle tissue has six main functions:

- It brings about body movement.
- It maintains body posture.
- It assists in stabilisation of the joints.
- It assists in the movement of substances in the body.
- It aids temperature control.
- It helps regulate breathing (the diaphragm).

Tendons and ligaments

Tendons and ligaments are two types of connective tissue with similar, but differing, functions. In essence, ligaments connect bone to bone, and tendons connect bone to muscle. Tendons are a tough yet flexible bands of fibrous tissue attached to the skeletal muscles that essentially allow movement by acting as intermediaries between the muscles and the bones. Ligaments, although similar to tendon, help to stabilise joints as they connect bone to bone. Their composition is mostly long, stringy collagen fibres that create short bands of tough fibrous connective tissue.

Joints

A joint, or articulation, is where two bones come together, for example in the knee. In terms of the amount of movement they permit, there are three main joint types: immovable (synarthrosis), slightly movable (amphiarthrosis) and freely movable (diarthrosis). Synovial joints (diarthroses) such as the hip or knee are by far the most common classification of joint within the human body. Additional examples of synovial joints include pivotal, ball and socket, and hinge (Figure 20.7).

Blood and nerve supply

The blood and nerve supply is a vast subject. Bones receive their blood supply from a number of different sources, all of which have their own importance. These sources include nutrient arteries, epiphyseal arteries, periosteal arteries and metaphyseal arteries. Most of the nerves supplying bones are sympathetic and vasomotor in function (Figure 20.8).

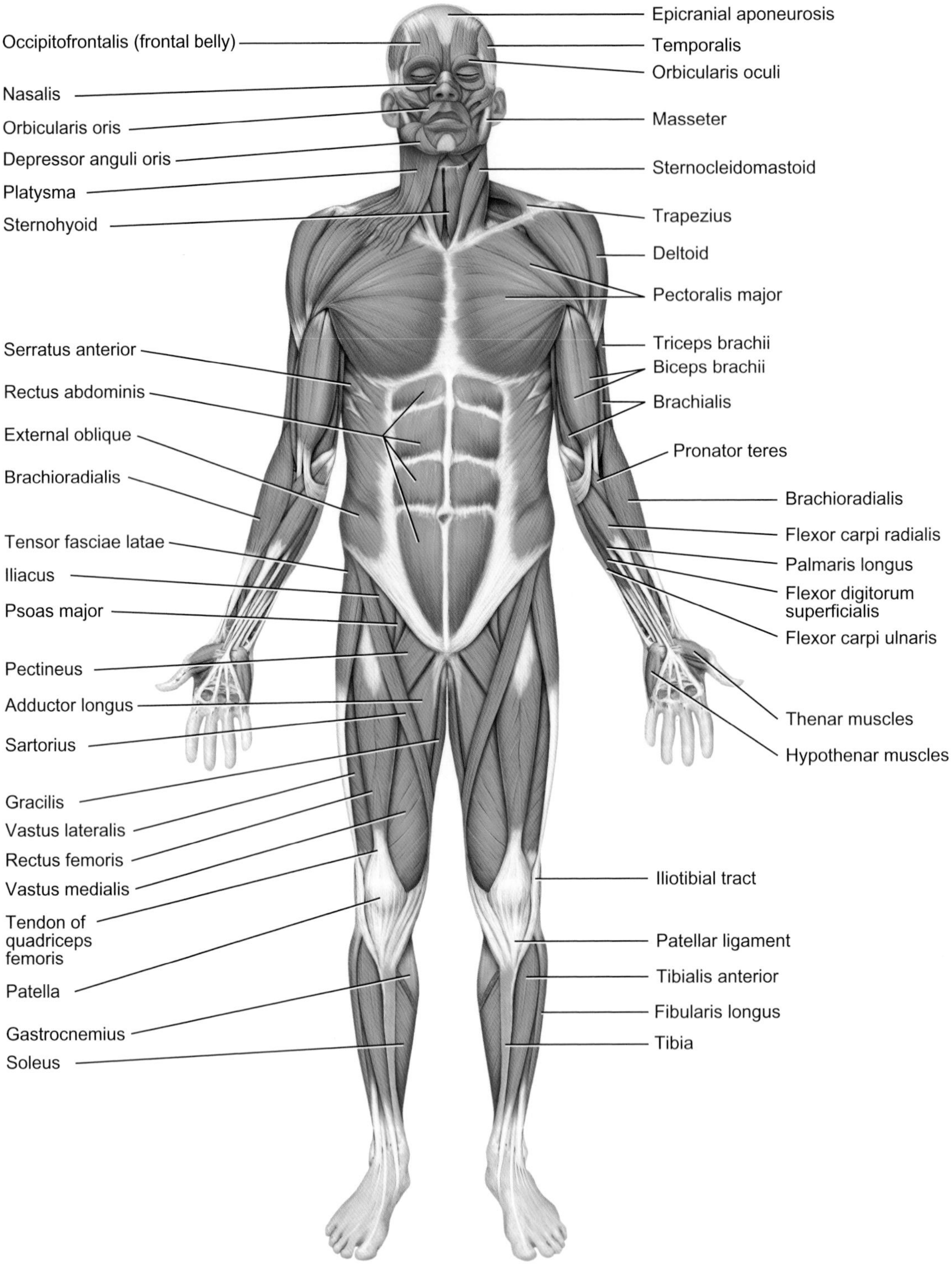

Figure 20.5 The principal superficial skeletal muscles, anterior view. Reproduced from Tortora, G.J. & Derrickson, B. (2011) *Principles of Anatomy & Physiology; Organization, Support and Movement, and Control Systems of the Human Body* (13th edition) Volume 2, John Wiley & Sons Ltd.

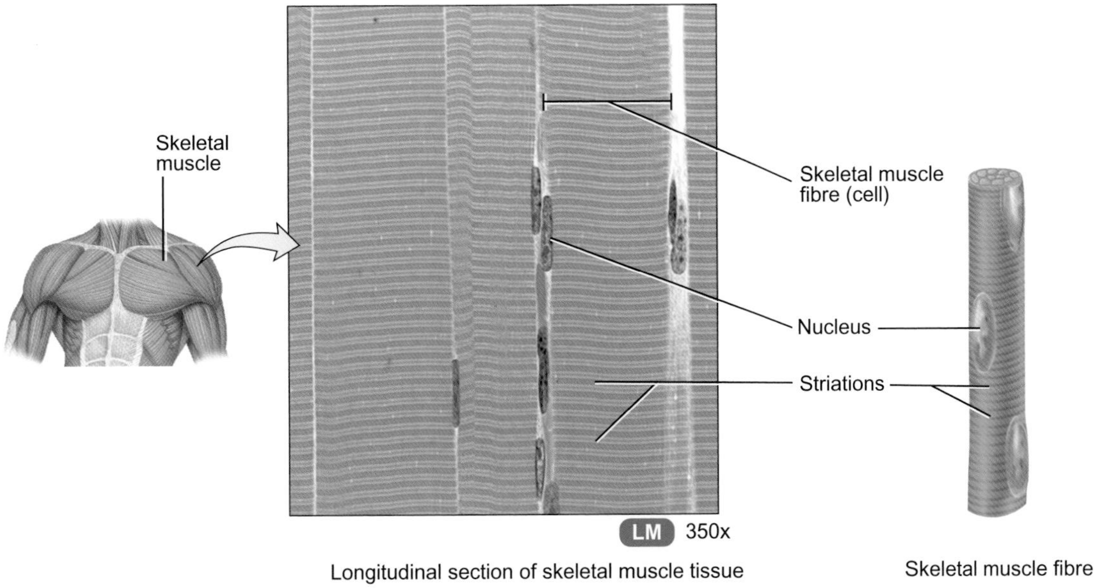

Figure 20.6 Skeletal muscle. LM, light microscope. Reproduced from Tortora, G.J. & Derrickson, B. (2011) *Principles of Anatomy & Physiology; Organization, Support and Movement, and Control Systems of the Human Body* (13th edition) Volume 2, John Wiley & Sons Ltd.

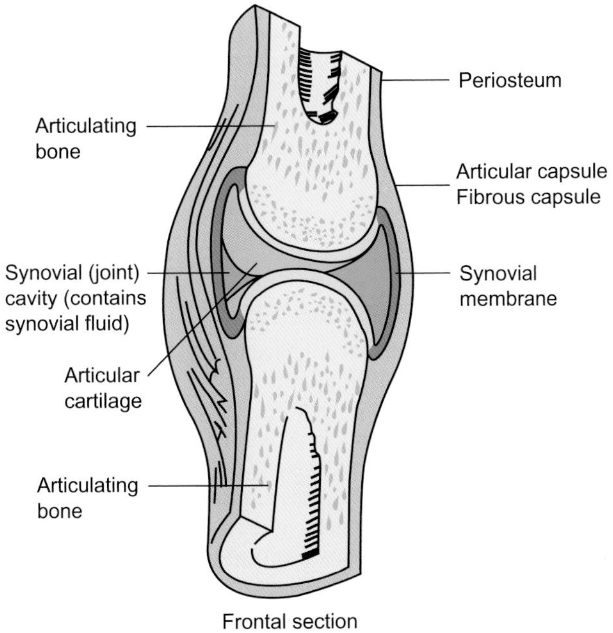

Figure 20.7 A synovial joint. Reproduced from Nair, M. & Peate, I. (2009) *Fundamentals of Applied Pathophysiology*, with kind permission from Wiley Blackwell.

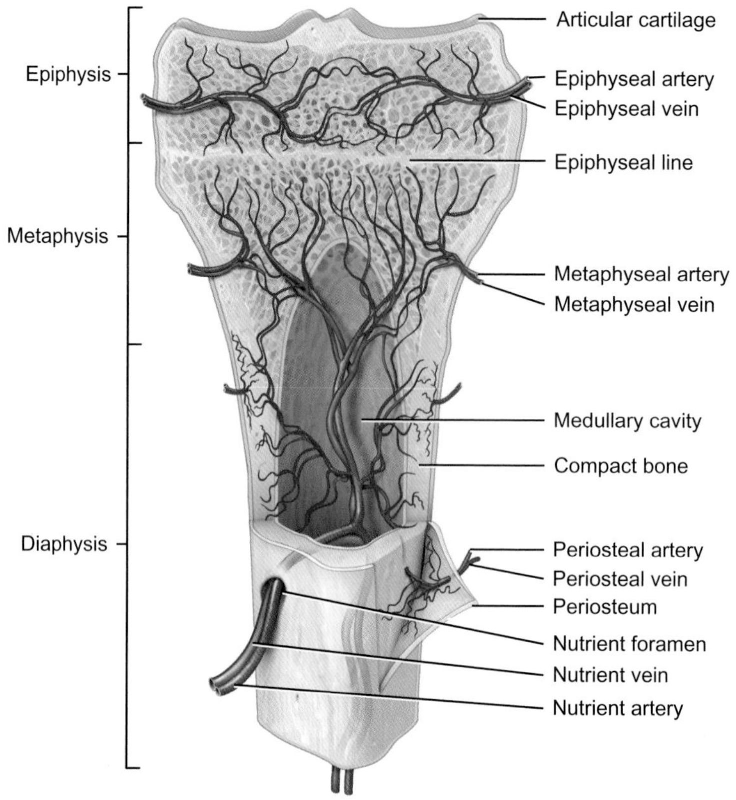

Figure 20.8 Partially sectioned tibia (shin bone). Reproduced from Tortora, G.J. & Derrickson, B. (2011) *Principles of Anatomy & Physiology; Organization, Support and Movement, and Control Systems of the Human Body* (13th edition) Volume 2, John Wiley & Sons Ltd.

Osteoarthritis

Osteoarthritis is a degenerative disease that usually initially affects a single joint, typically a hip, knee, hand, neck or lumbar spine joint, but further joints may be affected over time. Figure 20.9 shows the changes associated with a knee with osteoarthritis. In particular, articular cartilage and mechanical damage leads to problems with mobility and activities of daily living, with dependence on others occurring in severe cases. The disabling symptoms of pain, joint swelling, stiffness and restricted movement commonly cause patients to seek help. Individuals are further affected if they have to adapt or change their work or are unable to carry on working, have reduced social contact or are unable to participate in physical activities such as sports. This means that osteoarthritis is the most common cause of disability in the older person in the developed world (Jinks *et al.* 2002).

Notable osteoarthritic changes are seen in adults from 30 years of age onwards, with the incidence increasing in older age groups. These changes can result from a variety of causes (Box 20.2). The normal collagen fibres in the cartilage are broken down, causing a loss of resistance and a frayed appearance with loose bodies, and the underlying bone is exposed. A protective inflammatory reaction occurs, resulting in the synovium producing more synovial fluid. Eventually, both bones lose areas of cartilage. The two bone surfaces then come into contact owing to the loss of joint space and rub against each other. This leads to further abrasion, microfractures in the subchondral bone surface, the necrosis

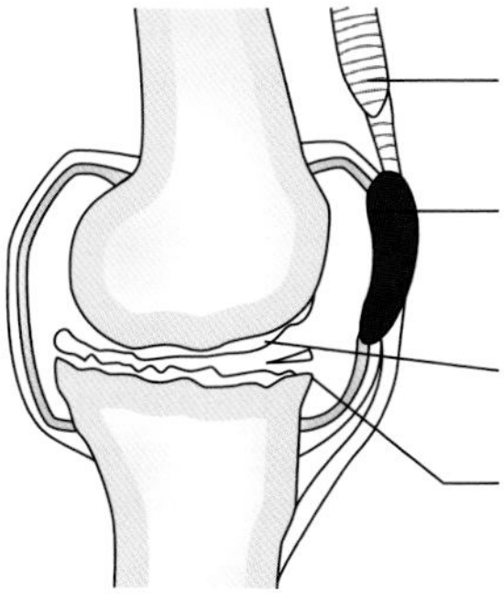

Figure 20.9 A knee joint with ostheoarthritis. Reproduced from Nair, M. & Peate, I. (2009) *Fundamentals of Applied Pathophysiology*, with kind permission from Wiley Blackwell.

Box 20.2 Factors predisposing to osteoarthritis

- Congenital joint deformities, e.g. developmental dysplasia of the hip
- Genetic disease affecting a joint, e.g. haemophilia or sickle cell anaemia
- Developmental changes in bone, e.g. Perthes' disease
- Metabolic changes, e.g. gout
- Infection of the bone or joint, e.g. osteomyelitis and septic arthritis due to tuberculosis or *Staphylococcus*
- Traumatic injury to bone or joint, e.g. a fracture damaging the articular cartilage, or a ligament tear causing joint instability
- Physically demanding activities, sports and repetitive joint injuries, e.g. farming and football
- Avascular necrosis, e.g. following a fracture
- Other skeletal changes, e.g. ankylosing spondylitis
- Hereditary factors, e.g. nodal arthritis affecting women's hands
- Ethnic origin – osteoarthritis is more common in the white European population

(death) of small areas of bone, and cyst formation from increased pressure in the joint forcing synovial fluid into the bone. The production of osteophytes (new bony projections) is evident at the joint margins, and the damage eventually causes distortion of the bone surfaces with potential for subluxation or dislocation.

The joint changes occur slowly over several years. In the early stages, one joint is affected, with the patient experiencing tenderness around the joint and pain that is often worse following exercise and initially relieved by rest. As the disease advances, surgery is considered when joint pain, for example hip pain radiating down towards the knee, is experienced at rest and at night.

Osteoarthritis is diagnosed by the symptom pattern, the exclusion of other conditions that can affect a joint and radiographic examination of the joint. An X-ray, magnetic resonance imaging (MRI) scan or computed tomography (CT) scan (Box 20.3) may show a combination of changes: a reduction or loss of the joint space, osteophytes, cysts in the subchondral bone, loose bodies, angulation, subluxation or dislocation of the joint. Even though the joint damage can be severe, this does not always equate to the patient's symptoms – some patients with moderate changes have severe pain and disability, whereas others with severe damage may only have mild discomfort.

Visit **www.wileyfundamentalseries.com/medicalnursing** and read **Reflective Question 20.1** to think more about this topic.

Table 20.1 reflects an adapted 'at-a-glance' summary of the 2008 guidance from the National Institute for Health and Clinical Excellence (NICE; now the National Institute for Health and Care Excellence) on the care and management of osteoarthritis in adults (see http://www.mims.co.uk/Guidelines/1087441/care-management-osteoarthritis-adults/).

Common surgical management

An **arthrodesis** (joint fusion), for example of the first metatarsal and first phalanx, creates a pain-free joint but there is a loss of all movement and there may be an increase in the stress on adjacent joints. An **osteotomy** is where the bones are cut and realigned to stop subluxation; this can reduce the level of pain and postpone the need for joint replacement surgery.

Box 20.3 Common radiological investigations

- **X-rays** use a type of high-energy ionising radiation to quickly create a two-dimensional picture. X-ray views include anteroposterior (AP) and lateral (from the side). The radiation doses used in medical X-rays are lower than those used in MRI and CT scans.
- **MRI scanning** uses a strong magnetic field to identify radio signals emitted by different tissues to create a three-dimensional picture of the bone and soft tissues. It is an expensive technique and many patients find the procedure claustrophobic. A MRI of an ankle could take 20–30 minutes.
- **CT scanning** uses high-dose radiation beams at multiple angles to create three-dimensional images of tissue structures or cross-sectional images of the tissues. It only shows bone tissue clearly, and not soft tissues. CT scanning is much quicker than MRI.

Put the term 'orthopaedic X-rays' into an online search engine to view some examples of X-rays

Table 20.1 Treatment protocol

Option	Intervention	Additional information
Pharmacological options	Paracetamol (given regularly if needed) Topical NSAIDs for OA of the knee or hand Topical capsaicin for OA of the knee or hand Intra-articular corticosteroid injections for moderate to severe pain	Identify drug allergies and check the medical history Injections can provide pain relief for several weeks but do not benefit all patients
If paracetamol and/or topical NSAIDs are ineffective	Add an opioid Prescribe an oral NSAID or COX-2 inhibitor in addition to paracetamol or instead of a topical NSAID Co-prescribe this with a proton pump inhibitor Use the lowest effective dose for the shortest possible duration Choose the agent and dose on the basis of risk factors for gastrointestinal, liver and cardiorenal toxicity, and monitor for any such effects If the patient is already taking low-dose aspirin for another condition, consider an alternative analgesic Do not prescribe etoricoxib 60 mg as first-line treatment	Review the patient's analgesic history to prevent complications such as falls Establish whether the patient is opioid-naive (i.e. does not take this type of analgesic) or alternatively has a tolerance Patients who are used to opioids may need a higher dose

Table 20.1 (*Continued*)

Option	Intervention	Additional information
Non-pharmacological options	Heat and cold packs TENS	Seek expert advice if needed
	Manipulation and stretching	Particularly for OA
	Assessment for bracing, joint supports or insoles	Assistive devices help with biomechanical joint pain or instability
	Assistive devices (e.g. walking sticks, tap turners) to address specific problems. Seek expert advice if needed	Assistive devices help with biomechanical joint pain or instability
Treatments not recommended	Rubefacients Intra-articular hyaluronan injections Electroacupuncture Chondroitin or glucosamine	
Self-management	Exercise Weight loss (if overweight) Suitable footwear Heat and cold packs TENS	Knee pain may decrease if the patient is obese and loses weight
Referral to joint surgery	Consider referral for joint surgery if symptoms continue to substantially affect quality of life despite medical treatment Arthroscopic lavage and debridement should be used only for patients with OA of the knee and a clear history of mechanical locking in the knee Scoring tools are not advocated to prioritise patients or to refuse referral on grounds of age, gender, smoking, obesity, etc.	

COX-2, cyclooxygenase-2; NSAID, non-steroidal anti-inflammatory drug; OA, osteoarthritis; TENS, transcutaneous electrical nerve stimulation.

An **arthroplasty** or joint replacement is an effective way of removing damaged bone and replacing it with an artificial joint (prosthesis), thus reducing or removing the pain and improving joint function and mobility (Croft *et al.* 2002). This is routinely done for the hip and knee joints, and 95% of replacements will last for 15 years (NICE 2008). Complications include loosening of the prosthesis and infection, which can lead to removal of the implant, either temporarily or permanently.

A total hip replacement is better for less mobile and older patients, and even though it can be effective surgically, not all patients will return to their premorbid level of fitness and quality of life (Montin *et al.* 2008). Hørdam *et al.* (2011) used telephone support at 2 and 10 weeks after discharge to assess their patients' health and activities of daily living, share information and provide education, support and counselling, with limited beneficial effect.

Nursing intervention in total hip replacement

Lucas (2008a, 2008b) explored key patient management for patients undergoing either a total hip or a knee replacement, both preparatory (Box 20.4) and postoperative (Box 20.5).

Box 20.4 Concepts relating to preparation for surgery (adapted from Lucas 2008a)

- Indications for surgery – why it is needed
- The importance of preoperative preparation – justify the need for the surgery and its impact on patient outcome
- Psychological preparation – informed consent, fasting, general anaesthetic versus spinal anaesthetic, preoperative information on pain assessment, analgesia, mobility, why routine investigations are important, etc.:
    - A Cochrane Review on preoperative education for hip and knee replacements (Donald *et al.* 2004) concluded that there may be beneficial effects when preoperative education is tailored accordingly to anxiety or targeted at those most in need of support (i.e. those who are particularly disabled or have limited social support structures)
- Physical preparation – the policy on going to theatre, the patient checklist, fasting, etc.
- Social preparation – identify difficulties with the home environment.
- Integrated preparation for procedures on both joint types
- Preparation before referral, progress from the waiting list to preoperative assessment, and then preoperative assessment clinic
- This clinic establishes the patient's medical history and comorbidities, confirms whether they have or carry methicillin-resistant *Staphylococcus aureus*, records the weight and vital signs, takes and tests blood samples, tests urine and completes an ECG and X-rays to produce baseline information that will establish the patient's level of risk
- Nursing interventions/management will be in the best interest of the patient

Box 20.5 Concepts related to postoperative care (adapted from Lucas 2008b)

Immediate recovery period – the first 5–7 days

- Recovery from anaesthetic (general or spinal)
- Pain relief
- Wound care
- Mobilisation
- Venous thromboembolism prophylaxis – to prevent deep venous thrombosis; use TED stockings and low molecular weight heparin (NICE 2010)
- Preparation for discharge – assess home circumstances and support
- First 6 weeks after discharge – patient education
- Long-term recovery and outcomes – review these and provide patient education

Osteomyelitis

Osteomyelitis is an infection of a bone usually caused by *Staphylococcus aureus*, *Pseudomonas* or *Mycobacterium tuberculosis*. This condition is considered to be an orthopaedic emergency. Patients at increased risk of osteomyelitis include those with diabetes mellitus, malnourished patients, immunosuppressed patients and those who have been on long-term steroid treatment.

A bone infection can occur from direct spread of the organism due to (Burden & Kneale 2005):

- direct inoculation from a penetrating injury or surgery to the bone;
- local spread from another infected bone, trauma or surgical wound or burn injury;
- haematogenous spread from elsewhere such as a lung or soft tissue infection.

Box 20.6 Local symptoms of acute osteomyelitis

- Pain at the site of infection
- Local tenderness
- Heat
- Swelling
- Redness over the area
- Later on, a sinus between bone and skin

An inflammatory response begins, and the increased pressure within the bone causes pain and local tenderness (Box 20.6). The increase in infected material towards the cortex of the bone causes the periosteum to lift, resulting in swelling. The affected bone tissues start to necrose and an abscess forms within the bone. If left untreated, the abscess can rupture and eventually form a sinus leading to the skin.

Diagnosis of the specific microorganism requires a needle aspiration bone biopsy at the site of infection. The infection will not be initially evident on an X-ray until changes in the bone have occurred, which can take several weeks. MRI, CT or bone scans will show the extent of the infection at an earlier stage. An elevation in the white cell count and positive blood cultures may also not initially be seen. The patient will develop systemic signs of an infection including pyrexia, lethargy and irritability (Zeller *et al.* 2008).

A prompt diagnosis and early treatment are essential. Treatment requires management of the patients' symptoms, the primary cause of infection if known and the bone infection. The degree of pain can be reduced by elevation, supporting the affected limb using a cast or splint and pre-emptive analgesia (Burden & Kneale 2005). Using a removable splint allows any wound to be treated and the area over the infection to be inspected. Paracetamol and aspirin are prescribed for their analgesic and antipyretic properties. If the pain is more severe, opiate analgesia is prescribed.

A broad-spectrum antibiotic such as flucloxacillin or vancomycin is prescribed until the causative microorganism has been isolated. Antibiotics are initially given intravenously and then orally. Patient compliance is essential as antibiotics are often prescribed for between 4 weeks and several months. Topical antibiotic therapy using antibiotic cement or removable beads in the affected area can be employed if the patient undergoes surgery (Chen *et al.* 2008; Sancineto & Barla 2008).

Surgical intervention is required if the pressure within the bone continues to increase, requiring the removal of necrotic tissues or draining of an abscess. Extensive debridement can be required and the wound left open for continued irrigation and removal of the exudate. Secondary wound closure is carried out once the area is clean and granulation is evident. A persistent organism, such as *Staphylococcus aureus* or *Mycobacterium tuberculosis*, can lie dormant in the tissues for years, leading to recurrence of the infection and creating a scenario of chronic osteomyelitis.

Rheumatoid arthritis

Rheumatoid arthritis affects about 1% of the population, with some patients having a family history of rheumatoid arthritis, psoriasis or another autoimmune disease (Bulstrode & Swales 2007). It is a chronic, systemic inflammatory disorder characterised by progressive joint changes leading to joint destructive, deformity and immobility.

Box 20.7 addresses the signs and symptoms of rheumatoid arthritis. These symptoms need generally to have lasted for more than 6 weeks to exclude postviral changes, which are likely to resolve. Although rheumatoid arthritis can occur at any age, the peak age for diagnosis is 35–45 years, and there is a higher incidence of rheumatoid arthritis in women. NICE (2009) provides guidance on determining a diagnosis of rheumatoid arthritis using X-rays to determine joint space, bone erosion and joint deformity, along with a serum test for rheumatoid factor, although this is not an absolute indicator as it may

Box 20.7 The joint changes seen with rheumatoid arthritis

- Swelling or inflammation of the affected joints
- Joint pain
- Erythema
- A joint that is warm to the touch
- Joint stiffness after a period of immobility
- Early morning stiffness
- Joint deformity
- Bilateral presentation with, for example, both hands or knees affected
- Restriction in movement from joint changes and ligaments being stretched
- Fixed flexion deformities; e.g. flexion of the proximal interphalangeal (PIP) joint and extension of the distal interphalangeal (DIP) joint causes a boutonnière deformity, whereas a fixed extension of the PIP joint and flexion of the DIP joint causes swan-neck deformity
- Subluxation of the joints, e.g. the metacarpophalangeal joints with or without palmar and ulnar deviation of the fingers, and subluxation and radial deviation of the wrist with prominence of the ulnar styloid process
- Instability of the cervical spine at the atlantoaxial (C1–C2) joint
- Tenosynovitis, i.e. inflammation of the synovium membrane covering the tendon
- Bursitis, which is the inflammation of the fluid-filled sac (bursa) that lies between a tendon and skin, or between a tendon and bone

Box 20.8 Systemic changes seen with advanced rheumatoid arthritis

- Cardiac system, e.g. pericarditis
- Circulatory system, e.g. Raynaud's phenomena
- Eyes, e.g. scleritis
- Haematological changes, e.g. anaemia
- Nervous system, e.g. sensorimotor neuropathy
- Respiratory system, e.g. pulmonary effusions or basal fibrosis
- Skin, e.g. vasculitis (ulcers or haemorrhages) and erythema
- Soft tissues, e.g. muscle wasting or nodules
- Other changes, e.g. weight loss, exhaustion, pyrexia and malaise

not be positive. The disabling effects of joint change are exacerbated by the range of systemic effects seen in patients with more advanced disease that have an impact on the psychosocial well-being of patients and their families (Box 20.8).

The multidisciplinary team, family and carers

Patients are regularly seen by other members of the health care team (NICE 2009). Physiotherapists will assess the patient's general fitness and encourage exercises to maintain joint function and muscle strength, and can help with pain relief. Occupational therapists can provide protective splints for joint protection and assist with hand problems, as well as giving advice on home, work and lifestyle adaptations. Referral to a podiatrist is essential for patients with foot problems as insoles or adapted footwear may be required. Patients are referred to an orthopaedic surgeon if a patient has persistent pain due to joint damage, worsening joint function, progressive joint deformity, persistent localised synovitis,

Table 20.2 Drugs commonly used in rheumatoid arthritis

Drug group	Patient type	Drug type/complications
Disease-modifying antirheumatic drugs (DMARDs)	Administered to newly diagnosed patients within the first 3 months of onset of symptoms	Aim to halt the progress of the disease and should include methotrexate and one other DMARD, e.g. hydroxychloroquine, sulphasalazine or leflunomide, plus a short-term glucocorticoid (NICE 2009). DMARDs can have severe side effects and should be reduced to a maintenance dose when the disease is under control
Oral steroid therapy Joint (intra-articular) steroid injections	Used to control symptoms when the disease is active Used for direct pain relief in an acute joint flare-up as they appear to have no long-term effect on the joint; however, drug action is short-lived	Steroids can have severe side effects so need close monitoring
Non-steroidal anti-inflammatory drugs	Short-term pain control	Cyclo-oxygenase-2 inhibitors, e.g. celecoxib, are favoured as they have fewer gastrointestinal side effects

tendon rupture, nerve compression or a stress fracture. Surgical options can include joint replacement surgery, arthrodesis (joint fusion), nerve decompression and tendon repairs.

Good communication and patients' education on and understanding of their condition and treatment options will ensure they are able to make informed decisions about their care (NICE 2009). Where possible, the family or carers should be involved in this as well. Care must be patient-centred, with a full multidisciplinary team involved. Most centres have a rheumatologist, as well as a rheumatoid specialist nurse who regularly sees each patient, assessing the progress of joint and systemic changes. Many specialist nurses provide patient education and support, and amend or prescribe drug regimens within agreed protocols.

The current recommendation is for aggressive early treatment to prevent or delay the onset of severe joint deformity and disability. Drugs will not reverse the damage that has already occurred to a joint but they will reduce the inflammation and pain and slow the progress of the disease (Table 20.2).

Fracture injuries

A bone becomes fractured when the force exerted on it is stronger than the strength of the bone, as, for example, when an adult is hit by a moving object such as a car. A fracture can occur when a normal force is exerted on a bone that has not developed correctly, as in osteogenesis imperfecta, or when a normal bone is weakened from changes to its structure, as with osteoporosis. A repeated force on a bone can also slowly damage the internal bone structure, leading to a fatigue or spontaneous fracture, as with the stress fractures of the tibia that are seen in runners.

Figure 20.10 demonstrates the four main fracture types, with Table 20.3 providing a more detailed classification of fractures.

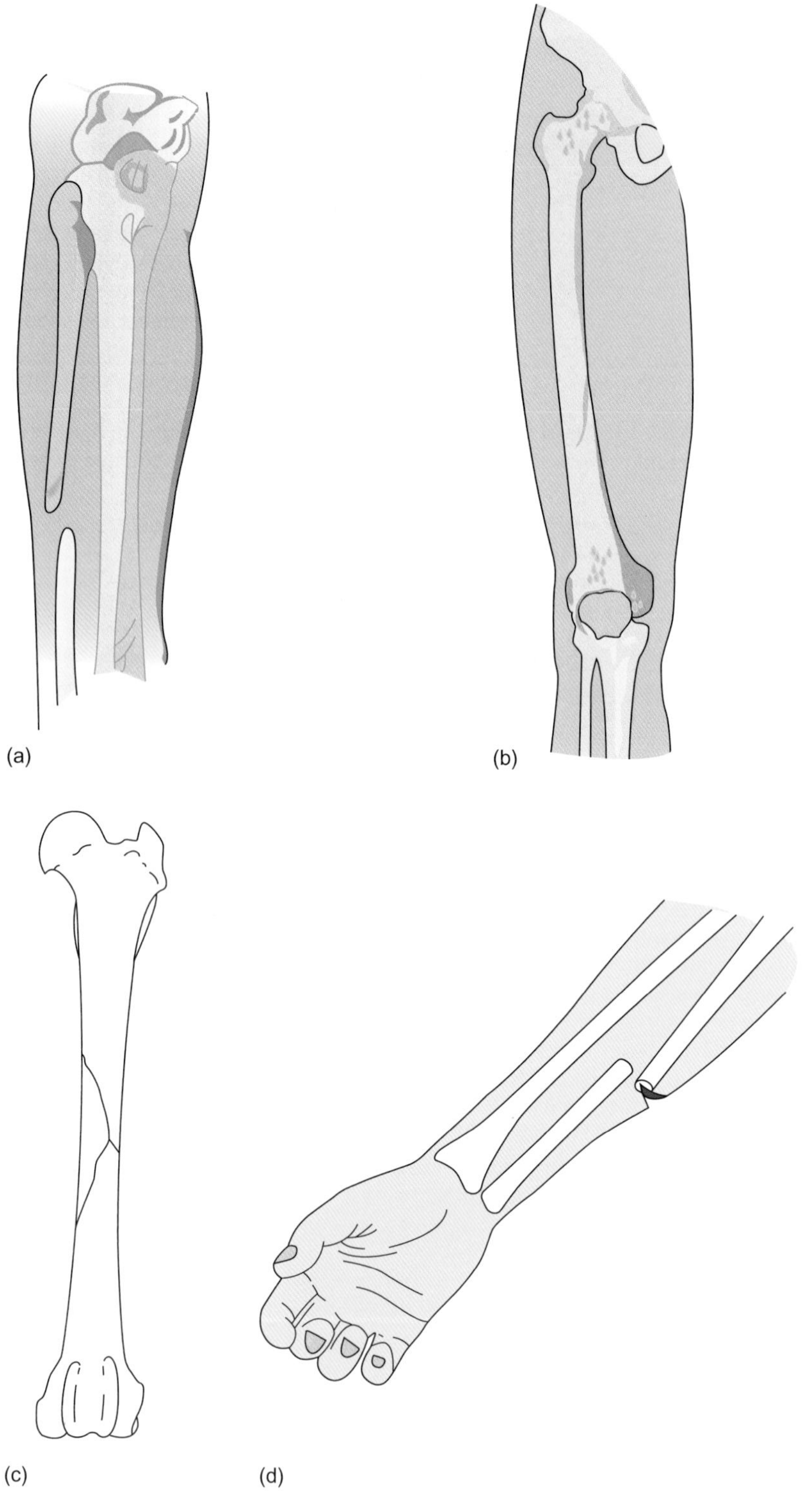

Figure 20.10 The four types of fracture: (a) simple, (b) incomplete (greenstick), (c) comminuted and (d) compound. Reproduced from Nair, M. & Peate, I. (2009) *Fundamentals of Applied Pathophysiology*, with kind permission from Wiley Blackwell.

Table 20.3 Classification of fractures

Fracture terms	Descriptions
Closed	Where there is no wound present over or near the fracture
Open or compound	A wound present, near or over the fracture site makes it an open or compound fracture. All wounds are assumed to be dirty and must be cleaned to reduce the risk of a bone infection (osteomyelitis) as an infection that occurs at a fracture site will stop the bone healing. Patients with an open fracture are generally given prophylactic antibiotics to prevent this
Stable or unstable	The fracture is stable if the bone ends do move without a significant additional force being applied
Extra-articular	Fractures away from a joint
Intra-articular	Fractures within a joint, which must be reduced with a high degree of accuracy to reduce the risk of further joint problems such as osteoarthritis
Pathological fracture	These injuries occur when the bone has been damaged by disease such as osteoporosis or bone metastases
Greenstick fracture	Seen in children; the malleable bone bends away from the direction of the force and is left at an angle but not broken
Avulsion fracture	Results from the sudden contraction of a muscle that results in a small area of bone being pulled away
Transverse fracture	The fracture occurs across the bone at 90°; these are usually stable as the surrounding muscles contract and hold the bones in place
Oblique fracture	The fracture is at 30° or more to the bone axis; these are often unstable as the bone is liable to slip when the muscles around it contract
Spiral fracture	Arises from a twisting force creating a spiral break around the bone
Impacted fracture	Caused by crushing of the bone where one part is driven into another; these are usually stable injuries
Comminuted fracture	Involves multiple bone fragments that arise from very high-impact or high-energy forces; such injuries often damage more than one bone or joint and there will be damage to other structures, e.g. skin, blood vessels and nerves

The bone healing process follows several clearly defined stages:

- **Stage 1, the inflammatory phase.** When the bone breaks, there is bleeding from the bone and surrounding tissues to create a fracture haematoma that seals the bone ends. An inflammatory response then occurs.
- **Stage 2, the reparative phase.** A capillary network forms within the haematoma and granulation tissue develops. Osteoblast cells that create new bone begin to form a bridge between the bone ends, and new bone (callus) is formed.
- **Stage 3, the remodelling stage.** There is gradual spread of callus, and the creation of the compact and cancellous bone structures occurs over several months to 2 years depending on the type and degree of damage to the bone. Osteoclast cells will absorb fragments of dead bone tissue and callus to reform the bone's internal and external structure.

Usually by 6 weeks, the bone can support movement and normal function, but in some areas where there is a compound and comminuted fracture of mainly compact bone, for example the femoral shaft, it can take 16 weeks for the bone to unite, and possibly longer before the bone can support weight and the patient mobilise unaided (McRae & Kinninmonth 1997).

When a patient with a suspected or actual joint or bone injury is admitted, the mechanism of injury that describes the incident is documented. However, immediate assessment of the patient's airway, breathing and circulation are essential, and these functions must be stabilised before other orthopaedic care is provided (see Chapter 10). Monitoring of vital signs, the pulses distal to the site of injury, skin

Box 20.9 Common interventions to treat fractures (Jester *et al.* 2011)

- **Splinting** – taping one finger or toe to its neighbour(s) (with mild analgesia)
- **Reduction** – manual manipulation to ensure correct positioning of the fractured bone (with or without analgesia and sedation)
- **Internal fixation** – (which is not usually visible to the patient) using metal screws, plates, wiring or intramedullary nails to ensure accurate reduction and allow early mobilisation (with analgesia dependent on fracture type)
- **External fixation** – visibly seen on the outside of the fractured limb and using either an Orthofix or Ilizarov fixator. Guidance on pin site care (a report and recommendations from the 2010 consensus) is available at www.rcn.org.uk/__data/assets/pdf_file/0009/413982/004137.pdf
- **Traction** – used to immobilise the fractured limb and reduce pain (with or without analgesia or sedation), e.g. a Thomas splint (see www.ossur.co.uk for a series of videos on how to apply a Thomas splint)

colour, sensory changes and movement of the limb or area distal to or around the injury is crucial. The corresponding limb is compared, with joints and muscles checked for their ligaments. X-rays are taken of potential and actual injury sites, along with an MRI or CT scan if a head or abdominal injury is suspected.

Common intervention in the treatment of fractures

The treatment of a fracture depends on the site, type and extent of injury. Pain relief is essential and based on a regular pain assessment. Box 20.9 lists the common interventions used in treating fractures.

Following treatment, patients will need information on how to look after their injury and how to protect it from further trauma (Table 20.4). Ideally, both verbal and written information will be given and where possible a relative or carer involved in the discussion in case the patient does not understand any of the information .

Complications of fractures

Complications can arise when a fracture occurs or later as healing takes place, and include:

- hypovolaemic shock from loss of blood at the time of injury;
- arterial and nerve trauma at the time of injury;
- tendon and muscle trauma at the time of injury;
- avascular necrosis, when a bone fragment does not have an adequate blood supply; the area then needs to be removed (debrided) and a new secure internal or external fixation created, possibly with bone graft materials applied to the area;
- compartment syndrome, in which swelling into a muscle increases the pressure within that muscle, causing extreme pain when it is touched or moved; if left untreated, this leads to muscle ischaemia and a permanent contraction of the distal limb. Any cast or bandages are removed in case they are preventing circulation, and if no improvement is seen, the patient is taken to theatre, where the muscle fascia is split and left open to allow the swelling to reduce. Secondary closure of the wound and any skin grafting is carried out later. Peripheral neurovascular assessment is pivotal to the patient's outcome (Judge 2007; Jester *et al.* 2011; Shields & Clarke 2011);
- non-union where the bone ends do not unite;
- malunion where the bone ends have united but at an inappropriate position or angle;
- joint or muscle stiffness of weakness, especially if the joint has been encased in a cast or the patient has not used their joints and muscles for a long time; physiotherapy can help to reduce the effect and enable full or near-full function to be restored;

Table 20.4 Patient information

Information topic	Why this is needed
Analgesia and anti-inflammatory drugs	To ensure the correct type and usage of analgesics and anti-inflammatory drugs
Elevating the limb	To reduce and prevent further swelling of the area; the area must be supported correctly
Sling	A high arm sling is used to reduce swelling of the fingers or wrist. A broad arm sling is used to take the weight and support the arm. Advice is needed on when to use or to remove the sling
Using a walking aid	If the leg is in a cast, or a ligament or muscle injury is affecting mobility, the patient must be taught how to use crutches, a walking stick or other walking aids correctly to prevent further falls and injury
Care of a plaster or fibreglass cast	A cast is used for immediate care of factures that do not require surgery or is used following surgery. It is often applied and then split. Alternatively, only a back slab is used and this is initially bandaged on to the limb to allow for swelling. This is replaced by a full plaster or fibreglass cast in the next 2–3 days once the swelling has subsided. Advice is essential to ensure it keeps the fracture stable and to protect the skin from damage

- wound infections, arising from an open injury and a contaminated wound, or in a surgical wound following surgery to stabilise the fracture;
- osteomyelitis, an infection in the bone, which must be suspected if the patient has pain and the bone is not healing.

Visit www.wileyfundamentalseries.com/medicalnursing and read Reflective Question 20.2 to think more about this topic.

Osteoporosis

Osteoporosis is a condition in which normal bone gradually loses mineral density. It is defined by the World Health Organization (1994) as a 'systemic skeletal disease characterised by low bone mass and microarchitectural deterioration of bone tissue with a consequent increase in bone fragility and susceptibility to fracture'. The bone mass or bone mineral density relies on the balance between osteoblast and osteoclast activity within the bone. Thus, the bone mass increases in childhood and plateaus at skeletal maturity until about 35 years of age, when it begins to decrease as part of the natural ageing process in both sexes (Bulstrode & Swales 2007). The whole skeleton is affected, but the condition may go unnoticed until the patient presents with one of three typical osteoporotic fractures:

- fracture of the distal radius (a Colles' fracture);
- fracture of the femoral neck (a hip fracture);
- a crush fracture of the vertebral body (commonly of a thoracic vertebra).

Box 20.10 addresses the main risk factors that accelerate the rate of bone density loss, while Table 20.5 outlines the drugs used in the prevention and treatment of osteoporosis. The key message is to:

Box 20.10 Risk factors for osteoporosis

- Female gender, age (over 60 years), Caucasian or Asian origin
- A maternal history of a hip fracture
- Oestrogen deficiency, e.g. due to early (premature) menopause, prolonged amenorrhoea or primary hypogonadism
- Corticosteroid therapy, e.g. prednisolone therapy of >7.5 mg per day for more than 6 months
- Low body mass index (<19 kg/m^2), owing to a combination of reduced oestrogen levels and a reduction in impact loading
- Low calcium levels and/or vitamin D deficiency
- Smoking
- Excess alcohol
- Sedentary lifestyle, lack of weight-bearing exercise and prolonged immobilisation
- Anorexia nervosa (low weight, menstrual irregularity and a low-calcium diet)
- Endocrine syndromes (hyperparathyroidism, hyperthyroidism and Cushing's syndrome)
- Inflammatory arthropathy
- A history of fractures in adulthood, especially a previous Colles', hip or vertebral fracture
- Breast cancer, especially for postmenopausal women

Table 20.5 Drugs used for the prevention or management of osteoporosis (Scottish Intercollegiate Guidelines Network 2011)

Drug	Rationale for use
Bisphosphonate group, e.g. risedronate, alendronate and etidronate Many patients will be advised to take with vitamin D and calcium supplementation	Inhibit osteoclast action and slow the rate of bone resorption to maintain the patient's current bone mass density and reduce the risk of a fracture. Known for their poor rate of absorption and potential gastrointestinal side effects: • Guidance on taking these include swallowing them on an empty stomach with a glass of water while standing, and then remaining upright and fasting for 30 minutes. Compliance is difficult to achieve and often poor
Selective oestrogen receptor modulators, e.g. raloxifene	Can reduce the rate of bone loss and reduce the risk of vertebral fractures. They are better tolerated but have an increased risk of deep vein thrombosis formation
Strontium	Stimulates bone formation in the natural cycle of remodelling of bone tissue. Has a beneficial effect in reducing vertebral and femoral neck fractures
Hormone replacement therapy	Currently used for management of menopause symptoms and has a role in maintaining bone mineral density
Testosterone	Used for men if hypogonadism is present or is the main cause of osteoporosis.
Teriparatide (synthetic parathyroid hormone)	Stabilises bone mineral density. Only used for the treatment of severe osteoporosis for 18 months due to a potential increased risk of osteosarcoma (bone cancer) with prolonged use

- have a healthy diet high in calcium and vitamin D or take alternative supplements;
- increase the level of activity, particularly weight-bearing exercise;
- stop or reduce their level of smoking;
- avoid excess levels of alcohol;
- seek medical advice about reducing or stopping taking steroid drugs.

The best approach to osteoporosis is that of prevention. The multidisciplinary team need to be involved in giving timely and appropriate advice on prevention, along with diagnosing and treating osteoporosis. Such health promotion would promote peak bone mass in adulthood and decrease the rate of loss of bone density with age. This should not be confined to the orthopaedic or trauma teams but include practitioners in primary care settings – physiotherapists, dietitians and occupational therapists all have a role in this area of health promotion (Horan & Timmins 2009). Schemes such as a nurse-led orthopaedic elderly care liaison service (Stephenson 2003), in which all elderly patients with a fragility fracture are assessed for their risk of osteoporosis and falling, are also able to give timely, relevant advice and make referrals to appropriate osteoporosis, fracture or falls clinics, thus improving care and reducing the risk of future fracture injuries and hospital admissions.

Hip fracture

Hip fracture or femoral neck fracture is normally seen in older women with osteoporosis, with the potential for such an injury to occur increasing in the over-85 years of age group. As many patients have one or more comorbid illnesses, the injury leads to a high level of complications, with a number of patients dying within 12 months of injury (Novack *et al.* 2007). Although the majority of hip fractures result from osteoporosis, they are also caused by the increased risk of falling that is seen with age (Department of Health 2001; see also Chapter 6).

> Visit www.wileyfundamentalseries.com/medicalnursing and read Reflective Question 20.3 to think more about this topic.

Once an elderly person has fallen and sustained a fracture, they are unable to get up and weight-bear, they experience tenderness or pain over the lateral aspect of the thigh and the leg is externally rotated and shortened due to contraction of the dominant muscles, but there is rarely any bruising evident. If the fracture is impacted, the patient may attempt to stand and walk, but the bone remains painful and the leg is shortened.

Classification and management of hip fracture

The patient is given opiate analgesia and an intravenous infusion is commenced in A&E. An X-ray of the hip will confirm the diagnosis of a hip fracture:

- An intra-articular fracture occurs within the joint capsule and presents as a subcapital fracture across the femoral neck high under the femoral head. This is the most common type of hip fracture, seen in more proportionally men than women (Jester *et al.* 2011).
- An extra-articular fracture occurs outside the joint capsule either at the base of the femoral neck or through the greater and/or lesser trochanter. These fractures have a better prognosis (Jester *et al.* 2011).

A full patient assessment is completed. The patient's pre-injury health status is recorded, and any medical issues such as those related to osteoporosis or a history of repeated falls are noted. Patients are then transferred to the orthopaedic trauma unit. Surgery will ideally take place within 24 hours because a worse health status prior to surgery and a delay in surgical intervention are known to affect recovery and possibly increase mortality risk (Novack *et al.* 2007; Scottish Intercollegiate Guidelines Network 2009) (Box 20.11). Additional benefits from early surgery are an increased ability to return to independent living (Al-Ani *et al.* 2008) and a reduced length of hospital stay (Lefaivre *et al.* 2009). The following points related to surgery should be remembered:

Box 20.11 Potential complications of a hip fracture pre- and post-surgery

Complications from the injury and the preoperative phase

- Hypovolaemic shock
- Pain
- Limb deformity – the limb is externally rotated and shortened
- Dehydration
- Avascular necrosis of the femoral head

Post-surgical and rehabilitation-related complications

- Complications of bed rest – pressure sores, chest infection, urinary tract infection
- Deep vein thrombosis and pulmonary embolism (NICE 2010)
- Joint dislocation if a hemi-arthroplasty has been used
- Loosening of fixation
- Non-union of the fracture
- Postoperative confusion
- Pressure sores

- The surgical procedure depends on the extent and type of injury.
- A subcapital fracture is liable to compromise the blood supply from the vascular ring outside the base of the femoral neck, which has several arterial entry points with vessels going up the femoral neck to the head.
- Trauma to these vessels risks avascular necrosis of the femoral head (bone death); therefore the femoral head is removed and replaced (a hemi-arthroplasty).
- No acetabular component is required unless there are severe osteoarthritic changes in the joint. With an extracapsular fracture, the blood supply is unaffected but this tends to be a more unstable fracture.
- An extracapsular fracture is treated with a dynamic hip screw going into the femoral neck and attached to a plate that is screwed on to the lateral surface of the femur below the greater trochanter.

Patients' length of stay overall is related to their comorbid conditions, where they were living before the injury, the timeliness of their transfer to rehabilitation and where they are discharged to. Unfortunately, many patients with comorbid conditions require an extensive rehabilitation period. Younger patients admitted from home who have a spouse to return to are more likely to return home (Titler *et al.* 2006).

Neurovascular assessment and plaster care

All patients who have a musculoskeletal injury or have undergone orthopaedic surgery or cast immobilisation of a limb are at risk of developing neurovascular compromise, which can lead to compartment syndrome (Judge 2007). Peripheral neurovascular assessment involves a systematic assessment of the neurological and vascular integrity of a limb, with the aim of promptly recognising any neurovascular deficit (Judge 2007). Damage to the tissues worsens as time passes, so prompt recognition and intervention are necessary (Jester et al. 2011).

Physiological indicators of vascular compromise are caused by a lack of oxygen within the muscles and all the tissues along with neurological compromise due to an interruption of the nerve supply to the tissue (Jester et al. 2011). Dykes' (1993) recognised '5Ps' approach to neurovascular assessment integrates assessment of the patient's limb with regard to pain, pulses, pallor, paraesthesia and paralysis. Shields and Clarke (2011) also highlight documentation on a dedicated chart noting pain intensity and type, warmth, sensation, colour, capillary refill time and the movement of the affected and unaffected limb key, in order to provide a baseline for comparison.

Pain is usually the earliest and most important presenting symptom of compartment syndrome (Judge 2007). Grottkau *et al.* (2005) undertook a retrospective study of 133 cases of compartment

Box 20.12 Key principles of plaster cast care (adapted from Clarke *et al.* 2003)

Patient education

- Keep the plastered arm or leg raised on a pillow for the first 12 hours and at rest as elevation aids the reduction of swelling. Continue to do this for another 12 hours if the cast still feels tight
- Don't get the plaster cast wet as this will weaken the cast, and the bone will no longer be fully supported and will become a source for infection (osteomyelitis or septic arthritis)
- Baths and showers should be avoided, but in reality a plastic bag can be used to cover the cast. Try using sticky tape or a rubber band to seal the bag at the top and bottom to make it as water-tight as possible. Alternatively, it is possible to buy special covers for plaster casts to keep them dry
- Always remove the bag as soon as possible to avoid sweating, which could also damage the cast
- Even if the plaster cast makes the skin feel very itchy, do not 'poke' anything down the cast to try to relieve the itch as it could cause a wound or source of infection. The itchiness should settle down after a few days (or contact your GP about taking an antihistamine)

Plaster cast tips

- Don't let any small objects fall inside the cast as they could irritate the skin
- Don't try to alter the length or position of the cast
- Don't lift anything heavy or drive until the cast has been removed and it has been agreed by a doctor that it is safe to lift or drive
- Use a sling, as advised by your health professional
- Don't write on the cast for at least 24 hours to prevent denting of the cast and skin problems – allow it to dry naturally

Plaster cast problems

- Contact A&E, the fracture clinic, the plaster unit or the ward if:
    - The plaster cast still feels too tight after keeping it elevated for 24 hours
    - The cast is rubbing or cutting into the skin
    - The fingers on the affected limb feel swollen, tingly, burning, painful (even after taking painkillers) or numb
    - The fingers turn blue or white
    - The cast feels too loose or slips
    - The cast is broken or cracked
    - The skin underneath or around the edge of the cast feels sore
    - There is an unpleasant smell, discharge or staining coming from the cast
- Document in the patient's notes when verbal and written advice has been given

syndrome and reported that 90% of patients complained of pain. Therefore a multidimensional approach should be applied, encompassing the use of a valid (ability to measure) and reliable (consistency) pain assessment tool (Clarke, 2003). Box 20.12 denotes key patient education for the patient in a plaster cast (Clarke 2003).

Bone metastases

As bone metastases are more commonly seen in adults than primary bone tumours, the latter are not discussed here. Although many primary tumours are known to result in bone metastases, they usually arise from primary breast, prostate, lung, kidney and thyroid tumours (Henry 2005). They occur in bones with a rich blood supply such as the vertebrae, humerus, acetabulum and femur. Patients generally present with dull, aching bone pain that increases during the day and may disturb the sleep at night (Henry 2005). Movement, especially weight-bearing, can increase the pain, leading to difficulty in weight-bearing and reduced mobility. A pathological fracture is identified by the sudden onset of severe pain. If bone metastases are suspected, a bone scan will identify the extent of the metastatic spread; if spread is shown, this should be followed by plain X-ray, CT or MRI scans to help plan patient care.

A diagnosis of bone metastases often indicates that the primary cancer has advanced or that treatment has been unsuccessful, causing a raised level of anxiety and fear in patients and their families. Psychological and social aspects of care are as essential for these patients, as is the management of their pain. Conservative management is essential to reduce the level of pain experienced, reduce the risk of a fracture occurring and ensure that a patient's level of health and quality of life are maintained. Options for pain relief include analgesia, radiotherapy, chemotherapy, surgery and bisphosphonate drugs (Henry 2005). For this reason, the oncology, orthopaedic and palliative care teams will collaborate to ensure appropriate care for the patient in relation to management of the primary cancer and any palliative care needs. Patients presenting with a fracture require symptomatic treatment including appropriate analgesia and management of the fracture, for example internal fixation, bed rest on traction and a plaster cast. The decision to operate on the fracture will depend on the patient's health and life expectancy.

Conclusion

This chapter has outlined some of the common conditions associated with the musculoskeletal system. The chapter should not be considered sufficient in itself and should be used in conjunction with other published material in order to ensure further development of knowledge gained.

References

Al-Ani, A., Samuelsson, B., Tidermark, J. *et al.* (2008) Early operation on patient with a hip fracture improved the ability to return to independent living. *Journal of Bone and Joint Surgery (American)*, **90**(7):1436–42.

Bulstrode, C. & Swales, C. (2007) *The Musculoskeletal System at a Glance*. Oxford: Blackwell Publishing.

Burden, J. & Kneale, J.D. (2005) Orthopaedic infections. In: Kneale, J.D. & Davis, P.S. (eds) *Orthopaedic and Trauma Nursing*, 2nd ed (pp. 215–36). Edinburgh: Churchill Livingstone.

Chen, L.H., Yang, S.C., Niu, C.C., Lai, P.L. & Chen, W.J. (2008) Percutaneous drainage followed by antibiotic-impregnated cement vertebroplasty for pyogenic vertebral osteomyelitis: a case report. *Journal of Trauma Injury, Infection and Critical Care*, **64**(1):E8–11.

Clarke, S. (2003) Orthopaedic paediatric practice: an impression of pain assessment. *Journal of Orthopaedic Nursing*, **7**:132–6.

Croft, P., Lewis, M., Wynn Jones, C., Coogan, D. & Cooper, C. (2002) Health status in patients awaiting hip replacement for osteoarthritis. *Rheumatology*, **41**:1001–7.

Department of Health (2001) *National Service Framework or Older People*. London: Department of Health.

Donald, S., Hetrick, S.E. & Green, S. (2004) Preoperative education for hip or knee replacement. *Cochrane Database of Systematic Reviews* (1):CD003526.

Dykes, P.C. (1993) Minding the five P's of neurovascular assessment. *American Journal of Nursing*, **6**:38–9.

Grottkau, B.E., Howard, R.E. & Scala, C. (2005) Compartment syndrome in children and adolescents. *Journal of Pediatric Surgery*, **140**:678–82.

Henry, C. (2005) Care of patients with bone tumours. In: Kneale, J.D. & Davis, P.S. (eds), *Orthopaedic and Trauma Nursing*, 2nd ed (pp. 265–85). Edinburgh: Churchill Livingstone.

Horan, A. & Timmins, F. (2009). The role of community multidisciplinary teams in osteoporosis treatment and prevention. *Journal of Orthopaedic Nursing*, **13**(2):85–96.

Hørdam, B., Pedersen, P.U, Søballe, K., Sabroe, S. & Ehlers, L.H. (2011) Quality adjusted life years gained in patients aged over 65 years after total hip replacement. *International Journal of Orthopaedic and Trauma Nursing*, **15**(1):11–17.

Jester, R., Santy, J. & Rodgers, J. (2011) *Oxford Handbook of Orthopaedic and Trauma Nursing*. Oxford: University Press.

Jinks, C., Jordan, K. & Croft, P. (2002) Measuring the population impact of knee pain and disability with the Western Ontario and McMaster Universities Osteoarthritis Index (WOMAC). *Pain*, **100**(1–2):55–64.

Judge, N.L. (2007) Neurovascular assessment. *Nursing Standard*, **21**(45):39–44.

Lefaivre, K., Macadam, S., Davidson, D., Gandhi, R., Chan, H. & Broekhuyse, H. (2009) Length, of stay, mortality, morbidity and delay to surgery in hip fractures. *Journal of Bone and Joint Surgery (British)*, **91**(7):922–7.

Lucas, B. (2008a) Total hip and total knee replacement: preoperative nursing management. *British Journal of Nursing*, **17**(21):1346–51.

Lucas, B. (2008b) Total hip and total knee replacement: postoperative nursing management *British Journal of Nursing*, **17**(22):1410–14.

McRae, R. & Kinninmonth, A.W.G. (1997) *Orthopaedics and Trauma: An Illustrated Colour Text*. New York: Churchill Livingstone.

Montin, L., Leino-Kilpi, T., Suominen, T. & Lepistö, J. (2008) A systematic review of empirical studies between 1966 and 2005 of patient outcomes of total hip arthroplasty and related factors. *Journal of Clinical Nursing*, **17**(1):40–5.

Nair, M. & Peate, I. (2009) *Fundamentals of Applied Pathophysiology: An Essential Guide for Nursing Students*. Basingstoke: Wiley Blackwell.

National Institute for Health and Clinical Excellence (2008) *Osteoarthritis: The Care and Management of Osteoarthritis in Adults*. Clinical Guideline No. 59. London: Department of Health.

National Institute for Health and Clinical Excellence (2009) *The Management of Rheumatoid Arthritis in Adults*. Clinical Guideline No. 79. London: Department of Health.

National Institute of Health and Clinical Excellence (2010) *Venous Thromboembolism: Reducing the Risk. Reducing the risk of venous thromboembolism (Deep Vein Thrombosis and Pulmonary Embolism) in Patients Admitted to Hospital*. Clinical Guideline No. 92. London: Department of Health.

Novack, V., Jotkowitz, A., Etzion, O. & Porath, A. (2007) Does delay in surgery after hip fracture lead to worse outcomes? A multicenter survey. *International Journal of Quality Health Care*, **19**(3):170–6.

Sancineto, C.F. & Barla, J.D. (2008) Treatment of long bone osteomyelitis with a mechanically table intramedullary antibiotic dispenser: nineteen consecutive cases with a minimum of 12 months follow-up. *Journal of Trauma*, **65**:1416–20.

Scottish Intercollegiate Guidelines Network (2009) *Management of Hip Fracture in Older People: A National Clinical Guideline*. Edinburgh: SIGN.

Scottish Intercollegiate Guidelines Network (2011) *Management of Osteoporosis: A National Clinical Guideline*. Edinburgh: SIGN.

Shields, C. & Clarke, S. (2011) Neurovascular observation and documentation for children within accident and emergency: a critical review. *International Journal of Orthopaedic and Trauma Nursing*, **15**:3–10.

Stephenson, S. (2003) Developing an orthopaedic elderly care liaison service. *Journal of Orthopaedic Nursing*, **7**(3): 150–5.

Titler, M., Dochterman, J., Xie, X.-J. *et al.* (2006) Nursing interventions and other factors associated with discharge disposition in older patients with hip fractures. *Nursing Research*, **55**(4):231–42.

World Health Organization (1994) *Assessment of Fracture Risk and its Application to Screening for Postmenopausal Osteoporosis. Report of a WHO Study Group*. World Health Organization Technical Report Series No. 843. Geneva: WHO.

Zeller, J.I., Burke, A.E & Glass, R.M. (2008) Osteomyelitis. *Journal of the American Medical Association*, **299**(7):858.

21

Nursing care of conditions related to the ear, nose, throat and eye

Dymphna Tuohy[1], Jane McCarthy[1], Carmel O'Sullivan[2] and Niamh Hurley[2]

[1]*University of Limerick, Limerick, Ireland*
[2]*Mid-Western Regional Hospital, Limerick, Ireland*

Contents

Introduction 449
Diagnostic investigations 449
The ear 451
The nose 455
The throat (pharynx) 460
The eye 469
Conclusion 477
References 477

Learning outcomes

Having read this chapter, you will be able to;

- Outline the anatomy and physiology of the ear, nose, throat and eye
- Define and describe common conditions affecting the ear, nose, throat and eye
- Describe the medical and nursing management of patients with ear, nose and throat and eye disorders

Fundamentals of Medical-Surgical Nursing: A Systems Approach, First Edition. Edited by Anne-Marie Brady, Catherine McCabe, and Margaret McCann.

Introduction

This chapter provides a concise account of the nursing care of individuals with conditions related to the ear, nose, throat and eye. A range of the more common conditions affecting the special senses are described, and the relevant nursing management is presented.

In today's rapidly changing healthcare environment, much of ear, nose and throat (ENT) and eye nursing is provided via:

- primary care;
- outpatient department appointments;
- day surgery;
- short-stay hospitalisation.

Nursing within these environments requires an ability to adapt in order to meet the different needs of various patient groups. Nurses are required to provide care, including health promotion and discharge planning, within an increasingly shorter time frame.

Diagnostic investigations

Individuals with ENT- and eye-related conditions require assessment and often specialised diagnostic investigations (Boxes 21.1–21.4).

Box 21.1 Assessment tools for ENT conditions

- An auriscope/otoscope – to examine the external ear
- A light:
  - A pen torch
  - A bull's eye lamp
  - A head mirror
- Tuning forks for the:
  - Weber test (for conduction deafness)
  - Rinne test (which compares air and bone conduction)
- Nasal and ear speculums
- Tongue depressors

Box 21.2 Assessment tools for eye conditions

- A pen torch – used to assess the gross structures of the eye
- A slit-lamp table – with a mounted binocular microscope for eye assessment
- A tonometer – used with the slit lamp to measure intraocular pressure
- An ophthalmoscope – a monocular instrument to view the inner eye, particularly the retina and fundus
- Relevant charts (e.g. Snellen chart) and forms

Box 21.3 Investigations for ENT conditions

- Audiometry tests, including the use of a Barany noise box for unilateral deafness
- Auriscopy/otoscopy to allow magnified inspection of the external auditory canal and tympanic membrane
- A barium swallow to rule out oesophageal problems
- Fibrescopic examination of the nose, pharynx, larynx, vocal cords and carina
- Laryngoscopy to examine the larynx and vocal cords:
  - Indirect – a mirror is used to examine the back of the throat
  - Direct – a fibreoptic instrument (flexible or rigid) is inserted into the throat, which may require general anaesthesia (especially with a rigid laryngoscope)
- Tissue biopsy
- Radiology examinations (for fractures, sinusitis, tumours, tissue damage, etc.) – X-ray, magnetic resonance imaging and computed tomography

Box 21.4 Investigations for eye conditions

- Fluorescein angiography visualises the retinal, choroidal and iris blood vessels in a two-part process involving:
  - Fluorescein dye injection
  - A series of photographs taken as the dye circulates in the blood vessels at the back of the eye
- Fluorescein staining identifies foreign bodies and corneal abrasions
- Fundoscopy views the fundus and optic nerve head to determine the damage
- Gonioscopy examines the anterior chamber to view the angle, structures and depth
- Keratometry measures corneal curvature; it is used in conjunction with biometry to calculate the strength of the intraocular lens in cataract surgery
- Optical coherence tomography:
  - Is non-invasive
  - Has a high resolution
  - Provides cross-sectional imaging of the eye's biological tissues
- Ophthalmoscopy detects haemorrhage in or trauma to the interior chamber
- Photodynamic therapy
- X-rays and computed tomography are used to identify orbital fractures or the presence of foreign bodies within the globe
- Ultrasonography is used to determine a detached retina or vitreous haemorrhage:
  - A-scan biometry measures the axial length of the eye and is necessary to calculate the intraocular lens to be used in cataract surgery
  - B-scanning determines the level of retinal detachment or vitreous haemorrhage
- Visual acuity testing:
  - A Snellen chart for distance vision
  - A Sheridan–Gardiner test chart, used for children and adults with reading difficulties
  - An E-chart
  - A pinhole for refractive errors
  - An Ishihara chart for colour vision
- A visual field analyser assesses for potential loss of the visual field due to glaucoma, optic neuritis, etc. and aids in mapping progression of the condition

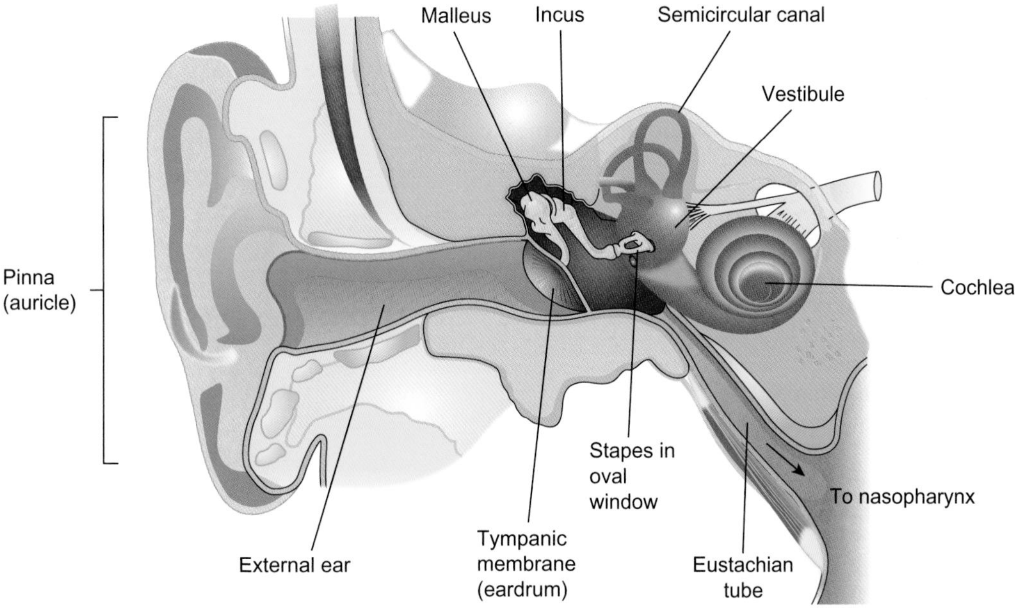

Figure 21.1 The ear. Reproduced from Nair, M. & Peate, I. (2009) Fundamentals *of Applied Pathophysiology*, with kind permission from Wiley Blackwell.

The ear

Anatomy and physiology

The functions of the ear relate to hearing and balance. The ear itself consists of three regions (Figure 21.1).

The **external ear** comprises the:

- cartilaginous pinna;
- external auditory canal;
- ceruminous glands;
- tympanic membrane.

The **middle ear** is in an air-filled space within the temporal bone. It is separated from the external ear by the tympanic membrane, and from the inner ear by bone. It is connected to the nasopharynx via the auditory tube, and contains three bones – the malleus, incus and stapes.

The **inner ear** contains a labyrinth canal structure comprising the outer bony labyrinth (containing perilymph) and the inner membranous labyrinth (which contains endolymph). It consists of three components:

- The vestibule.
- The cochlea. The organ of hearing (organ of Corti) is located in the cochlea and is innervated by the cochlear branch of vestibulocochlear nerve.
- The semicircular canals. The saccule, utricle and cristae located in the semicircular canals contain receptor cells involved in equilibrium and are innervated by the vestibular branch of the vestibulocochlear nerve.

Hearing impairment

Hearing impairment can be sensorineural (nerve), conductive (mechanical) or a mixture of both. Causes include:

- congenital, in which there is failure of the inner ear or nerves to develop properly as a result of intrauterine or perinatal damage;
- infection:
  - systemic, such as measles;
  - local, for example recurrent otitis media;
- disorders of the ear:
  - tinnitus;
  - Ménière's disease;
  - acoustic neuroma (see Chapter 17)
- ototoxic drugs:
  - aminoglycosides;
  - salicylates;
  - quinine;
  - loop diuretics;
  - platinum-based antineoplastic agents;
- foreign bodies;
- cerumen (earwax);
- trauma, for example to the ear, middle ear surgery or head injury;
- noise;
- presbycusis (ageing-related hearing loss).

The degree of impairment and loss, and whether it is transient or permanent, will have a bearing on management, treatment and patients' responses. Congenital or early childhood hearing loss adversely affects speech and language development. Not all individuals who are deaf consider this a disability as some consider it a cultural characteristic rather than a pathological condition (Lieu *et al*. 2007).

Hearing impairment and loss may, however, be problematic and can result in difficulty communicating. This is apparent if trying to communicate via telephone, as well as in situations where there is background noise or group conversation, or in noise-reverberant rooms. Individuals may experience social disengagement resulting in social isolation, loneliness, decreased self-esteem and depression. Individuals missing parts of a message can request its repetition, often leading to frustration and emotional distancing from the family (Preminger & Meeks 2010). There may also be safety issues, such as being unable to hear traffic.

Assessment

Assessment should take account of the following:

- A detailed history of the events leading to the hearing loss, including the medical history.
- Assessment of:
  - vital signs;
  - dizziness;
  - pain;
  - nausea;
  - vomiting, etc.
- Examination for:
  - discharge;
  - redness;
  - swelling;
  - cerumen (check for impaction).
- An assessment of hearing (see Box 21.3).
- Use of a hearing aid.

Nursing management

Nursing care is dependent on the type, cause, onset and duration of the hearing loss or impairment. Effective communication is paramount in caring for individuals with a hearing impairment (Box 21.5).

Box 21.5 Effective communication with individuals with impaired hearing

- Be aware of background noises within the healthcare environment
- Minimise background noises; for example, turn the radio or TV off when speaking with patients
- When talking to patients, face them at eye level (as this facilitates non-verbal communication by utilising facial cues)
- Speak clearly (but do not shout)
- Take time to communicate
- Do not exaggerate lip and mouth movements as this causes distortion and can adversely affect lip-reading
- Patients may be proficient in lip-reading, using sign language, writing, texting, etc. so these modes of communication need to be supported
- Check the patient's hearing is aid is working correctly

Nurses need to be aware that emotional support is required, especially if the hearing impairment has been newly diagnosed and will be permanent. Patients may require further support in the form of counselling to come to terms with the diagnosis and prognosis. Patient education includes:

- advice on prevention:
  - the use of earplugs at work;
  - reduction of exposure to excessive noise;
  - the management of cerumen;
  - the management of infections;
- information from relevant websites;
- home aids:
  - a flashing light for the door bell or phone;
  - adapters for the TV, radio or telephone;
  - hearing dogs;
  - pictographs (pictures of activities, common foods, etc.);
  - technology, such as computers and phone texting.

Ear trauma

Trauma to the ear can be caused by:

- the insertion of a foreign body (e.g. beads, toys or cotton wool buds) into the external auditory canal, which may result in a perforated tympanic membrane; this is usually seen in children;
- blunt trauma to the pinna, which may result in a subperichondrial haematoma.

The signs and symptoms include:

- with a foreign body, pain and discharge (indicative of a perforated tympanic membrane);
- blunt trauma:
  - redness;
  - tenderness;
  - swelling;
  - pain.
- with subperichondrial haematoma, the potential to lead to deformity (cauliflower ear) if untreated, because of cartilage necrosis due to a decreased blood supply.

Assessment will involve:

- a history;
- an examination of the ear's appearance, assessing for discharge, redness, swelling and any other abnormalities;
- pain.

Nursing management

Administer analgesia and antibiotics, as prescribed. Foreign objects will be removed by gentle irrigation (if they are non-expandable) or via a surgical procedure under general anaesthetic. A perforated tympanic membrane may heal without intervention or may require surgery, for example a myringoplasty. In trauma cases, lacerated ears require:

- aseptic cleaning;
- dressing;
- possibly suturing;
- application of an ice pack.

Otitis media

Otitis media is an infection of the middle ear. Patients diagnosed with serous otitis media may require a myringotomy and the insertion of grommet or tympanostomy tubes to facilitate drainage. Patients with chronic otitis media require antibiotic eardrops. Patients are educated on the condition and treatment, especially on the need to keep the ear dry if a perforation or tubes are present.

Ménière's disease

Ménière's disease is an imbalance in the production and absorption of endolymph within the inner labyrinth. The cause is unknown but it is thought to be associated with viral infections. The signs and symptoms are:

- vertigo;
- tinnitus;
- nausea and vomiting;
- sensorineural deafness;
- a feeling of fullness in the affected ear;
- bradycardia;
- sweating.

Assessment will involve a history and an assessment for dizziness, unsteadiness, nausea, vomiting and vital signs.

Nursing management

The patient's vital signs are monitored, especially for bradycardia. During an attack, assist patients to lie down and rest; they may vomit and will require assistance and oral hygiene. Intravenous therapy is necessary if patients become dehydrated and are unable to tolerate oral fluids. Symptoms are managed by a combination of medications, which includes:

- antiemetics;
- anticholinergic agents (to reduce autonomic nervous system activity);
- vasodilators and diuretics (which help to restore the fluid balance within the inner ear);
- sedatives.

Patients are educated on lifestyle, work, medication and diet (low salt with reduced caffeine and alcohol, and plenty of fluids). If surgery on the labyrinth (e.g. labyrinthectomy or decompression of fluid within the labyrinth) is indicated, patients will require perioperative care.

Box 21.6 Postoperative nursing management following ear surgery

- Assess the surgical site for discharge and bleeding
- Assess the patient's pain and administer analgesia as prescribed
- Monitor:
  - The patient's vital signs
  - Nausea and vomiting
  - Dizziness
- After mastoidectomy:
  - Patients should lie on the affected side with a pressure bandage *in situ*
  - There is danger of damage to the facial nerve with this procedure
  - Patients are asked to smile, shut their eyes tightly and wrinkle their noses (these being signs of intact nerve function)
- Discharge advice should cover:
  - Pain
  - Nausea
  - Dizziness
  - Removal of sutures (if any)
  - Swimming, showering and hair-washing, and how to prevent water entering the external auditory canal (after myringotomy and myringoplasty) by using cotton wool plugs

Ear surgery

Surgery on the ear includes:

- repair of a perforated tympanic membrane (myringoplasty);
- myringotomy – incision of the tympanic membrane, usually in both ears, allowing drainage of fluid; this can also include the insertion of ear tubes that are left in until they fall out or are removed by the physician;
- repair of the ossicles (ossiculoplasty):
- mastoidectomy;
- the excision of benign or malignant tumours.

Perioperative care

Patients requiring ear surgery may have the procedure undertaken as a day case or may require a short hospital stay. Postoperative nursing management is outlined in Box 21.6.

The nose

Anatomy and physiology

The nose has two components (Figure 21.2):

- The external component consists of bone, cartilage and two nostrils.
- The internal component comprises the nasal cavity (formed by the ethmoid, maxillae, lacrimal and palatine bones), the nasal septum and the paranasal sinuses.

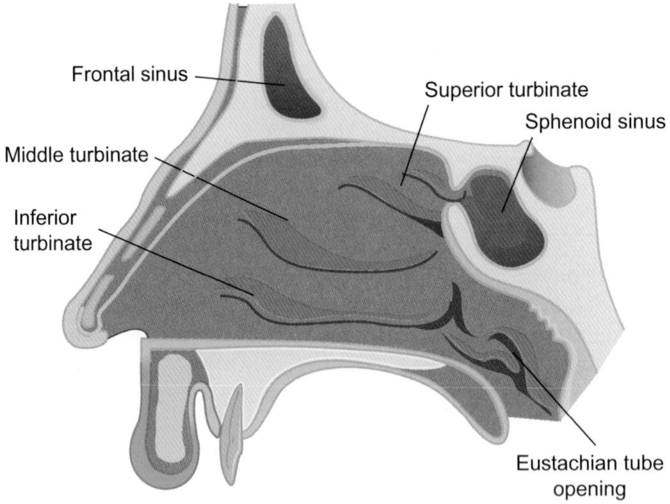

Figure 21.2 The nose. Reproduced from Nair, M. & Peate, I. (2009) *Fundamentals of Applied Pathophysiology*, with kind permission from Wiley Blackwell.

The nose, which leads to the pharynx, has four main functions:

- It facilitates the passage of air to and from the lungs.
- It warms, filters and moistens the incoming air.
- It is the sense organ for smell. The olfactory sense receptors are located on either side of the nasal septum in the superior part of the nasal cavity. These receptors are innervated by the olfactory nerve.
- The nasal cavity facilitates speech sounds.

Epistaxis

An epistaxis is a nose bleed, which usually occurs in Little's area in the nasal septum and ranges from mild to severe. Causes include:

- local:
  - idiopathic;
  - traumatic;
  - nasal septal perforation;
  - sinus tumours;
- general:
  - leukaemia;
  - thrombocytopenia;
  - anticoagulant therapy;
  - upper respiratory infection;
  - hereditary conditions (e.g. Osler–Weber–Rendu syndrome, haemorrhagic telangiectasia and haemophilia).

In epistaxis, blood flows from the nostrils or is passed back to the nasopharynx and is either swallowed or spat out. Severe bleeding may result in haemorrhage, hypotension, tachycardia or even hypovolaemic shock. Assessment involves:

- taking a history;
- examining the appearance of the nose, both external and internal, and assessing for swelling, bleeding, discharge, etc.;

- recording the vital signs;
- assessing the extent of the bleed.

Management

Advise patients to sit up with their head forward as this prevents swallowing of blood, which can cause nausea. Bleeding is controlled by applying pressure to the cartilaginous part of the nose, below the bridge; an ice pack can also be applied. For uncontrolled bleeding, and depending on the site of the bleeding, physicians insert either an anterior (Figure 21.3) or a posterior nasal pack. A nasal pack can be either gauze or an inflatable balloon, and as a result of its insertion patients will only be able to mouth-breathe. Nursing care following nasal pack insertion is outlined in Box 21.7. Further management includes:

- electrical or chemical cauterisation;
- arterial ligation surgery, for example septoplasty with ethmoidal ligation;
- radiological embolisation for patients with poor medical health.

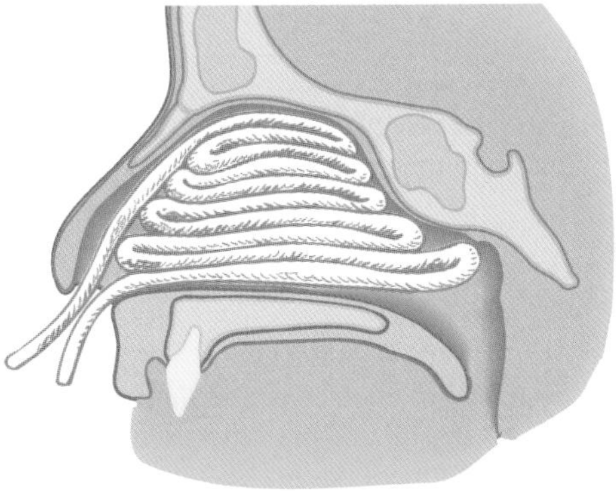

Figure 21.3 Anterior nasal packing. Reproduced from Bull, P.D. & Clarke, R. (2007) *Lecture Notes: Diseases of the Ear, Nose and Throat*, 10th Edition, with kind permission of Wiley Blackwell.

Box 21.7 Nursing care of patients following nasal pack insertion

- Reassure patients as they may fear suffocation
- A sedative may be required to relieve anxiety; administer this as prescribed
- Monitor for signs of hypoxia and airway occlusion:
  - Vital signs
  - Oxygen saturations
  - The position of the pack
- Nurse in a semi-Fowler's position
- Promote the patient's comfort by providing:
  - Oral hygiene
  - Eye care – as the pack may occlude the nasolacrimal duct, leading to tears
- Nutritional intake:
  - Provide cool fluids – hot fluids may cause local blood vessel dilatation and increase bleeding
  - A soft or liquid diet is recommended
- Antibiotics may be required as there is a risk of infection

Chronic sinusitis

Sinusitis is a sinus infection caused by a blockage, which prevents drainage. The blockage may be caused by a common cold, upper tooth root infection, poorly developed maxillary sinuses in some children or obstruction by muscosal oedema. Chronic sinusitis lasts longer than acute sinusitis despite frequent treatment attempts.

Patients initially present with symptoms similar to those of acute sinusitis but may experience headache and upper jaw toothache . They may also develop otitis media, chronic laryngitis, a postnasal drip and recurrent sore throats. The complications include:

- orbital cellulitis;
- orbital abscesses;
- blindness;
- cavernous sinus thrombosis;
- bacteraemia, septicaemia and osteomyelitis;
- a frontal lobe abscess.

Assessment involves:

- a history;
- vital signs;
- the level of pain;
- a nasal swab for culture and sensitivity;
- computed tomography (CT) and magnetic resonance imaging (MRI) scans and X-rays.

Management

The initial management is similar to that of acute sinusitis; however, unresolved nasal infection (determined by CT scanning) and orbital cellulitis that is unresponsive to antibiotic treatment may indicate a need for surgery such as functional endoscopic sinus surgery. This involves removing the damaged mucosal tissue and enlarging the nasal openings, which enhances drainage. Preoperative and postoperative nursing management includes:

- patient education;
- preparation for X-ray, CT or MRI scanning;
- nasal swabs for culture and sensitivity;
- perioperative care involving:
  - care of the nasal pack (Box 21.7);
  - monitoring for complications associated with the surgery, for example bleeding, haematoma or visual problems.

Deviated nasal septum

A deviated nasal septum can result from developmental problems of the septum and also from trauma. The condition may be asymptomatic, but signs and symptoms can be:

- unilateral nasal obstruction of varying degrees;
- sinus infection or otitis media;
- hypertrophy of the unaffected side of the nose.

Assessment involves taking the patient's history and examining the appearance of the nose.

Management

The main surgical procedures are:

- submucosal resection;
- septoplasty (straightening of the nasal septum).

Nursing management entails perioperative care, patient education and care of the nasal pack.

Nasal injuries

Nasal fractures and lacerations may be caused by trauma, while nasal airway obstruction may be caused by the insertion of a foreign body (e.g. paper, toys, beads, food) into the nasal cavity, which is most often seen in children. The signs and symptoms may encompass:

- fractures:
  - pain;
  - external deformity;
- septal haematoma;
  - septal deviation;
  - cerebrospinal fluid (CSF) rhinorrhoea (thin watery fluid escaping from the nose, in this instance CSF) if there is ethmoid involvement;
- laceration:
  - pain;
  - bleeding;
  - soreness;
- obstruction by a foreign body:
  - unilateral rhinorrhoea (a nasal cavity filled with significant amount of mucous fluid, commonly referred to as a runny nose), which may be bloodstained and is usually foul-smelling.

The assessment needs to take into account:

- the patient's history;
- an examination of the nose's appearance and a check of the airway;
- an X-ray to show any nasal fracture;
- the level of pain.

Management

For fractures:

- Administer the prescribed analgesia.
- Manage epistaxis; if the nose is badly damaged, there is a high risk of bleeding.
- Reduce oedema by applying an ice pack.
- Monitor the vital signs for complications, for example if there is a related head injury (see Chapter 17).
- Fractures may require manipulation. This is a day surgery procedure that is typically undertaken approximately 14 days after the injury to allow reduction of oedema. Perioperative care is needed.

With lacerations:

- Administer the prescribed analgesia.
- Staunch the bleeding with pressure. This may require steristrips or suturing using Prolene sutures (size 5-0), which remain *in situ* for 5 days.
- Clean and dress the laceration.
- Monitor the vital signs.
- A tetanus immunisation booster injection may be required.
- Further injury such as a nasal fracture needs to be ruled out, so an X-ray may be required.

If there is a foreign body:

- there may be some bleeding, which should be anticipated and managed;
- surgery is not usually required, although there may be some exceptions depending on the location of the foreign body and the length of time it has been *in situ*.

Nasal tumours (benign and malignant)

Tumours include:

- juvenile nasopharyngeal angiofibromas;
- inverting papillomas;
- malignant tumours of the paranasal sinus cavities.

The primary causes of nasal and sinus cancers are chemicals and carcinogenic substances such as those used in the furniture, textiles, shoe, paint and chemical industries. The signs and symptoms comprise:

- epistaxis;
- nasal obstruction;
- a polypoid mass in the nose.

Assessment involves:

- the patient's history;
- a CT scan to determine whether there is a mass, bony destruction or erosion;
- angiography to identify problems with the blood supply;
- nasal endoscopy;
- biopsy;
- a preoperative assessment.

Management

Surgical treatment includes:

- tumour embolisation (for a juvenile angiofibroma);
- excision of the tumour, which requires rhinotomy, subtotal maxillectomy or total maxillectomy;
- possibly also radiotherapy and chemotherapy.

Nursing management for nasal tumour surgery is outlined in Box 21.8.

The throat (pharynx)

Anatomy and physiology

The pharynx is a passageway for food and air and a resonating chamber for speech sounds. It extends from the nose to the cricoid cartilage and can be divided into three anatomical regions:

- The **nasopharynx**. This lies behind the nasal cavity and has openings to the auditory tubes and the internal nares. The adenoids are located in its posterior wall.
- The **oropharynx**. This forms the middle part of the pharynx and lies behind the oral cavity. It extends from below the soft palate to the level of the hyoid bone, and houses two pairs of tonsils (palatine and lingual).
- The **hypopharynx**. This forms the lower part of the pharynx, beginning at the level of the hyoid bone and at its lower portion continuing anteriorly into the larynx and posteriorly into the oesophagus (Figure 21.4).

Box 21.8 Nursing management of patients after removal of nasal/ sinus tumours

- Monitor the vital signs, especially for pyrexia
- Pain:
  - Assess for pain
  - Administer the prescribed analgesia
- Provide emotional support:
  - Patients may experience anxiety due to the diagnosis and altered body image (facial incision, sinus removal or facial disfigurement)
  - Introduce patients to individuals who have had similar surgery
  - Refer them to a counsellor, if needed
- Wound care:
  - Assess for crusting of the sinus and/or nasal cavity
  - Inspect the incision site
  - Monitor wound drainage – the amount, colour and presence of mucus
  - Monitor for signs of CSF leakage
- Assess for sensory and/or motor deficits:
  - Check for decreased vision, diplopia, epiphora (excessive tear production), trismus (jaw clenching) and facial paraesthesia or pain
- Assessment (especially of the palate) by a speech and language therapist is needed to determine:
  - The presence of speech difficulties
  - The need for a liquid or soft diet
- Patient education includes the following:
  - Patients should not blow their nose for 10 days postoperatively; instead, they should sniff the secretions in and either swallow or expectorate them
  - Humidification should be increased with a bedside humidifier, steam or nasal saline spray
  - Speech therapy may be needed
  - Depending on the type of surgery, patients may need to be informed how to remove, clean and reinsert the palate obturator, and how to camouflage defects with an eye patch or make-up

The larynx connects the pharynx with the trachea. The epiglottis covers the glottis during swallowing, preventing food and fluid entering the trachea. The larynx, through the vibration of its vocal cords and in conjunction with the pharynx, mouth, nasal cavity and paranasal sinuses, is responsible for voice production.

Laryngeal obstruction

Laryngeal obstruction is narrowing or closure of the airway due to oedema or blockage of the airway. It is an emergency life-threatening event and must be resolved immediately. Causes include:

- acute laryngitis;
- epiglottitis;
- an anaphylactic reaction;
- oedema following endotracheal intubation;
- laryngeal spasm;
- urticaria;
- inflammatory disease of the throat.

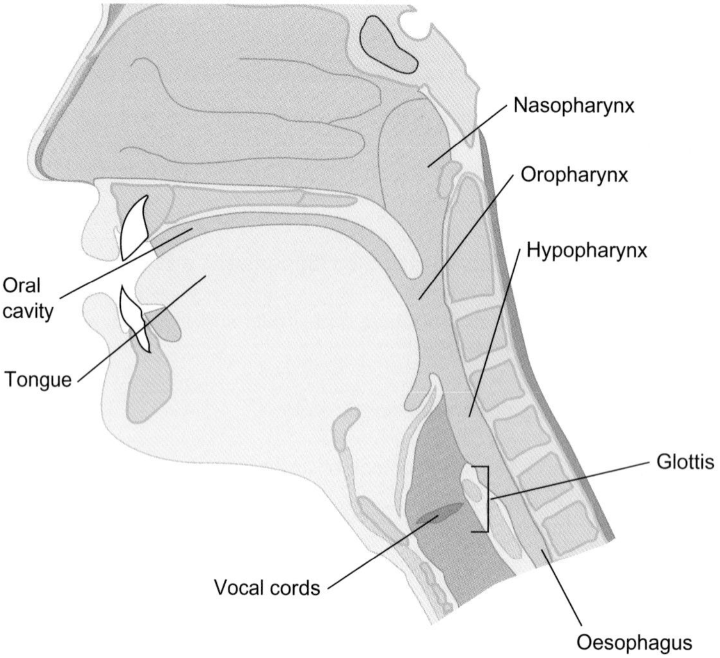

Figure 21.4 The throat. Reproduced from Nair, M. & Peate, I. (2009) *Fundamentals of Applied Pathophysiology*, with kind permission from Wiley Blackwell.

Signs and symptoms include:

- stridor;
- drooling;
- decreased breath sounds;
- cyanosis and cessation of breathing if the patient is not treated and managed immediately.

Assessment should involve inspecting the patient's ability to breath, identifying respiratory difficulties such as nasal flaring, the use of accessory muscles, cyanosis, decreased or absent breath sounds and movement of the chest, with resultant loss of consciousness.

Management

This is an emergency situation. Patients require oxygen and the administration of intravenous corticosteroids and adrenaline; they may also need endotracheal intubation and/or tracheostomy.

Throat tumours

Throat (pharyngeal) tumours can occur in the oropharynx, nasopharynx or hypopharynx and can be benign or malignant. Tumours are staged according to the TNM (tumour, node and metastasis) system. Primary causes of throat cancer are smoking, alcohol, carcinogens, nutrition and riboflavin deficiency. Signs and symptoms include:

- a painless mass;
- enlarged cervical nodes;
- hoarseness;
- pain on swallowing (odynophagia);
- referred pain (e.g. otalgia);

- dysphagia;
- weight loss.

Assessment needs to consider:

- the patient's history;
- an examination, for example for airway obstruction and weight loss;
- the swallow and gag reflex;
- the level of pain;
- the results of investigations:
  - laryngoscopy;
  - chest X-ray;
  - barium swallow;
  - endoscopy;
  - CT and MRI scans.

Management

Treatment includes:

- tumour resection;
- reconstruction (if radical neck dissection is undertaken for metastases);
- concurrent radiotherapy and chemotherapy.

The nursing management is outlined in Box 21.9.

Tonsillectomy

Tonsillectomy involves the removal of both tonsils and is indicated by tonsillar hypertrophy (causing speech and swallowing difficulties) and/or recurrent tonsillitis. It is a planned elective procedure, and patients should be asymptomatic at the time of surgery. Assessment and investigations should cover:

- the patient's history;
- an examination of the appearance of the throat for redness, inflammation and exudate;
- the vital signs, ruling out current infection.

Management

Preoperative care includes assessment and patient education related to the surgery. Box 21.10 outlines the postoperative care of patients following tonsillectomy.

Tracheostomy

A tracheostomy, which is the formation of a stoma within the trachea, is created to:

- maintain a patent airway;
- provide ventilatory assistance;
- protect the patient's airway;
- facilitate pulmonary suctioning.

A tracheostomy may be temporary (Figure 21.5) or permanent, and may be open (surgical), percutaneous or a cricothyroidotomy. A permanent tracheostomy is normally performed in conjunction with a total laryngectomy (Figure 21.6). The relevant nursing management is outlined in Box 21.11.

Box 21.9 Nursing management of patients after removal of throat tumours

- Monitor the vital signs, observing for postoperative haemorrhage
- Monitor for signs of respiratory distress:
  - Skin colour
  - Respiration rate, depth and pattern, and use of accessory muscles
  - Oxygen saturation levels
  - Level of consciousness
- Undertake tracheostomy care (the tracheostomy may be temporary or permanent)
- Administer prescribed oxygen therapy
- Pain:
  - Assess pain level
  - Administer prescribed analgesia
- Nutrition:
  - Intravenous fluids
  - Nasogastric feeding for 10 days, with assessment (including the gag reflex) by a speech and language therapist to determine when it is safe to commence an oral diet
- For wound management, assess and monitor:
  - The incision site
  - Skin integrity
  - Wound healing
  - Wound drains
  - Care of the skin flap
- Provide emotional support, especially in view of the diagnosis and possible altered body image
- Educate patients on treatment and self-care, including monitoring for signs of infection, and provide details on diet and nutrition

Laryngectomy

A laryngectomy involves the removal of all or part of the larynx, usually for laryngeal cancer. Risk factors for cancer include:

- heavy smoking;
- heavy alcohol consumption;
- family predisposition;
- chronic laryngitis;
- vocal abuse.

Laryngeal cancer affects more men than women and metastatic spread is common. The signs and symptoms include persistent hoarseness, otalgia and dysphagia. Signs of metastases include:

- a lump in the throat;
- otalgia;
- dysphagia;
- dyspnoea;
- a cough;
- enlarged lymph nodes.

Box 21.10 Nursing management of patients after tonsillectomy

- Place patients in the recovery position, and change this to the semi-Fowler's position when they regain consciousness
- Pain:
  - Assess the level of pain
  - Administer prescribed analgesia such as paracetamol (with or without codeine) or diclofenac
  - Encourage cold fluids and chewing gum (Scottish Intercollegiate Guidelines Network 2010) as increased swallowing decreases muscle spasms and therefore reduces pain
- Assess hydration:
  - Vital signs
  - Skin turgor
  - Fluid intake and output
- Administer prescribed intravenous fluids until there is an adequate oral intake
- An antiemetic may be prescribed
- Assess for signs of bleeding:
  - Restlessness
  - Excessive swallowing
  - Pallor
  - Vital signs – check for hypotension and tachycardia
  - Spitting up and aspiration of fresh blood, which is indicative of bleeding
- Reactionary bleeding:
  - Occurs with 24 hours of surgery
  - Is due to a ligature slipping or blood vessels opening spontaneously
  - May require surgery for resuturing
- Secondary haemorrhage:
  - Occurs within 5–10 days
  - Is due to infection or the separation of granulation tissue
  - The bleeding is less brisk than reactive bleeding
  - Admit to hospital for observation, antibiotic therapy, hydration, blood profiling and local clot debridement with hydrogen peroxide gargles or resuturing
- Discharge education includes:
  - Information on analgesia
  - Avoidance of strenuous exercise for a week or two
  - Drinking 2–3 L of fluid daily
  - Monitoring for complications such as dysphagia, secondary haemorrhage and infection and reporting these to the GP

Assessment involves:

- the patient's history;
- recording the vital signs;
- a laryngoscopy;
- a biopsy, chest X-ray and CT scan to determine metastases to the lung, lymph glands or surrounding tissue;
- a barium swallow to eliminate oesophageal cancer.

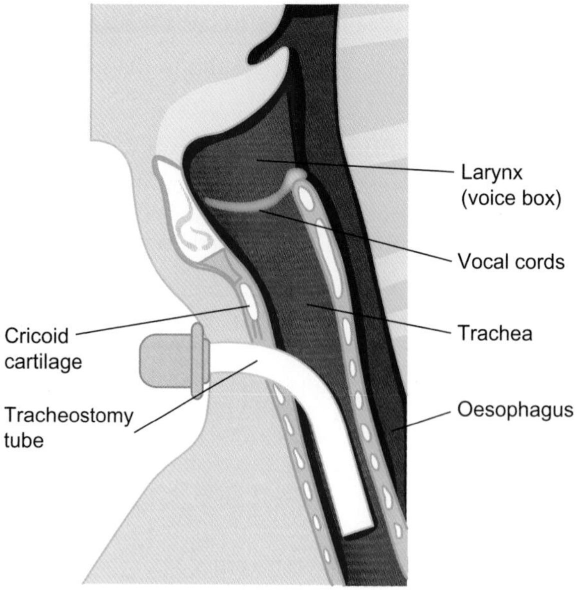

Figure 21.5 Temporary tracheostomy. Reproduced from Nair, M. & Peate, I. (2009) *Fundamentals of Applied Pathophysiology*, with kind permission from Wiley Blackwell.

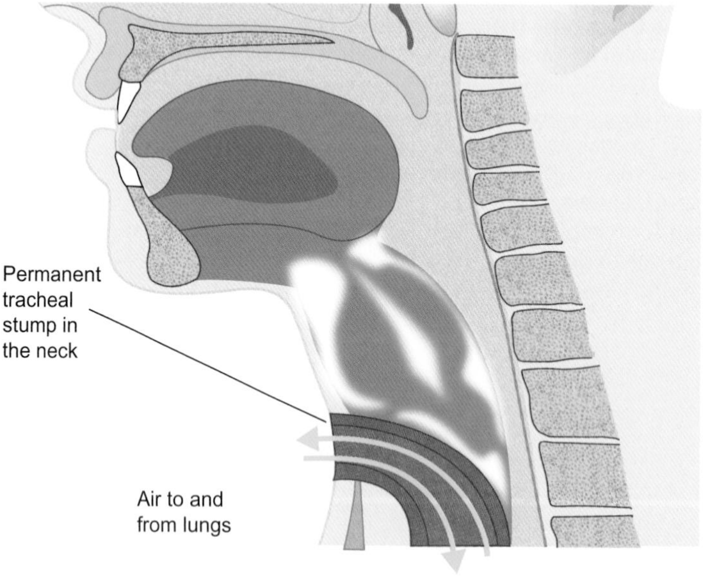

Figure 21.6 Laryngectomy. Reproduced from Nair, M. & Peate, I. (2009) *Fundamentals of Applied Pathophysiology*, with kind permission from Wiley Blackwell.

Box 21.11 Nursing management of patients with tracheostomy

- Nurse in a semi-Fowler's position as this:
  - Reduces oedema
  - Facilitates chest expansion
- Maintain a patent airway:
  - The stoma is maintained by the tracheostomy tube
  - Cuffed tubes are used in the immediate postoperative phase. A seal (via the cuff) is maintained between the tube and tracheal wall; this prevents the aspiration of food and fluid and facilitates optimal ventilation
  - Traction sutures are inserted to keep the stoma open in case of decannulation
- Monitor the cuff pressure to:
  - Ensure the seal
  - Prevent tracheal wall damage, which can occur if the pressure is too high
- A fenestrated tube may be inserted after 5–6 days to facilitate speech
- Ensure humidification:
  - Through nebulisers, heated humidifiers and exchange filters
  - This moistens the inhaled air and prevents crusting of secretions
- Suction:
  - Carry out as needed
  - The recommended suction time is less than 15 seconds with preoxygenation for 3 minutes, if the patient is oxygen-dependent
- An emergency tracheostomy pack is kept at the patient's bedside (Box 21.12)
- In the case of a respiratory or cardiac arrest, proceed to the emergency cardiac arrest technique
- If the tube is occluded:
  - Change the inner tube
  - Administer oxygen and suction
  - Should the occlusion remain, the tracheostomy tube needs to be changed
- Accidental decannulation:
  - A replacement tube is inserted or the stoma is kept open with tracheal dilators until specialised personnel arrive
  - Alleviate patient anxiety and fears during this time
- Tracheostomy care:
  - Maintain skin integrity at the stoma site by:
    - — cleaning the site, the tube and under the neck plate of the tube
    - — removing drainage and crusts
    - — using Velcro ties and Lyofoam dressings to avoid excoriation of the skin
    - — having two nurses involved to avoid accidental dislodgement of the tube, one to hold the tube and the second to undertake the dressing
- Monitor the vital signs and appearance for:
  - Bleeding
  - Airway obstruction
- Pain:
  - Monitor the vital signs
  - Assess the pain level
  - Administer prescribed analgesia
  - Maintain the patient's comfort

(*Continued*)

- Nutrition:
  - Administer intravenous fluid
  - Patients should be assessed on an individual basis for their ability to tolerate oral food and the appropriateness of inflating or deflating the tracheostomy tube cuff while eating
  - Impaired ability to swallow can cause food aspiration so there may be a need to:
    - — change to a thicker consistency of food
    - — commence nasogastric tube feeding
- The ability to speak is impaired. Alternative and augmentative methods of communication include:
  - Flashcards
  - A picture communication board
  - A 'magic slate'
  - Electronic devices
  - Writing
  - Gestures
  - Facial expressions
  - Therapeutic touch
- If the tracheostomy is present for an extended time period, speaking valves can be used:
  - A closed-position speaking valve (e.g. a Passy–Muir valve)
  - An open-position speaking valve (e.g. a Rusch valve)
  - Patients may be able to plug the tube with their finger and by breathing through their mouth and nose vibrate the vocal fold, which leads to speech
- The tracheostomy may adversely affect patients' body image so there is a need to provide emotional support
- Weaning patients off a tracheostomy incorporates four stages:
  - Cuff deflation
  - Downsizing of the tracheostomy tube
  - Tolerance of the speaking valve
  - The use of a decannulation cap

Box 21.12 Emergency tracheostomy tray

- Tracheal dilators
- Artery forceps
- A 10 mL syringe to remove air from the cuff
- Two cuffed tracheostomy tubes (one the same size as the patient already has in and the other a smaller size)
- Suction equipment
- A tracheostomy mask
- A suture cutter
- Neck ties

Box 21.13 Nursing management of patients following laryngectomy

Specific preoperative care

- Educate patients on:
  - The type and extent of the laryngectomy (partial or total)
  - The possibility of neck dissection and reconstructive surgery
- Provide emotional support to patients and their families
- Refer patients to the speech and language therapist
- Provide patients with information on support groups

Specific postoperative care

- Maintain a patent airway and effective airway clearance (see Box 21.11)
- Undertake tracheostomy care (see Box 21.11)
- Monitor for haemorrhage:
  - The wound
  - The drain
  - The vital signs
  - The patient's appearance
- Monitor the patient's pain:
  - Assess the pain level
  - Administer the prescribed analgesia
  - Provide comfort measures
- Monitor the wound:
  - Drains are removed when drainage has fallen to below 20 mL
  - Maintain skin integrity related to surgical incisions
  - Monitor for signs of infection
  - Monitor for the development of a pharyngocutaneous fistula
- Provide emotional support to patients in relation to the altered body image and anxieties associated with a diagnosis of cancer
- Provide additional support by introducing patients and their families to individuals who have had a laryngectomy and who are willing to provide advice and recount their personal experiences
- Care of patients:
  - Who are on chemotherapy and/or radiotherapy
  - Who have altered communication; e.g. with a total laryngectomy, patients will experience an initial lack of voice and later the creation of a new 'voice' through the use of oesophageal speech, special valves such as the Blom–Singer valve or the use of an electronic artificial larynx
- Patients may require radical neck dissection for metastases, which requires reconstructive surgery
- Patients are advised to wear a medical alert bracelet recording that they have a permanent tracheostomy

Management

The nursing management is outlined in Box 21.13.

The eye

Anatomy and physiology

The function of the eye is to achieve sight, and the eye contains the following structures:

- **Extraocular structures**:
  - An eyelid
  - A lacrimal system

- An orbit
- Extraocular muscles
- An optic nerve
- **Intraocular structures** (Figure 21.7):
  - The sclera
  - The cornea
  - The iris
  - The pupil
  - The lens
  - The retina
  - The vitreous humour.

Light is reflected by an object into the eye and passes through the lens. The lens then projects an inverted image of the object on to the retina at the back of the eye by accommodation (which focuses the image). The light rays are refracted (bent) as they pass through the cornea, aqueous humour, lens and vitreous humour, converging at a point in the retina.

The signals produced by the rod and cone cells in the retina travel to the brain via the optic nerve. The two optic nerves meet at the optic chiasma where axons from the nasal side of each retina cross to the opposite side and join axons from the temporal side of the retina of the other eye. These pairs continue as the left and right optic tracts. The crossing of the axons results in each optic tract carrying information from both eyes. The nerves continue to the thalamus, where projections extend to the visual areas in the occipital lobe of the cerebral cortex (Figure 21.8). The brain interprets the image so that the person perceives it as it occurs.

Visual impairment

Visual impairment can vary from mild to extreme, can be immediate or progressive and depends on the cause. It is broadly divided into sudden loss (trauma, retinal detachment, vitreous haemorrhage, acute angle closure glaucoma and retinal vein/artery occlusion) and gradual loss (cataracts, chronic angle closure glaucoma, age-related macular degeneration [AMD] and diabetic retinopathy).

Regardless of the degree of change, this can be a frightening and anxious time for patients, and their ability to cope depends largely on their experience of the staff they encounter. Nurses need to be aware of patients' specific concerns, fears and anxieties, and should discuss with them the level of assistance required and provide emotional support particularly for newly diagnosed patients. It is essential that visually impaired patients are treated with respect and their individual autonomy is acknowledged.

The National Council for the Blind (2012) recommends the following:

- Orientate patients to the ward environment (the position of the bed, toilet facilities, TV, call bell, etc.).
- Describe the activities going on around patients.
- Introduce yourself as you enter the room and inform patients when you are leaving.
- Identify potential hazards.
- Replace items in same place.
- Explain loud noises to avoid unnecessary worry and concern.
- Describe the position of food on the plate in terms of a clock face (potato at 3 p.m., etc.).
- Enable patients to hold your arm when assisting them with walking. Do not hold their arm. Describe the environment (e.g. 'There are two steps ahead').
- Ask patients if they require assistance.

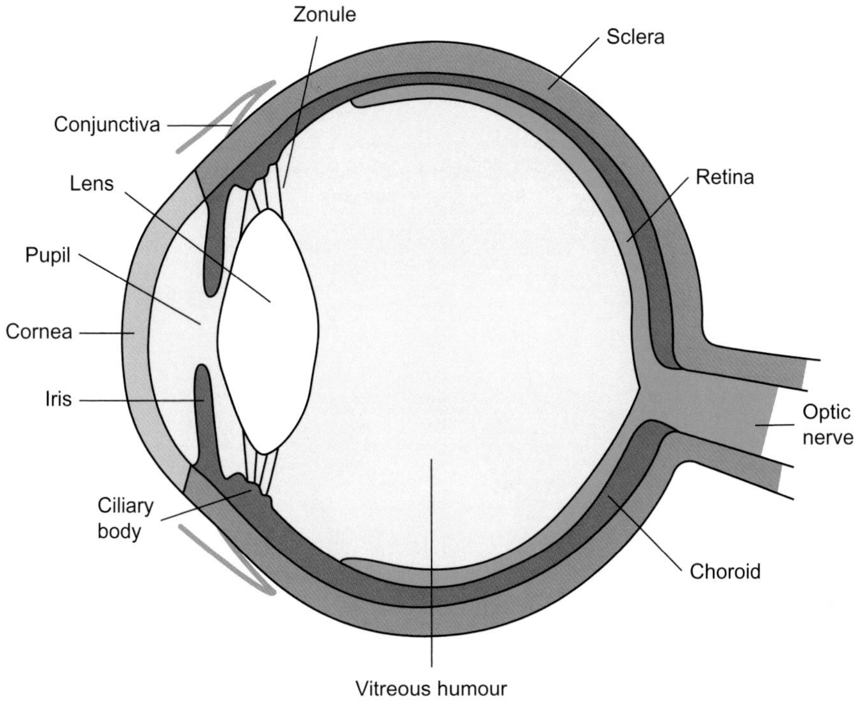

Figure 21.7 The eye. Reproduced from Nair, M. & Peate, I. (2009) *Fundamentals of Applied Pathophysiology*, with kind permission from Wiley Blackwell.

Glaucoma

Glaucoma is defined as optic nerve disease with changes on the optic disc and defects in the visual field associated with raised intraocular pressure (National Institute for Health and Clinical Excellence 2009). Glaucoma is broadly divided into acute and chronic forms.

Primary acute angle closure glaucoma

Primary acute angle closure glaucoma is an ocular emergency and involves the interruption of aqueous flow as a result of lens enlargement or a shallow anterior chamber. This leads to angle narrowing and prolonged raised intraocular pressure, resulting in unilateral ischemic optic nerve damage. The signs and symptoms are:

- severe pain;
- redness;
- blurring of vision;
- nausea;
- vomiting;
- a general feeling of being unwell.

Assessment will involve:

- the patient's history;
- tests:
  - tonometry;
  - fundoscopy;

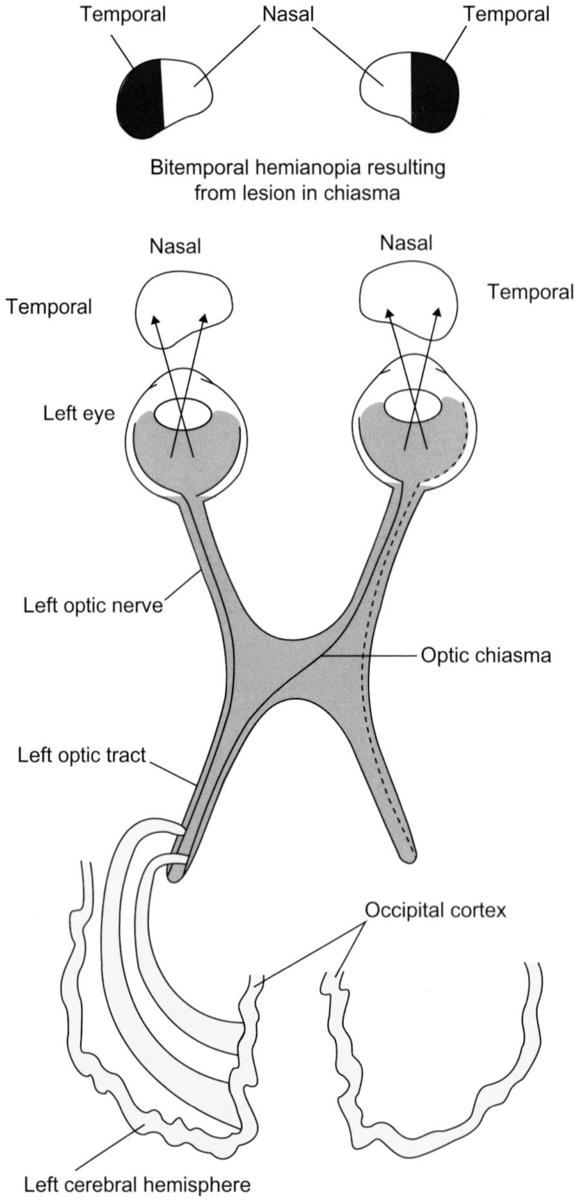

Figure 21.8 Visual pathways and visual fields. Reproduced from Dougherty & Lister, 2011, with kind permission of Wiley Blackwell.

  - gonioscopy;
  - visual field testing;
- the level of pain.

Management

The aim of medical management is to reduce intraocular pressure, thus limiting ischemic damage. Interventions include:

- the immediate administration of intravenous acetazolamide;
- an antiemetic;
- topical pilocarpine;
- anti-inflammatory eyedrops.

Nursing management includes the following:

- Ensure the patient's comfort.
- Monitor the intraocular pressure.
- Monitor the response to treatment.
- Alert medical staff if symptoms persist.

A peripheral iridotomy using YAG (yttrium–aluminium–garnet) laser therapy may be required once the inflammation has subsided; this creates an alternative drainage channel for the aqueous flow. It may also be performed prophylactically on the non-affected eye.

Chronic open angle glaucoma

This is a progressive disease with degeneration within the trabecular meshwork and is a leading cause of blindness. The signs and symptoms include:

- vague symptoms with peripheral visual loss;
- mild headaches;
- difficulty focusing on near objects;
- a lack of symptoms until the disease is advanced.

Management

The aim is to preserve vision and prevent deterioration. This requires life-long monitoring and treatment adherence (using prescribed eyedrops).

Diabetic retinopathy

This is a complication of diabetes that results from retinal blood vessel deterioration whereby the vessels leak and can damage or scar the retina. This leads to blurred vision or blindness if left untreated. It is preventable through early detection and treatment. Patients are referred to the diabetic eye clinic for:

- initial assessment of visual acuity;
- fluorescein angiography;
- regular follow-up.

Management

Following angiography:

- monitor for side effects of angiography; for example, the patient's skin will have a yellowish tinge for 24 hours and the urine will be bright green for 48 hours);
- educate patients on diabetic care and reporting visual changes.

Corneal disorders (corneal ulceration, keratitis and corneal exposure)

Disruption to corneal structure may result in:

- pain;
- the sensation of a foreign body;
- blurred or reduced vision;

- photophobia;
- watering of the eye;
- corneal scarring or perforation after long-term damage.

Causes include:

- bacterial infections, which may cause abrasion;
- contact lens issues:
  - poor hand hygiene;
  - leaving lenses in too long;
  - inadequate care of lenses;
- chronic blepharitis (dry eyes).

Assessment involves:

- the patient's history;
- the level of pain;
- a fluorescein stain;
- corneal swabs or scrapings to establish the causative factor.

Management

The treatment is dependent on the cause:

- Patients are cared for by an identified nurse and admitted to a single room to minimise the transmission of causative organism and ensure continuity of care.
- Antibiotic eye drops are administered every half hour for at least the first 24 hours.
- Oral or intravenous antibiotics may be prescribed.
- Ocular changes are noted and reported to the doctor.
- Analgesia is administered as required.
- Discharge education includes instillation of eyedrops and advice about wearing dark glasses, which helps to reduce glare and photophobia.

Eye trauma

The most common causes of eye trauma are:

- foreign bodies;
- abrasions;
- lacerations.

Other causes include:

- burns:
  - heat;
  - radiation;
  - explosions (which cause thermal burns);
  - chemical burns (acid or alkaline), which are the most common; it is important to identify the causative substance to ensure the correct treatment;
- penetrating objects:
  - metal flakes or particles produced by hammering or drilling;
  - glass shards;
  - gunshots and knives.
- blunt trauma to the eye caused during contact sports (football or boxing) or car accidents.

The signs and symptoms will be of:

- pain;
- partial or complete loss of vision;

- bleeding;
- extrusion of the eye contents.

Assessment involves the following:

- Examine the eye and surrounding areas.
- Assess the patient's sight.
- Undertake tests, including:
  - ophthalmoscopy;
  - ultrasonography;
  - fluorescein staining;
  - X-ray and CT scanning.
- Assess the pain level.

Management

Where possible, foreign bodies are removed using irrigation, a sterile cotton-tipped applicator or a sterile needle. Antibiotic ointment is applied after removal. Patients may have an eye patch applied after the antibiotic in order to keep the eye closed for approximately 24 hours.

Chemical burns are flushed with copious amounts of normal saline. Topical anaesthetic, applied initially, relieves the pain, making inspection and irrigation easier. During irrigation, the fluid is directed from the inner canthus of the eye to the outer canthus. The patient's head should be slightly tilted to the affected side to prevent contamination of the unaffected eye. Irrigation is continued until the pH of the eye is normal (use pH paper to test this and ensure the range is 7.2–7.4). A topical antibiotic ointment is applied following irrigation.

Penetrating wounds require surgery with immediate care focusing on relieving the patient's pain and protecting the eye from further injury. To prevent loss of the intraocular contents, do not place pressure on the eye itself; instead, gently cover it with sterile gauze or an eye pad. If a foreign body is embedded in the eye or sticking out, make no attempt to remove it. The object is immobilised and the eye protected until the patient can be seen by an ophthalmologist. Patients may require analgesia, sedation, an antiemetic and prophylactic intravenous antibiotics.

Blunt trauma may result in hyphaema (blood in the anterior chamber of the eye). Care of this includes bed rest and monitoring of intraocular pressure.

Age-related macular degeneration

There are two types of AMD that affect the macula. Dry AMD is the most common, developing slowly and leading to central loss of vision (Watkinson 2010). Wet AMD (which is less common) is caused by leaking blood vessels within the eye. The cause of AMD is unknown. The signs and symptoms include:

- lack of pain;
- blurring and distortion of vision;
- an inability to distinguish colour.

Assessment covers:

- a history;
- a test of visual acuity;
- a fundal examination by ophthalmologist.

Management

Patients and their families require education on living with visual impairment. There is no treatment available for dry AMD, but treatments for wet AMD include intravitreal injection (on an outpatient basis), photodynamic therapy and laser photocoagulation.

Surgery

Cataract

A cataract is a decrease in opacity (clouding) of the lens leading to interference with light transmission to the retina and decreased ability to perceive images clearly. Causes include:

- advancing age;
- congenital factors;
- eye trauma;
- inflammation;
- diabetes mellitus;
- medications (corticosteroids and chlorpromazine).

The signs and symptoms are:

- a variable density of the cataract;
- decreased visual acuity;
- difficulty adjusting between light and dark environments;
- a condition that may be bilateral unless it is related to eye trauma;
- sensitivity to glare;
- an inability to distinguish colour hues;
- pupil(s) that appear cloudy grey or white.

Assessment will take into account the patient's history and involve an examination with a Snellen test and slit lamp.

Management

Phacoemulsification is the most common surgical procedure and typically requires day surgery with local anaesthesia; however, some cases require general anaesthesia. Complications include:

- loss of vitreous humour;
- corneal oedema;
- increased intraocular pressure;
- haemorrhage;
- inflammation or infection;
- retinal detachment;
- displacement of the implanted lens.

Discharge education for patients and families is outlined in Box 21.14.

Box 21.14 Discharge education: Cataract care

- Medications and side effects
- Instillation of eye drops
- Ocular hygiene
- Follow-up appointments
- Not rubbing the operated eye
- Being alert for postoperative complications: pain, decreased visual acuity, headache, nausea and vomiting
- Avoidance of swimming and driving until advised otherwise
- Wearing an eye shield at night as advised

Retinal detachment

Retinal detachment is a medical emergency and involves retinal separation from the choroid. It may be precipitated by trauma but usually occurs spontaneously. The signs and symptoms are:

- floaters – irregular dark lines or spots in the visual field;
- flashing lights;
- blurred vision with progressive deterioration;
- a possible experience of a sensation of a curtain falling across the field of vision;
- if the macula is involved, a loss of central vision.

Assessment involves determining the extent and location of the detachment.

Management

Management focuses on early identification and treatment. Patients are admitted for bed rest, peri-operative care and surgery. Surgery may include:

- 'scleral buckling', which reattaches the retina);
- vitrectomy – replacement of the vitreous gel with gas, air or silicone oil, which restores normal pressure.

Discharge care is similar to that for other eye surgery.

Conclusion

Patients with ENT and eye conditions are cared for in a variety of healthcare settings, which means that nurses must have the necessary knowledge and skills in order to meet the different needs of this varied patient population. This chapter has provided an overview of the more common ENT and eye conditions encountered in everyday nursing practice.

Visit www.wileyfundamentalseries.com/medicalnursing and read Reflective Questions 21.1 and 21.2 to think more about this topic.

Now visit the companion website and test yourself on this chapter:
www.wileyfundamentalseries.com/medicalnursing

References

Lieu, C.C., Sadler, G.R., Fullerton, J.T. *et al*. (2007) Communication strategies for nurses interacting with patients who are deaf. *Dermatology Nursing*, **19**(6):541–51.

National Council for the Blind (2012) *Assisting Adults with Sight Loss in Hospital*. Retrieved 13th January 2012 from http://www.ncbi.ie/information-for/health-professionals/assisting-adults-with-sight-loss-in-hospital.

National Institute for Health and Clinical Excellence (2009) *Glaucoma: Diagnosis and Management of Chronic Open Angle Glaucoma and Ocular Hypertension.* Clinical Guideline No. 85. London: NICE.

Preminger, J.E. & Meeks, S. (2010) Evaluation of an audiological rehabilitation program for spouses of people with hearing loss. *Journal of American Academy of Audiology*, **21**(5):315–28.

Scottish Intercollegiate Guidelines Network (2010) *Management of Sore Throat and Indications for Tonsillectomy. A National Clinical Guideline*. Edinburgh: SIGN.

Watkinson, S. (2010) Management of older people with dry and wet age related macular degeneration. *Nursing Older People*, **22**(5):21–6.

22

Nursing care of conditions related to reproductive health

Debra Holloway and Louisa Fleure

Guy's Hospital, London, UK

Contents

Introduction 479
The female reproductive system 479
The male reproductive system 482
Disorders of the female reproductive system 482
Disorders of the male reproductive system 501
Conclusion 508
References 508

Learning outcomes

Having read this chapter, you will be able to:

- Identify the main components of the male and female reproductive system
- Discuss the medical and nursing management of conditions related to the male and female reproductive system
- Define the different types of pregnancy loss

Fundamentals of Medical-Surgical Nursing: A Systems Approach, First Edition. Edited by Anne-Marie Brady, Catherine McCabe, and Margaret McCann.

Introduction

Reproductive health is vital for men and women and affects sexuality, fertility and body image. Care is delivered within different settings including primary care, outpatients clinics and day surgery, with more complex conditions being managed in an inpatient hospital setting. This can impact on the psychological support that men and women receive, which is paramount within this speciality.

The female reproductive system

The main components of the reproductive system are shown in Figures 22.1 and 22.2.

The pelvic floor consists of muscles, pelvic fascia, ovarian ligaments and round ligaments. The vagina starts at the introitus and is a distensible muscular structure that is held in place by the levator ani muscles acting through the perineal body. The upper end of the vagina is attached to the cervix, which divides into the anterior, lateral and posterior walls. To the front of the vagina lie the urethra and bladder neck; to the back is the rectum.

The cervix (Figure 22.3) is cylindrical in shape and connects to the uterus, which is a pear-shaped organ with an inverted triangle-shaped cavity. The uterus is composed of three layers: the peritoneum – the outer serous layer; the myometrium – the middle muscular layer; and the endometrium – the inner functional layer. The uterus sits at right angles to the vagina and tilts forwards (anteversion); in 15% of women, the uterus tilts backward (retroversion).

Leading from the fundal portion of the uterus are the fallopian tubes, which are attached at both corners of the uterus. They are tubular structures containing small cilia that are responsible for the movement of the ovum from the ovary to the uterus. The fallopian tubes end at the fimbriae, where the ovaries can be found. Each ovary is attached to the cornu of the uterus by the ovarian ligament. The surface of the ovary is covered by a single layer of cuboidal cells called the germinal epithelium and has a central vascular medulla and an outer thicker cortex. In the young adult it is almond-shaped, solid and white in colour.

The menstrual cycle

The onset of menstruation is called the menarche and normally occurs at age 12–13 years, 2 years after the first signs of puberty. The first menstrual periods are generally anovulatory and irregular, but

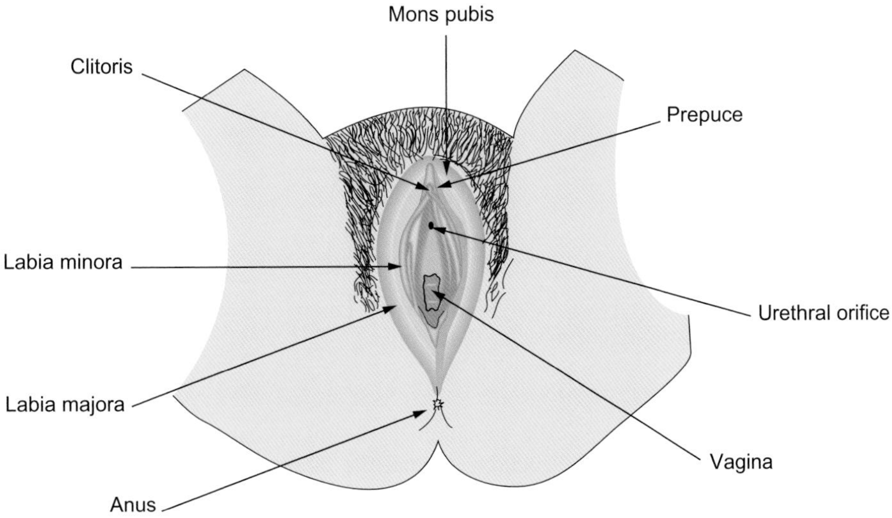

Figure 22.1 The female external genitalia. Reproduced from Nair, M. & Peate, I. (2009) *Fundamentals of Applied Pathophysiology*, with kind permission from Wiley Blackwell.

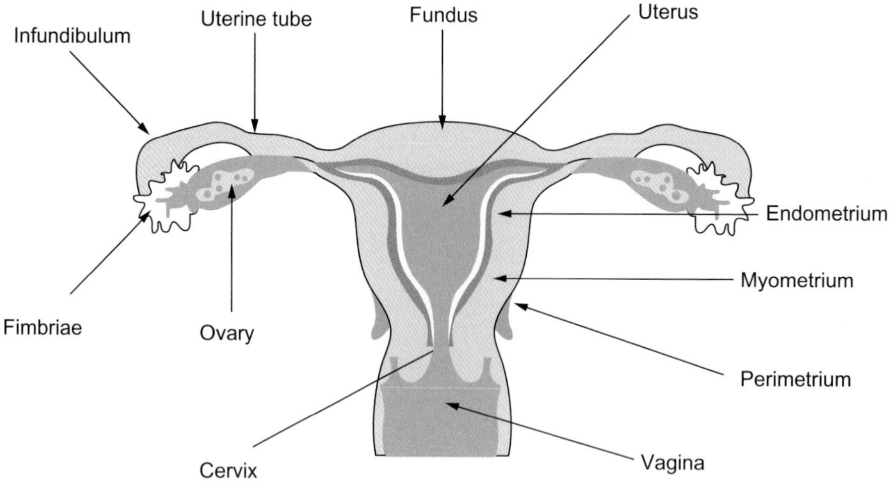

Figure 22.2 The uterus and associated structures. Reproduced from Nair, M. & Peate, I. (2009) *Fundamentals of Applied Pathophysiology*, with kind permission from Wiley Blackwell.

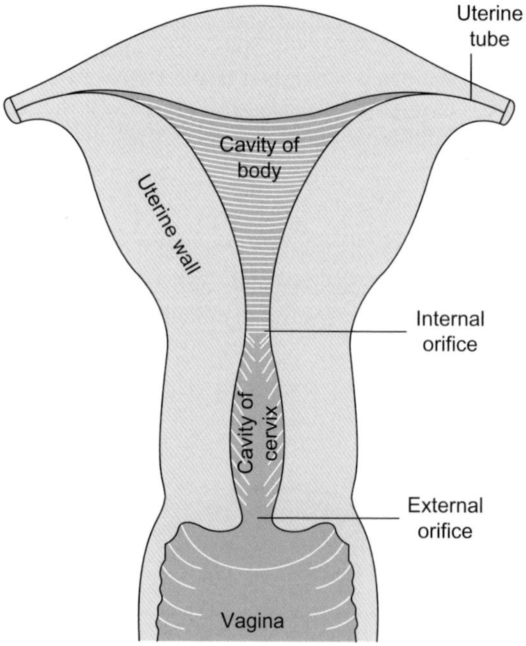

Figure 22.3 The cervix. Reproduced from Nair, M. & Peate, I. (2009) *Fundamentals of Applied Pathophysiology*, with kind permission from Wiley Blackwell.

they usually settle within 2 years. The cessation of the menstrual cycle is the menopause, which happens at an average age of 51. Around this time, the menstrual periods change frequency, with longer gaps between them until they stop completely.

The menstrual cycle (Figure 22.4) can range from 19 to 35 days in length. The proliferative phase is the first stage, which is governed by the production of follicle-stimulating hormone (FSH) from the

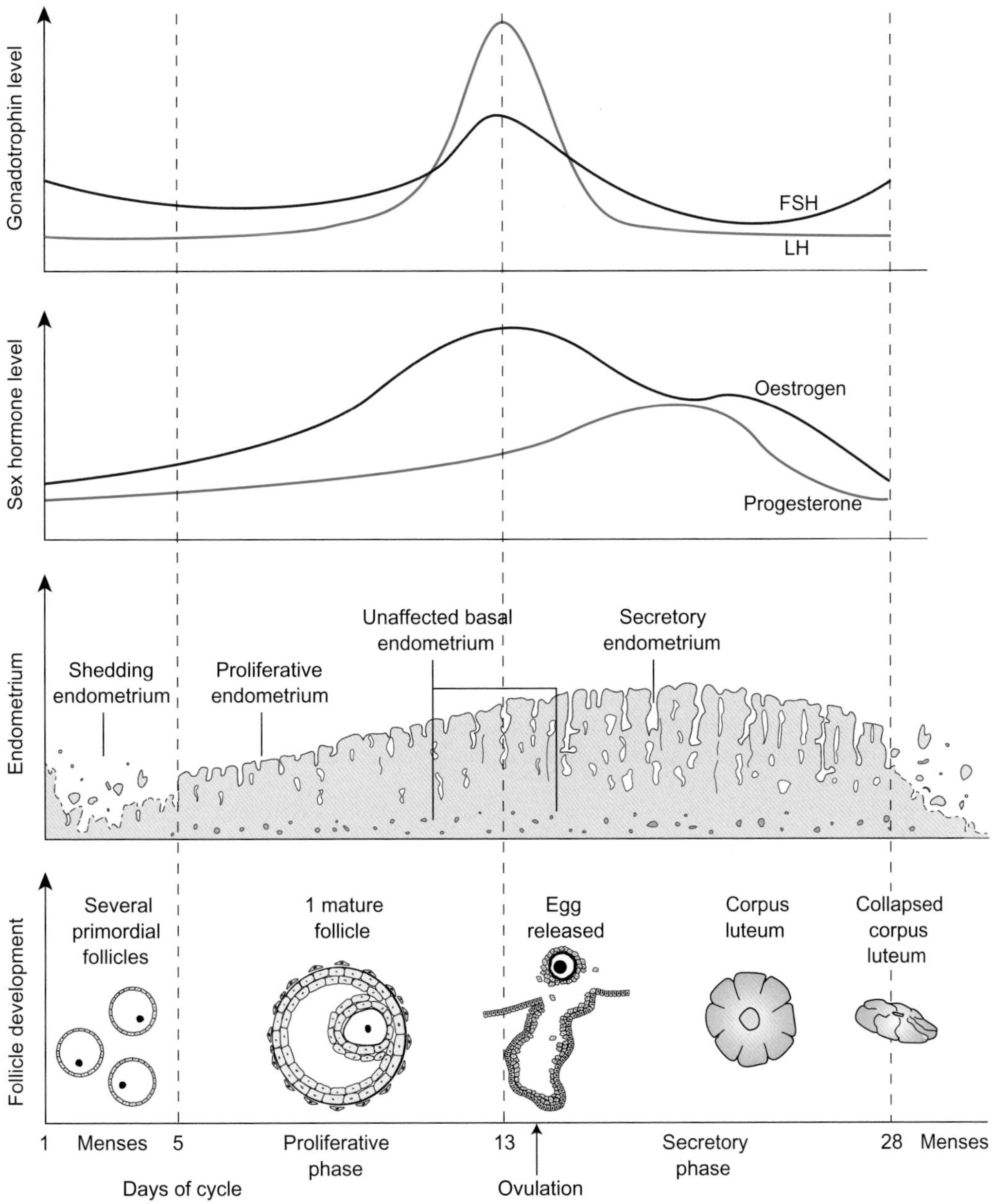

Figure 22.4 The menstrual cycle. Reproduced from Impey, L. (2004) *Obstetrics & Gynaecology*, 2e, with kind permission of Wiley Blackwell.

pituitary gland. The follicles within the ovary then develop under the influence of oestrogen. When oestrogen levels rise, there is suppression of the FSH via a negative feedback system, and one dominant follicle develops. Oestrogen also acts on the endometrium, causing the endometrial glands to grow and new blood vessels to form.

The second stage is the secretory phase, in which a surge of luteinising hormone (LH) from the anterior pituitary gland leads to maturation of the dominant follicle followed by a rise in progesterone release from the corpus luteum. A release of prostaglandins and cytokines leads to rupture of the follicle wall and ovulation, about 38 hours after the initiation of the LH surge. The empty follicle then becomes the corpus luteum. Progesterone is synthesised by the corpus luteum, its concentration rising to above 25 nmol/L, suggesting that the cycle is ovulatory. The endometrium thickens to become secretory, with an increased number of glands in readiness for a pregnancy to implant. The gradual fall of oestrogen and progesterone levels finally results in menses (loss of blood).

Menstruation refers to the shedding of superficial layers of the endometrium and is initiated by the fall in progesterone that follows the failure of the corpus luteum cyst as it starts to resolve. The amount of blood loss in a normal cycle is up to 80 mL, with menstruation starting on day one of a cycle and usually lasting up to 7 days.

Along with changes within the ovary and endometrium, other changes occur under the control of hormones at this time. Cyclical changes occur in the cervical mucus, which becomes thinner at the time of ovulation to facilitate penetration of the cervix by the sperm. It then becomes thicker under the influence of progesterone.

The male reproductive system

The male reproductive system (Figure 22.5) consists of the external organs (the penis and scrotum) and the internal organs (the testes, epididymes, vasa deferentia, ejaculatory ducts, seminal vesicles, prostate gland and bulbourethral glands). The purpose of the male reproductive system is the production, transport and discharge of sperm and the production and secretion of male sex hormones.

The testes sit within the scrotum and are responsible for producing sperm and testosterone. Testosterone production is regulated by the hypothalamus via the release of gonadatrophin-releasing hormone (GnRH), causing the pituitary gland to release LH and FSH. LH travels to the testes and triggers the production of testosterone. Testosterone initiates and maintains the development of the male sexual characteristics (such as development of the genitalia and pubertal changes) and governs the sex drive.

Each testis is surrounded by a fibrous capsule called the tunica albuginea, which is covered by the double-layered tunica vaginalis. Within each testis are small tubes (the seminiferous tubules) that lead to a coiled tube at the back of the testes called the epididymis.

FSH acts on the cells in the seminiferous tubules to stimulate the production of sperm. Specialised cells within the tubules divide many times to become the sperm; the sperm are released from the tubules and pass from the testis into the epididymis, where they mature and gain motility (the ability to move).

The vas deferens is part of the spermatic cord and leads from the epididymis to meet the seminal vesicle at the ejaculatory duct. Mature sperm are transported along the vas deferens during ejaculation, a process that is controlled by the autonomic nervous system and consists of two phases: the emission phase and the expulsion phase. During the emission phase, muscular contractions move the sperm, along with a little fluid, from the epididymis and along the vas deferens. Sperm move up to the ejaculatory ducts and through the prostate gland into the prostatic urethra. Fluid is added to sperm from the seminal vesicles and the prostate to make semen. Most of the volume of the semen is produced by the prostate and seminal vesicles.

During the expulsion phase, the bladder neck contracts to prevent semen entering the bladder, and the pelvic muscles contract rhythmically to propel the semen, which is discharged from the urethra through the urethral meatus.

Disorders of the female reproductive system

Menstrual disorders

There is a wide spectrum of menstrual disorders or disturbances, which are generally not life-threatening, although women with heavy menstrual bleeding (HMB) can experience chronic anaemia and decreased quality of life. Common menstrual disorders include:

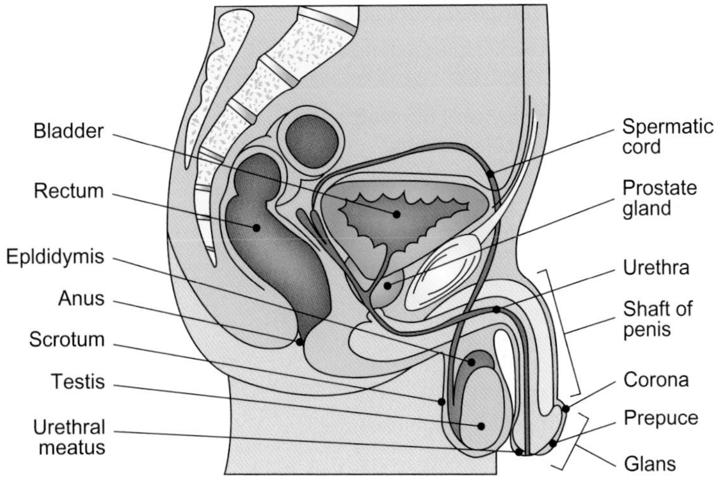

Figure 22.5 The male reproductive tract. Reproduced from Nair, M. & Peate, I. (2009) *Fundamentals of Applied Pathophysiology*, with kind permission from Wiley Blackwell.

- HMB;
- dysmenorrhoea (painful periods);
- premenstrual syndrome;
- intermenstrual postcoital bleeding;
- postmenopausal bleeding;
- amenorrhoea (lack of periods);
- menstrual dysfunction in the peri-menopause, which can cause changes in cycle length and flow;
- polycystic ovarian syndrome (PCOS).

Benign tumours of the female reproductive tract

Table 22.1 describes benign tumours and their management.

Fibroids

Fibroids are the most common benign tumours of the reproductive tract and arise from the smooth muscle of the uterus; their prevalence is hard to define as they can be asymptomatic. Their cause is unknown, but they are more common in African-Caribbean women and their growth is stimulated by oestrogen. Fibroids shrink after the menopause. Types of fibroid (Figure 22.6) include:

- intramural fibroids, contained within the wall of the uterus;
- submucosal fibroids, which lie inside the cavity of the uterus;
- subserosal fibroids, which are found outside wall of the uterus and can be pedunculated;
- cervical fibroids, positioned within the cervix.

The signs and symptoms include:

- HMB or irregular bleeding;
- pressure symptoms such as pain, swelling, pressure on the bowel or bladder (frequency of urination) and increased risk of thrombosis due to pressure on the venous return;
- reproductive problems due to pressure on the ostia or tubes and intracavity problems;
- pregnancy complications such as miscarriage, bleeding in pregnancy, degeneration of fibroids in pregnancy and pain.

Table 22.1 Benign tumours of the female reproductive tract

Site	Type	Cause and presentation	Management
Vulva	Lipoma	Arises from fibrofatty and muscular tissues	Surgical excision if it causes discomfort or interferes with sexual intercourse
	Bartholin's cyst	Blockage of duct by mucus Common Painful Can develop into an abscess	Marsupialisation of the cyst Stitching back of the cyst wall to allow drainage, followed by packing of the cavity Need to exclude infective causes
Vagina	Inclusion cysts	Trauma Imperfect repairs of the perineum	Surgical removal only if there is pain or discomfort
Cervix	Polyps	Small growths that arise from the: • Endocervical mucosa • Surface of the cervix May be asymptomatic Cause intermenstrual and postcoital bleeding Recur	Removal by avulsion or resection
	Nabothian cysts	Mucus retention cysts Seen on the surface of the cervix	No treatment unless there are signs of cervicitis, for which cryotherapy may help
Uterus	Polyps	A focal overgrowth of endometrial glands and stroma Cause irregular bleeding Approximately 1% are malignant More common after the menopause	Hysteroscopic resection
	Fibroids (leiomyomas)	Tumours that arise from the smooth muscle of the myometrium Their size and position define the symptoms	None Myomectomy Hysteroscopic resection Uterine artery embolisation Hysterectomy
Ovary	Ovarian cysts	Many different types	Nil Ovarian cystectomy Removal of ovary

If women are asymptomatic with fibroids and these are then found on routine pelvic examination, no further assessment or treatment is needed. If women have symptoms suspicious of fibroids, a pelvic examination should be undertaken. Ultrasound, either vaginal or abdominal, will also give information about the fibroid's size and position. If there is any doubt or difficulty, a magnetic resonance imaging (MRI) scan can be used, and in some cases hysteroscopy or saline sonography can be used to assess the cavity.

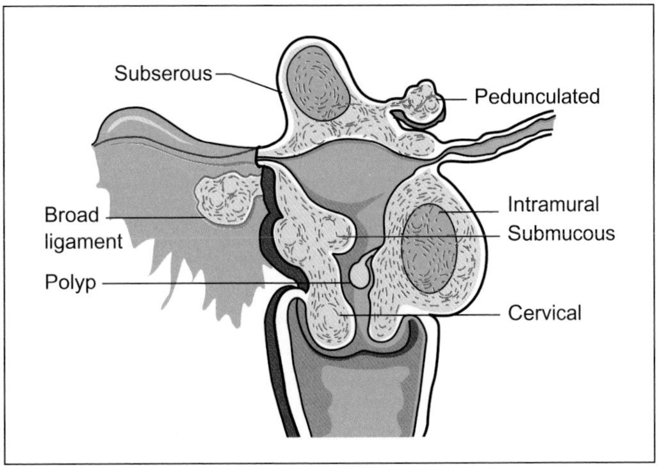

Figure 22.6 Fibroids. Reproduced from Hamilton-Fairley, D. (0000) *Lecture Notes: Obstetrics & Gynaecology*, with kind permission of Wiley Blackwell.

Management

Medical treatment, which is only really beneficial for women who have menstrual problems, includes:

- the combined oral contraceptive pill (COCP);
- tranexamic acid;
- an intrauterine system (IUS) of contraception, but only if there are no submucosal fibroids;
- GnRH analogues over a 3-month course to induce a temporary menopause, which can shrink the fibroids by up to 60%, although they will grow again once treatment has been discontinued; GnRH analogues should not be used as a long-term treatment as they can cause bone density loss, but they can be useful before surgical intervention;
- uterine artery embolisation (UAE), a procedure that aims to reduce the blood supply to the fibroids, causing them to shrink. The technique can be used on any fibroids except ones that are pedunculated. The procedure is carried out by an interventional radiologist and does not require a general anaesthetic. With a reduction in the size of the fibroids, there may be a reduction in the symptoms. Women should be advised that they are likely to have pain and bleeding after the procedure, as well as vaginal discharge, which may persist for several months. Other complications include further surgery due to sepsis, early ovarian failure and an up to 12% chance of having a hysterectomy within the first 2 years (NICE 2010).

The surgical treatment depends on the location, size and number of the fibroids. Myomectomy is the most common surgical treatment and can be carried out in different ways (Table 22.2).

Ovarian cysts

The majority of cysts are fluid-filled, although some have solid elements within them; 90% are likely to be benign. Ovarian cysts can arise from any cell type within the ovary:

- epithelium (mucinous cystadenomas, endometrioid tumours and Brenner tumours);
- germ cells (dermoid cysts, which may contain other materials such as hair, teeth and sebaceous matter);
- sex cord stroma (rarer granulosa cell tumours and theca cell tumours).

Some cysts may be functional, occurring during the menstrual cycle from corpus luteum cysts, and are generally asymptomatic. They arise during ovulation and resolve spontaneously.

Table 22.2 Myomectomy

Procedure	Advantages	Disadvantages	Suitable for
Laparoscopic myomectomy	Quicker recovery Smaller incisions	A limited number of fibroids can be treated Not all gynaecologists offer this procedure	Women with fibroids no larger than 7 cm Subserosal or intramural fibroids only
Abdominal myomectomy	Removes more and larger fibroids	1% risk of needing a hysterectomy Length of time in hospital May need a second operation	Large uterus Multiple fibroids
Hysteroscopic myomectomy	Day case procedure No abdominal cuts	Not suitable for all fibroids Risk of perforation If fibroids are large, may need a two-stage procedure Fluid overload	Submucosal only, with more than 50% in the uterine cavity
Hysterectomy	Cure	Length of stay Morbidity	All types

Cysts may be asymptomatic and discovered on examination or ultrasound for a different presenting complaint. Some women may complain of:

- pain;
- abdominal swelling;
- pain on intercourse;
- pressure symptoms such as a full feeling within the pelvis.

Progesterone-only contraception may also increase the risk of ovarian cysts. An acute onset of pain associated with nausea and vomiting may indicate torsion of the cyst, which will need immediate surgical intervention to prevent necrosis of the ovary. The assessment should include examination and ultrasonography. There are some tumour markers that can be helpful in distinguishing whether there is a risk of malignancy:

- CA-125, although this is also raised with endometriosis, adenomyosis and fibroids;
- alpha-fetoprotein (AFP), identified by a blood test;
- human chorionic gonadotropin (HCG).

Management

There is no medical management available for ovarian cysts, but many do not need any intervention. Benign cysts less than 5–6 cm in size can be monitored with regular ultrasound scans. If women are prone to recurrent cysts, the COCP may be helpful to prevent them.

For women experiencing symptoms, if there is any suspicion of malignancy or if the cysts are large (over 8 cm), surgical removal is recommended. This may be achieved by laparoscopy and aspiration of the cyst, laparoscopic or open removal of the cyst, or oopherectomy (removal of the ovary). For post-menopausal women, the routine practice should be removal of the ovary rather than just the cyst due to the risk of malignancy.

Cancers affecting the female reproductive tract

Cancer can occur in any part of the reproductive tract (Table 22.3).

Table 22.3 Gynaecological cancers

Type	Causes	Signs and symptoms	Diagnosis	Treatment
Vulval				
Accounts for less than 6% of gynaecological cancers Mainly squamous cell carcinomas More common in women >65 years On the increase in younger women	Has been linked to: ● HPV ● Smoking ● A history of precancerous changes ● Chronic skin conditions, e.g. lichen planus	Itching Ulceration Vulval pain Discharge Discoloration A mass	Vulval biopsy Check the vagina and cervix for coexisting disease EUA MRI to check the extent of disease for staging	If early stage, wide local excision With wide spread, vulvectomy and possibly removal of the groin lymph nodes Radiotherapy if the margins are not clear Chemotherapy for inoperable or recurrent disease and metastases Complications of surgery include sexual dysfunction and wound breakdown
Cervix				
Rates have dropped in countries where there is a screening programme The most common type is squamous cell (90%), adenocarcinomas making up the rest Most occur in the transformation zone as a result of dysplastic changes Cancers spread by direct invasion Spread in advanced cases is via lymph and blood	HPV types 16 and 18 Early sexual intercourse Multiple partners Non-use of barrier methods of contraception Smoking Immunosuppressants	None Vaginal discharge Postcoital bleeding Intermenstrual bleeding Back pain Late presentation – bladder and bowel dysfunction Fistula formation	Examination and colposcopy with biopsies EUA MRI/CT Assess local spread: ● Chest X-ray; ● Sigmoidoscopy ● Cystoscopy	Cervical screening HPV vaccination programmes are available in the UK and Ireland Treatment depends on stage If picked up in the precancerous stage (cervical screening), large loop excision Cone biopsy Trachelectomy (removal of the cervix) if fertility is an issue Early – radical hysterectomy Extensive – pelvic clearance Chemotherapy and radiotherapy; internal radiotherapy (brachytherapy) can be used with external beam radiotherapy

(Continued)

Table 22.3 (*Continued*)

Type	Causes	Signs and symptoms	Diagnosis	Treatment
Endometrial				
Second most common cancer and increasing in incidence Endometrioid adenocarcinoma is the most common type The majority are in postmenopausal women, with one-quarter being premenopausal	Oestrogen exposure No children and not breastfeeding Obesity Diabetes Tamoxifen Previous endometrial hyperplasia Unopposed oestrogen PCOS Family history	None Postmenopausal bleeding Vaginal bleeding Discharge Abnormal bleeding	Vaginal examination Ultrasound scan; a thin endometrium (under 4 mm) is normal in postmenopausal women If abnormal, a hysteroscopy and biopsy is undertaken Further imaging for assessment of stage	Total abdominal hysterectomy, bilateral salpingo-oophorectomy and possibly removal of lymph nodes Radical hysterectomy External or internal radiotherapy after surgery, depending on stage or if the patient is not fit for operation Progesterone if the patient is not fit for operation and in palliative settings
Ovarian				
The fourth most common cause of cancer in women Are many different types: • Serous • Mucinous • Endometrioid • Clear cell cystadenocarcinoma • Germ cell, and may be secondary	Related to ovulation The COCP and pregnancy have some protective effect *BRAC1* and *BRAC2* genetic mutations	Difficult to diagnose The patient may have no symptoms or may present with advanced disease Bloating Back and abdominal pain Tiredness Weight loss Urinary problems	Ultrasound MRI/CT Bloods for markers such as CA-125 (not always elevated and can also rise in other conditions, e.g. endometriosis) Royal College of Obstetricians and Gynaecologists has a risk of malignancy calculator to help distinguish tumours most at risk of being malignant (http://www.rcog.org.uk/files/rcog-corp/GTG3411022011.pdf)	Total abdominal hysterectomy and bilateral salpingo-oophorectomy with lymph node removal and staging of the disease at the same time Alternatively, debulking surgery, chemotherapy and more surgery Chemotherapy

CT, computed tomography; EUA, examination under anaesthesia; HPV, human papillomavirus.

Table 22.4 Preoperative patient education

Problem	Management
Loss of fertility	Preoperative counselling Fertility consultation (egg collection and storage)
Early menopause	Preoperative discussion Postoperative hormone replacement therapy, if indicated
Vaginal dryness	Dilators and lubrication
Changes in body image or sexuality and fertility	Specialist support
Unsure of the nature of the surgery	A full explanation of the operation: • What is removed • How the body will function postoperatively

Nursing management

The diagnosis of cancer affects both the women and their families. Some treatments affect body image, sexuality and fertility so referral to a psychosexual counsellor may be helpful. Treatment may also result in physical and functional changes that affect sexual function, such as vaginal problems after radiotherapy. All these changes will need to be discussed sensitively before and after treatment. Prior to surgery, fertility, plans for children, sexual activity and the nature of the surgery should be assessed and discussed (Table 22.4).

Depending on the type of cancer and the treatment, women may need to be educated to expect or monitor for ascites (especially with ovarian cancer). Hormonal changes such as hot flushes may occur if the ovaries have been removed; an induced menopause may also result following chemotherapy or radiotherapy. If surgery involves lymph node removal, resultant lower limb oedema may occur. Women may experience anxiety and fatigue. Support is available from various agencies including social services, the Irish Cancer Society and charities such as Macmillan Cancer Support and Cancer BACUP (UK only). Women should also have access to a clinical nurse specialist who can guide them on what specialist support is available locally.

Prolapse

A prolapse is a protrusion of an organ from its normal position. In the female reproductive system, the urethra (urethrocele), bladder (cystocele), rectum (rectocele) or uterus may prolapse into the vagina. Uterine prolapse may be first degree (still within the vagina), second degree (where the cervix is at the introitus) or third degree (where the entire uterus has come out of the vagina).

A prolapse generally occurs due to a weakness of the pelvic floor muscles, which may be due to:

- damage from pregnancy and labour;
- age-related changes;
- lack of oestrogen after the menopause;
- increased pressure in the abdomen due to heavily lifting, constipation or a pelvic mass.

Some women have no symptoms whereas others may complain of feeling a mass or lump within the vagina. Women may experience pain, a dragging sensation, urinary problems or defecation problems. Discharge and bleeding may be present if there is a third-degree uterine prolapse.

Table 22.5 Surgery for prolapse

Surgery	Type of prolapse	Comments
Anterior repair	Urethrocele and cystocele	There may be: • Urinary retention after surgery • Painful intercourse
Vaginal hysterectomy	Uterine prolapse	Can be combined with anterior and posterior repairs
Sacrospinus fixation	Vault repair	Risk of postoperative cystocele and stress incontinence
Posterior repair	Rectocele	Painful intercourse postoperatively

Management

Women with mild symptoms should be taught to perform pelvic floor exercises to strengthen the pelvic floor muscles. In some cases, the insertion of a ring pessary may also help to support the pelvic floor. If the symptoms are severe and not helped by these measures, surgery may be performed to correct the anatomical problem (Table 22.5).

Endometriosis

Endometriosis is a condition in which endometrial tissue is found outside the endometrial cavity but still responds to the influence of hormones. It can be found in the peritoneum over the uterosacral ligaments or in the ovaries, broad ligaments, fallopian tubes, pouch of Douglas, bowel and bladder. Less common sites include the diaphragm, the lungs and the brain. It is normally found in women of reproductive age, can be progressive and is linked with chronic pelvic pain, psychological problems and infertility. The symptoms will depend on the site of the endometriosis and may include:

- pelvic pain (which is not linked to the severity of the disease on laparoscopy);
- painful intercourse;
- dysmenorrhoea;
- infertility;
- painful bowel movements;
- painful micturition.

The exact aetiology of endometriosis is unknown. The endometrial deposits react to the influence of hormones and will bleed as if the tissue were in the uterine cavity. This bleeding can then cause inflammation, scarring and distortion of the pelvic anatomy. This may form as endometriomas, which are cysts on the ovary caused by endometriosis.

Management

Physical examination and ultrasound are used to assess and diagnose endometriosis, but the gold standard diagnostic tool is laparoscopy (Royal College of Obstetricians and Gynaecologists [RCOG] 2006a). Medical management will depend on the woman and her desired outcomes. Women who wish to avoid any hormonal treatment can be prescribed analgesia, which can be given during the menstrual period or when in pain (Allen *et al.* 2009). The aim of hormonal treatment is to suppress endometrial growth and proliferation. Treatment includes:

- COCPs, taken continuously;
- progesterone, taken continuously to cause atrophy of the endometriosis;
- an IUS for contraception;
- GnRH analogues with add-back hormone replacement therapy (HRT) to reduce the side effects of menopause and stop bone density loss.

Endometriosis can be treated surgically. Approaches include laparoscopy combined with laser therapy or diathermy, which destroys the endometrial deposits. In addition to surgery, a combined approach with medical management is often used; any adhesions that have formed can be divided to try to restore the pelvic anatomy. Ablation of the deposits can help to improve fertility, but this may not relieve the symptoms, and repeated laparoscopy may be needed. The definitive surgery for women who do not wish to retain their fertility is a total abdominal hysterectomy and bilateral salpingo-oopherectomy, although this may not cure long-standing pelvic pain. Continuous combined HRT may need to be prescribed to prevent the reactivation of any deposits.

Nurses need to provide patients with the following information:

- the impact the disease has on women's fertility;
- an explanation of the condition;
- the fact that many of the treatments are contraceptives;
- information on coping strategies or adequate analgesia regimens that can be used to manage the chronic pelvic pain that is often associated with this condition.

Unplanned pregnancy loss

Unplanned pregnancy loss refers to either miscarriage or an ectopic pregnancy. Women who present with pain and or bleeding in pregnancy will need the following investigations:

- a urinary pregnancy test;
- routine observations;
- urinalysis;
- a gentle bimanual and speculum examination to assess for pain and for whether the cervix is open;
- blood samples for a full blood count, group and save, and levels of βHCG (which reflects pregnancy) and progesterone;
- an ultrasound scan.

Risk factors for an ectopic pregnancy should be assessed, for example previous ectopic pregnancies or a history of *Chlamydia* infection or pelvic inflammatory disease (PID). Women should also be assessed for failed oral contraceptive pills or intrauterine contraceptive device, endometriosis and previous pelvic surgery.

Miscarriage

Miscarriage is defined as pregnancy loss before the 24th week of pregnancy and occurs in about 1 in 4 pregnancies. Miscarriage can be spontaneous, complete, incomplete, delayed or recurrent (which refers to more than three consecutive losses and occurs in 3% of the population) (RCOG 2003).

Causes of miscarriage can be:

- fetal, for example congenital malformations and genetic abnormalities (thought to be the most common cause and increasing with maternal age);
- maternal, for example acute illness, infections, trauma, antiphospholipid (APL) syndrome, diabetes, hypothyroidism, abnormalities of the uterus, cervical incompetence, smoking, alcohol and drugs.

A molar pregnancy occurs when there is overgrowth of the chorionic villi and is known as gestational trophoblastic disease. These are rare pregnancies and can be complete, partial or invasive; if left untreated, they can form choriocarcinomas.

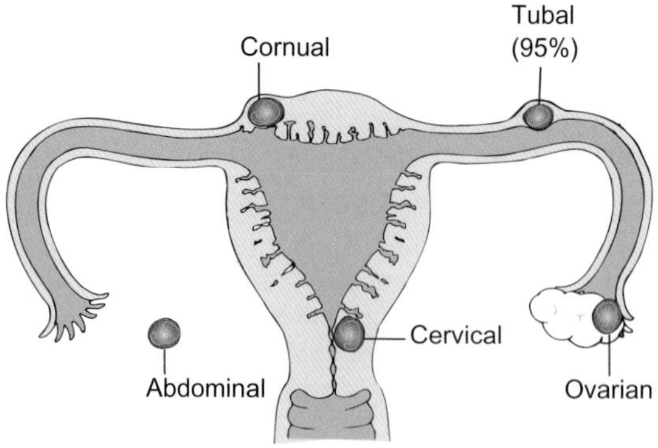

Figure 22.7 Ectopic pregnancy. Reproduced from Impey, L. (2004) *Obstetrics & Gynaecology*, 2e, with kind permission of Wiley Blackwell.

Management

The management of miscarriages can be medical or expectant (RCOG 2006b). Expectant management involves monitoring in order to wait and see whether pregnancy tissue will be passed naturally without the need for surgical intervention. Medical management involves giving medication to expel the fetus or any remaining pregnancy tissue. The usual regimen is a combination of mifepristone, an antiprogesterone, followed 35–48 hours later by a prostaglandin.

If women fail to progress with conservative or medical management, or are unsuitable for such management, surgical intervention involving the evacuation of retained products of conception (ERPC), may be needed. Depending on the length of gestation and the amount of retained products visible on a scan, the cervix can be primed with a prostaglandin. ERPC may also be necessary when a molar pregnancy is suspected to ensure that the products can be sent for histology, and when patients present with heavy bleeding and the condition is unstable.

Ectopic pregnancy

Ectopic pregnancies occur outside the uterus, predominantly in the fallopian tubes, but can also be ovarian, cervical or intra-abdominal (Figure 22.7). They occur when the fertilised ovum does not implant in the correct place, this generally being due to tubal damage from infections and other conditions such as endometriosis, although the cause is sometimes unknown. The incidence of ectopic pregnancy is about 1 in 200 in the UK, but is increasing with the rise in rate of *Chlamydia* infection.

Management

Ectopic pregnancies can be managed expectantly if the woman is stable and βHCG levels are decreasing, indicating a failing pregnancy. Medical management with methotrexate can be used; this interferes with cell growth and will prevent the egg or ectopic pregnancy-related tissue from growing. Methotrexate is effective in about 90% of cases. Most women require a single dose, but on occasions a second dose may be needed (RCOG 2004).

The woman's clinical condition will determine whether she needs urgent surgical intervention as an ectopic pregnancy can still cause death. In women who are haemodynamically unstable, a laparotomy may be needed. An ectopic pregnancy is generally managed with a laparoscopy and removal of the ectopic pregnancy by salpingostomy (opening the tube) or salpingectomy (removal of the tube).

Nurses need to support women with unplanned pregnancy loss by providing information on:

- bereavement counselling;
- local or national support groups or charities;
- future pregnancies;
- the timing of future pregnancies;
- the need for an early scan on the woman's next pregnancy;

- determination of rhesus factor level and administration of anti-D if the woman is rhesus negative; this may be necessary after surgical instrumentation of the uterus or after 12 weeks' gestation and acts to prevent rhesus incompatibility in any subsequent pregnancies;
- contraceptive advice (if necessary).

Termination of pregnancy

Many women will experience an unwanted and unplanned pregnancy. For some, the only solution is a termination of pregnancy (TOP), or abortion. This is a removal of the pregnancy from the uterus that does not lead to the survival of the pregnancy. The laws that govern TOP vary from country to country. TOP in the UK is governed by the 1967 Abortion Act, which was amended by the Human Fertilisation and Embryology Act 1990. Two doctors need to agree in good faith that one or more of five conditions apply and then complete the legal paperwork. The legal limit after which terminations may not be performed is 24 weeks, unless there is a severe threat to the women's life.

No practitioner in the UK has to take part in TOP unless there is a risk to the women's life. Women will be referred to a range of clinics to discuss the TOP. Investigations include:

- the patient's history;
- a full blood count;
- vaginal swabs;
- blood grouping for rhesus factor;
- ultrasound (if there is a doubt over the gestational age).

Medical management is undertaken for gestations up to 9 weeks. The current regimen is oral mifepristone, which inhibits progesterone and prevents the pregnancy progressing. This is followed by vaginal misoprostol, a prostaglandin analogue, which works to induce contractions. There is a 95% success rate for a complete TOP. Late medical TOP can be performed up to 24 weeks' gestation. This is normally with mifepristone and then gemeprost up to 2 days later, causing the abortion; women need to deliver the fetus.

Surgical management can be performed in the first trimester between 6 and 14 weeks of gestation. The procedure involves vacuum aspiration under general or local anaesthetic. The cervix may be dilated preoperatively with prostaglandin, and at the time of surgery an aspiration cannula is used to empty the uterus. Complications include perforation of the uterus and retained products of conception. After 15 weeks of gestation, dilatation and evacuation is used. This involves the removal of the pregnancy with forceps via the cervix.

Complications from all forms of TOP are rare but include:

- infections, which can be reduced by screening for sexually transmitted infections (STIs);
- haemorrhage;
- failed TOP needing a repeat procedure;
- uterine trauma such as perforation, which is more common with later gestations but lessened by using cervical preparations;
- cervical lacerations, which can be lessened by the use of cervical preparations;
- psychological problems – many women experience grief but also relief, and about 10% will experience long-term problems.

Women should have access to counselling both before and after the procedure if needed, and should be aware that there may be some bleeding and pain after the TOP. The rhesus factor should also be checked prior to discharge and anti-D given if needed. Women should be offered advice regarding adequate contraception after the procedure.

Pelvic inflammatory disease

PID is an acute infection that ascends from the endocervix or descends from the pelvis (as in appendicitis) and results in salpingitis, endometritis, tubo-ovarian abscess or pelvic peritonitis. PID is caused by:

- *Chlamydia* (60%);
- gonorrhoea;
- non-sexually transmitted infections such as *Escherichia coli*;
- instrumentation of the cervical canal in gynaecological procedures;
- TOP.

PID is more common in women under 25 years of age who have multiple partners and a history of STIs and can be associated with recent fitting of an IUC or IUS. The symptoms (British Association for Sexual Health and HIV 2011) include:

- a lack of symptoms;
- symptoms ranging from vague pain to peritonitis;
- lower abdominal pain;
- painful intercourse;
- deep pain;
- postcoital bleeding;
- intermenstrual bleeding;
- vaginal discharge.

On examination, women may present with:

- pyrexia;
- guarding on bimanual examination;
- cervical excitation (pain when the cervix is moved during examination);
- tenderness;
- an adnexal mass if there is an abscess;
- on speculum examination, discharge at the cervix (swabs and a midstream urine specimen will need to be obtained).

It is important to rule out the differential diagnoses of ectopic pregnancy, appendicitis, urinary tract infection, endometriosis and torsion of an ovarian cyst. This is done by ultrasound, blood tests (full blood count, C-reactive protein and erythrocyte sedimentation rate) and a pregnancy test.

Management

Treatment should be started if there is a suspicion of PID. If there is cervical excitation and tenderness on examination, the RCOG (2008) recommends prescribed (broad-spectrum) antibiotic treatment without having positive microscopy swabs. Women in severe pain may need admission to hospital and possibly a laparoscopy; intravenous antibiotics are the first line of management in this case. Women should be reviewed in 3 days and then after 2 weeks to check resolution of their symptoms and compliance with medication. If women do not respond to antibiotics within 24 hours, a laparoscopy and draining of any abscess may be needed.

Nurses need to provide women with the following information:

- Women may go on to develop chronic pelvic pain syndrome (possibly due to the formation of scar tissue).
- There is a risk of a second episode of PID.
- Women will have a sevenfold increased risk of ectopic pregnancy.
- There is a risk of infertility, with 20% of women having tubal damage after two episodes of PID (British Association for Sexual Health and HIV 2011).
- PID is generally sexually transmitted.
  - The woman's partner needs to be contacted and treated.
  - There should be no further sexual activity until both parties have completed the course of treatment.
  - Anxiety and relationship problems may arise if there has been infidelity.

Nursing care of women who have had gynaecological surgery

Surgery on the reproductive organs can be either diagnostic or therapeutic. The surgical approach can be vaginal, laparoscopic or via an open procedure depending on the type of operation. With changes in care procedures and advances in technology over the last decade, many women now do not require surgery. The developments in laparoscopic surgical techniques and the increase in the number of procedures being performed in outpatients or day units means that nurses must in a shorter space of time address the psychological care that is integral to women's health.

Preoperative nursing management for gynaecological surgery

In addition to carrying out standard preoperative checks and assessments, nurses should establish the date of the last menstrual period and check whether there is any chance of pregnancy before any operation that may have an impact on a woman's fertility proceeds. Most units ensure that a urinary HCG test is carried out before a gynaecological operation.

Preoperation anxiety is normal, but in the case of gynaecological surgery nurses must be aware that operations can be linked with fertility or infertility, loss of sexuality, loss of pregnancy and the onset of menopause. Women need additional support when undergoing operations, however minor they seem to the healthcare staff.

Postoperative nursing management following gynaecological surgery

Postoperative observations should be carried out to assess for signs of bleeding and infection. Bladder function should be monitored as there may be a risk of retention if catheterisation is not required. Wound sites should be regularly observed and vaginal bleeding assessed with each observation. Specific care related to gynaecological procedures is shown in Table 22.6.

Hysterectomy

One of the more common gynaecological operations is a hysterectomy (Box 22.1). This can be carried out in many different ways: as an open procedure, laparoscopically or via the vagina. The

Table 22.6 Nursing care for specific gynaecological procedures

Operation	Why	Where and anaesthetic	Specific care
ERPC	Removal of pregnancy tissue after miscarriage	Outpatient department, local anaesthetic Day surgery unit, general anaesthetic	Pregnancy loss Grief Check rhesus factor
Hysteroscopy	Diagnostic for bleeding Therapeutic, resection of: • Fibroids • Polyps Removal of lost IUS Sterilisation	Outpatient department, no anaesthetic or just local anaesthetic Day surgery unit, general anaesthetic Inpatient procedure, general anaesthetic	Can bleed up for to 2 weeks depending on the procedure

(*Continued*)

Table 22.6 (*Continued*)

Operation	Why	Where and anaesthetic	Specific care
Laparoscopy	Diagnostic for pain Therapeutic destruction of endometriosis Removal of cyst Ectopic pregnancy Sterilisation Removal of womb Fibroids	Day surgery unit, general anaesthetic Inpatient procedure, general anaesthetic	Pain under shoulder tip from carbon dioxide gas used in the procedure Dissolvable sutures or sutures that need to be removed after 5–7 days
Colposcopy	Large loop excision of transformation zone Cone biopsy	Outpatient department, local anaesthetic Day surgery unit, local or general anaesthetic	Risk of infection No sexual intercourse for up to 4 weeks No use of tampons for 4 weeks
Myomectomy	Removal of fibroids Can be: • Laparoscopic • Hysteroscopic • Via open laparotomy	Outpatient department, local anaesthetic Day surgery unit, general anaesthetic Inpatient procedure, general anaesthetic	As for laparotomy Wound care When to conceive will depend on the operation and whether the uterine cavity has been entered
Hysterectomy	Laparoscopic Open Vaginal	Day surgery unit, general anaesthetic Inpatient procedure, general anaesthetic	Psychological care Risk of early menopause If subtotal hysterectomy, stress need for future cervical screening See also Box 22.1
Bilateral salpingo-oopherectomy	Removal of both fallopian tubes and ovaries Laparotomy Laparoscopy	Day surgery unit, general anaesthetic Inpatient procedure, general anaesthetic	Same care as for hysterectomy Menopausal symptoms
Repairs	Anterior and posterior	Day surgery unit, general anaesthetic Inpatient procedure, general anaesthetic	Care of the wound Avoidance of constipation and straining
Transvaginal tape	Mesh to support the urethra	Outpatient department, local anaesthetic Day surgery unit, general anaesthetic Inpatient procedure, general anaesthetic	Avoidance of straining
TOP		Outpatient department, local anaesthetic Day surgery unit, general anaesthetic	Check rhesus factor and if negative give anti-D Contraception Psychological care

Box 22.1 Postoperative nursing care following hysterectomy

Risk of bleeding

- Monitor:
  - The wound and dressings
  - The wound drain, if used
  - The vital signs
  - Vaginal loss
- If there has been a vaginal hysterectomy:
  - Monitor the loss using a vaginal pack

Pain

- Provide regular analgesia

Risk of infection

- Monitor:
  - Temperature and pulse
  - The wound
- Remove clips and sutures at 5–10 days, as directed
- Remove the pack at 24 hours if vaginal hysterectomy has been carried out
- Monitor for vaginal discharge or wound haematomas

Urinary elimination

- A urinary catheter should be in place for 24–48 hours

Potential constipation

- Monitor the bowels
- Provide suppositories if the bowels have not opened by day 3

Profound change in body image and sexual function

- Allow the woman time to discuss her fears and concerns
- Warn of menopause if the ovaries have been removed
- Refer to a specialist counsellor

Discharge advice

- Seek medical help if signs of infection develop
- Access for ongoing psychological support if needed
- Carry out pelvic floor exercises
- Sexual activity can resume once it is comfortable to do so
- Housework and lifting should be limited for the first 6 weeks and gradually built up as is comfortable
- Driving can be resumed when the woman is comfortable enough to do an emergency stop
- Return to work at 6 weeks
- If the cervix has been removed and any smears were normal before surgery, no more cervical screening needs to be undertaken

approach used depends on the condition being treated and the surgeon's skills. Hysterectomy via a laparotomy – a cut in the abdomen (either transverse or longitudinal) – can involve:

- a radical hysterectomy (usually indicated for cancer): complete removal of the uterus, cervix, upper vagina, parametrium, lymph nodes, ovaries and fallopian tubes;
- a total hysterectomy: complete removal of the uterus and cervix;
- a subtotal hysterectomy: removal of the uterus, leaving the cervix *in situ*.

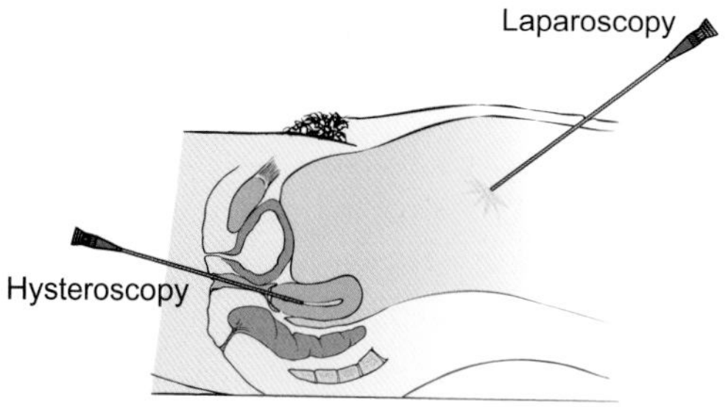

Figure 22.8 Laparoscopy. Reproduced from Impey, L. (2004) *Obstetrics & Gynaecology*, 2e, with kind permission of Wiley Blackwell.

A laparoscopic approach (Figure 22.8) can be used for a laparoscopic hysterectomy, alaparoscopically assisted vaginal hysterectomy or a robotic laparoscopic hysterectomy.

Health promotion

Sexually transmitted infections

STIs can be asymptomatic or can cause symptoms in the form of discharge. Nurses should encourage women to reduce the risk of STIs by using barrier methods of contraception, possibly in addition to other methods of contraception, as infections can impact on fertility and cause ectopic pregnancy and cervical cancer in later life.

Contraception

The aim of contraception is to prevent unplanned and unwanted pregnancies. Women's contraceptive needs change as they go through their reproductive life, and the use of contraception may also bring other health benefits, such as a reduction in menstrual loss with the COCP and IUS. For more information on methods of contraception, see http://www.fsrh.org/. Types of contraceptive include:

- male and female condoms;
- male and female sterilisation;
- female barrier methods (diaphragm/latex dome);
- the COCP;
- the progestogen-only pill;
- injections of progestrogen;
- implants, for example a progestrogen rod inserted subdermally into the arm;
- intrauterine contraceptive devices;
- IUSs.

Screening

Screening programmes for breast and cervical cancer are available in the UK via the National Health Service, now part of Public Health England (http://www.cancerscreening.nhs.uk), and in Ireland through the national cancer screening programme (http://www.cancerscreening.ie). These screening programmes have been shown to be specific and reliable; there is, however, no screening programme for ovarian cancer due to the low specificity of the tests.

In the UK, breast screening has been undertaken with 3-yearly mammograms in women aged between 50 and 70 (although this is now changing to 47–73); after this age, women may self refer. Screening in Ireland is for women aged 50–64 and takes place every 2 years. Women should be encouraged to examine their own breasts and be aware of any changes that might occur, such as lumps or nipple discharge.

Cervical screening in the UK is undertaken on women aged 25–65 years. The frequency is 3-yearly to the age of 50 and then 5-yearly; screening in Ireland occurs 3-yearly for women aged 25–44 and 5-yearly from 45 to 60 years. The timelines in both screening programmes depend on women having normal cervical screening results; if there has been any abnormality in the past, the screening frequency may change. It is thought that the cervical screening programme has been responsible for the decrease in mortality from cervical cancer.

Disorders of the breast

Breast problems are common (Table 22.7). Women are concerned and worried that they may have breast cancer if they discover a breast lump; however, the majority of lumps are benign. The incidence of breast cancer is increasing, with a lifetime risk of 1 in 8 women developing this condition.

Breast cancer

As with gynaecological cancers, the incidence of breast cancer is increasing and the condition has a profound psychological effect on women, their body image and their femininity. Risk factors include:

- age;
- onset of menstruation before the age of 11 years;
- menopause after 54 years of age;
- first pregnancy when aged over 35;
- a family history of breast cancer;
- a high fat and alcohol intake;
- obesity;
- HRT;
- possibly smoking.

The signs and symptoms include:

- any new lump;
- pain (although this is present in only 10% of women with cancer);
- newly occurring nipple retraction;
- nipple eczema;
- skin tethering or fixation;
- ulceration.

Management

Clinical examination, ultrasound and biopsy (core biopsy or needle aspiration) are the standard methods of investigating breast lumps. If the results are positive for cancer, surgery is the treatment of choice. A number of factors are taken into account when deciding what treatment is best:

- the stage and grade of the cancer (how big it is and how far has spread);
- the patient's general health;
- the menopausal status.

An MRI may give additional information about the extent of the disease. Women with cancer should be cared for by a multidisciplinary team consisting of a specialist cancer surgeon, an oncologist (a radiotherapy and chemotherapy specialist), a radiologist, a pathologist, a radiographer, a reconstructive surgeon and a specialist nurse. Treatment options are outlined in Table 22.8.

After surgery, breast cancers that are oestrogen and/or progestogen receptor positive are normally treated with antihormone medication such as tamoxifen or aromatase inhibitors to block the oestrogen receptors. Both of these medications have side effects similar to menopausal symptoms.

Table 22.7 Common breast problems

Condition	Signs and symptoms	Management
Mastalgia (breast pain)	Intermittent or cyclical In response to hormonal changes Can come from underlying structures such as ribs	A correctly fitting bra Analgesia Salt restriction Premenstrually, wearing a bra in bed Change hormonal contraception Evening primrose oil
Breast lumps (a variety of causes for non-cancerous lumps)	Fibroadenoma: • A firm oestrogen-sensitive nodule • Referred to as a breast mouse as it moves easily under the skin Cysts: • Can be large • Cause pain • More common in premenopausal women • Vary in number and size	No treatment unless >3 cm in size 20% will increase in size More common in younger women Ultrasound and possible aspiration
Nipple problems	Discharge Physiological Related to pregnancy	Reassurance
	Bloodstained discharge related to breast epithelial hyperplasia or ductal papilloma	Surgical excision
	Galactorrhoea, caused by medications (dopamine agonists), pituitary tumours or hypothyroidism	Treatment is based on cause
	Pituitary adenoma: increased prolactin levels are associated with visual disturbances and menstrual problems	MRI of the pituitary and medication such as bromocriptine or cabergoline
Mastitis	Infection related: • Lactation • Smoking	Antibiotics Possible aspiration and culture

After breast cancer, women need ongoing support and care and annual mammograms for at least 5 years. Follow-up includes:

- psychological care related to body image, fear of reoccurrence and fertility (as some treatments affects fertility);
- postoperative prosthetics following mastectomy; discussions with the patient may focus on reconstructive surgery;
- monitoring of fatigue and strategies to avoid tiredness.

Table 22.8 Breast cancer treatment options

Treatment	Description	Nursing care
Lumpectomy	Removal of the lump only	See Box 22.2
Wide local excision	Excision around the cancer	See Box 22.2
Simple mastectomy	Removal of the breast	See Box 22.2
Modified radical mastectomy	Removal of the breast and chest wall muscles	See Box 22.2
Lymph node clearance	Removal of the lymph nodes, used with any of the above options	Postoperative lymphoedema
Radiotherapy	Used with local excision Takes place after surgery Can be a course of 6 weeks	Monitor for fatigue, sore throat, dry cough, nausea and anorexia
Chemotherapy	Can be given: • Before surgery • After surgery • After radiotherapy	Monitor for adverse effects of chemotherapy: • Bone marrow suppression • Nausea and vomiting • Alopecia • Gain or loss of weight • Fatigue • Stomatitis • Anxiety • Depression Discuss changes in diet if needed
Hormone therapy	Used if tumours are oestrogen receptive positive; an example is tamoxifen Aromatase inhibitors Trastuzumab for HER-2-positive breast cancer	Menopausal symptoms Risk of deep vein thrombosis Risk of fractures

Disorders of the male reproductive system

Testicular disorders

Men may present with pain, swelling, infection, inflammation and lumps in the testis, which may have a variety of possible causes. Table 22.9 outlines the nursing care of common testicular disorders.

Testicular cancer

Testicular cancer accounts for 1–1.5% of all cancers in men and is the most common cancer in men between the ages of 15 and 44 years (Cancer Research UK 2011). The two main types of testicular cancer are seminomas and non-seminoma cancers, including teratomas, embryonal carcinomas, choriocarcinomas and yolk sac tumours. Between 40% and 45% of testicular cancers are pure seminomas (Cancer Research UK 2009a).

Box 22.2 Postoperative care following breast surgery

Risk of bleeding
- Observe the wound and dressings (the size of wound varies and depends on the surgical procedure that has been undertaken)
- Monitor:
  - The drain; if used, this may have been placed at the breast wound and/or in the axillary region
  - The vital signs

Pain
- Provide regular analgesia
- Numbness, pins and needles in the axilla are common – reassure the patient

Risk of infection
- Monitor:
  - Temperature and pulse
  - The wound for haematoma or signs of infection
- Remove clips and sutures after 5–10 days as directed
- Wound drains, if present, are removed after postoperative day 2

Profound change in body image and sexual function
- Allow the patient time to discuss fears and concerns
- Refer the patient to a specialist counsellor
- Provide advice on reconstruction or a prosthesis

Arm exercises following dissection of the axillary lymph nodes
- Women are at risk of developing problems with shoulder movement
- There is a need for specific arm exercises, usually taught by a physiotherapist; these can beginning on day 2 postoperatively

Lymphoedema of the arm
- Is a potential complication of axillary surgery and radiotherapy
- Educate patients on:
  - The cause of lymphoedema
  - The signs of lymphoedema
  - Preventing infection in the affected arm:
    - — signs of infection
    - — using gloves when gardening or doing household cleaning
    - — avoiding the use of razors other than electric razors
    - — cleaning any cuts and abrasions with antiseptic solutions
  - Moisturising the affected arm and hand
  - Carrying out arm and shoulder exercises
  - Elevating the affected arm, especially immediately postoperatively
  - Not carrying heavy objects with the affected arm
  - Not wearing heavy shoulder bags on the affected side
  - Avoiding injections, blood testing and the use of a blood pressure cuff on the affected arm

Discharge advice
- Seek medical help if signs of infection develop
- If needed, follow access for ongoing psychological support or support groups
- Attend outpatient follow-up appointments

Table 22.9 Care of common testicular disorders

Patient problems	Nursing care
Pain and swelling due to infection and inflammation	Regular analgesia Supportive underwear Antibiotics Observation for worsening of the condition Discharge advice: • Ensure the scrotum is well supported • Avoid trauma or long periods of standing • Seek medical advice if pain or inflammation worsens after discharge from hospital
Postoperative care following orchidectomy, orchidopexy or hydrocele repair	Risk of bleeding: • Monitor the vital signs, wound and wound drain if present • Observe for haematoma formation Pain: • Assess pain • Provide regular analgesia • Scrotal support or supportive underwear Psychological effects: • Testicular surgery (particularly orchidectomy) may cause fear and anxiety and a change in body image • Support should be offered along with information about local services • Men with a new diagnosis of testicular cancer should be given the details of the key worker, usually the clinical nurse specialist, who will take a lead role in coordinating their care. This promotes continuity of information and advice at different stages of the care pathway Discharge advice: • Check for signs of haematoma and infection and seek medical advice if necessary • Ensure the scrotum is well supported and avoid trauma and long periods of standing • Avoid sports and heavy lifting for 4 weeks or until comfortable • Avoid driving for 2 weeks (until able to safely perform an emergency stop)

Testicular cancer may present as:

- a lump in the testis, often painless;
- an ache in the testis or abdomen;
- breathlessness or backache if the cancer has spread.

Management

Testicular cancer is diagnosed using ultrasound and markers in the blood such as βHCG and AFP. If cancer is suspected, it is likely that the testicle will need to be removed (orchidectomy) (Table 22.9). Other tests such as MRI or computed tomography scans and chest X-rays will be needed to look for signs of spread to the lymph nodes or other organs.

Testicular cancer is primarily treated with orchidectomy (removal of the affected testis). Depending on the type of cancer and whether it has spread, chemotherapy and radiotherapy may also be used. Surgery may be required to remove tumours that have spread to other organs such as the lymph nodes and lungs. Men should be offered sperm storage as treatment may affect their future fertility. Testicular cancer has cure rates of over 95% (Cancer Research UK 2009b).

Testicular pain and swelling

Testicular torsion is a serious and painful condition in which the spermatic cord twists, causing disruption to the testicular blood supply, which may lead to the death of the testicular tissue. Quick surgical exploration is essential. If the testis is still viable, it may be untwisted and fixed to the scrotum (orchidopexy) to prevent recurrence. Otherwise the testis must be removed (orchidectomy).

Other causes of testicular pain and swelling include inflammation and infection. This may affect the epididymis (epididymitis), the testis (orchitis) or both (epididymo-orchitis). The symptoms are similar to those of torsion and a scan may be required to differentiate between the two. Unlike with torsion, the treatment involves analgesia, scrotal support and antibiotics. In severe cases, this will require admission for intravenous treatment.

A non-painful scrotal swelling may indicate a hydrocele, which is an accumulation of fluid between the layers of the tunica vaginalis. If this is painful or uncomfortable, the hydrocele can be drained or removed.

Penile disorders

The penis is made up of three columns of tissue. Two corpora cavernosa run along the dorsum (top) of the penile shaft, and below these two columns lies the corpus spongiosum. The corpus spongiosum surrounds the urethra along the ventral surface (underside) of the penis and forms the glans penis, which is the bulbous head of the penis. The glans is covered by a fold of retractable skin called the prepuce or foreskin, which is attached to the underside of the penis beneath the glans by a band of tissue called the frenulum.

A variety of disorders may affect the penis (Table 22.10). Some are congenital, for example hypospadias and epispadias, in which the urethral opening (meatus) is situated away from the tip of the glans and sometimes even on the shaft of the penis. Other disorders may be the result of trauma, infection, cancer or benign conditions that may develop later in life.

Men may find it difficult to seek help for penile problems due to fear or embarrassment. Changes in body image due to the condition or its treatment may lead to depression, social isolation and sexual and relationship difficulties.

Table 22.10 Care of common penile disorders

Patient problems	Nursing care
Paraphimosis	Be aware of the risk of paraphimosis Replace the foreskin after retraction Observe for paraphimosis after instrumentation (e.g. catheterisation and cystoscopy) or examination
Postoperative care for circumcision	Carries a risk of bleeding so monitor the vital signs and wound Pain: • Regular analgesia • Anaesthetic gel if needed Oedema may require a supportive pad or underwear with the penis held in an upright position Discharge advice • Counselling regarding sensitisation and later desensitisation of the glans • Most men can resume sexual intercourse after 4–6 weeks

Phimosis and paraphimosis

Phimosis describes the condition in which the foreskin cannot be fully retracted over the glans. In paraphimosis, the foreskin becomes stuck behind the glans and cannot be pulled back. This may occur after the foreskin has been retracted for a period of time, for example during catheterisation or other instrumentation, leading to the foreskin becoming swollen and oedematous. Care should always be taken to pull the foreskin forward following examination or catheterisation, and this should be routinely documented when such procedures are performed.

Peyronie's disease

Peyronie's disease is a condition in which scar tissue or plaques form in the tunica albuginea (the fibrous layer of tissue that covers the corpora cavernosa). These plaques can cause pain, an abnormal bend in the penis, erectile dysfunction (ED), indentations in the penis and penile shortening. If the penile bend is causing problems, either psychologically or with intercourse, an operation may be possible to correct it. In the Nesbit procedure, tissue is excised from the area opposite the plaque and the area is sutured. This has the effect of 'shortening' the opposite side and thereby straightening the bend. Alternatively, tissue from, for example, the saphenous vein (the Lue procedure) may be grafted over the incised plaque area, thereby 'lengthening' the side with the defect. A penile prosthesis may be offered to patients with Peyronie's disease and ED.

Penile cancer

Penile cancer is rare and mostly affects men over the age of 60. Symptoms may include growths or sores on the penis that do not heal, bleeding from under the foreskin and a rash or colour change on the penis. The majority of penile cancers (90%) are squamous cell cancers and tend to occur on the glans and foreskin. The likely outcome of treatment depends on how advanced the cancer is when diagnosed. Treatment may include radiotherapy, chemotherapy and surgery. The surgical options are shown in Table 22.11.

Table 22.11 Surgery for penile cancer (Cancer Research UK 2010)

Type of surgery	Description
Circumcision	Suitable if the cancer is only affecting the foreskin
Laser surgery or cryotherapy	Suitable for very early penile cancer Therapies use laser or liquid nitrogen to destroy the cancer cells
Wide local excision	The cancerous area is removed along with a border of healthy tissue This ensures complete removal of the tumour
Glansectomy (removal of the glans)	Removal of the glans followed by a skin graft to reconstruct the head of the penis Sexual function may remain
Penectomy (removal of all or part of the penis)	Performed for extensive cancer A full penectomy is necessary if the cancer is deep or at the base of the penis It may be possible to perform reconstructive surgery
Removal of the lymph nodes	Lymph nodes in the groin may be removed if the surgeon suspects the cancer may have spread

Box 22.3 Postoperative nursing care following penectomy

- Risk of bleeding:
  - Observe the wound and dressings
  - Monitor vital signs
- Risk of oedema – maintain a supportive dressing with mild compression for 24 hours
- Pain – provide regular analgesia
- Risk of infection – monitor temperature
- Inability to pass urine – a urinary catheter should be in place for 48 hours
- Profound change in body image and sexual function:
  - Allow patients time to discuss their fears and concerns
  - Refer to a specialist counsellor
- Discharge advice:
  - Seek medical help if signs of infection develop
  - Provide access for ongoing psychological support

Penile cancer and its treatment can affect sexual function, psychological well-being and quality of life, and may also result in post-traumatic stress disorder (Maddineni *et al.* 2009). The nursing care for men undergoing penectomy is described in Box 22.3. In the UK, men with penile cancer should be referred to specialist centres for treatment and care.

Erectile dysfunction

ED is the inability (persistent or recurrent) to attain and or maintain a penile ejection during sexual performance and is thought to affect around 1 in 10 men in the UK (Sexual Dysfunction Alliance 2011). ED may be due to physical or psychological causes, or a combination of the two.

An erection occurs when physical or psychological stimuli cause arousal and stimulate the parasympathetic nervous system. Neurochemicals act on the smooth muscle walls of the penile blood vessels, causing vasodilation. The flow of blood into the penis increases and fills the corpora cavernosa. This engorgement causes compression of the small veins that drain the blood from the corpora, allowing the corpora to fill and become rigid. The sympathetic nervous system controls ejaculation, after which the penis loses rigidity (detumescence).

Men may have problems attaining or maintaining erections for a number of reasons. An erection is a complex event requiring hormones, nerves and blood vessels to work together. In addition, a low sex drive or psychological issues may lower the ability to become aroused or respond to stimuli. Psychological issues and the stress response may also interfere with parasympathetic nerve pathways.

Management

Men often find it difficult to talk about sexual problems and often wait for months or years before discussing them with health professionals. Unfortunately, they often report that the response when they finally seek help is less than ideal. Nurses may be involved in the care and treatment of men with ED. As such, excellent communication and assessment skills and a non-judgemental attitude are essential. Given that ED is a common problem associated with many common diseases such as diabetes and cardiovascular disease, it is important that nurses are aware of the need to ask about these issues and provide an environment where men feel supported and safe to discuss them.

Management of ED includes lifestyle changes and a number of mechanical or pharmacological interventions to encourage erection (Table 22.12). Men should be counselled that some causes of ED are irreversible and that management options may be required for the long term. The nursing care of men with ED is outlined in Table 22.13.

Table 22.12 Managing ED

Treatment	Description
Lifestyle changes	Weight loss Smoking cessation Review of medication Stopping use of recreational drugs Relaxation Stress-relieving techniques
Oral medication	First-line treatment: • Phosphodiesterase type 5 inhibitors such as sildenafil (Viagra), tadalafil (Cialis) and vardenafil (Levitra) • Inhibition of phosphodiesterase type 5 increases nitrous oxide levels in the penile tissues, improves smooth muscle relaxation and facilitates erection This is contraindicated in men who take nitrate-based medications
Intracavernosal injections	Alprostadil is a prostaglandin that is injected directly into the corpus cavernosum via a fine-bore needle This causes vascular smooth muscle relaxation, inflow of blood into the corpora cavernosa and erection The injection technique can be taught to the man or his partner There is a risk of priapism (prolonged erection)
Intraurethral medication	Alprostadil may be administered via the medicated urethral system for erection This contains higher doses of alprostadil, delivered as a pellet into the urethra with an applicator The alprostadil is absorbed via the urethra and corpus spongiosum
Vacuum constriction device	Vacuum constriction devices are mechanical devices consisting of a cylinder, a manual or battery-powered pump and a constriction ring The man is taught to put the penis inside the cylinder, forming a good seal The pump is operated causing a vacuum inside the cylinder; negative pressure draws blood inside the penis to create an erection The constriction ring is applied at the base of the penis to maintain the erection once the cylinder has been removed
Psychosexual counselling	Techniques used may depend on the presenting factors Examples include behavioural techniques, cognitive techniques, psychotherapy and couple therapy An integrated approach combining medical and psychological therapies is the most effective treatment strategy
Penile prosthesis	A surgical procedure whereby implants are permanently inserted into the corpora cavernosum These may be semi-rigid silicone rods or inflatable sleeves that fill via a pump implanted in the scrotum This is only considered if the previous strategies fail It may also be useful in men with Peyronie's disease who have a severe curvature alongside ED

Table 22.13 Nursing care for men with ED

Area	Nursing care
General awareness and care	Be aware of the causes and risk factors for ED Encourage a sensitive and open discussion of sexual function Refer to specialist services if appropriate
Non-surgical treatments	Counsel regarding the availability and correct use of therapies
Penile prosthesis	Preoperative preparation to reduce risk of infection, as per local protocol Postoperative pain: • Elevate the penis with a scrotal support or pad and pants • Provide regular analgesia Risk of bleeding and infection: • Give prophylactic antibiotics, as per local protocol • Monitor the vital signs • Observe the wound site for bleeding and breakdown Discharge advice: • Seek medical advice if signs of infection, haematoma or erosion (where the prosthesis breaks through the skin) develop • Resume sexual intercourse after 4–6 weeks

Conclusion

The care of women and men with reproductive health issues is complex and multifaceted. This chapter has given an overview of the more common conditions that are seen in the hospital setting.

Visit www.wileyfundamentalseries.com/medicalnursing and read Reflective Questions 22.1 and 22.2 to think more about this topic.

Now visit the companion website and test yourself on this chapter:
www.wileyfundamentalseries.com/medicalnursing

References

Allen, C., Hopewell, S., Prentice, A. *et al.* (2009) Non-steroidal anti-inflammatory drugs for pain in women with endometriosis. *Cochrane Database of Systematic Reviews*, (2):CD004753.

British Association for Sexual Health and HIV (2011) *UK National Guideline for the Management of Pelvic Inflammatory Disease*. Retrieved June 2011 from http://www.bashh.org/guidelines.

Cancer Research UK (2009a) *Testicular Cancer*. Retrieved June 2011 from http://www.cancerhelp.org.uk/type/testicular-cancer/about/types-of-testicular-cancer.

Cancer Research UK (2009b). *Types of Testicular Cancer*. Retrieved June 2011 from http://info.cancerresearchuk.org/cancerstats/types/testis/survival.

Cancer Research UK (2010). *Penile Cancer*. Retrieved June 2011 from http://www.cancerhelp.org.uk/prod_consump/groups/cr_common/@cah/@gen/documents/generalcontent/treating-penile-cancer.pdf.

Cancer Research UK (2011) *Testicular Cancer: UK Incidence Statistics*. Retrieved June 2011 from http://info.cancerresearchuk.org/cancerstats/types/testis/incidence/.

Maddineni, S.B., Lau, M.M. & Sangar, V.K. (2009) Identifying the needs of penile cancer sufferers: a systematic review of the quality of life, psychosexual and psychosocial literature in penile cancer. *BMC Urology*, **8**(9):8.

National Institute for Health and Clinical Excellence (2010) *Uterine Artery Embolisation for Fidroids*. Retrieved June 2011 from http://www.nice.org.uk/nicemedia/live/11025/51706/51706.pdf.

Royal College of Obstetricians and Gynaecologists (2003) *The Investigation and Treatment of Couples with Recurrent Miscarriage*. Guideline No. 17. Retrieved June 2011 from http://www.rcog.org.uk/.

Royal College of Obstetricians and Gynaecologists (2004) *The Management of Tubal Pregnancy*. Retrieved June 2011 from http://www.rcog.org.uk/.

Royal College of Obstetricians and Gynaecologists (2006a) *The Investigation and Management of Endometriosis*. Retrieved June 2011 from http://www.rcog.org.uk/.

Royal College of Obstetricians and Gynaecologists (2006b) *The Management of Early Pregnancy Loss*. Retrieved June 2011 from http://www.rcog.org.uk/.

Royal College of Obstetricians and Gynaecologists (2008) *The Management of Acute Pelvic-Inflammatory Disease*. Green Top Guideline 32. Retrieved June 2011 from http://www.rcog.org.uk/.

Sexual Dysfunction Alliance (2011) *Impotence or Erectile Dysfunction (ED)*. Retrieved June 2011 from http://www.sda.uk.net/ed.

Index

5Ps approach, 444

ABCDE approach, 9, 127–8, 146, 219, 341
abdominal ultrasound, 246
ABGs *see* arterial blood gases
ACEIs *see* angiotensin-converting enzyme inhibitors
acid–base balance, 181
acne, 162–3
  aetiology, 163
  signs and symptoms, 163
  treatment, 163
acoustic neuromas, 345
acquired body defences, 365–6
ACSs *see* acute coronary syndromes
action potentials, 329
acute confusional state *see* delirium
acute coronary syndromes (ACSs), 222, 224–7
  clinical and nursing management, 226–7
  complications, 226
  diagnosis, 220
  differentiation, 225
  signs and symptoms, 225
acute HIV infection/syndrome, 377–8
acute kidney injury (AKI), 284–8, 289, 290
  causes, 285
  classification, 286
  clinical course, 286–7
  management, 287, 289
  nursing management, 287, 290
  signs and symptoms, 286
acute lymphoblastic leukaemia (ALL), 413, 415
acute myeloid leukaemia (AML), 413, 415
acute sinusitis, 458
Addison's crisis, 312
Addison's disease, 308, 310, 312
  causes, 308
  management, 310
  patients on corticosteroids, 312
  symptoms, 310
ADH *see* antidiuretic hormone
adrenal cortex, 308, 310, 311
adrenal glands, 308, 310–14
  disorders, 308, 310–14
  position, 310
adrenal medulla, 308, 310
adrenalectomy, 312, 314
  preoperative and postoperative care, 314
ADRs *see* adverse drug reactions
advanced life support (ALS), 145–6
  guidelines, 147
Advanced Trauma Life Support (ATLS) method, 148
Advanced Trauma Nursing Course, 148
adverse behavioural presentations, 152
adverse drug reactions (ADRs), 13, 24
AEDs, 352, 353
age-related macular degeneration (AMD), 475
  assessment, 475
  management, 475
  signs and symptoms, 475
ageing, 79
agranulocytes, 390–1
AIDS *see* HIV/AIDS
AIDS-associated illnesses, 379
airborne precautions, 73, 75
airway
  assessment, 127
  obstruction, 128
airway maintenance techniques, choice, 109
airway patency, 128–9
AKI *see* acute kidney injury
alcohol, guidelines, 320
ALERT®, 9, 125, 127
ALL, 413, 415
allergens, testing for, 190
allergy identification, 371
alpha cells (A cells), 315
ALS *see* advanced life support; amyotrophic lateral sclerosis
alternative technology, 72
Alzheimer's disease, 82, 359–62
  diagnosis, 360–1
  management, 360–2
  nursing management, 362
  person-centred care, 362
  stages, 361
ambulatory infusion devices, 35
ambulatory monitoring, 220
AMD *see* age-related macular degeneration
AML, 413, 415
amyotrophic lateral sclerosis (ALS), 357
anaemia, 402–8
  causative factors, 402
  management, 402–3
  see also iron deficiency anaemia; macrocytic anaemia; normocytic anaemia
anaesthesia, 108–13
  general, 111
  preparation of environment, 106
  regional, 111
  triad of, 108–9
analgesia, perioperative, 111
anaphylaxis, 21, 24, 370, 371
  prevention, 371
  signs and symptoms, 370, 371
  treatment, 370
angina, 222–4
  clinical and nursing management, 224
  diagnosis, 222
  unstable, 225
angiogenesis, 166
angiopathy, 324
angiotensin-converting enzyme inhibitors (ACEIs), 18, 24
antagonists, definition, 24
antibodies, 393
anticholinergic drugs, in death rattle management, 94
anticonvulsant medications (AEDs), 352, 353
antidiuretic hormone (ADH), 299, 302
  hypersecretion, 302
antigens, 393
antiseptic hand hygiene, 65
  see also aseptic technique
ANTT *see* aseptic non-touch technique
aortic aneurysm, 234–5
  causes, 234
  classification, 234
  clinical and nursing management, 234–5
  fusiform, 234, 235
  investigations, 234
  saccular, 234, 235
  signs and symptoms, 234

Fundamentals of Medical-Surgical Nursing: A Systems Approach, First Edition. Edited by Anne-Marie Brady, Catherine McCabe, and Margaret McCann.

aortic regurgitation, 230–1
aortic stenosis, 230
aplastic anaemia, 406–7
  causes, 406
  diagnosis, 406
  management, 407
appendicitis, 259
  diagnosis, 259
  symptoms, 259
  treatment, 259
appetite, problems affecting, 50, 53
aprons, 68
arachnoid mater, 333
arrhythmias, 227–8
  symptoms, 227
arterial blood gases (ABGs), 182
  analysis, 130, 189
  normal parameters, 130, 183
arterial disease, 235
  clinical and nursing management, 235
  investigations, 235
  signs and symptoms, 235
arteries, 214
arterioles, 214
arteriovenous fistula, 294, 295
arthrodesis, 432
arthroplasty, 433
  see also hip replacement
asepsis, 66
aseptic non-touch technique (ANTT), 66, 113
  points to remember, 70
aseptic technique, 113
assessment
  nursing *see* nursing assessment
  preoperative *see* preoperative assessment
asthma, 196–8
  assessment, 197–8
  clinical manifestations, 196–7
  definition, 196
  diagnosis, 197
  exacerbations management, 197
  management, 197–8
  nursing assessment and management, 198
  pathophysiology, 196
  pharmacological management, 197
  respiratory function tests, 197
  risk factors, 196
  triggers, 196
asystole, 228
atherosclerosis, 221, 222, 235
  development, 223
atherosclerosis obliterans, 235
ATLS *see* Advanced Trauma Life Support (ATLS) method
atrial fibrillation, 227
atrial flutter, 227
auscultation, 129, 133
autoimmunity, 372–5
  patient education, 375
  see also Goodpasture's syndrome; myasthenia gravis; systemic lupus erythematosus
autopsy, 153
AVPU framework, 128, 136
axons, 329

B cells, 366
bacteria, 62
  common sites of commensal, 59
  shapes, 62
bacterial phlebitis, 37
bacterial swabs, 160
bad news, Six Step Protocol for breaking, 97
bariatric surgery, 260
  categories, 260
  nursing management, 260
baseline data, 3, 9
basilic vein, 28
basophils, 390
BBB, 334–5
behavioural disturbance, 152
benign prostatic hyperplasia (BPH), 266, 270, 271
  management, 271
benzodiazepines, in dyspnoea management, 93
beta cells, 315
  destruction, 316
bile, 256
biliary system, 254–7
bilirubin, 389
binding properties, of drugs, 16
bioavailability, 13, 24
  food and, 15–16
biographical data, 5
bladder, 265
bladder cancer, 278–9
  management, 278–9
  muscle invasive, 278, 279
  non-muscle invasive, 278, 279
  risk factors, 278
  signs and symptoms, 278
bladder reconstruction, 279
blockers, definition, 24
blood
  cellular components, 387–90
  functions, 387
  overview, 387–95
blood–brain barrier (BBB), 334–5
blood clotting, 391–3
  clotting cascade, 392
  clotting factors, 393
blood film, 400
blood flow, and drug distribution, 17
blood groups, 393–5
blood plasma *see* plasma
blood pressure, 133, 214
  maintenance in diabetes, 319
  systolic, 133
  see also mean arterial blood pressure
blood products, 398
blood sampling, 396
blood spillage, management, 70
blood supply, 427
blood tests, 220, 249, 399, 400–1
blood transfusion, 39–40, 395–8, 399
  checklist for prescription, 39
  nursing management, 395–7
  reactions, 397, 399
blood vessels, 214
  arterial systems, 216
  layers, 214
  structure, 214, 218
  types, 214
  venous systems, 217
BMI *see* body mass index
body fluid spillage, management, 70
body mass index (BMI), 45–6, 190, 260
bone, 423, 426, 427
  healing stages, 439
  long, 427
  parts of long, 426
  sesamoid, 427
  types of tissue, 423
bone marrow aspiration, 399
  nursing management, 401
bone marrow transplant, 367
bone metastases, 445–6
  diagnosis, 446
  management, 446
bowel clearance, 244
BPH *see* benign prostatic hyperplasia
bradyarrhythmia, 228
  clinical and nursing management, 228
bradykinesia, 359
brain, 329, 331–4
  blood supply, 333, 334
  coverings, 333
  divisions, 331–3
  see also traumatic brain injury
brain abscesses, 354
brain tumours *see* intracranial tumours
brainstem, 333
  tumours, 347
breast disorders, 499–501
  cancer, 499–501
    follow-up, 500
    management, 499
    signs and symptoms, 499
    treatment options, 501
  postoperative care following surgery, 502
breast screening, 498–9
breath sounds
  abnormal, 187
  assessment, 187
breathing assessment, 127
breathing exercises, 190
breathlessness *see* dyspnoea
broad complex tachycardias, 227
bronchiectasis, 203–4
  assessment, 203–4
  clinical manifestations, 203
  diagnosis, 203
  management, 203–4
  pathophysiology, 203
bronchoscopy, 189
bullous pemphigoid, 164–5
  treatment, 165
burns, 148–51
  aetiology, 149
  assessment, 148–9
  depth, 148
  extent, 148
  major, 150
  minor, 151
  treatment, 150–1

CABG, 224, 229
CAD *see* coronary artery disease
cancer pain, management, 95

cancers of digestive system, 251–2
diagnosis, 251
treatment, 251–2
candidiasis, 164
Candida albicans, 380
capillaries, 214
capillary refill, 133
capsid, 62
carbon dioxide, transport, 180, 181–2
cardiac arrest
prevention, 127
rhythms, 228
cardiac pacing, 228
cardiac rhythm, 134
cardiac surgery, 229–30
clinical and nursing management, 229–30
complications, 229
cardiopulmonary resuscitation, 9
cardiovascular assessment, 132–5
history taking, 132
primary data, 132–3
secondary data, 133–4
cardiovascular disease (CVD), deaths from, 211
cardiovascular interventions, 134–5
cardiovascular risk factors, 218–20
assessment, 219
physical assessment, 218–19
cardiovascular system *see* circulatory system
cardioversion, 228
care bundles, 73
care planning, 4
cataract, 476
assessment, 476
discharge education, 476
management, 476
signs and symptoms, 476
CCrISP, 125
cellular immunity, 366
cellulitis, 164
central nervous system (CNS) 327, 328, 331
tumours, 347–9
central venous access devices, 29, 31
central venous catheter (CVC), 56
central venous pressure (CVP)
high, 134
low, 134
monitoring, 133–4
cephalic vein, 28
cerebellum, 332
cerebral angiography, 335
cerebral blood flow tests, 337
cerebrospinal fluid (CSF), 334
colour, 354
cerebrovascular disorders, 347–9
see also strokes
cerebrum, 332
cervical screening, 498, 499
cervix, 479, 480
benign tumours, 484
cancer, 487
CF *see* cystic fibrosis
chemical phlebitis, 37
chemoreceptors, 177
chest pain, assessment, 187
chest X-ray, in high-dependency unit, 130
cholecystectomy, 256
cholecystitis, 256
cholecystokinin, 256
cholelithiasis, 256
cholesterol, in diabetes patients, 319
cholinergic crisis, 373
chronic adrenocortical insufficiency *see* Addison's disease
chronic kidney disease (CKD), 288, 291–3
causes, 288
investigations, 288
management, 288, 293
physiological manifestations of end-stage kidney disease, 292
and renal replacement options, 291
stages of severity, 288, 291
chronic lymphocytic leukaemia (CLL), 413
chronic myeloid leukaemia (CML), 413, 415
chronic obstructive pulmonary disease (COPD), 198–203
acute exacerbations, 200
assessment, 199–203
classification, 198
clinical manifestations, 199
definition, 198
diagnosis, 199
exacerbations management, 200
management, 199–203
nursing assessment and management, 200
care plan, 201–3
palliative care, 200
pathophysiology, 199
risk factors, 199
chronic open angle glaucoma, 473
management, 473
signs and symptoms, 473
chronic sinusitis, 458
assessment, 458
complications, 458
management, 458
circle of Willis, 333, 334
circulating practitioner, role, 113
circulation, assessment, 127–8
circulatory overload, 38
circulatory system, 158, 210–37
anatomy, 211–13
assessment, 218–20
diagnostic investigation, 220–2
physiology, 211–14
see also arrhythmias; blood vessels; cardiac surgery; coronary artery disease; heart; heart failure; valvular heart disease; vascular disorders
circumcision, 504, 505
CJD, 354, 395
CKD *see* chronic kidney disease
claudication, 235
cleaning, 67, 72
definition, 70
clearance
accelerated, 17–18
reduced, 18
clinical observation, 7
clinical waste, 72
CLL, 413
Clostridium botulinum, 354
Clostridium difficile (C. diff), 63
Clostridium tetani, 354
clubbing of fingers, 187
CML, 413, 415
CNS *see* central nervous system
coagulation screen, 400
cohort isolation, 64
Colles' fracture, 441
colloids, 32, 134–5
colonisation, 60
colonoscopy, 248
colorectal cancer, 251
commensalism, 59
communication, at end of life, 96–8
compartment syndrome, 444–5
composite grafts, 169
computed tomography (CT) calcium scoring, 220–1
computed tomography (CT) scanning, gastrointestinal tract, 249
consciousness, disorders of, 342, 344
consent, 105
constipation, 249–50
contact precautions, 73, 74
contamination, definition, 70
continent urinary diversion, 279
continuous infusion, 32
continuous positive airway pressure (CPAP), 131
circuit, 132
continuous subcutaneous infusion (CSCI), 92, 93, 94–5
contraception, 498
Coomb's test, 400
COPD *see* chronic obstructive pulmonary disease
corneal disorders, 473–4
assessment, 474
causes, 474
management, 474
coronary angiography, 222
coronary artery disease (CAD), 222–7
coronary artery bypass grafting (CABG), 224, 229
corticosteroids, 312
nursing care of patients on long-term therapy, 313
corticotrophs, 301
cough, assessment, 184, 186
CPAP *see* continuous positive airway pressure
crackles, 187
cranial neurons, 336
cretinism, 303
Creutzfeldt–Jakob disease (CJD), 354, 395
critical care, 125
classification of critically ill patients, 125
in emergency department, 152–3
see also high-dependency care; intensive care
Crohn's disease, 257
cryoprecipitate, 398
Cryptococcus neoformans, 380
Cryptosporidium, 381
crystalloids, 32, 134–5
CSCI, 92, 93, 94–5
CSF *see* cerebrospinal fluid
CSF barrier, 334–5
CT angiography (CTA), 337
CT calcium scoring, 220–1
CT scanning *see* computed tomography (CT) scanning

CURB65 score, 194
Cushing's syndrome, 312, 314
  causes, 314
  management, 312, 314
  signs and symptoms, 312
CVC *see* central venous catheter
CVD *see* cardiovascular disease
CVP *see* central venous pressure
cyanosis, 129
cystectomy, 279
  management, 279
  postoperative nursing management, 282–3
  preoperative nursing management, 281
cystic fibrosis (CF), 204
  assessment, 204
  clinical manifestations, 204
  diagnosis, 204
  management, 204
  pathophysiology, 204
  respiratory-specific care, 204
cystitis, 280
  complicated, 284
  uncomplicated, 280, 284
cytomegalovirus (CMV), 381

damp dusting, 114
death rattle, 93–4
  nursing management, 93–4
  pharmacological management, 94
  type 1, 93
  type 2, 93
DECIDE model, 99, 100
decontamination, 66–72
  definition, 70
  of environment, 67
  of equipment, 67
deep vein thrombosis, perioperative risk, 107
defibrillators, 228
dehydration, 38
  prevention, 38
  treatment, 38
delirium, 82–3, 137
  definition, 82
  risk factors, 83
  types, 83
delta cells (D cells), 315
dementia, 81–3
  definition, 82
  with Lewy bodies, 82
  types, 82
  see also Alzheimer's disease
demyelination plaques, 355
dendrites, 329
dermis, 157–8
designated ward-specific precautions, 64
deviated nasal septum, 458–9
  assessment, 458
  management, 459
  signs and symptoms, 458
diabetes insipidus, 302
diabetes mellitus, 315–24
  diagnosis, 316
  type 1, 316–17, 318–19, 321
    characteristics, 318
    exercise modifications, 321
    medications, 321
  type 2, 317–24
    'ABC' of, 319
    characteristics, 318–19
    complications, 322–4
    dietary modifications, 320
    exercise modifications, 320–1
    goal-setting, 317, 319–20
    management, 317
    medications, 321
    nursing interventions, 319–20
    self-monitoring of blood glucose, 322
  see also hypoglycaemia
diabetic foot ulcers, classification, 167
diabetic ketoacidosis (DKA), 317, 322
diabetic retinopathy, 323, 473
  management, 473
dialysis *see* haemodialysis; peritoneal dialysis
diarrhoea, 250
diencephalon, 333
dietary advice, 192
dietary assessment, 47
dietary guidelines, 48
dietitian, referral to, 46
digestive system, 240–60
  conditions of, 249–53
  diagnostic investigations, 246–9
  functions, 241
  nursing assessment, 241–2
  nursing care, 242–6
    communication, 242
    elimination, 243
    hydration, 243
    mobilisation, 244
    nutrition, 243
    observations, 242
    pain relief, 243
    perioperative management, 244–5
    postoperative management, 244–5
    preparation for interventions, 243
    psychosocial support, 244
  organs, 241
  see also appendicitis; bariatric surgery; biliary system; irritable bowel disease
digital rectal examination (DRE), 266
direct intermittent injection, 32–3
disability, assessment, 128
discharge planning, 4
dishes, washing, 71
disinfectant, definition, 70
disinfection, 67
  definition, 70
disseminated intravascular coagulation, 410
disseminated sclerosis *see* multiple sclerosis
diverticulitis, 257
DKA, 317, 322
domestic waste, 72
Doppler ultrasonography, 160
dressings, 35
drop rate, 33
droplet precautions, 73, 75
drug absorption, 14
drug administration
  oral, 14–16
    crushing/breaking tablets, 15
    on empty stomach, 15
    with food, 15–16
  principles, 13–21
drug distribution, 16–17
drug elimination, 17–18
drug excretion, 18–20
drug–food interactions, 15–16
drug formulation, 13
  liquids vs solids, 13
drug metabolism, 17–18
duodenal ulcers, 252
dura mater, 333
dying
  nature of, 91
  see also end of life care
dyskinesia, 359
dyspnoea, 92–3
  assessment, 184, 186
  non-pharmacological management, 93
  oxygen, 92
  pharmacological interventions, 92–3
dystonia, 359

ear, 451–5
  anatomy, 451
  external, 451
  inner, 451
  middle, 451
  otitis media, 454
  perioperative care, 455
  physiology, 455
  postoperative nursing management, 455
  surgery, 455
  trauma, 453–4
    assessment, 454
    causes, 453
    nursing management, 454
    signs and symptoms, 453
  see also hearing impairment; Ménière's disease
Early Warning Score (EWS), 7–8, 118
  physiological parameters, 121
eating utensils, washing, 71
ECG *see* electrocardiogram
echocardiography, 221
ECM, 166
ectopic pregnancy, 492–3
  management, 492–3
  patient information, 492–3
eczema, 161
  aetiology, 161
  signs and symptoms, 161
  treatment, 161
ED *see* erectile dysfunction
EEG, 337–8
electrocardiogram (ECG), 212, 220
  ambulatory devices, 220
  electrode placement, 221
electroencephalogram (EEG), 337–8
electromyogram (EMG), 337
elimination half-life, 19
emergency care, 142–53
  adverse behavioural presentations, 152
  critically ill and dying patients, 152–3
  historical context, 143
  minor trauma, 148
  patient assessment, 145–6
  pre-hospital, 146

see also burns; emergency trauma; head injuries; medical emergencies; surgical emergencies
emergency trauma, 146
assessment, 148
treatment, 148
EMG, 337
emollients, 160
empiric precautions, 64
encephalitis, 353–4
end of life care, 90–101
comfort at end of life, 91–6
communication at end of life, 96–8
ethics and, 99–100
end-stage kidney disease, physiological manifestations, 292
endocrine system, 298–325
location of organs, 300
see also adrenal glands; hypothalamus; pancreas; pituitary gland; thyroid gland
endocrinology, 299
endometrial cancer, 488
endometriosis, 490–1
management, 490–1
patient information, 491
symptoms, 490
endoscopic retrograde cholangiopancreatography (ERCP), 248, 256
endoscopy, 246, 248–9
endotracheal intubation, 109
preparation, 110
ENT conditions
assessment tools, 449
diagnostic investigations, 449–50
see also ear; nose; throat
enteral, definition, 24
enteral tube feeding, 53–6
feeds, 55
gastrostomy tubes, 53, 54, 55
methods of providing feed, 55–6
nasogastric, 53
patient monitoring, 56
postpyloric, 53, 54, 55
enteric-coated preparations, 15, 24
enterococci, 63
glycopeptide-resistant, 63
eosinophils, 390
ependymal cells, 328
epidermis, 157
epidural anaesthesia, 111, 112
epiglottis, 461
epilepsy, 349–53
classification, 351
diagnosis, 352, 353
management, 352–3
signs of seizures, 351
see also seizures
epistaxis, 456–7
assessment, 456–7
causes, 456
management, 457
nursing care following nasal pack insertion, 457
epithelialisation, 166
EPs, 337–8
equipment, 67, 72
decontamination, 67
ERCP, 248, 256
erectile dysfunction (ED), 506–8
management, 275, 506–7
nursing care, 508
erythrocyte sedimentation rate (ESR), 400
erythrocytes (red blood cells), 388–9
reference values, 389
transfusion, 398
erythropoiesis, 389
ESR, 400
Ethical Grid Model, 99
ethics, and end of life care, 99–100
evoked potentials (EPs), 337–8
EWS see Early Warning Score
excipients, 13, 24
excretion, renal, 288, 302
see also drug excretion
exercise, and deep breathing, 190
exercise tolerance test, 220
exocrine glands, 299
exposure, assessment, 128
extracellular matrix (ECM), 166
extraocular structures, 469
extravasation, 37–8
eye, 469–77
anatomy, 469, 471
physiology, 469, 472
surgery, 476–7
trauma, 474–5
assessment, 475
causes, 474
management, 475
signs and symptoms, 474–5
see also age-related macular degeneration; cataract; corneal disorders; diabetic retinopathy; glaucoma; retinal detachment; visual impairment
eye conditions
assessment tools, 449
diagnostic investigations, 449–50
eye-opening, 136
eye protection, choice, 69

F cells, 315
face protection
choice, 69
masks, 69
face shields, 69
fading away, transition of, 98
falls, 86–7
definition, 86
interventions to prevent, 87
risk factors, 87
families, of dying patients, 98
FAST assessment, 348
FBC, 400
female reproductive system, 479–82
anatomy, 479, 480
disorders, 482–501
benign tumours, 483–6
see also breast disorders; endometriosis; gynaecological cancers; gynaecological surgery; menstrual disorders; pelvic inflammatory disease; prolapse; termination of pregnancy; unplanned pregnancy loss
health promotion, 498–9
FGHHI mnemonic, 146
fibrinogen clot formation, 391–2
fibrinolysis, 165
fibroids, 483–5
management, 485
signs and symptoms, 483
filtrate, 265
fingertip units (FTUs), 160
fluid replacement therapy, 99, 134–5
follicle stimulating hormone (FSH), 480–1, 482
folliculitis, 163
food, and bioavailability, 15–16
fracture injuries, 437–41
bone healing stages, 439
classification, 439
complications, 440–1
interventions to treat, 440
patient information, 441
types of fracture, 438
see also hip fracture
freezing, 359
FSH, 480–1, 482
full blood count (FBC), 400
fungal infections, 63
fungi, 62–3

gallbladder, 256
conditions affecting, 256
gallstones, 256
gamma knife surgery, 353
ganglia, 329
gas exchange, 180–1, 182
gastric ulcers, 252
gastrointestinal surgery, 244–6
gastrointestinal tract, body defences, 366
gastrostomy tubes, 53, 54, 55
GCS see Glasgow Coma Scale
genitourinary tract, body defences, 366
germ cell tumours, 346
gestational diabetes, 324
gestational trophoblastic disease, 491
GFR see glomerular filtration rate
Glasgow Coma Scale (GCS), 7, 128, 136–7, 151–2, 338–9
documentation, 338
Glasgow Coma Score, 339
glaucoma, 471–3
chronic open angle, 473
primary acute angle closure, 471–3
glia see neuroglia
gliomas, 345
glomerular filtration rate (GFR), 18, 25
glomerulus, 264–5
gloves, 68
glycated haemoglobin test, 319
glycopeptide-resistant enterococci, 63
glycopyrolate, in death rattle management, 94

goggles, 69
gonadotrophs, 299, 301
Goodpasture's syndrome, 372
  management, 372
  signs and symptoms, 372
gowns, 68
graft-versus-host disease, 367
Gram-negative microorganisms, 62
Gram-positive microorganisms, 60, 62, 63
Gram stain, 62
granulation tissue, 166
granulocytes, 390
Graves' disease, 306, 372
gravity infusion devices, 33
grey matter, 329
gynaecological cancers, 486–9
  nursing management, 489
  preoperative patient education, 489
gynaecological surgery
  nursing care, 495–6
  postoperative nursing management, 495
  preoperative nursing management, 495
  see also hysterectomy

H2-receptor antagonists, 15
haemangioblastomas, 345
haematological disorders, 395–421
  investigations, 397–401
  see also anaemia; blood transfusion; disseminated intravascular coagulation; haematopoietic stem cell transplant; haemophilia; leukaemia; lymphoma; multiple myeloma; polycythaemia; thrombocytopenia
haematological system, 387–95
  see also blood
haematopoietic stem cell transplant (HSCT), 417, 419–20
  complications, 420
  sources of cells, 419
  types, 417
haemodialysis, 291, 293, 294, 295
haemoglobin, 389
  measurement, 400
haemoglobin electrophoresis, 401
haemolysis, 389
haemolytic disease of the newborn, 394
haemolytic-uraemic syndrome, 409
haemophilia, 409
haemopoiesis, 388
haemoptysis, 184
haemorrhagic stroke, 348
hand hygiene, 64–5
  5 Moments for, 65, 66
  antiseptic/aseptic, 65, 113
  how to hand-rub, 68
  how to handwash, 67
  social, 64–5, 113
  surgical hand antisepsis, 65
HBGM, 322
HDU *see* high-dependency care
head injuries, 151–2
  classification, 151
  follow-up on discharge, 152
health history, obtaining, 5, 6–7
healthcare non-risk waste, 72
healthcare risk waste, 72
healthcare waste management, 72
hearing impairment, 451–3
  assessment, 452
  causes, 452
  communication with individuals with, 453
  nursing management, 452–3
heart, 211–14
  anatomy, 211–13
  blood flow through, 214, 215
  conduction system, 213
  coronary circulation, 212
  internal structures, 211
  physiology, 211–14, 215
  regulation, 214
  see also arrhythmias; cardiac surgery; coronary artery disease; valvular heart disease
heart failure, 232–4
  causes, 232
  clinical and nursing management, 233–4
    acute heart failure, 233
    chronic heart failure, 233–4
  diagnosis, 233
  investigations, 233
  medication, 233
  signs and symptoms, 232
heart rate, measurement, 133
Helicobacter pylori, and peptic ulcers, 252, 253
hepatitis, 255
herpes simplex type 1, 62
herpes zoster, 62, 164
HHS, 322–3
high-dependency care, 124–38
  current policy, 125
  environment, 125
  interdisciplinary team, 127
  monitoring equipment, 126
  nurse to patient ratio, 125
  nursing assessment and monitoring, 127–8
  role of nurse, 126
  technological developments, 126
  see also cardiovascular assessment; cardiovascular interventions; neurological assessment; neurological interventions; respiratory assessment; respiratory interventions
highly active antiretroviral therapy (HAART), 378–9
hip fracture, 443–4
  classification, 443
  complications, 444
  diagnosis, 443
  management, 443–4
hip replacement, 433
  nursing intervention, 434–5
HIV/AIDS, 375–84
  antiretroviral medication, 379
  family and patient education, 383
  management, 378–83
    body temperature, 382
    fatigue, 383
    impaired skin integrity, 383
    neurological status, 382
    nutritional status, 382–3
    psychological support, 381–2
    respiratory status, 382
  neurological system infections caused, 354
  nursing care, 379
  occupational infection, 377
  opportunistic infections in persons with, 380–1
  prevention, 384
  risk behaviours for contracting HIV, 376
  stages, 377–8
    AIDS, 378
    HIV asymptomatic stage, 378
    HIV symptomatic stage, 378
    primary infection, 377–8
  strains of HIV, 375
  transmission of HIV, 375–7
    sexual, 376
    vertical, 377
    via blood and body fluids, 376–7
HLAs *see* human leucocyte antigens
Hodgkin's disease, 415
holmium laser enucleation of the prostate (HoLEP), 271
Homan's sign, 236
home blood glucose monitoring (HBGM), 322
hormone deprivation therapy, 274, 275
HSCT *see* haematopoietic stem cell transplant
human immunodeficiency virus *see* HIV/AIDS
human leucocyte antigens (HLAs), 366, 367
  typing, 401
humoral immunity, 366
hydration
  artificial, withdrawal/withholding, 99–100
  and respiration, 192
hyoscine butylbromide, in death rattle management, 94
hyoscine hydrobromide, in death rattle management, 94
hyperactive delirium, 83
hypercapnia, 177
hyperglycaemia, 315
hyperkalaemia, management, 289
hyperosmolar hyperglycaemic syndrome (HHS), 322–3
hypersensitivity reactions, 13, 21, 25, 370, 371
  types, 371
hyperthyroidism, 306–7, 308, 309
  complications after surgery, 310
  effects, 307
  management, 307, 309
  treatment options, 308
hyphaema, 475
hypoactive delirium, 83
hypocapnia, 177
hypoglycaemia, 322, 323–4
  symptoms, 322
  treatment, 323–4
hypopharynx, 460
hypothalamus, 299–303
  hormones synthesised, 299
hypothermia, 134
  perioperative risk, 107

hypothyroidism, 303, 305–6
effects, 307
management, 305
patient education on, 306
primary, 305
secondary, 305
signs and symptoms, 305
hypoxaemia, 177
detection, 130
hysterectomy, 495, 496, 497–8
postoperative nursing care, 497

IBD *see* irritable bowel disease
ICP *see* intracranial pressure
ICU *see* intensive care
idiopathic diabetes, 316
idiopathic thrombocytopenic purpura (ITP), 409
immune system, 364–84
body defences preventing pathogenic organism entry, 366
parts, 365
see also anaphylaxis; autoimmunity; HIV/AIDS; hypersensitivity reactions; organ transplant
immunoglobin (Ig), 366
immunosuppressant medications, 369
infection
colonisation vs, 60
control
perioperative, 113–14
principles, 64–6
see also asepsis; care bundles; decontamination; isolation of patients
cycle of, 61
endemic/epidemic exogenous environmental, 60
endogenous, 60
exogenous/cross-, 60
fungal, 63
healthcare-associated, definition, 59
physiology associated, 59–62
presentation, 60
transmission, 60
infectious agents, 61
transmission, 61
infiltration, 37
infusion devices, 33–5
infusion rates, calculation, 35–6
innate body defences, 365
inotropic support, 135
inspection
in cardiovascular assessment, 132–3
in neurological assessment, 136
in respiratory assessment, 129
insulin therapy, 321
integrated care pathways, 107
intensive care, 125
nurse to patient ratio, 125
intermittent infusion, 32
International Prostate Symptom Score, 271
interviewing, 6–7
intima media, 27
intracoronary stenting, 224
intracranial pressure (ICP)
raised, 340–3
nursing management of patients with, 342–3
symptoms, 340
intracranial tumours, 343–7
classification, 344
examples, 345–6
management, 347
nursing management, 347
intraocular structures, 469, 471
intraoperative care plans, 107
intravenous drug (IVD) use, and HIV transmission, 377
intravenous therapy
administration, 30–5
methods, 31–3
nurse's responsibilities, 32
principles, 33
changing equipment, 36
infection prevention, 35–6
maintaining closed intravenous system, 36
maintaining patency, 36
managing complications, 36–9
preparation, 30–1
principles, 26–40
see also blood transfusion
intubation, 110
see also endotracheal intubation
iron deficiency anaemia, 404–5
causes, 404
diagnosis, 404
management, 405
irritable bowel disease (IBD), 257–9
complications, 258
diagnosis, 258
nursing management, 258
treatment, 258
ischaemic stroke, 348, 349
islets of Langerhans, 315
isolation of patients, 72–3, 74–5
cohort, 64
definition, 72
signage, 73
transmission-based precautions, 72–3, 74–5
ITP, 409

joints, 49, 427
synovial, 427, 429
types, 427

Kaposi's sarcoma, 381
keratitis, 473–4
key parts, 66
key sites, 66
kidney, 263–6
functions, 265, 266
macroscopic structure, 263–4
microscopic structure, 264–5
kidney cancer, 275–6
management, 275–6
signs and symptoms, 275
see also nephrectomy
knee, with osteoarthritis, 431

lactotrophs, 301
laparoscopy, 249
laryngeal cancer, 464–5
assessment, 465
risk factors, 464
signs and symptoms, 464
see also laryngectomy
laryngeal mask airway (LMA), 109–10
preparation, 110
laryngeal obstruction, 461–2
assessment, 462
causes, 461
management, 462
signs and symptoms, 462
laryngectomy, 464, 466, 470
nursing management following, 470
laryngoscopy, 110–11
larynx, 460–1
lateral position, 115
laundry, 71
left ventricular failure, 232
leucocytes (white blood cells), 390–1
leukaemia, 413–15, 418–19
causes, 414
classification, 413
diagnosis, 414
management, 415
nursing management, 418–19
signs and symptoms, 414
Lewy bodies, 358
LH, 481, 482
ligaments, 427
linen, 71
lipid solubility, 16
lithotomy position, 115
liver, 254–6
conditions affecting, 255–6
diagnosis, 255
nursing management, 255–6
treatment, 255
functions, 254
LMA *see* laryngeal mask airway
loading dose, 20, 25
lumbar puncture, 338, 354
Lund and Browder chart, 148, 150
lung cancer, 206–8
assessment, 207–8
classification, 207
clinical manifestations, 207
communication, 208
definition, 206
diagnosis, 207
epidemiology, 206
management, 207–8
nursing management, 208
palliative care, 208
risk factors, 207
lungs, anatomy, 179
lupus *see* systemic lupus erythematosus
luteinising hormone (LH), 481, 482
lymphatic system, 158, 365
lymphocytes, 366, 390
lymphoma, 415–17, 418–19
classification, 415, 416
diagnosis, 416
management, 417
nursing management, 418–19

signs and symptoms, 415
staging, 416, 417

macrocytic anaemia, 405–6
macroglia, 328
macrophages, 390–1
magnetic resonance angiography (MRA), 337
male reproductive system, 482, 483
disorders, 501–8
see also penile disorders; testicular disorders
malnutrition, 45–8
ongoing adverse effects, 48
Manchester Triage System, 143
MAP, 133
mask with Venturi valve, 190, 192
mastalgia, 500
mastitis, 500
mastoidectomy, 455
mean arterial blood pressure (MAP), 133
measles, 354
mechanical phlebitis, 35, 37
medical emergencies, 145
medications
assessment, 188
interventions to increase adherence, 86
non-adherence, 85
and older people, 83–6
'rights' of administration, 85
side effects, 49
memory B lymphocytes, 391
menarche, 479
Ménière's disease, 454–5
assessment, 454
nursing management, 454–5
signs and symptoms, 454
meninges, 333
meningiomas, 346
meningitis, 353, 354
menopause, 480
menstrual cycle, 479–82
menstrual disorders, 482–3
mesenchyme, 387
metabolic acidosis, management, 289
metacarpal veins, 28
methicillin-resistant *Staphylococcus aureus* (MRSA), 63
MEWS *see* modified early warning system
microcytic anaemia *see* iron deficiency anaemia
microglia, 328
microorganisms (microbes)
overview, 62–3
pathogenic, frequently encountered, 63
resident/endogenous, 59
transient/exogenous, 59
see also bacteria; viruses
micturition, 265
mini-strokes, 348, 349
miscarriage, 491–2
causes, 491
management, 492
mitral stenosis, 231
mitral valve prolapse, 231
mitral valve regurgitation, 231
mixed delirium, 83
MND *see* motor neuron disease
mobilisation, and chest clearance, 190
modified early warning system (MEWS), 118, 125, 126
monocytes, 391
morphine, in pain management at end of life, 96
motor neuron disease (MND), 356–8
diagnosis, 357–8
management, 357–8
nursing care, 358
types, 357
motor response, 136
MRSA, 63
MS *see* multiple sclerosis
multi-drug resistant (MDR) TB, 195
multiple myeloma, 410–12
medical management, 411
nursing priorities, 412
signs and symptoms, 411
multiple sclerosis (MS), 355–6
diagnosis, 355–6
management, 355–6
medical therapies, 356
nursing care, 356
signs and symptoms, 355
types, 355
muscle, 426–7, 428–9
functions, 427
skeletal, 426–7, 429
superficial skeletal, 428
types of tissue, 426–7
muscle biopsy, 338
musculoskeletal system, 422–46
anatomy, 423–30
physiology, 423–30
see also orthopaedic conditions; skeletal system
myasthenia gravis, 372–3
management, 373
signs and symptoms, 373
myasthenic crisis, 373
Mycobacterium avium, 380
Mycobacterium tuberculosis, 194
myelin sheath, 329
myocardial necrosis, 220
myocardial perfusion imaging, 222
myocardium, 211
myomectomy, 485, 486, 496
myringoplasty, 455
myringotomy, 455

nails, healthcare workers', 71
narrow complex tachycardias, 227
nasal cannula, 190, 191
nasal injuries, 459–60
assessment, 459
management, 459–60
signs and symptoms, 459
nasal packing, 457
nasal tumours, 460, 461
causes, 460
management, 460
nursing management after removal, 461
signs and symptoms, 460
nasogastric tubes (NGTs), 53, 54
risks of insertion, 53
nasojejunal tube, 55
nasopharynx, 460
national early warning score (NEWS), 126
nausea, 250–1
postoperative, 121
nebulisers, 190
nephrectomy, 276–8
postoperative care, 276–7
preoperative care, 276
nephrogenic diabetes insipidus, 302
nephrology, 263
nephron, 264–5
nephropathy, 324
nerve supply, 427
nerves *see* neurons
neurogenic diabetes insipidus, 302
neuroglia, 327, 328
neurological assessment, 135–7
history-taking, 135
primary data, 136–7
neurological interventions, 137–8
neurological system, 326–62
anatomy, 327–36
cells, 327–9
infections, 353–5
diagnosis, 354
management, 354–5
nursing management, 354–5
interventions, 337–8
nursing assessment, 338–40
physiology, 327–36
see also Alzheimer's disease; cerebrovascular disorders; epilepsy; intracranial tumours; motor neuron disease; multiple sclerosis; Parkinson's disease; traumatic brain injury
neurons, 327, 329, 330–1
components, 329, 330
types, 331
neuropathy, 324
neurophysiology tests, 337–8
neurostimulation therapy, 353
neurovascular assessment, 444–5
neutrophil count, 400
neutrophils, 390
NEWS, 126
NGTs *see* nasogastric tubes
NHL, 415, 416
nipple problems, 500
NIPPV *see* non-invasive positive-pressure ventilation
NIV *see* non-invasive ventilation
nocturia, 270
nodes of Ranvier, 329
non-Hodgkin's lymphoma (NHL), 415, 416
non-invasive positive-pressure ventilation (NIPPV), 131–2
non-invasive ventilation (NIV), 131–2
use assessment, 188
see also continuous positive airway pressure; non-invasive positive-pressure ventilation; oxygen therapy
non-shockable rhythms, 228
non-small cell lung cancer (NSCLC), 207
non-ST elevation myocardial infarction (NSTEMI), 225
clinical and nursing management, 226, 227

non-steroidal anti-inflammatory drugs (NSAIDs), 18, 25
CSCI administration, 95
normocytic anaemia, 406–8
see also aplastic anaemia; sickle cell anaemia
nose, 455–60
anatomy, 455–6
bleed *see* epistaxis
physiology, 455–6
see also chronic sinusitis; deviated nasal septum; nasal injuries; nasal tumours
NSAIDs *see* non-steroidal anti-inflammatory drugs
NSTEMI *see* non-ST elevation myocardial infarction
nuclear medicine scans, 247
nurse–patient relationship, 184
nursing action plans, 46
nursing assessment, 2–11
documenting, 9–10
frameworks, 4–6
in high-dependency unit, 127–8
methods, 6–8
and older adult, 80–1
purpose, 3–4
rapid, 8–9
tools, 7–8, 81
see also patient assessment
nutrition
artificial, withdrawal/withholding, 99–100
and pressure ulcer prevention/ management, 172
Nutrition Screening Week, 48
nutritional assessment, 46–7
nutritional care, 44–57
calculating nutritional requirements, 47–8
dietary guidelines, 48
effect of illness on nutrition, 48–9
effect of surgery on nutrition, 51
nursing action plans, 46
refeeding syndrome, 49–51
nutritional screening, 45
nutritional support, 51–6
nursing responsibility for oral nutrition, 52
parenteral feeding, 56
supplementing oral intake, 52
see also enteral tube feeding

obesity, 260
oesophago-gastroduodenoscopy, 248
oestrogen, 481–2
OLD CARTS mnemonic, 158
older people, 78–88
in acute care setting, 79–80
care of person with confusion, 81–3, 84
caring for people in later life, 79
falls *see* falls
health problem examples, 81
medications and, 83–6
nursing assessment and, 80–1
physiological changes, 84
rights, 79
'on-off' phenomenon, 359
opioids
in dyspnoea management, 92
in pain management at end of life, 95–6
optic neuritis, 355
oral hypoglycaemic agents, 321
oral nutrition, nursing responsibility for, 52
orchidectomy, 503
organ transplant, 367–70
graft rejection, 368–9
forms, 368
management, 368–9
signs and symptoms, 368–9
increased risk of infection, 367
management, 367–70
nursing interventions to prevent infection, 368
preparation for discharge, 370
psychological issues, 369
types, 367
see also bone marrow transplant
oropharynx, 460
orthopaedic conditions, 430–45
neurovascular assessment, 444–5
plaster cast care, 444–5
see also bone metastases; fracture injuries; hip fracture; osteoarthritis; osteoporosis; rheumatoid arthritis
ossiculoplasty, 455
osteoarthritis, 430–4
diagnosis, 431
factors predisposing to, 431
nursing intervention in total hip replacement, 433–4
postoperative care, 435
preparation for surgery, 435
radiological investigation, 432
surgical management, 432–4
treatment protocol, 432–3
osteogenesis imperfecta, 437
osteomyelitis, 434–5
diagnosis, 435
local symptoms, 435
surgical intervention, 435
treatment, 435
osteoporosis, 441–3
drugs used in prevention and treatment, 442
prevention, 443
risk factors, 442
osteotomy, 432
otitis media, 454
ovarian cancer, 488
ovarian cysts, 485–6
assessment, 486
management, 486
signs and symptoms, 486
ovaries, 479
benign tumours, 484
overfeeding, 47
overweight, definition, 260
oxygen
administration, 190, 191–2
transport, 180–1, 182
use assessment, 188
oxygen delivery systems
high-flow, 131
low-flow, 131
oxygen mask, 190, 192
oxygen therapy, 131
oxyhaemoglobin, 389
pacemakers, 228
PACU *see* post-anaesthetic care unit
pain, at end of life, 94–5
pain management
at end of life, 94–6
in high-dependency care, 137–8
in recovery, 121–2
pain thermometer, 8
palliative care
chronic obstructive pulmonary disease, 200
lung cancer, 208
palpation, 129, 133
pancreas, 256–7, 314–24
conditions affecting, 257
diagnosis, 257
nursing management, 257
treatment, 257
disorders, 315–24
see also diabetes mellitus
location, 315
pancreatitis, 257
papillary carcinoma, 306–7
paralytic ileus, 246
paraphimosis, 504, 505
parathyroid glands, 303, 304
parenteral feeding, 56
parenteral therapy, 27
see also intravenous therapy
Parkinson's disease, 358–9, 360
management, 359
nursing assessment, 359
pharmacological management, 360
signs and symptoms, 358–9
patch testing, 160
patency, 36
maintaining, 36
patient assessment, 5
in emergency department, 145–6
see also nursing assessment
patient movement, 64
patient placement, 64
patient self-assessment tools, 8
patient transfer, 64
PCI, 224
peak expiratory flow (PEF), measurement, 188
pelvic inflammatory disease (PID), 493–4
causes, 494
management, 494
patient information, 494
signs and symptoms, 494
penectomy, 505, 506
penile disorders, 504–8
cancer, 505–6
nursing care, 506
surgery for, 505–6
nursing care, 504
paraphimosis, 504, 505
Peyronie's disease, 505
phimosis, 505
see also erectile dysfunction
peptic ulcer disease, 252–3
clinical features, 252
common sites, 252
complications, 252–3
percussion, 129, 133

percutaneous coronary intervention (PCI), 224
percutaneous endoscopic gastrojejunostomy, 55
percutaneous endoscopic gastrostomy (PEG) tube, 53, 55
percutaneous nephrolithotomy, 270
percutaneous transluminal coronary angioplasty (PTCA), 224
perfusion (Q), 182
pericardium, 211
perikaryon, 329
perioperative care, 104–22
accountability, 114–15
circulating practitioner role, 113
diagnosis, 253
general issues, 105–7
infection control, 113–14
nursing management, 253
patient positioning, 115
patient safety, 107–8
risks, 111–13
scrub practitioner role, 113
temperature management, 107
treatment, 253
see also anaesthesia; preoperative assessment; recovery
peripheral devices, 29
peripheral nervous system (PNS), 327, 328, 331
peripheral vascular disease, 235–7
peritoneal dialysis (PD), 291, 293, 294, 296
peritonitis, 244, 253, 259
person-centred care, 362
personal protective equipment (PPE), 65–6, 114
how to choose, 68–9
Peyronie's disease, 505
pH regulation, 181
phacoemulsification, 476
pharmacokinetics, 13–21
pharynx *see* throat
phimosis, 505
phlebitis, 35, 36–7
bacterial, 37
chemical, 37
mechanical, 35, 37
see also thrombophlebitis
physical examination, 7
physiological changes, age-related, 84
pia mater, 333
PID *see* pelvic inflammatory disease
pitting oedema, 187
pituitary gland, 299–303
disorders, 302
hormones produced, 299, 301, 302
pituitary tumours, 345
plasma, 393
components, 394
transfusion, 398
plasma cells, 390–1
plasma protein binding, 16
plaster cast care, 444–5
platelet plug formation, 391
platelets (thrombocytes), 391
transfusion, 398
pleural friction, 187
PMA, 357
PNES, 352
Pneumocystis jiroveci, 380
pneumonia, 193–4
assessment, 194
classification, 193
clinical manifestations, 193
diagnosis, 194
management, 194
nursing assessment and management, 194
pathophysiology, 193
PNS *see* peripheral nervous system
polycythaemia, 408
polydendrocytes, 328
polypharmacy, 86
definition, 86
PONV *see* postoperative nausea and vomiting
portal of entry, 61
portal of exit, 61
positioning, and lung function, 190, 191
post-anaesthetic care unit (PACU), 117–18
postoperative care, nutrition, 52
postoperative nausea and vomiting (PONV), 121
postpyloric feeding, 53, 54, 55
PPE *see* personal protective equipment
PQRST chest pain assessment tool, 222, 223
preoperative assessment, 105–6
preoperative care, nutrition, 51
pressure ulcers, 170–2
categories, 167
definition, 170
impact of external mechanical forces on tissue viability, 170
nutrition in prevention/management, 172
prevention, 171–2
risk assessment, 171
tools, 8
skin care and, 172
primary acute angle closure glaucoma, 471–3
assessment, 471–2
management, 472–3
signs and symptoms, 471
primary assessment, 146, 148
primary cerebral lymphomas, 346
primary lateral sclerosis, 357
primitive neuroectodermal tumours, 346
proctoscopy, 248
progesterone, 481–2
progressive bulbar palsy, 357
progressive muscular atrophy (PMA), 357
prolapse, 489–90
management, 490
surgery, 490
prone position, 115
proprioceptors, 180
prostate, 265, 266
central zone, 266
conditions of, 270–75
peripheral zone, 266
transitional zone, 266
prostate cancer, 271–5
diagnosis, 272
management, 272–5
risk factors, 271
prostate-specific antigen (PSA), 266
pseudomembranous colitis, 63
psoriasis, 161–2
aetiology, 161, 163
signs and symptoms, 162
treatment, 162
psychogenic non-epileptic seizures (PNES), 352
psychogenic syncopes, 352
psychological status, and nutrition, 49
PTCA, 224
pulmonary rehabilitation, 193
pulse oximetry, 129–30, 188, 189
pulseless electrical activity, 228
punch biopsy, 160
pupillary reaction, 137
pyelonephritis, 280
complicated, 284
uncomplicated, 280, 284
pyrexia, 134

rabies, 354
radiological investigations
digestive system, 246, 247
neurological system, 337
respiratory system, 189
Ramsey Scale, 137
rashes, 161–5
endogenous, 161
exogenous, 161
rating scales, 7–8
RBCs *see* erythrocytes (red blood cells)
record-keeping, 9–10
recovery, 117
basic observations in, 120
pain management in, 121–2
red blood cells (RBCs) *see* erythrocytes
refeeding syndrome, 49–51
refined sugars, 320
renal cell carcinoma, 275
renal corpuscle, 264
renal replacement therapy (RRT), 293–6
renal system
anatomy, 263
see also kidney; urinary system
renal transplantation, 294, 296
renal tubule, 264
renin–angiotensin–aldosterone system, 266
repositioning, and pressure ulcer prevention, 171
reproductive health *see* female reproductive system; male reproductive system
reservoir, 61
respiration
control, 177, 180
mechanics, 177, 179
respirators, 69
respiratory assessment, 128–31, 183–8
general, 185
history-taking, 128
information collection, 184
primary data, 128–9
secondary data, 129–31
respiratory centre, 177
respiratory failure, 205–6
ABG values and, 205
assessment, 205–6
definition, 205
long-term oxygen therapy (LTOT), 206

management, 205–6
non-invasive ventilation, 206
nursing assessment and management, 206
oxygen therapy and ventilation, 206
pathophysiology, 205
respiratory function testing, 188–90, 197
respiratory interventions, 131–2, 190–3
see also continuous positive airway pressure; non-invasive positive-pressure ventilation; oxygen therapy
respiratory system, 176–209
anatomy, 177–9
function, 177
management of specific conditions, 193–209
nursing care, 183–4
physiology, 177–83
see also respiratory assessment; respiratory function testing; respiratory interventions
respiratory tract
anatomy, 177, 178
body defences, 366
resuscitation, family-witnessed, 153
reticulocyte count, 401
reticuloendothelial system, 391
retinal detachment, 477
assessment, 477
management, 477
signs and symptoms, 477
reverse Trendelenburg position, 115
reversibility testing, 189
rhesus factor, 393–5
rheumatoid arthritis, 435–7
drugs used in, 437
family and carers, 436
joint changes, 436
multidisciplinary team, 436–7
signs and symptoms, 435
systemic changes, 436
treatment, 437
rhonchi, 187
Richmond Agitation Sedation Scale, 137
RIFLE classification system, 286
right ventricular failure, 232
risk assessment, 3
rosacea, 163
aetiology, 163
signs and symptoms, 163
treatment, 163
RRT *see* renal replacement therapy
rubella, 354

salt, in diet, 320
saturated fats, 320
Schwann cells, 329
scleral buckling, 477
SCORE, 219
screening, 3, 498–9
scrub practitioner, role, 113
sebaceous glands, 299
secondary assessment, 146
securement, 35
sedation, 137
seizures, 349–53
absence ('petit-mal'), 351
generalized ('grand-mal'), 351
partial, 351
psychogenic non-epileptic (PNES), 352
signs, 351
tonic-clonic, 351, 352
see also epilepsy
selective serotonin-reuptake inhibitors (SSRIs), 20, 25
semen, 482
sepsis, 38
septicaemia, 38
Serious Hazards of Transfusion (SHOT) schemes, 397
serum creatinine level, 288–9
sexually transmitted infections (STIs), 498
sharps, definition, 72
sharps injury, 377
sharps waste management, 72
shingles *see* herpes zoster
shock-wave lithotripsy, 269
shockable rhythms, 228
SHOT schemes, 397
SIADH, 302
sickle cell anaemia, 408, 409
nursing management, 409
symptoms, 408
sickling test, 400
sigmoidoscopy, 248
'single use only' sign, 72
sinus bradycardia, 228
sinus tachycardia, 227
sinusitis, 458
Six Step Model (Purtilo), 99
Six Step Protocol, 97
skeletal system
bones, 423
divisions, 424
skin, 156–72
assessment, 158–60
diagnosis, 159
investigations, 160
patient history, 158
physical examination, 159
setting and equipment, 158
bullous pemphigoid, 164–5
treatment, 165
cleaning, 35
common diseases, 161–5
examination, 7
function, 157–8
infections, 163–4
treatment, 164
infestations, 164
treatment, 164
maintaining tissue integrity, 158
structure, 157–8
treatments, 160–1
tumours, 165
diagnosis, 165
treatment, 165
see also pressure ulcers; surgical wounds; wound assessment; wound healing; wound management
skin grafts, 169
types, 169
skin prick testing, 190
skin scrapings, 160
SLE *see* systemic lupus erythematosus
small cell lung cancer (SCLC), 207
smoking
cessation, 193
history assessment, 187–8
and lung cancer, 207
social assessment, 6
social hand hygiene, 64–5, 113
somatotrophs, 301
speech and language therapist, referral to, 46
speed shock, 39
sperm, 482
spillages, management, 70
spinal anaesthesia, 111, 112
spinal cord, 335
coverings, 333
tumours, 346
spinal nerves, 335
spiritual needs, at end of life, 95
spirometry, 189, 197
splinting, 440
spongiform encephalopathies, 354
sputum, analysis, 189
SSRIs *see* selective serotonin-reuptake inhibitors
ST elevation myocardial infarction (STEMI), 225
clinical and nursing management, 226
stable angina *see* angina
standard precautions, 64
Staphylococcus aureus, 63
and folliculitis, 163
methicillin-resistant (MRSA), 63
starvation, process of, 49–51
status epilepticus, 351
steady-state concentration, 20
STEMI *see* ST elevation myocardial infarction
stereotactic radiotherapy, 353
sterile field, 115
sterilisation, definition, 70
STIs, 498
stoma formation, 244
stool analysis, 249
stretch receptors, 180
stridor, 187
strokes, 347–9
diagnosis, 348
management, 348
nursing management, 349–50
risk factors, 347
types, 348
subacute sclerosing panencephalitis, 354
suctioning, oropharyngeal, 94
sugars, refined, 320
supine position, 115
support surfaces, 171–2
surgical drains, 116
types, 117
surgical dressings, 116
types, 117
surgical emergencies, 144–5
surgical hand antisepsis, 65
surgical instruments, 116, 118
surgical jejunostomy, 55
surgical needles, 116
surgical positions, 115
Surgical Safety Checklist, 107–8
surgical scrub, 113, 114

surgical specialties, 117, 119
surgical sutures, 116
absorbable, 116
non-absorbable, 116
surgical swabs, 114
surgical wounds, 169–70
closure methods, 169–70
susceptible hosts, 61
synapses, 329
syndrome of inappropriate ADH hypersecretion (SIADH), 302
syringe pumps, 34–5
Systemic Coronary Risk Estimation (SCORE), 219
systemic lupus erythematosus (SLE), 372, 373–5
management, 374–5
signs and symptoms, 374

T cells, 366
tachyarrythmias, 227–8
categorisation, 227
clinical and nursing management, 228
TBI *see* traumatic brain injury
temperature
monitoring, 134, 339
perioperative management, 107
tendons, 427
termination of pregnancy (TOP), 493, 496
complications, 493
management, 493
testes, 482
testicular disorders, 501, 503–4
cancer, 501, 503
management, 503
nursing care, 503
pain and swelling, 504
testosterone, 482
tetanus, 354
therapeutic failure, 13, 25
therapeutic range, 19, 25
therapeutics, 21
throat
anatomy, 460, 462
physiology, 460–1
tumours, 462–3, 464
assessment, 463
management, 463
nursing management after removal, 464
signs and symptoms, 462–3
see also laryngeal cancer; laryngeal obstruction; laryngectomy; tonsillectomy; tracheostomy
thrombocytes *see* platelets
thrombocytopenia, 409–10
causes, 410
management, 410
signs and symptoms, 410
types, 409
thrombophlebitis, 237, 313
thrombosis, 38
symptoms, 38
thrombotic thrombocytopenic purpura, 409
thyroid crisis, 307
thyroid gland, 303–8
disorders, 303–8
thyroid neoplasm, 306–7
thyroid-stimulating hormone (TSH), 303
thyroid storm, 307
thyrotoxicosis *see* hyperthyroidism
thyrotrophs, 301
thyroxine (T_4), 303, 305, 306
TIAs, 348, 349
tibia, partially sectioned, 430
tissue flaps, 169–70
free, 169
local, 169–70
TNM system, 462
tonsillectomy, 463, 465
assessment, 463
management, 463
nursing management after, 465
TOP *see* termination of pregnancy
topical antimicrobials, 168
topical steroids, 160
toxic multinodular goitre, 306
toxicity, 18, 25
Toxoplasma gondii, 381
tracheostomy, 463, 466–8
emergency tray, 468
nursing management, 467–8
permanent, 463
temporary, 463, 466
Track and Trigger, 3, 9, 126
traction, 440
transient ischaemic attacks (TIAs), 348, 349
transmission-based precautions, 72–3, 74–5
transporters, in cell membranes, 16
transurethral resection of the prostate (TURP), 271
nursing management, 272
traumatic brain injury (TBI), 340–2, 344
classification, 340
disorders of consciousness, 342, 344
grading, 341–2
management, 340–3
non-physical problems associated, 344
nursing management, 342–3
tremor, 187
Trendelenburg position, 115
triage, 143–4
mental health, 152
steps, 144
triiodothyronine (T_3), 303, 306
troponin, 220
TSH *see* thyroid-stimulating hormone
tuberculosis (TB), 194–6
aetiology, 194
assessment, 195
clinical manifestations, 195
diagnosis, 195
directly observed therapy, 195
HIV/AIDS and, 380
management, 195–6
nursing management, 195–6
tunica adventitia, 27
tunica intima, 27
TURP *see* transurethral resection of the prostate

ulcerative colitis, 257
uniforms, 71
'universal donor', 393
unplanned pregnancy loss, 491–3
see also ectopic pregnancy; miscarriage
uraemia, management, 289
ureteroscopy, 269
urethra, 265
urethritis, 280
urinalysis, 7
urinary diversion, 279–80
management, 279
postoperative nursing management, 282–3
preoperative nursing management, 281
urinary output, monitoring, 134
urinary system, 262–96
anatomy, 263–5
physiology, 263–9
see also acute kidney injury; bladder cancer; chronic kidney disease; kidney; kidney cancer; prostate; renal replacement therapy; urinary tract infections
urinary tract infections (UTIs), 280, 284–5, 286
complicated, 284, 286
management, 284, 286
risk factors, 284
uncomplicated, 280, 284
management, 284
prevention of recurrent, 285
risk factors, 280
signs and symptoms, 280, 284
urinary tact stones and, 266–7
urinary tract stones, 266–9
classification, 267
management, 267–9
nursing management for removal procedures, 269
signs and symptoms, 267
urology, 263
urostomy, 279
uterus, 479, 480
benign tumours, 484
UTIs *see* urinary tract infections

V/Q imbalance, 182
causes, 183
V/Q ratio, 182, 183
VADs *see* vascular access devices
vagina, benign tumours, 484
valvular heart disease, 230–2
clinical and nursing management, 231–2
investigations, 231
surgery, 231–2
variant CJD, 354
varicose veins, 237
clinical and nursing management, 237
investigations, 237
vascular access devices (VADs), 29–30
vascular dementia, 82
vascular disorders, 234–7
vasoconstriction, 391
veins, 214
anatomy, 27–9
of central venous circulation, 28–9
of peripheral circulation, 28
physiology, 27–9

venous disease, 236–7
venous thromboembolism (VTE), 236–7
  clinical and nursing management, 237
  diagnosis, 236
  factors predisposing to, 236
  symptoms, 236
ventilation (V), 182
ventricular fibrillation, 228
ventricular tachycardia, 227, 228
venules, 214
verbal response, 136
vertebral column, 335, 425
viruses, 62
visual fields, 472
visual impairment, 469–70
  gradual loss, 469
  sudden loss, 469
visual pathways, 472
vital signs
  measurement, 7, 339
  nursing assessment, 339
vitamin B_{12} deficiency, 405–6
  management, 406
  signs and symptoms, 405
vitrectomy, 477
volumetric pumps, 34
vomiting, 250
  postoperative, 121
VTE *see* venous thromboembolism
vulva
  benign tumours, 484
  cancer, 487

Wallace Rule of Nines, 148, 149
WBCs *see* leucocytes (white blood cells)
weight, recording, 7
wheezing, 187
white blood cells *see* leucocytes
white matter, 329
wound assessment, 167–8
  depth of tissue, 167
  location, 167
  odour, 168
  pain/discomfort amount, 168
  size, 167
  stage of wound, 167
  wound bed, 167–8
  wound drainage nature, 168
  wound edges, 167–8
wound healing, 165–7
  angiogenesis, 166
  contraction, 166
  early inflammation, 165
  epithelialisation, 166
  granulation tissue production, 166
  late inflammation, 166
  primary intention, 169, 170
  remodelling, 167
  secondary intention, 169, 170
wound management, 168
  principles, 170
wrong-site surgery, 107–8

zona fasciculata, 311
zona glomerulosa, 311
zona reticularis, 311